Opioids and Their Receptors

Opioids and Their Receptors

Present and Emerging Concepts in Opioid Drug Discovery

Editors

Mariana Spetea
Helmut Schmidhammer

MDPI • Basel • Beijing • Wuhan • Barcelona • Belgrade • Manchester • Tokyo • Cluj • Tianjin

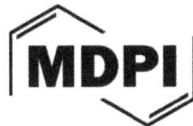

Editors
Mariana Spetea
University of Innsbruck
Austria

Helmut Schmidhammer
University of Innsbruck
Austria

Editorial Office
MDPI
St. Alban-Anlage 66
4052 Basel, Switzerland

This is a reprint of articles from the Special Issue published online in the open access journal *Molecules* (ISSN 1420-3049) (available at: https://www.mdpi.com/journal/molecules/special_issues/Opioid_Drug).

For citation purposes, cite each article independently as indicated on the article page online and as indicated below:

LastName, A.A.; LastName, B.B.; LastName, C.C. Article Title. *Journal Name* **Year**, *Volume Number*, Page Range.

ISBN 978-3-0365-0046-1 (Hbk)
ISBN 978-3-0365-0047-8 (PDF)

© 2020 by the authors. Articles in this book are Open Access and distributed under the Creative Commons Attribution (CC BY) license, which allows users to download, copy and build upon published articles, as long as the author and publisher are properly credited, which ensures maximum dissemination and a wider impact of our publications.

The book as a whole is distributed by MDPI under the terms and conditions of the Creative Commons license CC BY-NC-ND.

Contents

About the Editors ix

Mariana Spetea and Helmut Schmidhammer
Opioids and Their Receptors: Present and Emerging Concepts in Opioid Drug Discovery
Reprinted from: *Molecules* 2020, 25, 5658, doi:10.3390/molecules25235658 1

Łukasz Sobczak and Krzysztof Goryński
Pharmacological Aspects of Over-the-Counter Opioid Drugs Misuse
Reprinted from: *Molecules* 2020, 25, 3905, doi:10.3390/molecules25173905 7

**Meining Wang, Thomas C. Irvin, Christine A. Herdman, Ramsey D. Hanna,
Sergio A. Hassan, Yong-Sok Lee, Sophia Kaska, Rachel Saylor Crowley,
Thomas E. Prisinzano, Sarah L. Withey, Carol A. Paronis, Jack Bergman, Saadet Inan,
Ellen B. Geller, Martin W. Adler, Theresa A. Kopajtic, Jonathan L. Katz,
Aaron M. Chadderdon, John R. Traynor, Arthur E. Jacobson and Kenner C. Rice**
The Intriguing Effects of Substituents in the N-Phenethyl Moiety of Norhydromorphone:
A Bifunctional Opioid from a Set of "Tail Wags Dog" Experiments
Reprinted from: *Molecules* 2020, 25, 2640, doi:10.3390/molecules25112640 21

**Noriki Kutsumura, Yasuaki Koyama, Tsuyoshi Saitoh, Naoshi Yamamoto,
Yasuyuki Nagumo, Yoshiyuki Miyata, Rei Hokari, Aki Ishiyama, Masato Iwatsuki,
Kazuhiko Otoguro, Satoshi Ōmura and Hiroshi Nagase**
Structure-Activity Relationship between Thiol Group-Trapping Ability of Morphinan
Compounds with a Michael Acceptor and Anti-*Plasmodium falciparum* Activities
Reprinted from: *Molecules* 2020, 25, 1112, doi:10.3390/molecules25051112 53

**Chiharu Iwamatsu, Daichi Hayakawa, Tomomi Kono, Ayaka Honjo, Saki Ishizaki,
Shigeto Hirayama, Hiroaki Gouda and Hideaki Fujii**
Effects of N-Substituents on the Functional Activities of Naltrindole Derivatives for the δ
Opioid Receptor: Synthesis and Evaluation of Sulfonamide Derivatives
Reprinted from: *Molecules* 2020, 25, 3792, doi:10.3390/molecules25173792 63

Dagmara Tymecka, Piotr F. J. Lipiński, Piotr Kosson and Aleksandra Misicka
β^2-*Homo*-Amino Acid Scan of μ-Selective Opioid Tetrapeptide TAPP
Reprinted from: *Molecules* 2020, 25, 2461, doi:10.3390/molecules25102461 81

Maria Dumitrascuta, Marcel Bermudez, Steven Ballet, Gerhard Wolber and Mariana Spetea
Mechanistic Understanding of Peptide Analogues, DALDA, [Dmt^1]DALDA, and KGOP01,
Binding to the Mu Opioid Receptor
Reprinted from: *Molecules* 2020, 25, 2087, doi:10.3390/molecules25092087 99

**Robert J. Cassell, Krishna K. Sharma, Hongyu Su, Benjamin R. Cummins, Haoyue Cui,
Kendall L. Mores, Arryn T. Blaine, Ryan A. Altman and Richard M. van Rijn**
The Meta-Position of Phe^4 in Leu-Enkephalin Regulates Potency, Selectivity, Functional
Activity, and Signaling Bias at the Delta and Mu Opioid Receptors
Reprinted from: *Molecules* 2019, 24, 4542, doi:10.3390/molecules24244542 111

**Ariana C. Brice-Tutt, Sanjeewa N. Senadheera, Michelle L. Ganno, Shainnel O. Eans,
Tanvir Khaliq, Thomas F. Murray, Jay P. McLaughlin and Jane V. Aldrich**
Phenylalanine Stereoisomers of CJ-15,208 and [D-Trp]CJ-15,208 Exhibit Distinctly Different
Opioid Activity Profiles
Reprinted from: *Molecules* 2020, 25, 3999, doi:10.3390/molecules25173999 127

Banulata Gopalsamy, Jasmine Siew Min Chia, Ahmad Akira Omar Farouk,
Mohd Roslan Sulaiman and Enoch Kumar Perimal
Zerumbone-Induced Analgesia Modulated via Potassium Channels and Opioid Receptors in
Chronic Constriction Injury-Induced Neuropathic Pain
Reprinted from: *Molecules* **2020**, *25*, 3880, doi:10.3390/molecules25173880 . . . . **147**

Ferenc Zádor, Amir Mohammadzadeh, Mihály Balogh, Zoltán S. Zádori, Kornél Király,
Szilvia Barsi, Anna Rita Galambos, Szilvia B. László, Barbara Hutka, András Váradi,
Sándor Hosztafi, Pál Riba, Sándor Benyhe, Susanna Fürst and Mahmoud Al-Khrasani
Comparisons of In Vivo and In Vitro Opioid Effects of Newly Synthesized 14-
Methoxycodeine-6-O-sulfate and Codeine-6-O-sulfate
Reprinted from: *Molecules* **2020**, *25*, 1370, doi:10.3390/molecules25061370 . . . . **173**

Susanna Fürst, Zoltán S. Zádori, Ferenc Zádor, Kornél Király, Mihály Balogh,
Szilvia B. László, Barbara Hutka, Amir Mohammadzadeh, Chiara Calabrese,
Anna Rita Galambos, Pál Riba, Patrizia Romualdi, Sándor Benyhe, Júlia Timár,
Helmut Schmidhammer, Mariana Spetea and Mahmoud Al-Khrasani
On the Role of Peripheral Sensory and Gut Mu Opioid Receptors: Peripheral Analgesia
and Tolerance
Reprinted from: *Molecules* **2020**, *25*, 2473, doi:10.3390/molecules25112473 . . . . **195**

Helmut Schmidhammer, Filippo Erli, Elena Guerrieri and Mariana Spetea
Development of Diphenethylamines as Selective Kappa Opioid Receptor Ligands and Their
Pharmacological Activities
Reprinted from: *Molecules* **2020**, *25*, 5092, doi:10.3390/molecules25215092 . . . . **217**

Lyes Derouiche, Florian Pierre, Stéphane Doridot, Stéphane Ory and Dominique Massotte
Heteromerization of Endogenous Mu and Delta Opioid Receptors Induces Ligand-Selective
Co-Targeting to Lysosomes
Reprinted from: *Molecules* **2020**, *25*, 4493, doi:10.3390/molecules25194493 . . . . **241**

Karol Wtorek, Anna Adamska-Bartłomiejczyk, Justyna Piekielna-Ciesielska,
Federica Ferrari, Chiara Ruzza, Alicja Kluczyk, Joanna Piasecka-Zelga, Girolamo Calo'
and Anna Janecka
Synthesis and Pharmacological Evaluation of Hybrids Targeting Opioid and
Neurokinin Receptors
Reprinted from: *Molecules* **2019**, *24*, 4460, doi:10.3390/molecules24244460 . . . . **255**

Abdelfattah Faouzi, Balazs R. Varga and Susruta Majumdar
Biased Opioid Ligands
Reprinted from: *Molecules* **2020**, *25*, 4257, doi:10.3390/molecules25184257 . . . . **269**

Joaquim Azevedo Neto, Anna Costanzini, Roberto De Giorgio, David G. Lambert,
Chiara Ruzza and Girolamo Calò
Biased versus Partial Agonism in the Search for Safer Opioid Analgesics
Reprinted from: *Molecules* **2020**, *25*, 3870, doi:10.3390/molecules25173870 . . . . **303**

Wolfgang Sadee, John Oberdick and Zaijie Wang
Biased Opioid Antagonists as Modulators of Opioid Dependence: Opportunities to Improve
Pain Therapy and Opioid Use Management
Reprinted from: *Molecules* **2020**, *25*, 4163, doi:10.3390/molecules25184163 . . . . **317**

Sabina Podlewska, Ryszard Bugno, Lucja Kudla, Andrzej J. Bojarski and Ryszard Przewlocki
Molecular Modeling of μ Opioid Receptor Ligands with Various Functional Properties: PZM21, SR-17018, Morphine, and Fentanyl—Simulated Interaction Patterns Confronted with Experimental Data
Reprinted from: *Molecules* **2020**, *25*, 4636, doi:10.3390/molecules25204636 . . . . **331**

About the Editors

Mariana Spetea earned her M.Sc. degree in Biochemistry (1993) from the University of Bucharest (Romania) and her Ph.D. degree in Biology (1998) from József Attila University and the Biological Research Center (Szeged, Hungary). She spent two years (1998–1999) as a post-doctoral fellow at the Karolinska Institute (Stockholm, Sweden), with research fellowships awarded by the Swedish Institute and the Wenner-Gren Center Foundation. In 2000, she joined the Opioid Research Group led at that time by Prof. Helmut Schmidhammer at the University of Innsbruck (Austria), as a research associate and assistant professor, where she has habilitated in Pharmacology (2010). Since 2011, she is the head of the Opioid Research Group and holds a senior lecturer position at the University of Innsbruck. In 2013, she was a visiting scientist at The Scripps Research Institute (Jupiter, FL, USA) in the laboratory of Dr. Laura Bohn, and in 2014, she spent a sabbatical at the Torrey Pines Institute for Molecular Studies (Port St. Lucie, FL, USA) with Dr. Laurence Toll and Dr. Jay P. McLaughlin. An important focus of her research is directed to opioid drug discovery and development, with main interests in pain research and opioid pharmacology. Central topics of her research include structure–activity relationships of new opioid ligands, modulation of the ligand/opioid receptor system in pathological pain, and molecular mechanisms of opioid actions. Since she joined the Opioid Research Group, she put the basis of screening platforms for opioid compounds, including state-of-the-art biochemical assays, as well as pharmacological and disease animal models. She has been a research leader and associate researcher of several research projects, as well as the scientific coordinator of a European Union research project. In addition to her research, Prof. Spetea is devoted to the Pharmaceutical Sciences education of undergraduate and graduate students at the Faculty of Chemistry and Pharmacy, University of Innsbruck. Her scientific achievements have been published in numerous peer-reviewed articles, reviews, conference proceedings and patents, and have been disseminated in popular science reports. She is Editorial Board Member of Frontiers (Frontiers in Neuroscience, Pharmacology, Neurology and Psychiatry) and Molecules, and was a Guest Editor of Special Issues of Current Pharmaceutical Design (2013) and Molecules (2020).

Helmut Schmidhammer earned his M.Sc. degree in Pharmacy (1972) and a Ph.D. in Organic Chemistry (1975) from the University of Innsbruck (Austria), where he continued to work as an assistant professor and habilitated in Pharmaceutical Chemistry (1985). He joined as a visiting scientist from 1980–1982 the laboratory of Dr. Arnold Brossi and Dr. Kenner C. Rice at the Section on Medicinal Chemistry, Laboratory of Chemistry, NIDDK, National Institutes of Health (NIH), Bethesda, MD, USA. During his research stay at the NIH, he became interested in morphinan chemistry and opioid drug design. After his return to the University of Innsbruck, he established the Opioid Research Group at the Institute of Organic and Pharmaceutical Chemistry, which he headed until his retirement in 2011. In 1995, he was visiting professor at the Department of Chemistry, Astra Pain Research Unit, Montreal, Canada. From 2000–2010, Prof. Schmidhammer was the head of the Department of Pharmaceutical Chemistry, Institute of Pharmacy, University of Innsbruck, and since 2004 he has been a full member of the Center for Molecular Biosciences (CMBI), University of Innsbruck. He constantly pursued basic and translational research in the opioid field, with a focus on the development of new synthetic methodologies, and the development of active opioid ligands as potential drugs for the treatment of pain, immunological and neurodegenerative diseases, and addiction. More than 2000 compounds have been synthesized, and numerous opioid compounds developed by Prof. Schmidhammer are cited in medicinal chemistry and pharmacological journals as reference compounds, and are used as research tools. His research has been continuously and generously supported by several funding agencies (FWF, TWF, OEAD, BMWFW, EU, and NIDA-USA). He also has extensive pharmaceutical and biotech experience. In addition to numerous awards, he was also the recipient of the "Science4Life Venture Cup 2003". His more than 40 years of expertise in medicinal chemistry, particularly in opioid drug development, is reflected by the large number of peer-reviewed manuscripts, reviews, book chapters, and patents he has published.

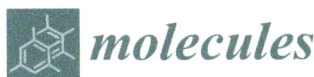

Editorial

Opioids and Their Receptors: Present and Emerging Concepts in Opioid Drug Discovery

Mariana Spetea * and Helmut Schmidhammer

Department of Pharmaceutical Chemistry, Institute of Pharmacy and Center for Molecular Biosciences Innsbruck (CMBI), University of Innsbruck, 6020 Innsbruck, Austria; helmut.schmidhammer@uibk.ac.at
* Correspondence: mariana.spetea@uibk.ac.at

Received: 26 November 2020; Accepted: 27 November 2020; Published: 1 December 2020

The interest in opioids such as morphine, the prototypical opioid ligand, has been maintained throughout the years. Identification of endogenous opioid peptides and their receptors (µ, mu (MOR); δ, delta (DOR); κ, kappa (KOR); nociceptin (NOP)), along with molecular cloning and elucidation of crystal structures of opioid receptors represent key milestones in opioid research. With its ubiquitous distribution in the central and peripheral nervous systems (CNS and PNS), the opioid system has a central role in modulating pain and other physiological functions and pharmacological responses, with therapeutic as well as unwanted side effects. The dramatic increase in medical use and misuse of opioids with the rising number of opioid-related overdose deaths and diagnoses of opioid-use disorder has led to the 21st century opioid crisis.

The Special Issue, "Opioids and Their Receptors: Present and Emerging Concepts in Opioid Drug Discovery", includes 11 research articles, one communication and six reviews, with authors from 12 different countries, giving insight into ongoing subjects that span the opioid research field. This issue presents recent advances in medicinal chemistry and pharmacology of new ligands targeting the opioid receptors. Moreover, it highlights current concepts in opioid drug discovery together with strategies to mitigate the deleterious effects of opioids. Central topics of this Special Issue include drug design, structure–activity relationships (SAR), biochemistry of the receptors, understanding of ligand specific actions and the link between therapeutic effects, side effects and molecular mode of action.

The review by Sobczak and Goryński [1] addresses the present opioid epidemic with literature showing that over-the-counter (OTC) opioids are misused as an alternative for illicit narcotics or prescription-only opioids. Three OTC opioid drugs, codeine, dihydrocodeine and loperamide, are discussed, including pharmacology, interactions, safety profiles and how pharmacology is being manipulated to misuse, focusing on abuse prevention and prevalence rates. Relatively easy access to OTC opioids is alarming and requires further attention and discussion on the rescheduling of their availability.

The imperative need for safer therapies for pain and other human disease states involving the opioid system continues to drive the search for novel lead molecules and the development of new mechanism-based treatment strategies. Since the structural elucidation of morphine, its skeleton and its conversion to new analogues has been constantly in the attention of medicinal chemists, aiming to discover therapeutically useful drugs and research tools. Three reports present new research in the field of opioid morphinans [2–4].

In their study, Wang et al. [2] elaborated on extended SARs in (−)-*N*-phenethyl analogs of *N*-nor-hydromorphone. Within the designed series, *N*-*p*-chloro-phenethylnorhydromorphone was a bifunctional MOR-DOR ligand with a potent partial agonism at the MOR and a full potent agonism at the DOR. This favorable combination of MOR and DOR activities in vitro was translated in vivo by potent antinociception without respiratory depression in squirrel monkeys after subcutaneous administration. In their communication, Kutsumura et al. [3] reported on SARs between the thiol group-trapping ability of morphinans with a Michael acceptor and anti-*Plasmodium falciparum* activities. Using the

DOR antagonist 7-benzylidenenaltrexone (BNTX) as a lead structure, new derivatives were designed and a correlation between the antimalarial activity and the chemical reactivity of the BNTX derivatives with 1-propanethiol was established. Using naltrindole (NTI), the indolo-morphinan DOR antagonist, as a lead, Iwamatsu et al. [4] designed sulfonamide-type NTI derivatives by targeting the effect of the N-substituent on functional activities at the DOR. They revealed SARs among the ligands with activities at the DOR ranging from full inverse agonists to full agonists, with cyclopropyl-sulfonamide (SYK-83) as the most potent full inverse agonist. The new NTI derivatives are expected to be useful tools for investigating interactions of ligands with the DOR, conformational changes of the DOR and induced functional activities.

Endogenous and naturally occurring opioid peptides have continuously served as important leads for the design of peptide analogues, with a repertoire of structural modifications that can be targeted when exploring SARs or focusing on the improvement of their pharmacodynamics and the pharmacokinetics of peptide active compounds. Four research articles [5–8] focused on this subject.

In their report, Tymecka et al. [5] performed a β^2-*Homo*-amino acid (β^2hAA) scan of the selective MOR peptide agonist TAPP (H-Tyr-D-Ala-Phe-Phe-NH$_2$) sequence, an analogue of endomorphin-2 and enkephalin-derived DAMGO. Derivatives with (R)- or (S)-β^2hPhe^4 bound the MOR with affinities equal to that of TAPP. Combining design strategies, synthesis, binding assays and molecular modeling, they provided additional understanding of SARs of the TAPP sequence. Using a structure-based docking at the MOR and three-dimensional interaction pattern analysis, Dumitrascuta et al. [6] rationalized the experimental results on binding and activation of the MOR by three synthetic analogues of the naturally occurring dermorphin and effective analgesics, DALDA, [Dmt^1]DALDA and KGOP01. The Dmt (2',6'-dimethyl-L-Tyr) moiety of [Dmt^1]DALDA and KGOP01 represented the driving force for the high potency and agonist activity at the MOR. The findings of Tymecka et al. [5] and Dumitrascuta et al. [6] offer significant structural insights into flexible peptide ligand-MOR interactions that are important for further understanding of MOR function and pharmacology, and the future design of peptide-based analgesics.

Cassell et al. [7] explored SAR trends, at the meta-position of Phe^4, of the endogenous DOR peptide Leu^5-enkephalin, demonstrating that substitution at this position variously regulated DOR and MOR affinity and G protein activity, enabled the fine-tuning of β-arrestin2 recruitment to both receptors, and increased the plasma stability of the derived peptides. The resulting peptide analogues should be useful tools for studying the role of DOR in cardiac ischemia and the importance of DOR mediated β-arrestin2 signaling in the peptides cardioprotective effects.

The SAR study by Brice-Tutt et al. [8] studied the influence of the Phe residues' stereochemistry in the macrocyclic tetrapeptide CJ-15,208 (*cyclo*[Phe-D-Pro-Phe-Trp]), from the fungus *Ctenomyces serratus*, and its analogue [D-Trp]CJ-15,208 (*cyclo*[Phe-D-Pro-Phe-D-Trp]) on opioid activity profiles. Unlike the parent peptides, KOR antagonism was exhibited by only one stereoisomer, while another isomer produced DOR antagonism. They identified the stereoisomer [D-Phe^{1,3}]CJ-15,208 as a potent antinociceptive after oral administration lacking respiratory depression and locomotor impairment and without preference or aversion in mice.

Natural product medicines have a long history of use in the treatment and prevention of many human diseases. Zerumbone, a sesquiterpene from the wild ginger plant *Zingiber zerumbet* (L.) Smith, produces allodynia and hyperalgesia in animals. Gopalsamy et al. [9] reported on the involvement of potassium channels and opioid receptors (MOR, DOR and KOR) in zerumbone-induced antinociception in a mouse model of chronic constriction injury neuropathic pain after intraperitoneal administration.

As the ongoing worldwide opioid crisis is the result of the use of centrally-acting opioids for controlling pain, the idea of peripheralization of opioids to minimize the activation of central opioid receptors, and as a consequence the unwanted CNS side effects, has stimulated the development of peripherally selective opioid ligands, discussed in a research article [10] and a review [11].

In their study, Zádor et al. [10] reported on a new analogue of codeine, 14-methoxycodeine-6-O-sulfate (14-OMeC6SU), as a potent, peripheral MOR agonist. It was more effective than codeine, and equipotent to morphine in inducing antinociception in acute nociceptive pain, and it produced peripherally-mediated anti-hyperalgesic effects in inflammatory pain after subcutaneous administration in rats. Additionally, 14-OMeC6SU showed an improved in vitro and in vivo activity profile compared to codeine-6-*O*-sulfat. Fürst et al. [11] reviewed the consequence of the activation of peripheral MORs in analgesia and analgesic tolerance, along with approaches that enhanced analgesic efficacy and decreased the development of tolerance to opioids at the peripheral sites. They also addressed the advantages and drawbacks of the activation of peripheral MORs on the sensory neurons and gut (leading to dysbiosis) in the development of central and peripheral analgesic tolerance. The reviewed data suggest that the development of peripheral analgesic tolerance to opioids is largely dependent on the pain entity, animal pain model, and the route of administration, local versus systemic.

With the awareness that narcotic addiction is derived from the MOR, the KOR is emerging as a promising target for developing safer therapeutics without the common side effects associated with classical opioids, such as rewarding effects, respiratory depression and overdose. Schmidhammer et al. [12] reviewed recent chemical developments of SARs on diphenethylamines, a new class of structurally distinct and selective KOR ligands, with diverse profiles ranging from potent and selective agonists to G protein-biased agonists and selective antagonists. The first lead molecules in the series included the selective KOR full agonist HS665 and the partial agonist HS666. The combination of target drug design, synthetical efforts and pharmacology of diphenethylamines has enabled the identification of structural elements that determine distinct activity profiles, with the potential as candidates for future drug development for the treatment of pain and neuropsychiatric diseases.

Increasing evidence on the heteromerization of native opioid receptors in discrete brain neuronal circuits with selective targeting of heteromers as a tool to modulate receptor activity, and multifunctional ligands, which simultaneously activate two or more targets to produce a more desirable drug profile, are emerging concepts for the development of novel therapeutic drugs and strategies, presented in the earlier cited report [2] and in two additional research articles [13,14].

Using double-fluorescent knock-in mice co-expressing functional MOR and DOR, Derouiche et al. [13] demonstrated that co-expression of native MOR and DOR in hippocampal neurons alters the intracellular fate of the MOR in a ligand-selective manner, with MOR-DOR co-internalization induced by the MOR-DOR biased agonist CYM51010, the MOR agonist DAMGO and the DOR agonist deltorphin II, but not the MOR agonists morphine and methadone or the DOR agonist SNC80. Their observations pointed out to MOR-DOR heteromerization as a means to fine-tune MOR signaling and neuronal activity with the potential for developing novel innovative therapeutics.

The study by Wtorek et al. [14] targeted the concept of multifunctional ligands, specifically novel hybrids combining opioid pharmacophores with either substance P (SP) or neurokinin receptor (NK1) antagonist fragments, as a strategy for developing effective and safer medications for pain treatment. They reported on opioid agonist/NK1 antagonist Tyr-[D-Lys-Phe-Phe-Asp]-Asn-D-Trp-Phe-D-Trp-Leu-Nle-NH$_2$ and opioid agonist/NK1 agonist Tyr-[D-Lys-Phe-Phe-Asp]-Gln-Phe-Phe-Gly-Leu-Met-NH$_2$ peptide hybrids with antinociceptive efficacy without inducing analgesic tolerance or constipation in mice after intraperitoneal administration. Research approaches to diminish opioid liabilities take advantage of the current concept of functional selectivity, with biased ligands (agonists and antagonists) as innovative opportunities for opioid pain therapy and use management, subjects reviewed in [12,15–17] and explored in a research article [18].

In their review, Faouzi et al. [15] presented the design and pharmacological outcomes of biased agonists of all opioid receptor types (MOR, DOR, KOR and NOP), aiming at achieving functional selectivity. They described a large number of structurally diverse biased agonists, with the focus on the understanding of the limitations and advantages both in vitro and in vivo that they can provide. Azevedo Neto et al. [16] discussed the accumulated literature on the potential of biased MOR agonists for the development as safer analgesics. They presented the pharmacology of three G protein-biased MOR agonists, oliceridine (TRV130), very recently approved for pain treatment, and PZM21 and

SR-17018, in relationship to that of morphine and fentanyl, and proposed that their improved safety profile could be likely attributable to low efficacy partial agonism rather than G protein-bias.

A review by Sadee et al. [17] addressed the less explored area of biased opioid antagonism, where biased MOR antagonists, such as 6β-naltrexol, could serve as modulators of opioid dependence, for improved pain therapy and opioid use management. They proposed a novel receptor model that can account for diverse pharmacological effects of MOR ligands, including biased antagonists.

Using molecular docking and molecular dynamics (MD) simulations at three crystal structures of the MOR, Podlewska et al. [18] explored the distinct activity profiles at the MOR of morphine (unbiased ligand), PZM21 and SR-17018 (G protein-biased MOR agonists) and fentanyl (β-arrestin2-biased MOR agonist). Several shared and distinct receptor-ligand interaction patterns were identified, and specific amino acids were proposed to be of particular interest when designing new G protein-biased MOR agonists.

The diversity among the topics in this Special Issue in the up-to-date reports is a testimony to the complexity of the opioid system that results from the expression, regulation and functional role of ligands and receptors. Moreover, the array of multidisciplinary research areas illustrates the rapidly developing research and translational activities in the opioid drug discovery.

We wish to thank all the authors for their contribution to this Special Issue. It is beyond any doubt that it will serve as a useful reference while also stimulating continued research in the chemistry and pharmacology of opioids and their receptors, with the prospective for developing improved therapies of human diseases, but also improving health and quality of life in general.

Funding: The authors thank the Austrian Science Fund (FWF: I2463, P30433, P30592, and I4697), and the University of Innsbruck.

Conflicts of Interest: The authors declare no conflict of interest.

References

1. Sobczak, Ł.; Goryński, K. Pharmacological Aspects of Over-the-Counter Opioid Drugs Misuse. *Molecules* **2020**, *25*, 3905. [CrossRef] [PubMed]
2. Wang, M.; Irvin, T.C.; Herdman, C.A.; Hanna, R.D.; Hassan, S.A.; Lee, Y.-S.; Kaska, S.; Crowley, R.S.; Prisinzano, T.E.; Withey, S.L.; et al. The Intriguing Effects of Substituents in the *N*-Phenethyl Moiety of Norhydromorphone: A Bifunctional Opioid from a Set of "Tail Wags Dog" Experiments. *Molecules* **2020**, *25*, 2640. [CrossRef] [PubMed]
3. Kutsumura, N.; Koyama, Y.; Saitoh, T.; Yamamoto, N.; Nagumo, Y.; Miyata, Y.; Hokari, R.; Ishiyama, A.; Iwatsuki, M.; Otoguro, K.; et al. Structure-Activity Relationship between Thiol Group-Trapping Ability of Morphinan Compounds with a Michael Acceptor and Anti-*Plasmodium falciparum* Activities. *Molecules* **2020**, *25*, 1112. [CrossRef] [PubMed]
4. Iwamatsu, C.; Hayakawa, D.; Kono, T.; Honjo, A.; Ishizaki, S.; Hirayama, S.; Gouda, H.; Fujii, H. Effects of *N*-Substituents on the Functional Activities of Naltrindole Derivatives for the δ Opioid Receptor: Synthesis and Evaluation of Sulfonamide Derivatives. *Molecules* **2020**, *25*, 3792. [CrossRef] [PubMed]
5. Tymecka, D.; Lipiński, P.F.J.; Kosson, P.; Misicka, A. β^2-*Homo*-Amino Acid Scan of μ-Selective Opioid Tetrapeptide TAPP. *Molecules* **2020**, *25*, 2461. [CrossRef] [PubMed]
6. Dumitrascuta, M.; Bermudez, M.; Ballet, S.; Wolber, G.; Spetea, M. Mechanistic Understanding of Peptide Analogues, DALDA, [Dmt^1]DALDA, and KGOP01, Binding to the Mu Opioid Receptor. *Molecules* **2020**, *25*, 2087. [CrossRef] [PubMed]
7. Cassell, R.J.; Sharma, K.K.; Su, H.; Cummins, B.R.; Cui, H.; Mores, K.L.; Blaine, A.T.; Altman, R.A.; van Rijn, R.M. The Meta-Position of Phe^4 in Leu-Enkephalin Regulates Potency, Selectivity, Functional Activity, and Signaling Bias at the Delta and Mu Opioid Receptors. *Molecules* **2019**, *24*, 4542. [CrossRef] [PubMed]
8. Brice-Tutt, A.C.; Senadheera, S.N.; Ganno, M.L.; Eans, S.O.; Khaliq, T.; Murray, T.F.; McLaughlin, J.P.; Aldrich, J.V. Phenylalanine Stereoisomers of CJ-15,208 and [D-Trp]CJ-15,208 Exhibit Distinctly Different Opioid Activity Profiles. *Molecules* **2020**, *25*, 3999. [CrossRef] [PubMed]

9. Gopalsamy, B.; Chia, J.S.M.; Farouk, A.A.O.; Sulaiman, M.R.; Perimal, E.K. Zerumbone-Induced Analgesia Modulated via Potassium Channels and Opioid Receptors in Chronic Constriction Injury-Induced Neuropathic Pain. *Molecules* **2020**, *25*, 3880. [CrossRef] [PubMed]
10. Zádor, F.; Mohammadzadeh, A.; Balogh, M.; Zádori, Z.S.; Király, K.; Barsi, S.; Galambos, A.R.; László, S.B.; Hutka, B.; Váradi, A.; et al. Comparisons of In Vivo and In Vitro Opioid Effects of Newly Synthesized 14-Methoxycodeine-6-*O*-sulfate and Codeine-6-*O*-sulfate. *Molecules* **2020**, *25*, 1370. [CrossRef] [PubMed]
11. Fürst, S.; Zádori, Z.S.; Zádor, F.; Király, K.; Balogh, M.; László, S.B.; Hutka, B.; Mohammadzadeh, A.; Calabrese, C.; Galambos, A.R.; et al. On the Role of Peripheral Sensory and Gut Mu Opioid Receptors: Peripheral Analgesia and Tolerance. *Molecules* **2020**, *25*, 2473. [CrossRef] [PubMed]
12. Schmidhammer, H.; Erli, F.; Guerrieri, E.; Spetea, M. Development of Diphenethylamines as Selective Kappa Opioid Receptor Ligands and Their Pharmacological Activities. *Molecules* **2020**, *25*, 5092. [CrossRef] [PubMed]
13. Derouiche, L.; Pierre, F.; Doridot, S.; Ory, S.; Massotte, D. Heteromerization of Endogenous Mu and Delta Opioid Receptors Induces Ligand-Selective Co-Targeting to Lysosomes. *Molecules* **2020**, *25*, 4493. [CrossRef] [PubMed]
14. Wtorek, K.; Adamska-Bartłomiejczyk, A.; Piekielna-Ciesielska, J.; Ferrari, F.; Ruzza, C.; Kluczyk, A.; Piasecka-Zelga, J.; Calo', G.; Janecka, A. Synthesis and Pharmacological Evaluation of Hybrids Targeting Opioid and Neurokinin Receptors. *Molecules* **2019**, *24*, 4460. [CrossRef] [PubMed]
15. Faouzi, A.; Varga, B.R.; Majumdar, S. Biased Opioid Ligands. *Molecules* **2020**, *25*, 4257. [CrossRef] [PubMed]
16. Azevedo Neto, J.; Costanzini, A.; De Giorgio, R.; Lambert, D.G.; Ruzza, C.; Calò, G. Biased versus Partial Agonism in the Search for Safer Opioid Analgesics. *Molecules* **2020**, *25*, 3870. [CrossRef] [PubMed]
17. Sadee, W.; Oberdick, J.; Wang, Z. Biased Opioid Antagonists as Modulators of Opioid Dependence: Opportunities to Improve Pain Therapy and Opioid Use Management. *Molecules* **2020**, *25*, 4163. [CrossRef] [PubMed]
18. Podlewska, S.; Bugno, R.; Kudla, L.; Bojarski, A.J.; Przewlocki, R. Molecular Modeling of μ Opioid Receptor Ligands with Various Functional Properties: PZM21, SR-17018, Morphine, and Fentanyl—Simulated Interaction Patterns Confronted with Experimental Data. *Molecules* **2020**, *25*, 4636. [CrossRef] [PubMed]

Publisher's Note: MDPI stays neutral with regard to jurisdictional claims in published maps and institutional affiliations.

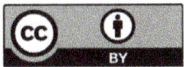

© 2020 by the authors. Licensee MDPI, Basel, Switzerland. This article is an open access article distributed under the terms and conditions of the Creative Commons Attribution (CC BY) license (http://creativecommons.org/licenses/by/4.0/).

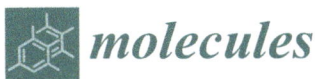 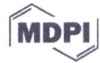

Review

Pharmacological Aspects of Over-the-Counter Opioid Drugs Misuse

Łukasz Sobczak and Krzysztof Goryński *

Bioanalysis Scientific Group, Faculty of Pharmacy, Collegium Medicum in Bydgoszcz at Nicolaus Copernicus University in Toruń, 87-100 Toruń, Poland; lukasz.sobczak@cm.umk.pl
* Correspondence: gorynski@cm.umk.pl; Tel.: +48-52-585-3921

Received: 31 July 2020; Accepted: 24 August 2020; Published: 27 August 2020

Abstract: Several over-the-counter (OTC) drugs are known to be misused. Among them are opioids such as codeine, dihydrocodeine, and loperamide. This work elucidates their pharmacology, interactions, safety profiles, and how pharmacology is being manipulated to misuse these common medications, with the aim to expand on the subject outlined by the authors focusing on abuse prevention and prevalence rates. The reviewed literature was identified in several online databases through searches conducted with phrases created by combining the international non-proprietary names of the drugs with terms related to drug misuse. The results show that OTC opioids are misused as an alternative for illicit narcotics, or prescription-only opioids. The potency of codeine and loperamide is strongly dependent on the individual enzymatic activity of CYP2D6 and CYP3A4, as well as P-glycoprotein function. Codeine can also be utilized as a substrate for clandestine syntheses of more potent drugs of abuse, namely desomorphine ("Krokodil"), and morphine. The dangerous methods used to prepare these substances can result in poisoning from toxic chemicals and impurities originating from the synthesis procedure. OTC opioids are generally safe when consumed in accordance with medical guidelines. However, the intake of supratherapeutic amounts of these substances may reveal surprising traits of common medications.

Keywords: over-the-counter drugs; misuse; abuse; opioid drugs; pharmacology; codeine; dihydrocodeine; loperamide

---

1. Introduction

Over-the-counter (OTC) drugs are medicines sold without medical prescription to treat common and temperate medical conditions. Unfortunately, the misconception that OTC drugs are devoid of any harm to users has become established as a commonly held belief. While it is true that most of them are relatively safe, if administered with moderation, misuse is usually associated with the intake of excessive amounts and is burdened with life-threatening consequences. Due to the acknowledged misuse liability, or associated health risks, some countries have already restricted access to several OTC drugs by introducing an intermediate category of pharmacy-only (or pharmacist-only) medicines (POMs). While the purchase of POMs does not require a prescription from a physician, they may only be purchased in a pharmacy. Other restrictions, such as age limit or maximal purchase quotas, may also be in place for the sale of POMs and OTC drugs.

This matter is further complicated by the differences in local regulations. For example, codeine is available as an OTC medicine in countries such as Denmark [1], Poland (up to 240 mg per single purchase—since December 2016) [2], the UK (up to 12.8 mg per single tablet), and several other European states [3], as well as in Japan. At the same time, it is classified as prescription only medicine in Australia (where it has been recently up-scheduled from the OTC category) [4], or USA [5]. Dihydrocodeine, a stronger opioid drug, is generally not available as an OTC medicine. However, few exceptions exist—e.g., in the UK or Japan. Loperamide on the other hand, is usually available without prescription and without almost any restrictions regarding its sale.

All of the aforementioned drugs are classified as opioid agents, and the evidence exists that they are misused, either unintentionally, or for non-medical intents. Several authors have already investigated the issue of misuse and abuse of OTC drugs from the perspective of pharmacology; however, these reports usually address single drugs, and few reports that are focused on a broader picture are regretfully still not fully comprehensive. This especially concerns the opioid drugs that tend to be omitted from such reviews. Out of four of the most extensive works investigated by the authors, only two discuss codeine, and none discuss either dihydrocodeine or loperamide [6–9].

This review is focused on three opioid drugs—codeine, dihydrocodeine, and loperamide—that can still be purchased without medical prescription in numerous parts of the world, addressing their pharmacology, interactions, safety profiles, and how pharmacology is manipulated in non-medical applications. This work intends to elucidate the reasons behind the misuse or abuse of these common medications. As such, it adds to numerous works regarding abuse prevention and prevalence rates that are already published.

2. Results and Discussion

2.1. Introduction to Opioid Drugs

From a chemical standpoint, opioids comprise a diverse group of drugs, but they all share a common affinity towards µ, δ, and κ opioid receptors. Most of the opioids used in clinical practice, including those available as OTC medicines, are agonists of opioid receptors that are predominantly selective for µ type receptors. Receptor type specific effects, as well as some examples of the drugs that are selective ligands for those receptors, are presented in Table 1 [10,11].

Therapeutically beneficial analgesia results from diminished nociceptor excitability and the reduced release of pro-inflammatory peptides at nerve terminals [12]. However, effects, such as euphoria resulting from the agonism of µ receptors (described as sudden rush), mood modulation contributed by the agonism of δ receptors, or hallucinations caused by agonism of κ receptors [10,11], are often credited with the interest in these drugs with non-medical intents. Opioids also possess synergic effects with GABAergic receptor agonists, such as alcohol, barbiturates, or benzodiazepines.

Table 1. Receptor type specific effects of opioid drugs (agonists).

Receptor Type	Main Effects of Receptor Agonism	Receptor Agonist	Receptor Type Selectivity [1]	Ref.
µ (mu)	• analgesia • bradycardia • cough suppression • euphoria (rush) • miosis (pupil constriction) • physical dependence • reduced gastrointestinal motility (constipation, cramps) • respiratory depression (including decrease in sensitivity of respiratory center for CO_2) • sedation	morphine (reference)	µ/δ: 0.006–0.040 µ/κ: 0.023–0.059	[13–16]
		codeine (OTC drug)	µ/δ: 0.049–0.051 µ/κ: 0.033–0.044	[13,15]
		dihydrocodeine (OTC drug)	µ/δ: 0.036–0.055 µ/κ: 0.018–0.023	[13,15]
		loperamide (OTC drug)	µ/δ: 0.003	[17]
δ (delta)	• cough suppression (disputed) • gastrointestinal dysmotility • mood modulation • respiratory depression • spinal analgesia (pain control)	morphine (reference)	δ/µ: 25.000–159.091	[13–16]
		SNC80 [2]	δ/µ: 0.002	[18,19]
		BW373U86 [3]	δ/µ: 0.120	[20]
κ (kappa)	• cough suppression • dysphoria (profound sensation of dissatisfaction and unease) • gastrointestinal dysmotility • hallucinations • peripheral analgesia • physical dependence • pupil constriction • sedation	morphine (reference)	κ/µ: 16.950–42.636	[13–16]
		butorphanol [4]	κ/µ: 0.545	[21,22]
		pentazocine [4]	κ/µ: 0.564–0.772	[14]
		nalorphine [5]	κ/µ: 0.667–0.895	[14]

[1] Ratio of Ki-values (lower value = more selective); [2] experimental drug (convulsant/antidepressant/anxiolytic); [3] experimental drug (convulsant/antidepressant/analgesic); [4] therapeutic analgesic; [5] opioid overdose antidote.

Typical opioid overdose is associated with a characteristic triad of symptoms: decreased consciousness (or coma), abnormally slow or ceased respiration, and pinpoint pupils. Respiratory depression can manifest as cyanosis and have severe (neural damage caused by cerebral hypoxia) or even fatal consequences [10]. Paraesthesia (abnormal dermal sensations), urinary retention, and histamine-mediated reactions (emesis, flushing, itching, and nausea) have been also reported for opiate use [23]. Prolonged abuse results in physical and psychological dependence, the development of tolerance (possibly due to the desensitization and internalisation of µ receptors [24], and probable formation of opiate antibodies [25]), and is associated with the onset of withdrawal syndrome (symptoms include: agitation, diarrhoea, insomnia, muscle cramps, panic attacks, and sweating), when dosing is abruptly discontinued [26,27].

2.2. Codeine

Codeine is a natural alkaloid of opium poppy (an opiate), with affinity to µ, δ and κ receptors acting as their agonist. Codeine is approximately 20 times more selective towards the µ receptors than towards δ type, and even less selective (ca. 20–30 times) towards κ receptors (see Table 1). It is marketed as a cough suppressant and analgesic and is available for patients as tablets and syrups. In medications indicated for mild to moderate pain control, codeine is often paired with paracetamol (acetaminophen) or ibuprofen, and in medications indicated for cough and cold with promethazine or salicylic acid. The drug is generally not perceived as harmful by the patients [28,29], and this lenient attitude has perhaps resulted in increased worldwide consumption within the last 20 years and also in increased codeine dependency rates. In this regard, codeine is the world's most consumed opioid (based on drug quantity [30]), and codeine-dependent individuals account for approximately 2% of all admissions to some substance abuse centers [31].

The pharmacological profile of codeine as therapeutic drug, as well as a misused substance, is an outcome of active metabolite formation. The complex biotransformation pathways leading to prescription-only opioids, such as hydrocodone (up to 11% of parent drug), morphine (5–30%), and its more potent metabolites (hydromorphone and morphine-6-glucuronide), are presented in Figure 1 [6,12,32]. Such pharmacokinetics result in codeine potency being approximately one tenth the potency of morphine and resulting equianalgesic dose of codeine being 6.67–10 times larger than with morphine (both administered orally) [33,34].

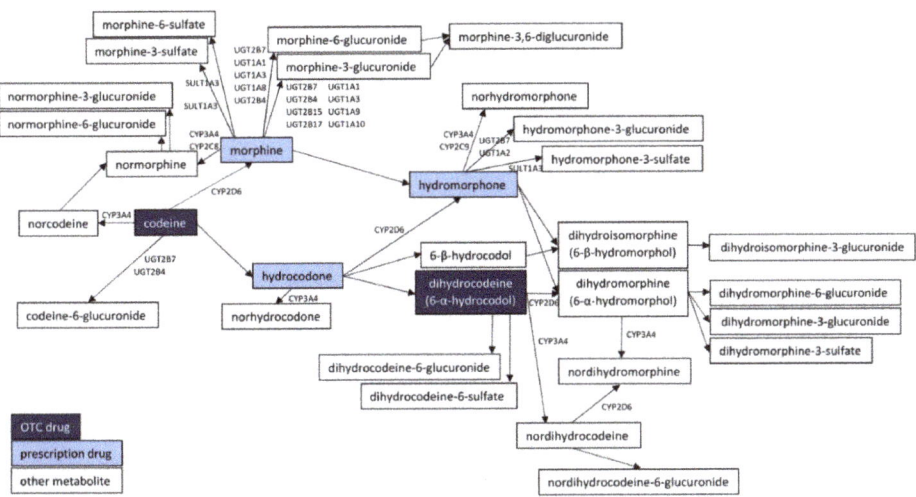

Figure 1. Metabolic pathways of codeine and dihydrocodeine. Abbreviations used: CYP = cytochrome P450, SULT = sulfotransferase, UGT = uridine diphosphate glucuronosyltransferase.

Although codeine is almost completely absorbed from the gastrointestinal tract (94 ± 4%), the pharmacokinetics of the drug may vary significantly between individuals due to genetic polymorphisms of *CYP2D6* and *CYP3A4* genes [6]. The transformation of codeine to morphine is especially dependent on CYP2D6 functionality, a factor firmly associated with one's ethnicity. In poor metabolizers (with two non-functional alleles of the *CYP2D6* gene), codeine may not express the desired effect at all, while in ultra-rapid metabolizers (with three or more functional alleles), poisoning is possible even within the recommended dose [12,32,35,36]. Other factors, such as a fat-rich diet and contents of grapefruit juice (especially bergamottin, an inhibitor of CYP3A4), are proven to potentialize the drug. In addition, P-glycoprotein (P-gp)—an efflux pump preventing certain drugs from penetrating the blood–brain barrier (BBB)—has been shown to have significant impact on brain concentration of the morphine [37].

As a cough suppressant, codeine (through active metabolites) acts in sub-analgesic doses at the μ_2 and κ receptors by inhibiting the medullary cough center. The analgesic action is mediated by μ receptors, with the complementary contribution of other opioid receptor types [6,38]. Codeine-containing OTC medications are often misused to achieve euphoria, relaxation, and feeling of warmth (described as recurrent waves of pleasurable sensations), or as a substitute for illicit narcotics [26]. In a single dose, codeine is generally described by its misusers as sedating, but repetitive doses tend to be energizing [27]. Positive reinforcement is an effect of μ_2 receptor stimulation. Misuse has also been reported as a means to escape persistent pain or achieve a state of disconnection or dissociation. This dissociative state is described as a dream-like floating sensation accompanied by slight hallucinations (e.g., seeing geometric shapes), or even out-of-body experiences [26].

The symptoms of codeine overdose are mostly consistent with typical opioid poisoning, but the drug originating from OTC formulations is often accompanied by non-opioid analgesics. Thus, hepatotoxicity from paracetamol, or gastrointestinal damage (haemorrhages, ulcerations, hypokalaemia, metabolic acidosis) and nephrotoxicity caused by ibuprofen are common consequences of its misuse [27,39–41]. In effort to evade these harms, various homemade extraction methods are used to separate codeine from the abovementioned drugs—for example, the so-called cold water extraction that exploits solubility differences between ingredients [35,42,43]. Lately, some pharmaceutical companies begun to incorporate physical or chemical barriers to their products as a means to combat such practices [26].

OTC codeine tablets are available in doses up to 15 mg, with guidelines recommending 15 mg every 4–6 h (maximally 45 mg a day) as an antitussive, and up to 15–30 mg every 6h (maximally 90 mg a day) for pain control. Drug misusers propose 30–60 mg as a starting dose (to test individual reaction for the drug), and further doses of 100–250 mg in order to achieve euphoria [27,28,44]. While a quantity of 500–1000 mg is usually considered lethal [45], as much as 1536 mg a day has been reported as dependent individuals' routines [6,26,39,40,46–48]. Due to the large doses consumed, codeine used for non-medical purposes is more dangerous than morphine used for anesthesia. The safety ratio of misused codeine is ca. 20 [45] (ratio of usual lethal dose to the usual effective dose), while the therapeutic index of morphine is 70 [49] (ratio of lethal dose (LD_{50}) to the therapeutic effective dose (ED_{50})). The safety ratio of codeine is equal to that of methadone (when both drugs are administered orally for non-medical purposes), but this is more than three times larger than for the injected heroin [45]. Based on animal studies it is possible to compare the safety of codeine with morphine, and also with fellow OTC opioid loperamide (all drugs administered orally; see Table 2). Experimental data show that, despite its reputation as a safe drug [28,29], codeine is in fact dangerous and is characterized by a narrow therapeutic index.

Table 2. Efficacy and toxicity of selected opioids in animal studies.

Drug	Mouse				Rat			
	LD_{50} (mg/kg)		ED_{50} (mg/kg)		Therapeutic Index	LD_{50} (mg/kg)		ED_{50} [1] (mg/kg)		Therapeutic Index
Morphine (reference)	524 610	[50] [52]	28.8	[51]	18.2–21.2	335	[50]	N/A	N/A
Codeine	250	[45,53]	43.2 139.9	[54] [51]	1.8–5.8	266 427	[45] [53]	69.3 [55]	3.8–6.2
Loperamide	105	[56]	N/A		N/A	185	[56]	0.15 [57] 0.61 [58] 1.81 [57,58]	102–1233

[1] Morphine and codeine tested as analgesics, loperamide tested as antidiarrheal.

The effects of opioids such as codeine are known to be potentialized by the non-selective H_1 histaminergic receptor antagonists such as promethazine. Usually, therapeutic doses of first-generation antihistamines cause sedation by blocking the H_1 receptors located in the central nervous system (CNS), sometimes to such extent that diphenhydramine is even marketed as an OTC sleeping aid. Surprisingly, supratherapeutic doses may cause paradoxical CNS stimulation (euphory, hallucinations), mainly due to anticholinergic poisoning [59]. Promethazine misuse is either related to its calming effect or ability to induce paradoxical euphoria and occasional hallucinations (auditory and visual), when administered in larger amounts [60]. Such effects are further enhanced by the simultaneous consumption of alcohol. To exploit these features, promethazine–codeine containing syrup is mixed with alcohol, candy, and soft drinks to create "purple drank". The concoction is probably named after the color of the syrup's dye and pursued in order to achieve euphoric and relaxing sensations [6,61]. Arrhythmia (manifesting as a prolongation of the QT interval in electrocardiogram), delirium, psychoses, substance dependence, and withdrawal syndrome are some of the known consequences of its misuse, as well as tardive dyskinesia resulting from the antagonism of D_2 dopaminergic receptors [62].

Another alarming trend entails clandestine syntheses of more potent opioids with codeine used as a substrate. The "homebake" method results in the demethylation of codeine to morphine, while with a slightly more complex protocol [63–66] it is possible to obtain desomorphine—a drug with an 8–10 times stronger analgesic effect (up to 80–100 times stronger than the precursor codeine) and three times the toxicity of morphine [42,65]. Structural differences between these opioids are presented in Figure 2.

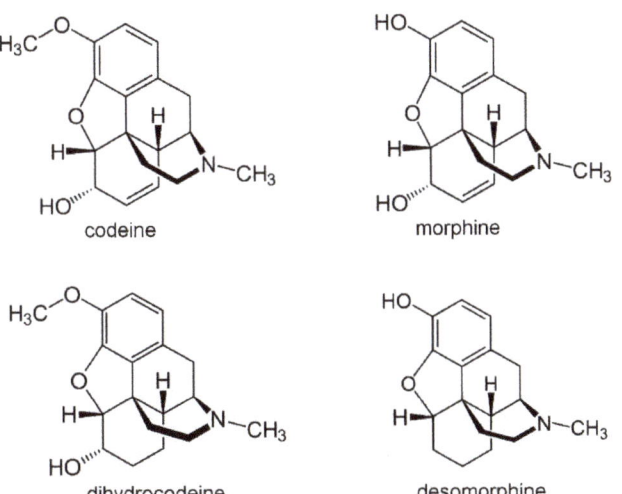

Figure 2. Chemical structures of selected opioid drugs.

Desomorphine is commonly known as "Krokodil", allegedly due to consequences of its injectable use, which presents as discoloured (green/black), flaking, and scale-like skin with ulcerations, somewhat resembling crocodile scale [11,23,63]. Although the drug is dated back to 1920s, it remained on the sidelines until its non-medical use spread across Russia, Ukraine, and neighbouring countries as a shocking new menace, reaching its apex just several years ago. Harm caused by "Krokodil" seems to be mostly related to reagents and contaminants introduced during the synthesis process, and include jaw osteonecrosis caused by red phosphorus, heavy metal poisoning (concentration, memory, motor, and speech impairments) due to corroded laboratory equipment, and skin infections with vascular damage that often leads to necrosis/gangrene, sometimes requiring limb amputation [23]. As an opioid, desomorphine has the same µ receptor affinity as morphine (but weaker to δ and κ type receptors), but is more addictive due a to faster onset of action and shorter elimination time, while also not inducing the emetic effects related to the use of morphine [64,67]. Damage to liver and kidneys has also been reported, as well as hallucinations [23].

2.3. Dihydrocodeine

Twice as strong as codeine, dihydrocodeine is a cough suppressant and analgesic used for mild to moderate pain control [68]. Slight euphoria, reported as a therapeutic side effect, increases further with supratherapeutic doses. Other adverse effects include constipation, drowsiness, dry mouth, headaches, nausea, respiratory depression, urinary retention, and substance dependence.

Dihydrocodeine, an agonist of µ, δ, and κ opioid receptors, is highly selective for µ type (µ/δ selectivity ratio is ca. 20–25; µ/κ selectivity ratio is ca. 45–55; see Table 1). As with codeine, dihydrocodeine acts through the formation of active metabolites. A small percentage of parent drug (1.3–9%) is transformed to dihydromorphine (1.2 times as potent as morphine) by CYP2D6. However, the formation of this metabolite is not solely responsible for the analgesic effect of dihydrocodeine [69]. Other metabolites include nordihydrocodeine, which has the same µ, δ, and κ receptors affinity as dihydrocodeine (16% of parent drug, mediated by CYP3A4), and dihydrocodeine-6-glucuronide (28% of parent drug) [68,70,71].

Over-the-counter dihydrocodeine medicines are available as syrups and tablets with doses up to 20 mg, and often contain paracetamol, or non-steroidal anti-inflammatory drugs (NSAIDs), as opposed to prescription-only medications, in which dihydrocodeine is generally the sole active ingredient, which is also present in higher dose and in controlled release formulation. Typical dihydrocodeine dosing as an OTC analgesic is ca. 7.5–15 mg every 4–6 h, not surpassing ca. 60 mg a day. Reports on drug misuse point at single doses of 300–900 mg, and up to 1350 mg a day [72]. A single dose of 70 mg is usually sufficient to induce a euphoric state. The lowest published toxic dose (oral) is 28 mg/kg (what corresponds to approximately 2000 mg for an average adult) [73].

2.4. Loperamide

Is a synthetic opioid antidiarrheal characterized by poor bioavailability and substantial metabolism due to a first pass effect and only a fraction of ingested drug crossing the blood–brain barrier. These traits have contributed to a long-lasting belief that, although a potent opioid (with structural similarity to fentanyl), loperamide is devoid of a central mechanism of action and perfectly safe to use [58,74–76]. However, recent reports on its misuse and a sudden increase in number of poisonings recorded since 2014, have led to a re-evaluation of its safety, and prompted a warning from the Food and Drug Administration (FDA) issued in 2016 and regarding arrhythmogenic potential of loperamide when taken in high doses [77–79]. The minimal BBB penetration and subsequent insignificant effects on the central nervous system, despite the lipophilic nature of the compound (logP value is estimated to be in the range 4.44–5.5 [80,81]), are a result of P-gp's activity [82,83]. However, the ingestion of massive amounts, so called megadosing, can lead to drug concentration surpassing P-gp's processing capacity. Additionally, common agents, such as piperidine (present in black pepper), proton-pump inhibitors (including fellow OTC drug omeprazole), as well as loperamide itself, are P-gp inhibitors with considerable potential to increase the amount of loperamide that is crossing the BBB [78,84]. Additionally, the inhibition of CYP3A4 and CYP2C8 by cimetidine or ranitidine (OTC medications from H$_2$-antihistamine class) and the contents of grapefruit juice, have been shown to hinder loperamide's metabolism, increasing bioavailable drug concentration [75,76,83,84].

Loperamide is an agonist of the μ, δ, and κ opioid receptors. The drug shows strong selectivity towards μ receptors (μ/δ selectivity >300; see Table 1). In therapeutic doses, it almost exclusively binds to a fraction of these receptors located along the gastrointestinal tract. However, when taken in supratherapeutic doses it can manifest its central mechanism of action. Loperamide is also an inhibitor of voltage-dependent P/Q$_{(1A)}$ calcium channels, calcium channels in the intestines, sodium channels in the heart, and calmodulin [75,82,83].

Cardiotoxicity in large doses is visible as a widening of the QRS complex. This is caused by a prolongation in depolarization due to a blockade of sodium channels, and the widening of the QT interval due to prolonged repolarization, which is caused by a blockade of potassium ion channels regulating delayed rectifier currents [74,78,82,85–88].

Therapeutic dosing typically involves an initial dose of 4 mg, followed by 2 mg after every loose stool (but not exceeding 16 mg a day). A quantity corresponding to 5–10 times the therapeutic dose (20–40 mg) is allegedly enough to alleviate symptoms of opioid withdrawal syndrome, and larger doses of 60–800 mg, or 1600 mg a day, can cause euphoria. However, regardless of consumed amount, loperamide seems to be without an analgesic effect [76,89]. While misuse is more often intended to aid opioid withdrawal rather than for other non-medical purposes, most of the reported poisonings (almost half of them) have been associated with suicide attempts [77,79,90]. As with other opioids, withdrawal syndrome and dependence have also been described with prolonged use of loperamide.

2.5. Alternative (Non-Opioid) Antitussives Used to Treat Unproductive Cough

Cough medications stand as one of the most misused drugs, not only within the OTC drugs category, but also among all psychoactive substances [91]. The misuse of antitussives is often associated with the aforementioned opioids, such as codeine or dihydrocodeine, but non-opioid dextromethorphan and zipeprol also gained some recognition as recreational drugs, owing to their hallucinogenic properties when taken in supratherapeutic doses. Several cases of fatal poisonings have since led to a withdrawal of zipeprol. However, dextromethorphan-based cough medicines remain available as one of the most popular antitussive medicines worldwide.

Structurally, dextromethorphan is an isomer of the opioid levorphanol, but due to its marginal affinity to opioid receptors, it is not classified as an opioid. Pharmacologically, dextromethorphan is an agonist of σ receptors (formerly classified as opioid receptors) and, in higher doses, an antagonist of excitatory N-methyl-D-aspartate glutamate receptors (NMDARs). Dextromethorphan is metabolized to dextrophan by the CYP2D6 [92] and, given that this metabolite is credited for the dissociative effects of the drug, in the case of its misuse, dextromethorphan can be considered a prodrug [8].

According to the reports, dextromethorphan is usually misused in quantities of 225–2500 mg [7,93], while a lethal dose is considered to be within the 50–500 mg/kg range (approximately 3500–35,000 mg for an adult) [8]. Such a wide range is mainly an outcome of significant differences to the CYP2D6 activity found across populations, caused by the polymorphism of a related gene [6]. Nevertheless, the aforementioned values result in a drug safety ratio of approximately 15 (other authors state it to be ca. 10 [45]), which is less than a corresponding value for codeine (safety ratio = 20) [45]. This shows that dextromethorphan, although not an opioid itself, is no safer than codeine if not used accordingly.

3. Conclusions

The misuse of opioid drugs is an important issue burdening the modern world more than ever before. The scale of this phenomenon, called the 21st century opioid crisis, is clearly illustrated by an ever-increasing involvement of opioids in the total number of all substance overdoses. The number of opioid overdoses has increased nearly 6-fold over the course of the last 20 years, and their contribution to fatal intoxications grew from approximately one half to over two thirds of all cases [94].

While it is generally agreed upon that this problem concerns mainly prescription-only opioids and illicit narcotics (such as novel analogues of fentanyl), the involvement of OTC opioids should not be overlooked as there is sound evidence that such substances are being misused. Relatively easy access to OTC opioids is alarming and perhaps requires additional consideration and debate on the rescheduling of their availability (some countries already undertaken such steps and limited access to codeine or dihydrocodeine [4]). However, as discussed, drugs are among the most popular medicines worldwide, their sudden disappearance from over-the-counter sale could prove problematic for patients. At the moment, codeine and loperamide are both considered essential medicines according to the WHO [95]. However, their misuse liability is an important stimulus for research on new, less-addictive candidates to replace them (both opioid and non-opioid).

4. Materials and Methods

4.1. Data Source

Study material was identified and retrieved from the Medline database, accessed via the PubMed website [96], and the full-text databases of the following publishers: Elsevier [97], Springer Nature [98], and Wiley [99]. The search was conducted with phrases created by combining the international non-proprietary names of opioid drugs (codeine, dihydrocodeine, and loperamide), or the word OTC, with terms such as abuse, misuse, addiction, dependence, intoxication, poisoning, and toxicity. An additional search was conducted with the Nicolaus Copernicus University search engine, and references from already included items were screened for previously omitted records. The complete workflow is presented in Figure 3, showing flow diagram prepared according to the PRISMA guidelines [100].

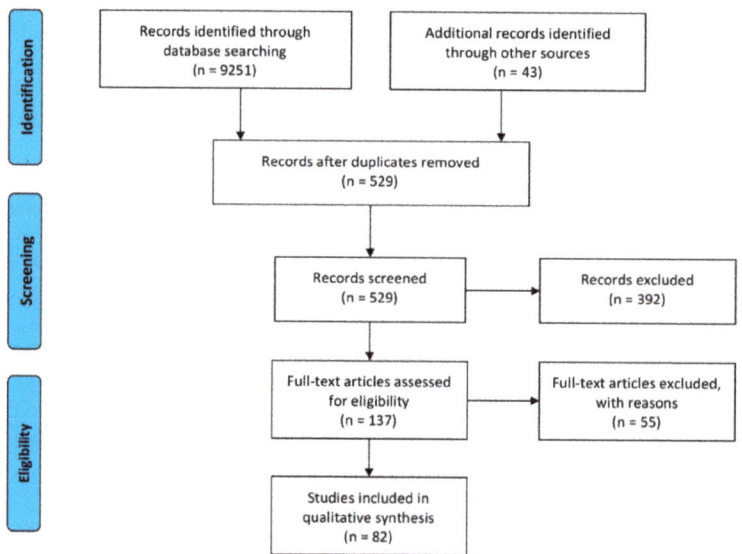

Figure 3. PRISMA Flow Diagram.

Initially, 9182 items were identified, specifically 5477 for codeine, 393 for dihydrocodeine, 836 for loperamide, and 2476 records discussing OTC drugs in general. Eventually, 137 items were assessed, 43 for codeine, 19 for dihydrocodeine, 20 for loperamide, 41 for opioids, and 14 for OTC drugs.

4.2. Inclusion and Exclusion Criteria

As pharmacology was the main focus of this review, no territorial criteria were used. Therefore, records from both counties where disclosed drugs are available without prescription, and those where they are only available with a prescription were included. No limitations regarding publication date were in place; however, when available, recent (less than 5-years-old) and primary literature was prioritized to display the current state of knowledge on the subject. Only papers written in the English and Polish languages were assessed.

4.3. Additional Limitations of the Work

The abuse-related substance consumption amounts disclosed in this work are based on user self-reports or toxicological case reports. Thus, presented values only hint at the most popular patterns, and are not establishing the definitive boundaries of this phenomenon. Furthermore, it should be noted that most pharmaceuticals containing the herein discussed substances are formulated using salts of active pharmaceutical ingredients, not their free base or acid forms. As many investigated records failed to mention the exact chemical form, this review further disregarded them, using instead a simplified nomenclature for the sake of unification and clarity.

Author Contributions: The manuscript was written through contributions of all authors. CRediT statement: Conceptualization, Ł.S.; Methodology, Ł.S.; Formal Analysis, Ł.S.; Investigation, Ł.S.; Resources, K.G.; Data Curation, Ł.S.; Writing—Original Draft Preparation, Ł.S.; Writing—Review & Editing, Ł.S. and K.G.; Visualization, Ł.S.; Supervision, K.G.; Project Administration, K.G.; Funding Acquisition, K.G. All authors have read and agreed to the published version of the manuscript.

Funding: This research was funded by The National Centre for Research and Development grant number LIDER/44/0164/L-9/17/NCBR/2018. The APC was funded by The National Centre for Research and Development grant number LIDER/44/0164/L-9/17/NCBR/2018.

Conflicts of Interest: The authors declare no conflict of interest.

References

1. Foley, M.; Breindahl, T.; Hindersson, P.; Deluca, P.; Kimergård, A. Misuse of 'Over-The-Counter' Codeine Analgesics: Does Formulation Play a Role? *Public Health* **2016**, *130*, 95–96. [CrossRef]
2. DZIENNIK USTAW RZECZYPOSPOLITEJ POLSKIEJ, Poz. 2189, ROZPORZĄDZENIE MINISTRA ZDROWIA z dnia 16 grudnia 2016 r. w sprawie wykazu substancji o działaniu psychoaktywnym oraz maksymalnego poziomu ich zawartości w produkcie leczniczym, stanowiącego ograniczenie w wydawaniu produktów leczniczych w ramach jednorazowej sprzedaży. Available online: http://isap.sejm.gov.pl/isap.nsf/download.xsp/WDU20160002189/O/D20162189.pdf (accessed on 20 August 2020).
3. Foley, M.; Harris, R.; Rich, E.; Rapca, A.; Bergin, M.; Norman, I.; Van Hout, M.C. The Availability of Over-The-Counter Codeine Medicines Across the European Union. *Public Health* **2015**, *11*, 1465–1470. [CrossRef] [PubMed]
4. Mishriky, J.; Stupans, I.; Chan, V. Pharmacists' Views on the Upscheduling of Codeine-Containing Analgesics to 'Prescription Only' Medicines in Australia. *Int. J. Clin. Pharm* **2019**, *41*, 538–545. [CrossRef] [PubMed]
5. Tay, E.M.Y.; Roberts, D.M. A Spotlight on the Role, Use, and Availability of Codeine and the Implications Faced. *Expert Rev. Clin. Pharmacol.* **2018**, *11*, 1057–1059. [CrossRef] [PubMed]
6. Burns, J.M.; Boyer, E.W. Antitussives and substance abuse. *Subst. Abuse Rehabil.* **2013**, *4*, 75–82. [CrossRef]
7. Motyka, M.; Marcinkowski, J.T. New methods of narcotization. Part I. Drugs available without a prescription used for psychoactive purposes. *Probl. Hig. Epidemiol.* **2014**, *95*, 504–511.
8. Piątek, A.; Koziarska-Rościszewska, M.; Zawilska, J.B. Recreational use of over-the-counter drugs: The doping of the brain. *Alcohol. Drug Addict.* **2015**, *28*, 65–77. [CrossRef]
9. Jakubowski, P.; Puchała, Ł.; Grzegorzewski, W. Recreational use of popular OTC drugs—Pharmacological review. *Farmacia* **2018**, *66*, 209–215.
10. Oelhaf, R.C.; Azadfard, M. Opioid Toxicity. In *StatPearls [Internet]*; StatPearls Publishing: Treasure Island, FL, USA, 2020.

11. Van Hout, M.C. Kitchen chemistry: A scoping review of the diversionary use of pharmaceuticals for non-medicinal use and home production of drug solutions. *Drug Test. Anal.* **2014**, *6*, 778–787. [CrossRef]
12. DePriest, A.Z.; Puet, B.L.; Holt, A.C.; Roberts, A.; Cone, E.J. Metabolism and Disposition of Prescription Opioids: A Review. *Forensic Sci. Rev.* **2015**, *27*, 115–145.
13. Mignat, C.; Wille, U.; Ziegler, A. Affinity profiles of morphine, codeine, dihydrocodeine and their glucuronides at opioid receptor subtypes. *Life Sci.* **1995**, *56*, 793–799. [CrossRef]
14. Toll, L.; Berzetei-Gurske, I.P.; Polgar, W.E.; Brandt, S.R.; Adapa, I.D.; Rodriguez, L.; Schwartz, R.W.; Haggart, D.; O'Brien, A.; White, A.; et al. Standard binding and functional assays related to medications development division testing for potential cocaine and opiate narcotic treatment medications. *NIDA Res. Monogr.* **1998**, *178*, 440–466. [PubMed]
15. Schmidt, H.; v Vormfelde, S.; Klinder, K.; Gundert-Remy, U.; Gleiter, C.H.; Skopp, G.; Aderjan, R.; Fuhr, U. Affinities of dihydrocodeine and its metabolites to opioid receptors. *Pharmacol. Toxicol.* **2002**, *91*, 57–63. [CrossRef] [PubMed]
16. Peng, X.; Knapp, B.I.; Bidlack, J.M.; Neumeyer, J.L. Synthesis and preliminary in vitro investigation of bivalent ligands containing homo- and heterodimeric pharmacophores at mu, delta, and kappa opioid receptors. *J. Med. Chem.* **2006**, *49*, 256–262. [CrossRef]
17. Breslin, H.J.; Miskowski, T.A.; Rafferty, B.M.; Coutinho, S.V.; Palmer, J.M.; Wallace, N.H.; Schneider, C.R.; Kimball, E.S.; Zhang, S.P.; Li, J.; et al. Rationale, design, and synthesis of novel phenyl imidazoles as opioid receptor agonists for gastrointestinal disorders. *J. Med. Chem.* **2004**, *47*, 5009–5020. [CrossRef]
18. Bilsky, E.J.; Calderon, S.N.; Wang, T.; Bernstein, R.N.; Davis, P.; Hruby, V.J.; McNutt, R.W.; Rothman, R.B.; Rice, K.C.; Porreca, F. SNC 80, a selective, nonpeptidic and systemically active opioid delta agonist. *J. Pharmacol. Exp. Ther.* **1995**, *273*, 359–366.
19. Saitoh, A.; Kimura, Y.; Suzuki, T.; Kawai, K.; Nagase, H.; Kamei, J. Potential anxiolytic and antidepressant-like activities of SNC80, a selective delta-opioid agonist, in behavioral models in rodents. *J. Pharmacol. Sci.* **2004**, *95*, 374 380. [CrossRef]
20. Chang, K.J.; Rigdon, G.C.; Howard, J.L.; McNutt, R.W. A novel, potent and selective nonpeptidic delta opioid receptor agonist BW373U86. *J. Pharmacol. Exp. Ther.* **1993**, *267*, 852–857.
21. Fulton, B.S.; Knapp, B.I.; Bidlack, J.M.; Neumeyer, J.L. Synthesis and Pharmacological Evaluation of Hydrophobic Esters and Ethers of Butorphanol at Opioid Receptors. *Bioorg. Med. Chem. Lett.* **2008**, *18*, 4474–4476. [CrossRef]
22. Zhang, B.; Zhang, T.; Sromek, A.W.; Scrimale, T.; Bidlack, J.M.; Neumeyer, J.L. Synthesis and Binding Affinity of Novel Mono- and Bivalent Morphinan Ligands for κ, μ and δ Opioid Receptors. *Bioorg. Med. Chem.* **2011**, *19*, 2808–2816. [CrossRef]
23. Florez, D.H.Â.; Dos Santos Moreira, A.M.; da Silva, P.R.; Brandão, R.; Borges, M.M.C.; de Santana, F.J.M.; Borges, K.B. Desomorphine (Krokodil): An overview of its chemistry, pharmacology, metabolism, toxicology and analysis. *Drug Alcohol. Depend.* **2017**, *173*, 59–68. [CrossRef] [PubMed]
24. Ueda, H.; Inoue, M.; Mizuno, K. New approaches to study the development of morphine tolerance and dependence. *Life Sci.* **2003**, *74*, 313–320. [CrossRef] [PubMed]
25. Kim, H.; Oh, S.; Sung, B.; Tian, Y.; Yang, L.; Wang, S.; Mao, J. Anti-morphine antibody contributes to the development of morphine tolerance in rats. *Neurosci. Lett.* **2010**, *480*, 196–200. [CrossRef] [PubMed]
26. Van Hout, M.C. Nod and wave: An Internet study of the codeine intoxication phenomenon. *Int. J. Drug Policy* **2015**, *26*, 67–77. [CrossRef] [PubMed]
27. Van Hout, M.C.; Horan, A.; Santlal, K.; Rich, E.; Bergin, M. 'Codeine is my companion': Misuse and dependence on codeine containing medicines in Ireland. *Ir. J. Psychol. Med.* **2018**, *35*, 275–288. [CrossRef] [PubMed]
28. Peechakara, B.V.; Gupta, M. Codeine. In *StatPearls [Internet]*; StatPearls Publishing: Treasure Island, FL, USA, 2020.
29. Wells, J.S.; Bergin, M.; Van Hout, M.C.; McGuinness, P.; De Pleissisc, J.; Rich, E.; Dada, S.; Wells, R.; Gooney, M.A. Purchasing Over-The-Counter (OTC) Medicinal Products Containing Codeine—Easy Access, Advertising, Misuse and Perceptions of Medicinal Risk. *J. Pharm. Pharm. Sci.* **2018**, *21*, 286–295. [CrossRef]
30. Narcotic Drugs—Estimated World Requirements for 2020. Available online: https://www.incb.org/documents/Narcotic-Drugs/Technical-Publications/2019/Narcotic_Drugs_Technical_Publication_2019_web.pdf (accessed on 20 August 2020).

31. Parry, C.D.H.; Rich, E.; Van Hout, M.C.; Deluca, P. Codeine misuse and dependence in South Africa: Perspectives of addiction treatment providers. *S. Afr. Med. J.* **2017**, *107*, 451–456. [CrossRef]
32. Smith, H.S. Opioid Metabolism. *Mayo. Clin. Proc.* **2009**, *84*, 613–624. [CrossRef]
33. Opioid Equivalence Chart. Available online: https://www.gloshospitals.nhs.uk/gps/treatment-guidelines/opioid-equivalence-chart/ (accessed on 20 August 2020).
34. OPIATE CONVERSION DOSES. Available online: https://www.wales.nhs.uk/sites3/Documents/814/OpiateConversionDoses%5BFinal%5DNov2010.pdf (accessed on 20 August 2020).
35. Nielsen, S.; Van Hout, M.C. Over-the-Counter Codeine-from Therapeutic Use to Dependence, and the Grey Areas in Between. *Curr. Top. Behav. Neurosci.* **2017**, *34*, 59–75. [CrossRef]
36. Gasche, Y.; Daali, Y.; Fathi, M.; Chiappe, A.; Cottini, S.; Dayer, P.; Desmeules, J. Codeine intoxication associated with ultrarapid CYP2D6 metabolism. *N. Engl. J. Med.* **2004**, *27*, 2827–2831. [CrossRef]
37. Lam, J.; Woodall, K.L.; Solbeck, P.; Ross, C.J.; Carleton, B.C.; Hayden, M.R.; Koren, G.; Madadi, P. Codeine-related deaths: The role of pharmacogenetics and drug interactions. *Forensic Sci. Int.* **2014**, *239*, 50–56. [CrossRef] [PubMed]
38. Roussin, A.; Bouyssi, A.; Pouché, L.; Pourcel, L.; Lapeyre-Mestre, M. Misuse and Dependence on Non-Prescription Codeine Analgesics or Sedative H1 Antihistamines by Adults: A Cross-Sectional Investigation in France. *PLoS ONE* **2013**, *8*, e76499. [CrossRef] [PubMed]
39. Frei, M.Y.; Nielsen, S.; Dobbin, M.D.H.; Tobin, C.L. Serious morbidity associated with misuse of over-the-counter codeine-ibuprofen analgesics: A series of 27 cases. *Med. J. Aust.* **2010**, *193*, 294–296. [CrossRef] [PubMed]
40. Robinson, G.M.; Robinson, S.; McCarthy, P.; Cameron, C. Misuse of over-the-counter codeine-containing analgesics: Dependence and other adverse effects. *N. Z. Med. J.* **2010**, *123*, 59–64. [PubMed]
41. Mill, D.; Johnson, J.L.; Cock, V.; Monaghan, E.; Hotham, E.D. Counting the cost of over-the-counter codeine containing analgesic misuse: A retrospective review of hospital admissions over a 5-year period. *Drug Alcohol. Rev.* **2018**, *37*, 247–256. [CrossRef] [PubMed]
42. Kimergård, A.; Deluca, P.; Hindersson, P.; Breindahl, T. How Resistant to Tampering are Codeine Containing Analgesics on the Market? Assessing the Potential for Opioid Extraction. *Pain Ther.* **2016**, *5*, 187–201. [CrossRef]
43. Pascali, J.P.; Fais, P.; Vaiano, F.; Pigaiani, N.; D'Errico, S.; Furlanetto, S.; Palumbo, D.; Bertol, E. Internet pseudoscience: Testing opioid containing formulations with tampering potential. *J. Pharm. Biomed. Anal.* **2018**, *153*, 16–21. [CrossRef]
44. Van Hout, M.C.; Rich, E.; Dada, S.; Bergin, M. "Codeine Is My Helper": Misuse of and Dependence on Codeine-Containing Medicines in South Africa. *Qual. Health Res.* **2017**, *27*, 341–350. [CrossRef]
45. Gable, R.S. Comparison of acute lethal toxicity of commonly abused psychoactive substances. *Addiction* **2004**, *99*, 686–696. [CrossRef]
46. Evans, C.; Chalmers-Watson, T.A.; Gearry, R.B. Medical image. Combination NSAID-codeine preparations and gastrointestinal toxicity. *N. Z. Med. J.* **2010**, *1324*, 92–93.
47. Nielsen, S.; MacDonald, T.; Johnson, J.L. Identifying and treating codeine dependence: A systematic review. *Med. J. Aust.* **2018**, *208*, 451–461. [CrossRef] [PubMed]
48. Van Hout, M.C.; Delargy, I.; Ryan, G.; Flanagan, S.; Gallagher, H. Dependence on Over the Counter (OTC) Codeine Containing Analgesics: Treatment and Recovery with Buprenorphine Naloxone. *Int. J. Ment. Addict.* **2016**, *14*, 873–883. [CrossRef]
49. Stanley, T.H. Anesthesia for the 21st century. *Proc. Bayl. Uni. Med. Cent.* **2000**, *13*, 7–10. [CrossRef] [PubMed]
50. Morphine SAFETY DATA SHEET. Available online: https://www.caymanchem.com/msdss/15464m.pdf (accessed on 20 August 2020).
51. Cichewicz, D.L.; Martin, Z.L.; Smith, F.L.; Welch, S.P. Enhancement of μ Opioid Antinociception by Oral Δ^9-Tetrahydrocannabinol: Dose-Response Analysis and Receptor Identification. *J. Pharmacol. Exp. Ther.* **1999**, *289*, 859–867. [PubMed]
52. La Barre, J. The pharmacological properties and therapeutic use of dextromoramide. *Bull. Narc.* **1959**, *4*, 10–19.
53. Codeine SAFETY DATA SHEET. Available online: https://www.caymanchem.com/msdss/ISO60140m.pdf (accessed on 20 August 2020).

54. Eddy, N.B.; Friebel, H.; Hahn, K.J.; Halbach, H. Codeine and its Alternates for Pain and Cough Relief, 2. Alternates for Pain Relief. *Bull. Wld. Hlth. Org.* **1969**, *40*, 1–53.
55. Schellekens, K.H.L.; Awouters, F.; Artois, K.S.K.; Frederickx, R.E.J.; Hendrickx, H.M.R.; van Bruggen, W.; Niemegeers, C.J.E. R 62 818, a new analgesic: A comparative study with codeine. *Drug Dev. Res.* **1986**, *8*, 353–360. [CrossRef]
56. Loperamide (hydrochloride) SAFETY DATA SHEET. Available online: https://www.caymanchem.com/msdss/14875m.pdf (accessed on 20 August 2020).
57. Niemegeers, C.J.; McGuire, J.L.; Heykants, J.J.; Janssen, P.A. Dissociation between opiate-like and antidiarrheal activities of antidiarrheal drugs. *J. Pharmacol. Exp. Ther.* **1979**, *210*, 327–333.
58. Baker, D.E. Loperamide: A pharmacological review. *Rev. Gastroenterol. Disord.* **2007**, *7*, S11–S18.
59. Halpert, A.G.; Olmstead, M.C.; Beninger, R.J. Mechanisms and abuse liability of the anti-histamine dimenhydrinate. *Neurosci. Biobehav. Rev.* **2002**, *26*, 61–67. [CrossRef]
60. Jensen, L.L.; Rømsing, J.; Dalhoff, K. A Danish Survey of Antihistamine Use and Poisoning Patterns. *Basic Clin. Pharmacol. Toxicol.* **2017**, *120*, 64–70. [CrossRef] [PubMed]
61. Agnich, L.E.; Stogner, J.M.; Miller, B.L.; Marcum, C.D. Purple drank prevalence and characteristics of misusers of codeine cough syrup mixtures. *Addict. Behav.* **2013**, *38*, 2445–2449. [CrossRef] [PubMed]
62. Parker, S.D.; De Gioannis, A.; Page, C. Chronic promethazine misuse and the possibility of dependence: A brief review of antihistamine abuse and dependence. *J. Subst. Use* **2013**, *18*, 238–241. [CrossRef]
63. Grund, J.P.; Latypov, A.; Harris, M. Breaking worse: The emergence of krokodil and excessive injuries among people who inject drugs in Eurasia. *Int. J. Drug Policy* **2013**, *24*, 265–274. [CrossRef] [PubMed]
64. Katselou, M.; Papoutsis, I.; Nikolaou, P.; Spiliopoulou, C.; Athanaselis, S. A "krokodil" emerges from the murky waters of addiction. Abuse trends of an old drug. *Life Sci.* **2014**, *102*, 81–87. [CrossRef]
65. Alves, E.A.; Grund, J.P.; Afonso, C.M.; Netto, A.D.; Carvalho, F.; Dinis-Oliveira, R.J. The harmful chemistry behind krokodil (desomorphine) synthesis and mechanisms of toxicity. *Forensic Sci. Int.* **2015**, *249*, 207–213. [CrossRef]
66. Alves, E.A.; Soares, J.X.; Afonso, C.M.; Grund, J.C.; Agonia, A.S.; Cravo, S.M.; Netto, A.D.P.; Carvalho, F.; Dinis-Oliveira, R.J. The harmful chemistry behind "krokodil": Street-like synthesis and product analysis. *Forensic Sci. Int.* **2015**, *257*, 76–82. [CrossRef]
67. Gahr, M.; Freudenmann, R.W.; Hiemke, C.; Gunst, I.M.; Connemann, B.J.; Schönfeldt-Lecuona, C. "Krokodil": Revival of an old drug with new problems. *Subst. Use Misuse* **2012**, *47*, 861–863. [CrossRef]
68. Leppert, W.; Woroń, J. Dihydrocodeine: Safety concerns. *Expert Rev. Clin. Pharmacol.* **2016**, *9*, 9–12. [CrossRef]
69. Jurna, I.; Kömen, W.; Baldauf, J.; Fleischer, W. Analgesia by dihydrocodeine is not due to formation of dihydromorphine: Evidence from nociceptive activity in rat thalamus. *J. Pharmacol. Exp. Ther.* **1997**, *281*, 1164–1170.
70. Ammon, S.; Hofmann, U.; Griese, E.U.; Gugeler, N.; Mikus, G. Pharmacokinetics of dihydrocodeine and its active metabolite after single and multiple oral dosing. *Br. J. Clin. Pharmacol.* **1999**, *48*, 317–322. [CrossRef] [PubMed]
71. Al-Asmari, A.I.; Anderson, R.A. The role of dihydrocodeine (DHC) metabolites in dihydrocodeine-related deaths. *J. Anal. Toxicol.* **2010**, *34*, 476–490. [CrossRef] [PubMed]
72. Marks, P.; Ashraf, H.; Root, T.R. Drug dependence caused by dihydrocodeine. *Br. Med. J.* **1978**, *1*, 1594. [CrossRef] [PubMed]
73. Dihydrocodeine SAFETY DATA SHEET. Available online: https://www.caymanchem.com/msdss/15460m.pdf (accessed on 20 August 2020).
74. Borron, S.W.; Watts, S.H.; Tull, J.; Baeza, S.; Diebold, S.; Barrow, A. Intentional Misuse and Abuse of Loperamide: A New Look at a Drug with "Low Abuse Potential". *J. Emerg. Med.* **2017**, *53*, 73–84. [CrossRef] [PubMed]
75. Hughes, A.; Hendrickson, R.G.; Chia-Chi Chen, B.; Valentod, M. Severe loperamide toxicity associated with the use of cimetidine to potentiate the "high". *Am. J. Emerg. Med.* **2018**, *36*, 1527.e3–1527.e5. [CrossRef] [PubMed]
76. Schifano, F.; Chiappini, S. Is there such a thing as a 'lope' dope? Analysis of loperamide-related European Medicines Agency (EMA) pharmacovigilance database reports. *PLoS ONE* **2018**, *13*, e0204443. [CrossRef]
77. Lasoff, D.R.; Koh, C.H.; Corbett, B.; Minns, A.B.; Cantrell, F.L. Loperamide Trends in Abuse and Misuse over 13 Years: 2002–2015. *Pharmacotherapy* **2017**, *37*, 249–253. [CrossRef]

78. Miller, H.; Panahi, L.; Tapia, D.; Tran, A.; Bowman, J.D. Loperamide misuse and abuse. *J. Am. Pharm. Assoc.* **2017**, *57*, S45–S50. [CrossRef]
79. Vakkalanka, J.P.; Charlton, N.P.; Holstege, C.P. Epidemiologic Trends in Loperamide Abuse and Misuse. *Ann. Emerg. Med.* **2017**, *69*, 73–78. [CrossRef]
80. DrugBank. Available online: https://www.drugbank.ca/drugs/DB00836 (accessed on 20 August 2020).
81. PubChem. Available online: https://pubchem.ncbi.nlm.nih.gov/compound/3955#section=Chemical-and-Physical-Properties (accessed on 20 August 2020).
82. Stanciu, C.N.; Gnanasegaram, S.A. Loperamide, the "Poor Man's Methadone": Brief Review. *J. Psychoact. Drugs* **2017**, *49*, 18–21. [CrossRef]
83. Wu, P.E.; Juurlink, D.N. Clinical Review: Loperamide Toxicity. *Ann. Emerg. Med.* **2017**, *70*, 245–252. [CrossRef] [PubMed]
84. Montesinos, R.N.; Moulari, B.; Gromand, J.; Beduneau, A.; Lamprecht, A.; Pellequer, Y. Coadministration of P-glycoprotein modulators on loperamide pharmacokinetics and brain distribution. *Drug Metab. Dispos.* **2014**, *42*, 700–706. [CrossRef] [PubMed]
85. Marraffa, J.M.; Holland, M.G.; Sullivan, R.W.; Morgan, B.W.; Oakes, J.A.; Wiegand, T.J.; Hodgman, M.J. Cardiac conduction disturbance after loperamide abuse. *Clin. Toxicol.* **2014**, *52*, 952–957. [CrossRef] [PubMed]
86. Kang, J.; Compton, D.R.; Vaz, R.J.; Rampe, D. Proarrhythmic mechanisms of the common anti-diarrheal medication loperamide: Revelations from the opioid abuse epidemic. *Naunyn. Schmiedebergs. Arch. Pharmacol.* **2016**, *389*, 1133–1137. [CrossRef] [PubMed]
87. Upadhyay, A.; Bodar, V.; Malekzadegan, M.; Singh, S.; Frumkin, W.; Mangla, A.; Doshi, K. Loperamide Induced Life Threatening Ventricular Arrhythmia. *Case Rep. Cardiol.* **2016**, *2016*, 5040176. [CrossRef]
88. Eggleston, W.; Clark, K.H.; Marraffa, J.M. Loperamide Abuse Associated with Cardiac Dysrhythmia and Death. *Ann. Emerg. Med.* **2017**, *69*, 83–86. [CrossRef]
89. MacDonald, R.; Heiner, J.; Villarreal, J.; Strote, J. Loperamide dependence and abuse. *BMJ Case Rep.* **2015**, *2015*, bcr2015209705. [CrossRef]
90. Daniulaityte, R.; Carlson, R.; Falck, R.; Cameron, D.; Perera, S.; Chen, L.; Sheth, A. "I Just Wanted to Tell You That Loperamide WILL WORK": A Web-Based Study of Extra-Medical Use of Loperamide. *Drug Alcohol. Depend.* **2013**, *130*, 241–244. [CrossRef]
91. Trends in Annual Prevalence of Use of Various Drugs for Grades 8, 10, and 12 Combined. Available online: http://monitoringthefuture.org/data/19data/19drtbl6.pdf (accessed on 20 August 2020).
92. Monte, A.A.; Chuang, R.; Bodmer, M. Dextromethorphan, chlorphenamine and serotonin toxicity: Case report and systematic literature review. *Br. J. Clin. Pharmacol.* **2010**, *70*, 794–798. [CrossRef]
93. Linn, K.A.; Long, M.T.; Pagel, P. "Robo-tripping": Dextromethorphan abuse and its anesthetic implications. *Anesth. Pain Med.* **2014**, *4*, e20990. [CrossRef]
94. Overdose Death Rates, Drug Overdoses Data Document.xls. Available online: https://www.drugabuse.gov/drug-topics/trends-statistics/overdose-death-rates (accessed on 20 August 2020).
95. World Health Organization Model List of Essential Medicines. Available online: https://apps.who.int/iris/bitstream/handle/10665/325771/WHO-MVP-EMP-IAU-2019.06-eng.pdf?ua=1 (accessed on 20 August 2020).
96. PubMed.gov. Available online: https://pubmed.ncbi.nlm.nih.gov/ (accessed on 20 August 2020).
97. ScienceDirect.com, Science, Health and Medical Journals, Full Text Articles and Books. Available online: https://www.sciencedirect.com/ (accessed on 20 August 2020).
98. Springer Link. Available online: https://link.springer.com/ (accessed on 20 August 2020).
99. Wiley Online Library, Scientific Research Articles, Journals, Books, and Reference Works. Available online: https://onlinelibrary.wiley.com/ (accessed on 20 August 2020).
100. Prisma Transparent Reporting of Systematic Reviews and Meta-Analyses. Available online: http://www.prisma-statement.org/ (accessed on 20 August 2020).

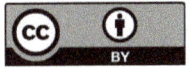

© 2020 by the authors. Licensee MDPI, Basel, Switzerland. This article is an open access article distributed under the terms and conditions of the Creative Commons Attribution (CC BY) license (http://creativecommons.org/licenses/by/4.0/).

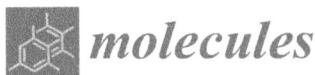

Article

The Intriguing Effects of Substituents in the *N*-Phenethyl Moiety of Norhydromorphone: A Bifunctional Opioid from a Set of "Tail Wags Dog" Experiments

Meining Wang [1], Thomas C. Irvin [1], Christine A. Herdman [1], Ramsey D. Hanna [1], Sergio A. Hassan [2], Yong-Sok Lee [2], Sophia Kaska [3], Rachel Saylor Crowley [3], Thomas E. Prisinzano [3], Sarah L. Withey [4], Carol A. Paronis [4], Jack Bergman [4], Saadet Inan [5], Ellen B. Geller [5], Martin W. Adler [5], Theresa A. Kopajtic [6], Jonathan L. Katz [6], Aaron M. Chadderdon [7], John R. Traynor [7], Arthur E. Jacobson [1,*] and Kenner C. Rice [1,*]

[1] Department of Health and Human Services, Drug Design and Synthesis Section, Molecular Targets and Medications Discovery Branch, Intramural Research Program, National Institute on Drug Abuse and the National Institute on Alcohol Abuse and Alcoholism, National Institutes of Health, 9800 Medical Center Drive, Bethesda, MD 20892-3373, USA; wangmeining8911@163.com (M.W.); Tom.irvin8@gmail.com (T.C.I.); caherdman@gmail.com (C.A.H.); Ramsey.hanna1@gmail.com (R.D.H.)

[2] Department of Health and Human Services, Center for Molecular Modeling, Office of Intramural Research, Center for Information Technology, National Institutes of Health, Bethesda, MD 20892, USA; hassan@mail.nih.gov (S.A.H.); leeys@mail.nih.gov (Y.-S.L.)

[3] Department of Medicinal Chemistry, School of Pharmacy, University of Kansas, Lawrence, KS 66045-7582, USA; sophia.kaska@uky.edu (S.K.); crowleyrachels@gmail.com (R.S.C.); prisinzano@uky.edu (T.E.P.)

[4] Behavioral Biology Program, McLean Hospital/Harvard Medical School, 115 Mill Street, Belmont, MA 02478, USA; swithey@mclean.harvard.edu (S.L.W.); cparonis@mclean.harvard.edu (C.A.P.); jbergman@hms.harvard.edu (J.B.)

[5] Center for Substance Abuse Research, Lewis Katz School of Medicine of Temple University, 3500 N. Broad St., Philadelphia, PA 19140, USA; sinan@temple.edu (S.I.); gellerellen@gmail.com (E.B.G.); baldeagl@temple.edu (M.W.A.)

[6] Department of Health and Human Services, Psychobiology Section, Molecular Neuropsychiatry Research Branch, Intramural Research Program, National Institute on Drug Abuse, National Institutes of Health, Baltimore, MD 21224, USA; theresa.kopajtic@gmail.com (T.A.K.); jkatzzz@gmail.com (J.L.K.)

[7] Department of Pharmacology and Edward F Domino Research Center, University of Michigan Medical School, Ann Arbor, MI 48109, USA; Aaron.Chadderdon@gmail.com (A.M.C.); jtraynor@umich.edu (J.R.T.)

* Correspondence: arthurj@nida.nih.gov (A.E.J.); kennerr@nida.nih.gov (K.C.R.); Tel.: +1-301-451-5028 (A.E.J.); +1-301-451-4799 (K.C.R.)

Academic Editor: Mariana Spetea
Received: 24 April 2020; Accepted: 3 June 2020; Published: 6 June 2020

Abstract: (−)-*N*-Phenethyl analogs of optically pure *N*-norhydromorphone were synthesized and pharmacologically evaluated in several in vitro assays (opioid receptor binding, stimulation of [^{35}S]GTPγS binding, forskolin-induced cAMP accumulation assay, and MOR-mediated β-arrestin recruitment assays). "Body" and "tail" interactions with opioid receptors (a subset of Portoghese's message-address theory) were used for molecular modeling and simulations, where the "address" can be considered the "body" of the hydromorphone molecule and the "message" delivered by the substituent (tail) on the aromatic ring of the *N*-phenethyl moiety. One compound, *N*-*p*-chlorophenethynorhydromorphone ((7a*R*,12b*S*)-3-(4-chlorophenethyl)-9-hydroxy-2,3,4,4a,5,6-hexahydro-1*H*-4,12-methanobenzofuro[3,2-e]isoquinolin-7(7a*H*)-one, **2i**), was found to have nanomolar binding affinity at MOR and DOR. It was a potent partial agonist at MOR and a full potent agonist at DOR with a δ/μ potency ratio of 1.2 in the ([^{35}S]GTPγS) assay. Bifunctional opioids that interact with MOR and DOR, the latter as agonists or antagonists, have been reported to have fewer side-effects than

MOR agonists. The *p*-chlorophenethyl compound **2i** was evaluated for its effect on respiration in both mice and squirrel monkeys. Compound **2i** did not depress respiration (using normal air) in mice or squirrel monkeys. However, under conditions of hypercapnia (using air mixed with 5% CO_2), respiration was depressed in squirrel monkeys.

Keywords: opioid; bifunctional ligands; (−)-*N*-phenethylnorhydromorphone analogs; [^{35}S]GTPgammaS assay; forskolin-induced cAMP accumulation assays; β-arrestin recruitment assays; MOR and DOR agonists; respiratory depression; bias factor; molecular modeling & simulation

1. Introduction

It is well-known that various *N*-substituents in the classical opioid-type of structure (e.g., 4,5-epoxy morphinans, morphinans, 6,7-benzomorphans, 5-phenylmorphans) can change prototypical *N*-methyl substituted agonist opioids to opioid antagonists. Most familiar, replacement of the *N*-methyl with an *N*-allyl moiety in morphine and oxymorphone converted them to the antagonists nalorphine and naloxone (Scheme 1).

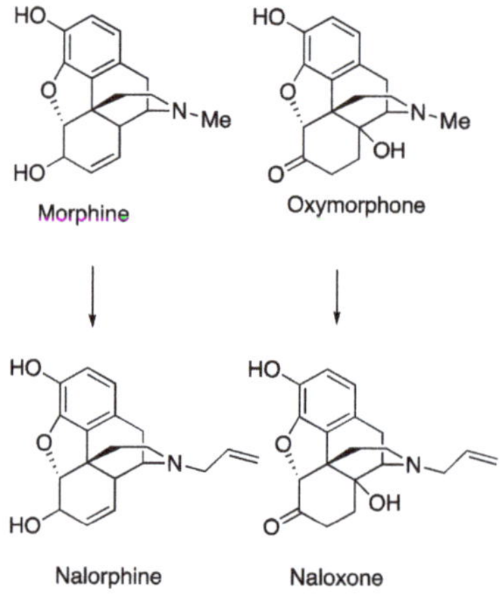

Scheme 1. Prototypical 4,5-epoxymorphinan agonists and antagonists.

Exactly how the *N*-substituent interaction with amino acid residues in the receptor induces that change remains uncertain. The *N*-methyl substituent in morphine and oxymorphone either permits or does not prevent the ligand from receptor interactions that result in analgesia and the well-known panoply of opioid side-effects. Concurrent with their interaction with G-proteins, potent clinically utilized opioids also recruit β-arrestin2. This recruitment has been hypothesized to underly the undesirable effects of opioids, including respiratory depression, inhibited gastrointestinal transport, and tolerance [1–4], although recent data using β-arrestin2 knockout mice cast doubt on that hypothesis [4].

Replacement of an *N*-methyl group with a different substituent, the *N*-phenethyl moiety, has also been shown to change an opioid agonist to an antagonist in at least one of the types of classical opioids; however, that outcome is not consistent for all opioid structures. Most *N*-phenethyl-substituted opioids, such as *N*-phenethylnormorphine [5], *N*-phenethylnoroxymorphone [6], and 2'-hydroxy-5,9-dimethyl-*N*-phenethylbenzomorphan [6] have been found to be potent μ-opioid receptor (MOR) agonists, but *N*-phenethyl-5-phenylmorphan acts as a MOR antagonist [7]. In that 5-phenylmorphan series, we found that the agonist vs antagonist activity of the compound was dependent on chirality.

The 1*R*,5*R*,9*S*-enantiomer of the *N*-*p*-nitrophenethyl-5-phenylmorphan was found to be a potent MOR agonist, and the 1*S*,5*S*,9*R*-enantiomer acted as a MOR antagonist [8].

N-Phenethylnorhydromorphone (**S11**, Scheme S1 in the Supplementary Material) was first synthesized in 2001 by Lo and McErlane in 1.3% yield; it was not further examined at that time because their synthesis did not provide the quantity of **S11** necessary for in vitro or in vivo assays [9]. It could be anticipated that it, like *N*-phenethylnormorphine and all other classical opioids, would display the side-effects displayed by morphine. We obtained **S11** through an improved synthesis (see Scheme S1 in the Supplementary Material), and we found that **S11** acts as a bifunctional ligand, with a DOR-MOR δ/μ ratio = 39 in a functional assay (Table 2). It displayed extremely high MOR potency (EC_{50} = 0.04 nM) compared to morphine (EC_{50} = 4.7 nM), DOR potency (EC_{50} = 1.54 nM), and also κ-opioid receptor (KOR) activity (EC_{50} = 23 nM). This interesting pharmacology prompted our use of **S11** as a template for modifying its activity with the addition of different substituents on the nitrogen atom. We hypothesized that relatively small changes in, for example, the *N*-phenethyl group, hereafter referred to as the "tail" of the molecule, e.g., by adding substituents in various positions on the aromatic ring (Table 1), might modify the ligand's activity and, perhaps, enhance its therapeutic potential. This "tail wags dog" experiment can be considered a subset of the message-address concept [10] as applied to opioids, where the "address" can be considered the bulk of the hydromorphone molecule and the "message" delivered by the substituent on the aromatic ring of the *N*-phenethyl moiety. We needed to modulate (decrease) the agonist potency of the **S11** compound at MOR and KOR without disturbing its DOR activity. Since we were unaware of a theoretical model that could predict which substituent would be able to tweak the molecule in that way, we decided to begin our exploration with the design and synthesis and evaluation of compounds with varied substituents on the nitrogen atom and on the aromatic ring of the phenethyl moiety, followed by rationalization of their activity using molecular modeling and dynamics simulations.

A bifunctional compound that acted as a MOR agonist and DOR antagonist would be of the greatest interest, since that combination of receptor interactions is believed to produce antinociceptive activity with fewer of the unfortunate side-effects of opioids [11–13]. The receptor interaction induced by ligands with MOR agonist and DOR agonist activity would also be of interest because that type of combination of MOR and DOR occupancy has also been noted to produce fewer of the undesirable side-effects caused by MOR agonist opioids [14–16]. For example, Su et al., have found that one of the DOR functions was to modulate or counteract the respiratory depression caused by the MOR and, most importantly, further noted that both DOR agonists and DOR antagonists acted similarly in counteracting respiratory depression [17]. It has been found that deaths due to opioid overdose are directly related to an opioid's effect on respiratory depression [18]. It is theoretically possible that a potent agonist with the "correct" δ/μ potency ratio would have diminished effects on respiration or not depress respiration at all. The question of what that "correct" δ/μ ratio might be has not as yet been answered. Our previous attempts to determine this in the 5-phenylmorphan series failed due to their lack of potency [19,20]. There have been many reports of lessened side-effects induced by bifunctional ligands, mostly reduced gastrointestinal effects, a few equivocal results on reduced tolerance and dependence, and other reports have indicated reduced respiratory depression [21–27].

2. Results and Discussion

2.1. Chemistry

To prepare the necessary quantity of *N*-norhydromophone base (**S10** in Scheme S1, see Supplementary Material) we used a previously reported efficient process (hydromorphone synthesis, Scheme S1) for the conversion of (−)-tetrahydrothebaine (**S1**) to dihydromorphine (**S3**) [28]. We found that using the HCl salt of compound **S3** as the reactant instead of the hydrate (product of the basic hydrolysis of **S2**) could dramatically increase the yield of the oxidation [29], achieving hydromorphone hydrochloride (**S4**) in 90% yield. Transformation of hydromorphone **S4** into one of our key intermediates, **S7**, was performed in four steps [30]. Optically pure (−)-N-substituted hydromorphone analogs with different substituents on the N-phenethyl moiety were obtained by N-alkylation of the secondary amine **S10** (Scheme 2).

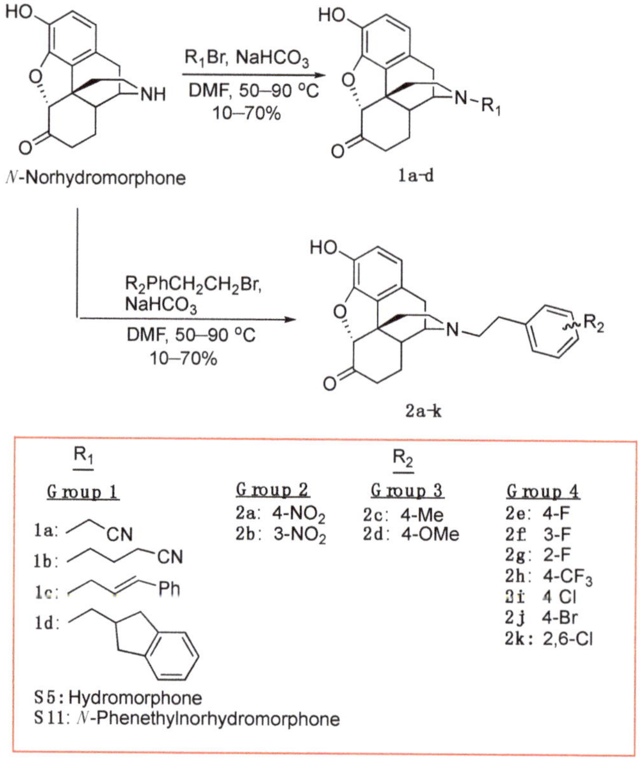

Scheme 2. Synthesis of N-substituted hydromorphones.

2.2. In Vitro Studies

We prepared four groups of compounds (Scheme 2); two cyano analogs (**1a**, **1b**) and two aromatic ring compounds without substituents (**1c**, **1d**) in group 1, two N-nitrophenethyl compounds (**2a**, **2b**) in group 2, N-p-methylphenethyl and p-methoxyphenethyl compounds (**2c**, **2d**) in group 3, and three fluorophenethyl-substituted compounds (**2e**, **2f**, **2g**), a p-trifluoromethylphenethyl (**2h**), and a p-chlorophenethyl (**2i**) compound in group 4. Opioid receptor binding data (Ki, nM) and stimulation of ([^{35}S]GTPγS) binding were obtained for all of these compounds (Table 1). Two additional compounds were added to group 4 in Table 2 (forskolin-induced cAMP accumulation assay), a 4-bromo (**2j**) and a 2,6-dichlorophenethyl compound (**2k**), and two additional compounds were added to group 1, hydromorphone (**S5**) and N-phenethylnorhydromorphone (**S11**). These four compounds were only examined using the forskolin-induced cAMP accumulation assay. The ability of all of the compounds to recruit β-arrestin was also determined (Table 2).

Opioid receptor binding data (Ki, nM) and stimulation of ([^{35}S]GTPγS) binding were obtained for all of these compounds (Table 1). Two additional compounds were added to group 4 in Table 2 (forskolin-induced cAMP accumulation assay), a 4-bromo (**2j**) and a 2,6-dichlorophenethyl compound (**2k**), and two additional compounds were added to group 1, hydromorphone (**S5**) and N-phenethylnor hydromorphone (**S11**). These four compounds were only examined using the forskolin-induced cAMP accumulation assay. The ability of all of the compounds to recruit β-arrestin was also determined (Table 2).

Table 1. Opioid Receptor Binding Data [a] (Ki, nM) and Stimulation of [^{35}S]GTPγS [b] Binding at MOR (μ), DOR (δ) and KOR (κ) opioid receptors.

Compound	Structure	Receptor Binding (Ki, nM)			[^{35}S]GTPγS		
		MOR Binding	DOR Binding	KOR Binding	MOR EC50 [c], nM (% Stimulation)	DOR EC50 [c], nM (% Stimulation)	KOR EC50 [c], nM (% Stimulation)
Group 1. N-Cyanoalkyl Compounds and Compounds Lacking Substituents on the Aromatic Ring							
1a		4.51 ± 0.27	141 ± 2.8	90.3 ± 6.6	425 ± 133 (47.1 ± 3.3)	NT	NT
1b		4.25 ± 0.29	72.2 ± 1.2	2.7 ± 0.22	DNS	NT	24.3 ± 5.0 (89.6 ± 0.9)
1c		90.5 ± 11.0	NT	NT	NT	NT	NT
1d		40.1 ± 5.9	844 ± 107	NT	NT	NT	NT
Group 2. Nitro Substituents							
2a		0.52 ± 0.01	6.07 ± 0.86	56.0 ± 8.2	1.9 ± 0.5 (26.6 ± 1.4)	227 ± 53 (64.3 ± 3.3)	NT

Table 1. *Cont.*

Compound	Structure	Receptor Binding (Ki, nM)			[35S]GTPγS		
		MOR Binding	DOR Binding	KOR Binding	MOR EC50 c, nM (% Stimulation)	DOR EC50 c, nM (% Stimulation)	KOR EC50 c, nM (% Stimulation)
2b		5.88 ± 0.38	92.5 ± 7.3	65.4 ± 7.7	DNS	NT	NT
Group 3. Alkyl and Alkoxy Substituents							
2c		0.86 ± 0.12	6.34 ± 0.65	44.0 ± 3.8	1.9 ± 0.7 (55.6 ± 2.1)	23.1 ± 6.9 (95.4 ± 3.8)	38.1 ± 10.6 (31.4 ± 4.2)
2d		0.67 ± 0.05	5.43 ± 0.47	26.3 ± 1.9	DNS	33.6 ± 6.4 (48.9 ± 3.2)	5.9 ± 1.7 (21.8 ± 0.8)
Group 4. Halides and Trifluromethyl Substituents							
2e		0.87 ± 0.10	13.4 ± 0.9	44.3 ± 6.0	2.5 ± 0.3 (42.6 ± 2.9)	64.2 ± 9.9 (243 ± 49)	DNS
2f		0.49 ± 0.07	4.48 ± 0.43	30.2 ± 2.3	2.4 ± 0.3 (56.8 ± 7.5)	54.1 ± 4.7 (86.7 ± 8.0)	DNS

Table 1. *Cont.*

Compound	Structure	Receptor Binding (Ki, nM)			[35S]GTPγS		
		MOR Binding	DOR Binding	KOR Binding	MOR EC50 [c], nM (% Stimulation)	DOR EC50 [c], nM (% Stimulation)	KOR EC50 [c], nM (% Stimulation)
2g		0.32 ± 0.04	3.57 ± 0.49	23.2 ± 2.8	2.1 ± 0.7 (100 ± 0.3)	92.7 ± 17.0 (83.0 ± 3.3)	DNS
2h		2.70 ± 0.17	16.4 ± 0.4	NT	3.4 ± 1.2 (72.2 ± 5.5)	35.7 ± 12.3 (82.3 ± 2.3)	NT
2i		1.09 ± 0.06	7.89 ± 1.10	NT	2.0 ± 1.0 (39.0 ± 2.1)	2.4 ± 0.7 (83.8 ± 3.7)	NT
Standard							
-	Morphine	3.26 ± 0.39	NT	145 ± 15	194 ± 21 (57 ± 5) [31]	NT	NT

[a] Binding assays were typically conducted in at least three independent experiments, each performed with triplicate observations using whole rat brains excluding cerebellum; *Ki* ± SEM (nM); NT = not tested—inactive (<50% activity at 100 nM concentration in exploratory binding assays (displaced less than half of radioligand). Also, compounds with low binding affinity (>50 nM) were not further examined in functional assays); [b] [35S]GTPγS functional assays: % stimulation compared to standard maximal at each receptor MOR = DAMGO; DOR = DPDPE; KOR = U69593) in C6 cells expressing MOR or DOR or CHO cells expressing KOR. All experiments were repeated on three separate occasions in duplicate. Values are given as means ± SEM; DNS = no stimulation (indicates antagonist activity when coupled with high receptor binding affinity); [c] EC50 = Effective dose for 50% maximal response.

Table 2. Opioid Receptor Activity Measured in the Forskolin-induced cAMP Accumulation Assay [a].

Compound	Structure	MOR cAMP Agonist Potency ± SEM (nM) (% Efficacy)	MOR Mediated β-arrestin Recruitment (% Control, Emax DAMGO), nM	Bias Factor	DOR cAMP Agonist Potency ± SEM (nM) (% Efficacy)	KOR cAMP Agonist Potency ± SEM (nM) (% Efficacy)
Group 1. N-Cyanoalkyl Compounds and Compounds Lacking Substituents on the Aromatic Ring						
1a		4.16 ± 0.64 (101.6 ± 1.1)	424 ± 69 (33.4 ± 0.25)	2.18	254 ± 167 (77 ± 4)	109.4 ± 45.4 (99.3 ± 4.0)
1c		76.7 ± 7.4 (103 ± 0.9)	584 ± 286 (4.1 ± 0.1)	1.35	1699 ± 847 (96.5 ± 5.4)	>10,000
1d		18.29 ± 4.70 (95.2 ± 1.2)	130.4 ± 37.5 (1.9 ± 0.4)	2.53	596 ± 92 (94.4 ± 1.4)	>10,000
S5 Hydromorphone		1.67 ± 0.30 (102 ± 1)	159 ± 28 (19.8 ± 3)	3.48	134.3 ± 31.4 (95.4 ± 0.8)	176.1 ± 32.7 (80.4 ± 3.9)
S11 N-Phenethylnor-hydromorphone		0.04 ± 0.01 (102.1 ± 0.8)	1.71 ± 0.66 (61.9 ± 5.2)	0.47	1.54 ± 0.22 (95.1 ± 0.8)	22.7 ± 4.8 (80.6 ± 18.3)

Table 2. *Cont.*

Compound	Structure	MOR cAMP Agonist Potency ± SEM (nM) (% Efficacy)	MOR Mediated β-arrestin Recruitment(% Control, Emax DAMGO), nM	Bias Factor	DOR cAMP Agonist Potency ± SEM (nM) (% Efficacy)	KOR cAMP Agonist Potency ± SEM (nM) (% Efficacy)
		Group 2. Nitro Substituents				
2a		0.05 ± 0.02 (102 ± 0.4)	6.38 ± 0.59 (26.2 ± 2.8)	4.51	0.53 ± 0.03 (96 ± 1.5)	74.6 ± 5.6 (63 ± 1.5)
2b		5.22 ± 1.20 (102.3 ± 0.6)	116 ± 21 (6 ± 0.1)	3.38	46.7 ± 17.6 (95.3 ± 1.3)	>10,000
		Group 3. Alkyl and Alkoxy Substituents				
2c		0.08 ± 0.02 (101.5 ± 0.2)	5.6 ± 1.4 (46.5 ± 3)	1.12	1.0 ± 0.3 (95.0 ± 1.3)	8.71 ± 0.09 (99.4 ± 0.8)
2d		0.13 ± 0.04 (103 ± 2)	11.2 ± 1.8 (23 ± 2.2)	2.69	2.71 ± 0.93 (97.5 ± 0.7)	7.38 ± 2.10 (96.2 ± 1.0)
		Group 4. Halides and Trifluromethyl Substituents				
2e		0.17 ± 0.08 (100.8 ± 1.1)	15.5 ± 2.1 (45.8 ± 2.4)	1.39	2.58 ± 1.60 (98.1 ± 1.1)	19.9 ± 1.3 (80.0 ± 3.8)

Table 2. *Cont.*

Compound	Structure	MOR cAMP Agonist Potency ± SEM (nM) (% Efficacy)	MOR Mediated β-arrestin Recruitment (% Control, Emax DAMGO), nM	Bias Factor	DOR cAMP Agonist Potency ± SEM (nM) (% Efficacy)	KOR cAMP Agonist Potency ± SEM (nM) (% Efficacy)
2f	(3-F phenethyl)	0.06 ± 0.01 (101.7 ± 0.3)	6.2 ± 1.1 (40.3 ± 2.3)	1.94	1.64 ± 0.11 (96.9 ± 1.6)	56.5 ± 21.1 (58.0 ± 8.4)
2g	(2-F phenethyl)	0.010 ± 0.003 (101.2 ± 0.1)	1.7 ± 0.6 (73.2 ± 2.1)	1.37	0.26 ± 0.13 (93.8 ± 2.1)	19.9 ± 0.6 (74.0 ± 5.2)
2h	(4-CF3 phenethyl)	0.21 ± 0.04 (102 ± 0.2)	10.3 ± 1.8 (62.4 ± 1.5)	0.56	2.41 ± 0.47 (94.3 ± 1.8)	98.2 ± 7.7 (95.7 ± 0.6)
2i	(4-Cl phenethyl)	0.05 ± 0.03 (98.8 ± 2.1)	2.44 ± 0.45 (44.8 ± 1.8)	0.82	0.53 ± 0.18 (84.8 ± 5.6)	55.2 ± 26.1 (76.6 ± 11.3)
2j	(4-Br phenethyl)	0.15 ± 0.04 (103 ± 1.5)	4.9 ± 0.3 (53 ± 3.4)	0.43	0.97 ± 0.22 (96 ± 1.1)	20.1 ± 3.3 (99.04 ± 3.74)
2k	(2,6-diCl phenethyl)	0.37 ± 0.09 (101.3 ± 0.5)	13.13 ± 0.19 (24.6 ± 3.9)	1.04	21.89 ± 0.87 (95.8 ± 1.1)	1881 ± 687 (73.97 ± 5.49)

Table 2. Cont.

Compound	Structure	MOR cAMP Agonist Potency ± SEM (nM) (% Efficacy)	MOR Mediated β-arrestin Recruitment (% Control, Emax DAMGO), nM	Bias Factor	DOR cAMP Agonist Potency ± SEM (nM) (% Efficacy)	KOR cAMP Agonist Potency ± SEM (nM) (% Efficacy)
			Standards			
-	DAMGO	0.3 ± 0.04 (101.5 ± 0.5)	44.1 ± 3.9 (103 ± 0.4)	1.0	-	-
-	U-69593	-	-	-	-	0.7 ± 0.3 (101.2 ± 1.4)
-	Leu-Enkephalin	-	-	-	0.04 ± 0.10 (95 ± 2)	-
-	Morphine	4.7 ± 0.6 (102.9 ± 0.6)	378 ± 41 (25.7 ± 0.6)	2.27	-	-

[a] Inhibition of forskolin-induced cAMP accumulation; DAMGO ([D-Ala^2, N-MePhe^4, Gly-ol]-enkephalin); U-69593 ((+)-(5α,7α,8β)-N-methyl-N-[7-(1-pyrrolidinyl)-1-oxaspiro[4.5]dec-8-yl]-benzeneacetamide); Leu-Enkephalin (Tyr-Gly-Gly-Phe-Leu). To determine % efficacy of MOR-mediated β-arrestin recruitment, the highest dose(s) of DAMGO were used as 100% and the respective data were converted to percentages based on the response of DAMGO and analyzed using GraphPad Prism. To determine % efficacy in forskolin-induced cAMP assays, data were normalized to the vehicle control, followed by the forskolin control. Data were then analyzed in GraphPad Prism using nonlinear regression.

2.2.1. Opioid Receptor Binding, Ligand Efficacy and Potency ([^{35}S]GTPγS Binding Assays)

The MOR binding affinity, in the receptor binding assay, of N-cyanomethyl (**1a**) and N-cyanopropyl compounds (**1b**) in group 1 (Table 1), both without an aromatic ring on the nitrogen atom, were comparable to the affinity of morphine (Ki = 4.51 and 4.25 vs 3.26 for morphine). However, **1a** had only partial MOR agonist activity (47% stimulation) and very low potency (EC$_{50}$ = 425 nM) in the [^{35}S]GTPγS assay (Table 1), and **1b**, in contrast, was a MOR antagonist in that assay (antagonist activity was assumed given the high MOR binding affinity, and lack of [^{35}S]GTPγS stimulation at MOR). All of the compounds in group 1 (Table 1) that were assessed at DOR had relatively low receptor binding affinity (Ki > 70 nM). At KOR, **1a** had a Ki of about 90 nM, whereas **1b** had a higher binding affinity at KOR than MOR, a > 30-fold increase in KOR agonist affinity due to the extension of the carbon chain from N-cyanomethyl to N-cyanopropyl. Compounds in group 1 with an extended and rotationally restricted N-substituent (compound **1c**) or a bulky N-substituent (compound **1d**) showed little binding affinity or potency at any opioid receptor. Compounds were considered inactive and were not tested (NT) in functional assays when they were found to displace <50% of the radioligand at a 100 nM concentration in an exploratory binding assay (not described in the Material and Methods Section).

The m-(**2b**) and p-N-nitrophenethylnorhydromorphone (**2a**) in group 2 in Table 1 showed a >10-fold difference in MOR binding affinity in the receptor binding assay and a remarkable change from potent MOR agonist **2a** to MOR antagonist **2b** (Table 1) was observed in the [^{35}S]GTPγS assay, apparently induced by the change in the position of the aromatic ring's substituent. This bolstered our hypothesis that we could influence and considerably alter activity by substitution on the phenyl ring.

The group 3 alkyl and alkoxy compounds had very high MOR affinity (Ki < 1 nM) and high DOR affinity (Ki = 5–6 nM) in the receptor binding assay, and while **2c** was a potent partial MOR agonist in the [^{35}S]GTPγS assay, the methoxy compound **2d** appeared to be a MOR antagonist in that assay. Both of these compounds had EC$_{50}$ < 35 nM at DOR with **2c** acting as a full agonist (95% stimulation) and **2d** a partial agonist (49% stimulation). Compound **2d** was also a potent KOR agonist (EC50 = 5.9 nM), although it was not efficacious at KOR (21.8% stimulation).

The halides in group 4 (Table 1) harbored the most interesting compound **2i**, from the perspective of having a desirable δ/μ potency ratio. All of the halides had high affinity at MOR and DOR (Ki ranged from 0.3 to 2.7 nM at MOR and 4 to 16 nM at DOR), and less affinity at KOR (Ki > 20 nM), in the receptor binding assays. Additionally, all group 4 compounds had nanomolar MOR potency in the [^{35}S]GTPγS assay (EC50 = 2.0–3.4 nM) and all except **2i** and **2h** had lower DOR agonist potency (EC50 > 50 nM). The trifluoromethyl compound **2h** had moderate DOR potency (EC$_{50}$ = 36 nM), whereas **2i** had nanomolar potency at DOR (EC50 = 2.4 nM), with a δ/μ potency ratio of 1.2.

2.2.2. Ligand Potency and Efficacy Using the Forskolin-induced cAMP Accumulation Assay

As seen in the forskolin-induced cAMP accumulation assay (group 1, Table 2), **1a** had morphine-like potency, as it did in the [^{35}S]GTPγS assay. In contrast, compounds **1a**, **1c** and **1d** had relatively low potency for DOR or KOR cAMP stimulation.

Again, as in the [^{35}S]GTPγS assay, **1c** with restricted rotation and **1d** with a bulky side-chain were less potent than the cyanomethyl compound **1a**. The standard compounds for comparison purposes, **S5** and **S11**, hydromophone and N-phenethylnorhydromorphone in group 1, were relatively potent at MOR (EC$_{50}$ = 1.67 and 0.04 nM, respectively) and **S11** was potent at DOR (EC$_{50}$ = 1.54 nM) and somewhat less potent at KOR (EC$_{50}$ = 22.7 nM). The parent compound hydromorphone (**S5**) was essentially inactive at DOR and KOR (EC$_{50}$ > 130 nM). The N-phenethylnorhydromorphone (**S11**), had an EC$_{50}$ δ/μ ratio = 38.5, and that was possibly too high for the mitigation of side-effects that might be provided by interaction with DOR.

The bias factor of all of the tested compounds ranged between ca. 0.4 and 3.5 (Table 2). Examination of the MOR β-arrestin recruitment for **S11** and **2i** indicated that they both had a lower bias factor than morphine (indicating their greater ability to recruit β-arrestin). All of these G-protein biased ligands recruit β-arrestin almost as well, or better than morphine. If recruitment of β-arrestin correlated with the side-effects of these compounds, they should all cause, for example, respiratory depression, as well as other side-effects caused by interaction with MOR. As noted previously, however, the ability of MOR ligands to recruit β-arrestin may not have any bearing on whether they will or will not display opioid-like side-effects [4].

The MOR antagonist profile of **2a** in group 2 (Table 1), the *p*-nitro compound, that was seen in the [^{35}S]GTPγS assay was not observed in the forskolin-induced cAMP accumulation assay (Table 2). In the cAMP assay, both **2a** and **2b** had MOR agonist activity (EC_{50} = 0.05 and 5.2 nM, respectively); a >100-fold potency change due to a positional shift of an aromatic substituent.

In group 3 in Table 2, the alkyl and alkoxy compounds, **2c** and **2d**, were found to have relatively high potency (EC_{50} = 0.08 and 0.13 nM, respectively) at MOR and at DOR (EC_{50} = 1.0 and 2.7 nM, respectively). They were also KOR agonists (EC_{50} = 8.7 and 7.4 nM, respectively). In the cAMP assay (Table 2), **2d** was not found to have MOR antagonist activity.

In group 4 (Table 2), the most interesting compound was again found to be **2i**. It had extremely high agonist potency at MOR and DOR (EC_{50} = 0.05 and 0.53 nM, respectively), and was efficacious at both receptors. It was much less potent at KOR (EC_{50} = 55 nM). The *o*-fluoro compound **2g** was notable for its relatively high MOR agonist potency (0.01 nM), with full (101%) efficacy. The *p*-bromo compound **2j** also appeared to be of interest in that its EC_{50} δ/μ ratio = 6.5 was less than the ratio found for **2i** in the cAMP assay (δ/μ ratio = 10 for **2i**). Compound **2j** was also potent at both MOR and DOR in the cAMP assay (EC_{50} < 1 nM), but it had moderate agonist potency at KOR (20 nM). Although KOR agonists have therapeutic potential, they also have undesirable CNS-mediated side-effects (e.g., dysphoria, hallucinations) [32].

We hypothesized that a compound with a δ/μ potency ratio of less than 7 in the [^{35}S]GTPγS assay would be desirable if the compound were to display other than the full array of undesirable effects that clinically used analgesics manifest. Recent work on bifunctional compounds explored compounds with δ/μ potency ratios of 5 to 7 in [^{35}S]GTPγS assay assays, and found that those compounds had a less disruptive effect on locomotor activity than morphine or oxymorphone [33].

2.2.3. Molecular Modeling and Simulations.

Specifically placed moieties at the tail end of the *N*-phenethyl substituent changed the compound from a MOR partial agonist in the [^{35}S]GTPγS assay (e.g., *N*-*p*-nitrophenethyl-norhydromorphone, **2a**) to a MOR antagonist (e.g., *N*-*m*-nitrophenethylnorhydromorphone, **2b**). In the forskolin-induced cAMP accumulation assay, that same positional shift of the substituent in the aromatic ring in **2a** to **2b** caused a >100 fold change in potency. We used quantum chemical calculations and molecular dynamics simulations to determine if a moiety in precise positions on the aromatic ring in the *N*-phenethyl moiety of norhydromorphone would display sufficient differences in their interaction with MOR to induce the change in activity and/or potency. More generally, our simulations allowed us to identify the critical residues interacting with the body (Figure 1) and the tail (Figure 2) of the ligands that are responsible for the differences in receptor properties. Together, the experimental and simulation data led us to propose a set of general rules for the *N*-phenethyl-substitutions to impart specific behaviors, such as partial or full agonist or possible antagonist activities, which may help design compound with novel properties (see details in the Supplementary Materials).

Body-Opioid Receptor (OR) interactions

All the compounds considered in our simulations have similar body-OR interaction patterns regardless of the substituents on the N-phenethyl ring; the interactions are consistent with those reported recently for a series of phenethyl oxymorphone compound bound to the active MOR [33]. These are shown in Figure 1 for both the MOR and the DOR, and involve polar/charged residues in transmembrane helix (TMH) 3, 5 and 6, and hydrophobic residues in TMH 5, 6, and 7. A contact is deemed significant if it persists for at least 50% of the time (see example in Table S2), although not necessarily all the interactions are seen at a given time. Different substituents, however, lead to different statistics of the individual interactions due to modest repositioning of the ligands resulting from different tail-OR interactions. All the residues in direct contact with the body are conserved in both receptors. Three additional, non-conserved residues, each belonging to TMH 5, 6, and 7 interact indirectly with -O- and -OH groups of the body via short water chains. Thus, suitable substitutions that engage these residues more directly (e.g., polar or H-bond interactions) may help modulate the MOR and DOR activity, potency and affinities independently.

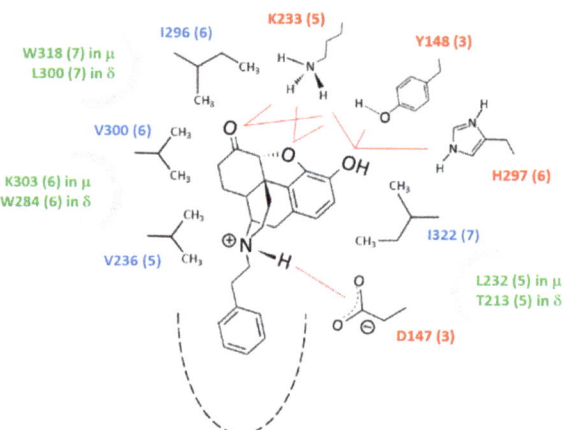

Figure 1. Conserved polar/charged residues (in red; numbering as in MOR) that interacted with the -O and -OH groups of the *N*-phenethylnorhydromorphone body through H-bonds; the body was also stabilized by close packing with four conserved nonpolar residues (blue) through hydrophobic forces. Although not in direct interactions, a few non-conserved residues (green) were seen to interact with the ligands indirectly through short water chains. These residues may thus be important to modulate the behavior of MOR and DOR independently, which may be accomplished through specific substituents that can engage them more directly. Frequencies of contacts were deemed statistically relevant if they were observed at least 25% of the time, except for the critical -NH—D147 distance (MOR) and -NH—D128 distance (DOR) that was required to persist for at least 75% of the time for the conformer to be considered (see details of the analysis in Table S2).

Tail-OR interactions

Because the tail is located deep inside the pocket, relatively small changes in the *N*-phenylethyl ring via substitutions perturb residues located in different regions of the ORs and engage different TMHs (Figure S1). The constrained environment of the tail suggests that these interactions can induce major changes in the OR structure and/or dynamics, as confirmed by preliminary data from principal component analysis (to be published). Unlike the relatively rigid ligand body, the tail has several energetically similar conformers (Figure S2). Some of these conformers can be ruled out based on unfavorable steric interactions (cf. Computational Section 5). However, the simulations show that all of the conformers selected by the pocket can be stabilized because each substituent can always find favorable interactions through polar/nonpolar or H-bond interactions. It is noted that none of these conformers lose the critical polar/H-bond interaction between the protonated nitrogen of the ligands and the carboxylate of the anchoring aspartic acid D147 (MOR) or D128 (DOR) (cf. Table S2). The multiplicity of binding modes may explain, in part, the tendency of most ligands in the Table 1 series to display partial agonist activity, i.e., with some modes leading to agonist and others to antagonist activity. This scenario may coexist with the more traditional view of partial activity as the result of multiple substates of the receptor stabilized by a single conformer (not observed in the simulations). We carried out a comparative analysis of the experimental observations summarized in Table S1. Here we focused on the results pertaining to the effects of F and Cl substitution at the *p*-position of the *N*-phenethyl moiety on both receptors (Figure 2A, additional details in SI). The *p*-F (**2e**) was found to be a potent partial MOR agonist and weak partial DOR agonist, whereas *p*-Cl (**2i**), although still a potent partial MOR agonist, becomes a potent full DOR agonist, an unexpected result with therapeutic potential.

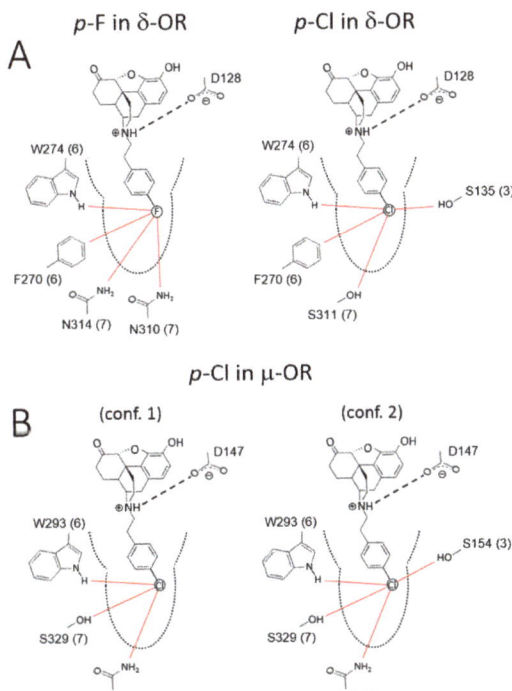

Figure 2. Critical tail-OR interactions of *p*-F (**2e**) and -Cl (**2i**) substituents. (**A**) *p*-F (weak partial DOR agonist) vs. *p*-Cl (potent full DOR agonist); only one of the two conformers of each ligands are shown (see text); (**B**) *p*-Cl (potent partial MOR agonists); the two conformers shown. The red lines represent frequent, statistically significant interactions that were obtained from the dynamic simulations. Sequence numbering as in the corresponding ORs.

One of the conformers of **2e** and of **2i** showed the same pattern of interactions with the DOR, engaging both TMH 6 (W274) and 7 (N310, S311, N314); this conformer (not shown) was expected to elicit the same dynamic behavior of the receptor and was unlikely to be responsible for the observed partial vs. full agonist activities. The second conformer did show qualitative differences (Figure S2A); when compared to **2e**, **2i** partially disengaged TMH 7 and engaged TMH 3. On the one hand, Cl is larger than F, resulting in higher polarizability together with a longer C-Cl bond distance, and is less electronegative, resulting in a less negative partial charge and weaker electric field at the atom surface. These differences appeared to be enough for **2i** to interact more favorably with both S135 and S311, which were in opposite sides across the pocket; **2e** instead interacted more closely with the polar groups of adjacent N310 and N314 on the same TMH 7. In both cases, the ligands interacted with TMH 6, showing persistent interactions with the -NH group of W274 and with the H atoms on the F270 ring via weak polar interactions. Although halogen-bonding interactions were not included in the forcefield [34,35], it could be predicted that the incipient σ-hole and equatorial negative charge of the Cl atom (Figure S2) would further stabilize this pattern of interactions. There may be other qualitative differences between **2e** and **2i** if the latter interacts with the aromatic ring via C-Cl/π interactions [36]; in this case, the side-chain may adopt a different conformation and affect the dynamics of TMH 6. Despite the differences in the pattern of interactions, the type and frequency of polar and non-polar contacts were fundamentally the same in both ligands, which may explain their similar K_i values. When all the interactions were considered, only two residues of DOR show unique interactions with these ligands: N314 (only with **2e**) and S135 (only with **2i**). Therefore, substituents that interacted with S135 (or engaged TMH 3 near this residue) and interacted less strongly with N314 (or disengaged TMH 7) may confer potent full DOR agonism. The difference in atomic size, polarizability, and electronegativity, as well as the putative C-Cl/π interactions, appear to play a role in the difference between **2e** and **2i**. Accordingly, it would be of interest to see the effects of *p*-Br and *p*-I on DOR behavior. In MOR, the patterns of interactions of **2i** were similar to those in DOR (Figure 2B): one conformer interacted with TMH 6 and 7 and the other with TMH 3 and 7. This may be enough to impart potent agonism, as in the DOR, but only partial agonist activity in MOR. When all the interactions were considered, F289 is the only residue that was unique in the interaction patterns of **2i** with the receptors. The present investigation indicated that changing the balance of interactions of the phenethyl ring with S154, N332, and F289 by a suitable substituent may help design potent, full DOR agonists.

The constrained environment of the tail substituent on the aromatic ring of the *N*-phenethyl moiety located deep inside the receptor pocket suggested that these interactions can induce major changes in the OR structure or dynamics. The consequences of such effects were already observed in a previous study where a *p*-NO$_2$ substitution in the ring elicited significant changes in OR activity and efficacy [8]; computational studies of other GPCRs have also shown the importance of the lower strata of the binding pocket to affect function [37]. Thus, moieties in specific positions on the phenyl ring in *N*-phenethylnorhydromorphone might convert a potent MOR agonist to MOR antagonist or significantly change its potency. This was shown using in vitro assays with the nitro substituent on the phenyl ring (in **2a** and **2b**, Table 1). Depending on the position of the nitro substituent in the phenyl ring, one of the compounds (with a *p*-nitro substituent, **2a**) was a potent low efficacy MOR agonist with subnanomolar affinity and the other (with a *m*-nitro substituent, **2b**) was a high-affinity MOR antagonist in the [^{35}S]GTPγS assay (Table 1), a minor positional change inducing a significant change in activity. In the forskolin-induced cAMP accumulation assay, a major difference in potency was observed with these compounds.

2.3. In Vivo Data

2.3.1. Respiratory Depression Assays in Mice

The *p*-chlorophenyl compound **2i** was among the most interesting of the compounds in that it exhibited high MOR and DOR affinity and potency and was a potent efficacious DOR agonist and a partial MOR agonist in the [^{35}S]GTPγS assay (Table 1). It was an exceptionally potent MOR agonist in the forskolin-induced cAMP accumulation assay (Table 2). Few compounds have been noted in the literature that combine potent MOR partial agonist and potent DOR full agonist activity in a δ/μ ratio of about 7 in opioid receptor binding studies and in a δ/μ ratio of about 1 from potency studies in the [^{35}S]GTPγS assay (Table 1). We thought that it would be of interest to further examine that compound in vivo.

In mice, **2i** did not depress respiration rate in the presence of normal air. Figure 3A shows time courses of saline, morphine (10 mg/kg), and different doses of **2i** on respiration rate. Figure 3B shows the calculated area under the curve (AUCs) from 6 min to 45 min post injection. As seen in Figure 3B, 10 mg/kg morphine significantly reduced ($p < 0.0001$) respiration rate compared to saline (One-way ANOVA revealed a significant effect for treatment $F(5,38) = 18.34$, $p < 0.0001$).

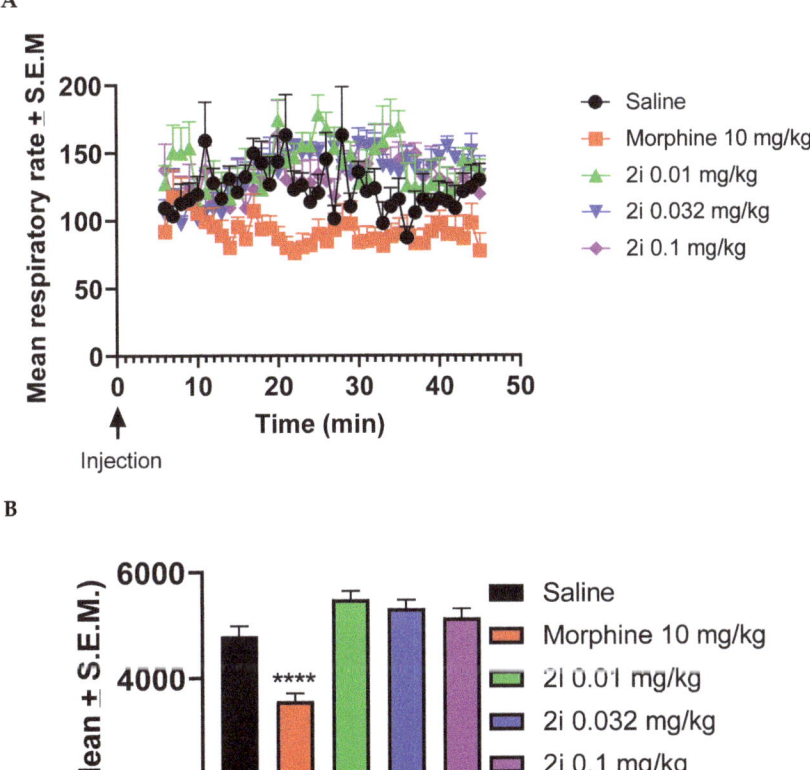

Figure 3. Effects of morphine and **2i** on respiratory rate in mice. After acclimation in observation boxes, mice were injected with either saline, morphine 10 mg/kg, or **2i** and connected to a throat sensor. Five min later, the recording was started and respiratory rate was measured from 6 min to 45 min post-injection (**A**). Area under the curve (AUC) was calculated from 6 min to 45 min. Morphine significantly reduced respiratory rate compared to saline (**B**). Data are expressed as mean ± standard error of the mean (SEM.) (n = 6–8) (**** p < 0.0001). One-way ANOVA followed by Dunnett's multiple comparison test.

The doses chosen were based on the squirrel monkey tail withdrawal latency assay and the highest dose (0.1 mg/kg) was about 5 or 6 times higher than the ED_{50} values at 50 and 52 °C from the tail withdrawal latency assay (the usual dose studied to observe side-effects is about 4× the ED50). Compound **2i** (0.01–0.1 mg/kg) had no effect on respiration rate in this assay in mice although morphine, as expected, significantly decreased respiratory rate. Results for oxygen saturation (SpO_2) indicated that neither morphine nor **2i** had any effect on SpO_2 from 6 min to 45 min post-injection (data not shown).

2.3.2. Antinociceptive Studies and Respiratory Depression Studies in Squirrel Monkeys

Further studies evaluated the effects of **2i** and, for comparison, morphine, in assays of antinociception and respiratory depression in nonhuman primates. In a squirrel monkey tail withdrawal latency assay, the *p*-chlorophenethyl compound **2i** exhibited the observed partial MOR agonist in vitro characteristics (in the [^{35}S]GTPγS assay) by having a full effect at moderate (50 °C) and hot (52 °C) but not at very hot (55 °C) water temperatures. In comparison, morphine elicited full antinociceptive effects at all three water temperatures. The compound **2i**, like morphine, also produced dose-related behavioral impairment, evident as decreases in operant performance and, consequently, the number of reinforcers obtained during an operant task interspersed between tail-withdrawal tests. The doses of **2i** that produced behavioral impairment were similar to those that produce antinociception in 50 °C and 52 °C water (Figure 4).

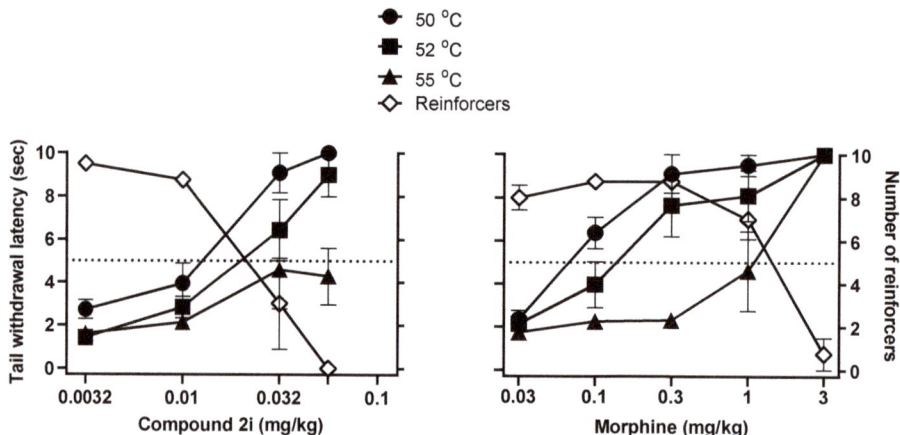

Figure 4. Effects of **2i** on tail withdrawal latency from different temperatures of water (filled symbols) and operant behavior disruption (open symbols) in squirrel monkeys (*n* = 4). Data are expressed as mean ± SEM (*n* = 4).

The ED$_{50}$ doses for producing antinociception at 50 °C or 52 °C were, respectively, 0.010 and 0.015 mg/kg, and the ED50 dose for reducing the number of reinforcers earned (behavioral impairment), was 0.022 mg/kg, resulting in ED$_{50}$ ratios (behavioral impairment/antinociception) that were about 2 or less. Ratio values greater than 1 imply some behavioral selectivity in observed effects although, as can be seen in Table 3, morphine had an even greater behavioral impairment/antinociception potency ratio than did **2i**. Further studies evaluated whether **2i** differed from morphine in its capacity to produce respiratory depression in squirrel monkeys.

The results from a respiratory depression assay in squirrel monkeys correlated somewhat with data obtained using mice. As shown in Figure 5 during exposure to air alone, neither **2i** (0.003–0.1 mg/kg) nor morphine (0.03–3.0 mg/kg) had effects on respiratory rate or overall ventilation (minute volume) in squirrel monkeys, whereas in mice morphine (10 mg/kg), but not **2i** (0.01–0.1 mg/kg), depressed ventilation. In contrast, during exposure to 5% CO_2 mixed in air (hypercapnia), both **2i** and morphine significantly decreased ventilation in squirrel monkeys, resulting from respiratory depressant effects (Figure 5).

Table 3. ED50 values and ratios of ED50 values for effects measured in squirrel monkeys.

Behavioral Measures	2i	Morphine
	ED_{50} (mg/kg)	
Antinociception (52 °C) [a]	0.015	0.14
Behavioral Disruption [b]	0.022	1.30
Respiratory Depression [c]	0.057	1.06
	Potency Ratios	
Behavioral Disruption: Antinociception	1.5	9.0
Respiratory Depression: Antinociception	3.9	7.3
Respiratory Depression: Behavioral Disruption	2.6	0.8

[a] Dose required to increase tail withdrawal latency to 5 s; [b] dose required to reduce the number of reinforcements earned to 5 per cycle; [c] dose required to decrease minute volume in 5% CO_2 to 50% of the baseline value.

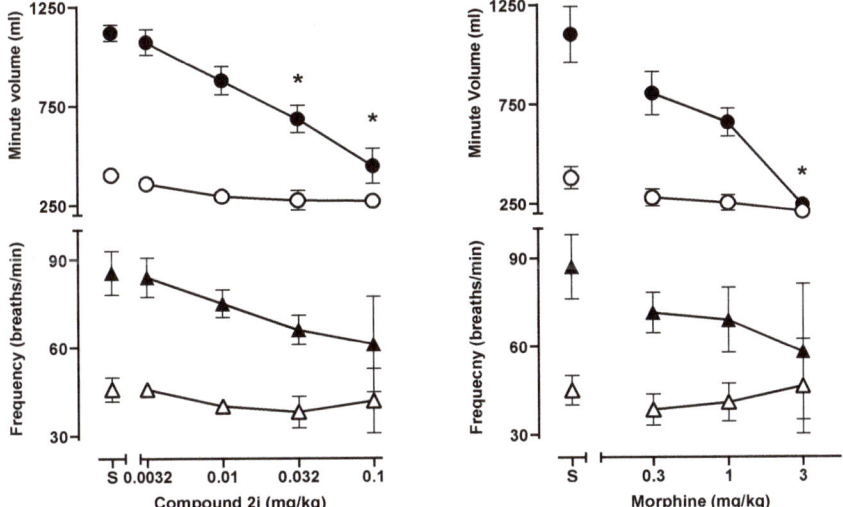

Figure 5. Effects in squirrel monkeys of **2i** and morphine on respiratory rate (bottom panels) or on minute volume (top panels) in the presence of normal air (open symbols) or air mixed with 5% CO_2 (filled symbols). **2i** and morphine significantly reduced minute volume in 5% CO_2 without significantly altering respiratory rate. Data are expressed as mean ± SEM. (n = 4); (*) indicates the difference from saline ($p \leq 0.01$; one-way ANOVA followed by Dunnett's multiple comparison test.

The ED_{50} values for producing antinociception in 52 °C water, decreasing the number of reinforcers earned in an operant behavioral task, and decreasing ventilation in 5% CO_2, as well as calculated potency ratios across the procedures, are summarized in Table 3. Here, a complicated picture emerges in which morphine has a larger, and hence more favorable, potency ratio for antinociceptive and behaviorally disruptive effect than does **2i**, whereas **2i** has a higher ratio for behaviorally disruptive and respiratory depressant effects. Indeed, the potency ratio for morphine for behavioral disruption and respiratory depression was ≤ 1, indicating that breathing was decreased at similar doses to those that decreased behavior, whereas 2-fold higher doses of **2i** were needed to decrease CO_2-stimulated breathing (Figure 5).

The ED_{50} values for producing antinociception in 52 °C water, decreasing the number of reinforcers earned in an operant behavioral task, and decreasing ventilation in 5% CO_2, as well as calculated potency ratios across the procedures, are summarized in Table 3. Here, a complicated picture emerges in which morphine has a larger, and hence more favorable, potency ratio for antinociceptive and behaviorally disruptive effect than does **2i**, whereas **2i** has a higher ratio for behaviorally disruptive and respiratory depressant effects. Indeed, the potency ratio for morphine for behavioral disruption and respiratory depression was ≤1, indicating that breathing was decreased at similar doses to those that decreased behavior, whereas 2-fold higher doses of **2i** were needed to decrease CO_2-stimulated breathing.

3. Material and Methods

3.1. General Information

Melting points were determined on a B-545 instrument (Büchi, Labortechnik AG, Flawii, Switzerland) and are uncorrected. Proton and carbon nuclear magnetic resonance (^{1}H and ^{13}C-NMR) spectra were recorded on a Gemini-400 spectrometer (Varian, Palo Alto, CA, USA) with the values given in ppm (TMS as internal standard) and *J* (Hz) assignments of ^{1}H resonance coupling. Mass spectra (HRMS) were recorded on a VG 7070E spectrometer (VG Analytical Ltd., Altrincham, Cheshire, England, UK) or a SX102a mass spectrometer (JEOL, Tokyo, Japan) 41 polarimeter (PerkinElmer, Shelton, CT, USA) at room temperature. Gas chromatography (GC) was performed on a 6850 GC system (Agilent Technologies, Santa Clara, CA, USA) equipped with a VL MSD detector. Thin layer chromatography (TLC) analyses were carried out on prepackaged plates using various gradients of $CHCl_3$/MeOH containing 1% of 28% NH_4OH (CMA) or gradients of EtOAc:*n*-hexane. Visualization was accomplished under UV light or by staining in an iodine chamber. Flash column chromatography was performed using RediSep Rf normal phase silica gel cartridges. Atlantic Microlabs, Inc. (Norcross, GA, USA) or Micro-Analysis, Inc. (Wilmington, DE, USA) performed elemental analyses, and the results were within ± 0.4% of the theoretical values. All spectra were obtained on the free base.

3.2. Synthesis. General Procedure for Formation of Tertiary Amines.

(7aR,12bS)-3-(4-Chlorophenethyl)-9-hydroxy-2,3,4,4a,5,6-hexahydro-1H-4,12-methanobenzofuro[3,2-e]-isoquinolin-7(7aH)-one (**2i**): To a stirred solution of *N*-norhydromorphone (**S10** in the Supplementary Materials, 0.406 g, 1.5 mmol) in DMF (10 mL) were added $NaHCO_3$ (0.504 g, 6 mmol) and 1-(2-bromoethyl)-4-chlorobenzene (0.480 mL, 3.3 mmol). The mixture was heated at 90 °C overnight, cooled to room temperature, filtered through Celite, and concentrated in vacuo. Water (10 mL) was added and the mixture extracted with $CHCl_3$ (3 × 20 mL). The combined organics were washed with H_2O (5 × 20 mL), dried over Na_2SO_4, filtered through Celite, and concentrated in vacuo to afford **2i** free base as a crude colorless oil. Purification of this oil by SiO_2 column chromatography with 10% NH_4OH in MeOH/$CHCl_3$ (gradient, 0 → 4% of 10% NH_4OH) afforded **2i** (0.420 g, 70%) as a colorless oil. ^{1}H-NMR (DMSO-d_6): δ 9.09 (s, 1H), 7.30 (d, *J* = 8.4 Hz, 2H), 7.26 (d, *J* = 8.4 Hz, 2H), 6.51 (d, *J* = 8.0 Hz, 1H), 6.46 (d, *J* = 7.6 Hz, 1H), 4.78 (s, 1H), 3.17 (s, 1H), 2.79 (d, *J* = 18.4 Hz, 1H), 2.71–2.56 (m, 5H), 2.52 (dd, *J* = 14.4 Hz, 4.8 Hz, 1H), 2.48–2.40 (m, 1H), 2.23 (dd, *J* = 18.2 Hz, 5.4 Hz, 1H), 2.11 (d, *J* = 13.6 Hz, 1H), 2.04–1.93 (m, 2H), 1.76–1.71 (m, 1H), 1.47 (d, *J* = 10.0 Hz, 1H), 1.01–0.91 (m, 1H); ^{13}C-NMR (DMSO-d_6): δ 209.2, 144.3, 140.1, 139.6, 131.0, 130.8, 128.5, 127.9, 124.9, 119.6, 117.3, 90.7, 57.3, 56.4, 47.1, 44.8, 41.8, 40.1, 35.3, 33.4, 25.5, 21.2; HRMS (TOF MS ES$^+$) calcd for $C_{24}H_{25}ClNO_3$ (M + H$^+$) 410.1523, found 410.1527. **2i HCl**: An HCl salt was prepared by dissolving **2i** free base in hot *i*-PrOH (5.0 mL) followed by the addition of 37% HCl (0.10 mL, 3 equiv). It was concentrated in vacuo to afford the salt. Anal. Calcd for $C_{24}H_{24}ClNO_3 \cdot 0.5H_2O \cdot 0.5C_3H_8O$ (**2i HCl**·$0.5H_2O$·$0.5C_3H_8O$): C, 63.29; H, 6.11; N, 2.77; found: C, 63.09; H, 6.23; N, 2.89%. $[\alpha]_D^{20}$ − 138.5 (*c* 0.65, MeOH, HCl·$0.5H_2O$·$0.5i$-PrOH).

2-((7aR,12bS)-9-Hydroxy-7-oxo-1,2,4,4a,5,6,7,7a-octahydro-3H-4,12-methanobenzofuro[3,2-e]isoquinolin-3-yl)acetonitrile (**1a**): The general procedure with **S10** (0.406 g, 1.5 mmol), 2-bromoacetonitrile (0.230 mL, 3.3 mmol), $NaHCO_3$ (0.504 g, 6 mmol), and DMF (10 mL) at room temperature. Purification by column chromatography afforded **1a** free base (0.250 g, 50%) as a white solid. ^{1}H-NMR (CD$_3$OD): δ 6.61 (d, *J* = 8.0 Hz, 1H), 6.56 (d, *J* = 8.4 Hz, 1H), 4.76 (s, 1H), 3.74 (d, *J* = 17.2 Hz, 1H), 3.63 (d, *J* = 17.2 Hz, 1H), 3.36 (dd, *J* = 5.2 Hz, 2.8 Hz, 1H), 2.99 (d, *J* = 18.4 Hz, 1H), 2.69 (dd, *J* = 11.6 Hz, 3.6 Hz, 1H), 2.62 (dt,

J = 12.6 Hz, 3.4 Hz, 1H), 2.53 (td, J = 14.0 Hz, 4.4 Hz, 1H), 2.46-2.35 (m, 2H), 2.28 (dt, J = 14.0 Hz, 3.0 Hz, 1H), 2.13 (td, J = 12.4 Hz, 4.8 Hz, 1H), 1.89–1.83 (m, 1H), 1.72 (ddd, J = 12.4 Hz, 3.2 Hz, 1.6 Hz, 1H), 1.14 (ddd, J = 27.2 Hz, 13.2 Hz, 2.8 Hz, 1H); ^{13}C-NMR (CD$_3$OD): δ 210.0, 144.1, 139.4, 126.7, 124.4, 119.7, 117.4, 117.0, 90.9, 58.3, 46.7, 44.4, 42.2, 41.8, 39.2, 34.5, 25.1, 21.1; HRMS (TOF MS ES$^+$) calcd for C$_{18}$H$_{19}$N$_2$O$_3$ [M + H]$^+$ 311.1396, found 311.1397. Anal. Calcd for C$_{18}$H$_{18}$N$_2$O$_3$·0.1CHCl$_3$·0.25H$_2$O (**1a**·0.1CHCl$_3$·0.25H$_2$O): C, 66.48; H, 5.42; N, 8.46; found: C, 66.52; H, 5.74; N, 8.57%. $[\alpha]_D^{20}$ −190.5 (*c* 0.43, CHCl$_3$/MeOH (20/1)).

2-((7aR,12bS)-9-Hydroxy-7-oxo-1,2,4,4a,5,6,7,7a-octahydro-3H-4,12-methanobenzofuro[3,2-e]isoquinolin-3-yl)butanenitrile (**1b**): The general procedure with **S10** (0.406 g, 1.5 mmol), 4-bromobutanenitrile (0.344 mL, 3.3 mmol), NaHCO$_3$ (0.504 g, 6 mmol), and DMF (10 mL). Purification by column chromatography afforded **1b** free base (0.350 g, 70%) as a colorless oil. ^{1}H-NMR (CD$_3$OD): δ 6.59 (d, J = 8.0 Hz, 1H), 6.54 (d, J = 8.4 Hz, 1H), 4.74 (s, 1H), 3.22 (dd, J = 5.6 Hz, 2.8 Hz, 1H), 2.91 (d, J = 18.4 Hz, 1H), 2.72–2.48 (m, 7H), 2.37 (dd, J = 18.4 Hz, 5.6 Hz, 1H), 2.28 (dt, J = 13.6 Hz, 3.2 Hz, 1H), 2.19 (td, J = 12.0 Hz, 3.2 Hz, 1H), 2.09 (td, J = 12.0 Hz, 4.4 Hz, 1H), 1.88–1.77 (m, 3H), 1.66 (ddd, J = 12.4 Hz, 3.0 Hz, 1.8 Hz, 1H), 1.14 (ddd, J = 27.4 Hz, 13.0 Hz, 2.8 Hz, 1H); ^{13}C-NMR (CD$_3$OD) δ 210.4, 144.1, 139.1, 127.1, 125.0, 119.9, 119.6, 117.3, 91.0, 57.7, 52.8, 47.3, 44.5, 41.7, 39.4, 34.8, 25.3, 22.9, 20.8, 13.8; HRMS (TOF MS ES$^+$) calcd for C$_{20}$H$_{23}$N$_2$O$_3$ [M + H]$^+$ 339.1709, found 339.1711. An HCl salt was prepared by dissolving **1b** free base in hot *i*-PrOH (5.0 mL) followed by the addition of concentrated aq HCl (0.10 mL, 3 equiv) and cooling to 5 °C. The crystals were filtered and air-dried to give **1b** as its HCl salt. Anal. Calcd for C$_{20}$H$_{22}$N$_2$O$_3$·HCl·1.5H$_2$O·0.25C$_3$H$_8$O (**1b**·HCl·1.5H$_2$O·0.25C$_3$H$_8$O): C, 59.65; H, 6.74; N, 6.49; found: C, 59.78; H, 6.77; N, 6.72%. $[\alpha]_D^{20}$ − 188.3 (*c* 0.6, CHCl$_3$/MeOH (1/10), HCl·1.5H$_2$O·0.25C$_3$H$_8$O salt).

(7aR,12bS)-3-Cinnamyl-9-hydroxy-2,3,4,4a,5,6-hexahydro-1H-4,12-methanobenzofuro[3,2-e]isoquinolin-7(7aH)-one (**1c**): The general procedure with **S10** (0.406 g, 1.5 mmol), (*E*)-(3-bromoprop-1-en-1-yl)benzene (0.650 mg, 3.3 mmol), NaHCO$_3$ (0.504 g, 6 mmol), and DMF (10 mL). Purification by column chromatography and crystallization from MeOH afforded **1c** free base (0.180 g, 31%) as a white solid. ^{1}H-NMR (DMSO-d$_6$) δ. 9.10 (s, 1H), 7.41 (d, J = 7.6 Hz, 2H), 7.29 (t, J = 7.4 Hz, 2H), 7.20 (t, J = 7.4 Hz, 1H), 6.57–6.49 (m, 3H), 6.26 (dt, J = 15.6 Hz, 6.4 Hz, 1H), 4.80 (s, 1H), 3.32–3.28 (m, 1H), 3.21–3.14 (m, 2H), 2.86 (d, J = 18.4 Hz, 1H), 2.57–2.48 (m, 3H), 2.23 (dd, J = 18.2 Hz, 5.4 Hz, 1H), 2.12 (dt, J = 14.0 Hz, 2.8 Hz, 1H), 2.01 (d, J = 7.2 Hz, 2H), 1.77–1.72 (m, 1H), 1.48 (d, J = 9.2 Hz, 1H), 0.97 (ddd, J = 27.2 Hz, 12.8 Hz, 2.2 Hz, 1H); ^{13}C-NMR (DMSO-d$_6$): δ 209.2, 144.4, 139.7, 137.2, 131.8, 129.0, 128.5, 127.9, 127.8, 126.6, 124.9, 119.6, 117.3, 90.8, 57.2, 56.9, 47.1, 45.0, 41.9, 40.1, 35.3, 25.5, 20.9; HRMS (TOF MS ES$^+$) calcd for C$_{25}$H$_{26}$NO$_3$ [M + H]$^+$ 388.1913, found 388.1906. Anal. Calcd for C$_{25}$H$_{25}$NO$_3$·0.25H$_2$O (**1c**·0.25H$_2$O): C, 76.60; H, 6.56; N, 3.57; found: C, 76.28; H, 6.42; N, 3.62%. $[\alpha]_D^{20}$ − 214.0 (*c* 0.4, CHCl$_3$/MeOH (1/10)).

(7aR,12bS)-3-((2,3-Dihydro-1H-inden-2-yl)methyl)-9-hydroxy-2,3,4,4a,5,6-hexahydro-1H-4,12-methanobenzofuro[3,2-e]isoquinolin-7(7aH)-one (**1d**): The general procedure with **S10** (0.406 g, 1.5 mmol), 2-(bromomethyl)-2,3-dihydro-1H-indene (0.470 mL, 3.3 mmol), NaHCO$_3$ (0.504 g, 6 mmol), and DMF (10 mL). Purification column chromatography and crystallization from chloroform afforded **1d** (0.190 g, 32%) as white solid. ^{1}H-NMR (CD$_3$OD): δ 7.16–7.14 (m, 2H), 7.08–7.05 (m, 2H), 6.60 (d, J = 8.0 Hz, 1H), 6.55 (d, J = 8.0 Hz, 1H), 4.75 (s, 1H), 3.24 (dd, J = 5.0 Hz, 2.6 Hz, 1H), 3.07–2.99 (m, 2H), 2.93 (d, J = 18.4 Hz, 1H), 2.76–2.59 (m, 5H), 2.56–2.49 (m, 3H), 2.35–2.26 (m, 2H), 2.20 (td, J = 12.0 Hz, 3.0 Hz, 1H), 2.11 (td, J = 12.0 Hz, 4.2 Hz, 1H), 1.86–1.80 (m, 1H), 1.65 (d, J = 12.0 Hz, 1H), 1.13 (ddd, J = 27.2 Hz, 13.2 Hz, 2.2 Hz, 1H); ^{13}C-NMR (CD$_3$OD): δ 210.6, 144.1, 142.7, 142.6, 139.1, 127.2, 125.7, 125.2, 124.1, 119.6, 117.2, 91.1, 59.6, 57.5, 45.1, 41.8, 39.5, 37.2, 37.1, 37.0, 34.9, 25.4, 20.7; HRMS (TOF MS ES$^+$) calcd for C$_{26}$H$_{28}$NO$_3$ [M + H]$^+$ 402.2069, found 402.2068. Anal. Calcd for C$_{26}$H$_{27}$NO$_3$·CHCl$_3$ (**1d**·CHCl$_3$): C, 62.30; H, 5.12; N, 2.68; found: C, 62.26; H, 5.42; N, 2.69%. $[\alpha]_D^{20}$ −137.0 (*c* 0.77, CHCl$_3$/MeOH (10/1)).

(7aR,12bS)-9-Hydroxy-3-(4-nitrophenethyl)-2,3,4,4a,5,6-hexahydro-1H-4,12-methanobenzofuro[3,2-e]isoquinolin-7(7aH)-one (**2a**): The general procedure with **S10** (0.406 g, 1.5 mmol), 1-(2-bromoethyl)-4-nitrobenzene (759 mg, 3.3 mmol), NaHCO$_3$ (0.504 g, 6 mmol), and DMF (10 mL). Purification by column chromatography afforded **2a** (0.070 g, 10%) as a colorless oil. ^{1}H-NMR (CD$_3$OD): δ 8.16 (d,

J = 8.4 Hz, 2H), 7.51 (d, J = 8.4 Hz, 2H), 6.61 (d, J = 8.4 Hz, 1H), 6.56 (d, J = 8.0 Hz, 1H), 4.77 (s, 1H), 3.32–3.30 (m, 1H), 2.99–2.72 (m, 6H), 2.61–2.49 (m, 2H), 2.38 (dd, J = 18.6 Hz, 5.8 Hz, 1H), 2.29 (dt, J = 14.0 Hz, 3.0 Hz, 1H), 2.24 (td, J = 12.2 Hz, 3.4 Hz, 1H), 2.11 (td, J = 12.4 Hz, 4.8 Hz, 1H), 1.88–1.81 (m, 1H), 1.69 (d, J = 12.0 Hz, 1H), 1.15 (ddd, J = 27.2 Hz, 13.2 Hz, 2.0 Hz, 1H); ^{13}C-NMR (100 MHz, CD$_3$OD): δ 210.4, 148.6, 146.5, 144.1, 139.2, 129.5, 127.0, 124.9, 123.0, 119.6, 117.3, 91.0, 57.5, 55.6, 47.2, 44.7, 41.6, 39.4, 34.7, 33.4, 25.3, 20.6; HRMS (TOF MS ES$^+$) calcd for C$_{24}$H$_{25}$N$_2$O$_5$ [M + H]$^+$ 421.1763, found 421.1762. An HCl salt was prepared by dissolving **2a** free base in hot *i*-PrOH (5.0 mL) followed by the addition of concentrated aqueous HCl (0.10 mL, 3 equiv) and cooling to 5 °C. The crystals were filtered and air-dried to give **2a** as its HCl salt. Anal. Calcd for C$_{24}$H$_{24}$N$_2$O$_5$·HCl·1.75H$_2$O (**2a**·HCl·1.75H$_2$O): C, 58.99; H, 5.69; N, 5.56; found: C, 59.02; H, 5.88; N, 5.74%. $[α]_D^{20}$ −107 (*c* 0.4, MeOH, HCl·1.75H$_2$O salt).

(7aR,12bS)-9-Hydroxy-3-(3-nitrophenethyl)-2,3,4,4a,5,6-hexahydro-1H-4,12-methanobenzofuro[3,2-e]-0isoquinolin-7(7aH)-one (**2b**): The general procedure with **S10** (0.406 g, 1.5 mmol), 1-(2-bromoethyl)-3-nitrobenzene (759 mg, 3.3 mmol), NaHCO$_3$ (0.504 g, 6 mmol), and DMF (10 mL). Purification by column chromatography afforded **2b** free base (0.035 g, 5%) as a colorless oil. ^{1}H-NMR (CD$_3$OD): δ 8.16 (t, J = 3.0 Hz, 1H), 8.05 (ddd, J = 8.0 Hz, 2.4 Hz, 0.8 Hz, 1H), 7.66 (d, J = 7.6 Hz, 1H), 7.51 (t, J = 7.8 Hz, 1H), 6.59 (d, J = 8.0 Hz, 1H), 6.55 (d, J = 8.0 Hz, 1H), 4.75 (s, 1H), 3.28–3.27 (m, 1H), 2.97–2.84 (m, 4H), 2.82–2.71 (m, 2H), 2.60–2.47 (m, 2H), 2.37 (dd, J = 18.6 Hz, 5.8 Hz, 1H), 2.30–2.21(m, 2H), 2.09 (td, J = 12.2 Hz, 4.6 Hz, 1H), 1.86–1.79 (m, 1H), 1.68 (ddd, J = 12.4 Hz, 3.2 Hz, 1.6 Hz, 1H), 1.13 (ddd, J = 27.4 Hz, 13.0 Hz, 2.8 Hz, 1H); ^{13}C-NMR (CD$_3$OD): δ 210.3, 148.2, 144.1, 142.8, 139.2, 134.9, 129.0, 127.0, 125.0, 123.2, 120.6, 119.6, 117.3, 91.0, 57.5, 55.7, 47.3, 44.7, 41.7, 39.4, 34.8, 33.1, 25.3, 20.7; HRMS (TOF MS ES$^+$) calcd for C$_{24}$H$_{25}$N$_2$O$_5$ [M + H]$^+$ 421.1763, found 421.1762. An HCl salt was prepared by dissolving **2b** free base in hot *i*-PrOH (5.0 mL) followed by the addition of concentrated aqueous HCl (0.10 mL, 3 equiv) and cooling to 5 °C. The crystals were filtered and air-dried to give **2b** as its HCl salt. Anal. Calcd for C$_{24}$H$_{24}$N$_2$O$_5$·HCl·1.5H$_2$O (**2b**·HCl·1.5H$_2$O): C, 59.64; H, 5.55; N, 5.49; found: C, 59.56; H, 5.83; N, 5.79%. $[α]_D^{20}$ −137.9 (*c* 0.6, CHCl$_3$/MeOH (1/20), HCl·1.5H$_2$O).

(7aR,12bS)-9-Hydroxy-3-(4-methylphenethyl)-2,3,4,4a,5,6-hexahydro-1H-4,12-methanobenzofuro[3,2-e]-isoquinolin-7(7aH)-one (**2c**): The general procedure with **S10** (0.406 g, 1.5 mmol), 1-(2-bromoethyl)-4-methylbenzene (0.502 mL, 3.3 mmol), NaHCO$_3$ (0.504 g, 6 mmol), and DMF (10 mL). Purification by SiO$_2$ column chromatography afforded **2c** free base (0.330 g, 65%) as a colorless oil. ^{1}H-NMR (CD$_3$OD): δ 7.11 (d, J = 8.4 Hz, 2H), 7.08 (d, J = 8.4 Hz, 2H), 6.61 (d, J = 8.4 Hz, 1H), 6.56 (d, J = 8.4 Hz, 1H), 4.77 (s, 1H), 3.36 (dd, J = 5.2 Hz, 2.4 Hz, 1H), 2.97 (d, J = 18.4 Hz, 1H), 2.80–2.65 (m, 5H), 2.62 (dt, J = 12.8 Hz, 3.2 Hz, 1H), 2.53 (td, J = 14.0 Hz, 4.8 Hz, 1H), 2.36 (dd, J = 18.4 Hz, 5.6 Hz, 1H), 2.29 (dt, J = 13.2 Hz, 3.0 Hz, 1H), 2.28 (s, 3H), 2.21 (td, J = 12.0 Hz, 2.1 Hz, 1H), 2.12 (td, J = 12.0 Hz, 4.0 Hz, 1H), 1.88–1.82 (m, 1H), 1.68 (d, J = 12.4 Hz, 1H), 1.15 (ddd, J = 27.0 Hz, 13.4 Hz, 2.4 Hz, 1H); ^{13}C-NMR (CD$_3$OD): δ 210.3, 144.1, 139.2, 136.9, 135.2, 128.6, 128.2, 127.0, 124.8, 119.6, 117.3, 91.0, 57.0, 56.7, 47.2, 45.1, 41.4, 39.4, 34.6, 33.2, 25.4, 20.2, 19.7; HRMS (TOF MS ES$^+$) calcd for C$_{25}$H$_{28}$NO$_3$ [M + H]$^+$ 390.2069, found 390.2071. An HCl salt was prepared by dissolving **2c** free base in hot MeOH (5.0 mL) followed by the addition of concentrated aq HCl (0.10 mL, 3 equiv) and cooling to 5 °C. The crystals were filtered and air-dried to give **2c** as its HCl salt. Anal. Calcd for C$_{25}$H$_{27}$NO$_3$·HCl·1.5H$_2$O·0.5CH$_4$O (**2c**·HCl·1.5H$_2$O·0.5CH$_4$O): C, 65.56; H, 6.78; N, 2.92; found: C, 65.37; H, 7.09; N, 2.99%. $[α]_D^{20}$ − 139.5 (*c* 0.63, MeOH, HCl·1.5H$_2$O·0.5CH$_4$O).

(7aR,12bS)-9-Hydroxy-3-(4-methoxyphenethyl)-2,3,4,4a,5,6-hexahydro-1H-4,12-methanobenzofuro[3,2-e]-isoquinolin-7(7aH)-one (**2d**): The general procedure with **S10** (0.406 g, 1.5 mmol), 1-(2-bromoethyl)-4-methoxybenzene (0.520 mL, 3.3 mmol), NaHCO$_3$ (0.504 g, 6 mmol), and DMF (10 mL). Column chromatography afforded **2d** free base (0.370 g, 64%) as a colorless oil. ^{1}H-NMR (DMSO-d$_6$): δ 9.09 (s, 1H), 7.13 (d, J = 8.4 Hz, 2H), 6.81 (d, J = 8.4 Hz, 2H), 6.51 (d, J = 8.0 Hz, 1H), 6.46 (d, J = 8.4 Hz, 1H), 4.79 (s, 1H), 3.69 (s, 3H), 3.20 (s, 1H), 2.80 (d, J = 18.4 Hz, 1H), 2.63–2.53 (m, 5H), 2.51–2.44 (m, 2H), 2.23 (dd, J = 18.4 Hz, 5.6 Hz, 1H), 2.12 (d, J = 13.6 Hz, 1H), 2.01–1.97 (m, 2H), 1.76–1.72 (m, 1H), 1.47 (d, J = 9.2 Hz, 1H), 1.02–0.91 (m, 1H); ^{13}C-NMR (DMSO-d$_6$): δ 209.3, 157.9, 144.3, 139.6, 132.8, 130.0,

128.0, 124.9, 119.6, 117.3, 114.0, 90.8, 57.2, 57.1, 55.4, 47.1, 44.9, 41.8, 40.1, 35.3, 33.4, 25.5, 21.0; HRMS (TOF MS ES+) calcd for $C_{25}H_{28}NO_4$ [M + H]+ 406.2018, found 406.2014. An HCl salt was prepared by dissolving **2d** free base in hot i-PrOH (5.0 mL) followed by the addition of concentrated aqueous HCl (0.10 mL, 3 equiv) and cooling to 5 °C. The crystals were filtered and air-dried to give **2d** as its HCl salt. Anal. Calcd for $C_{25}H_{27}NO_4 \cdot HCl \cdot 0.5H_2O \cdot 0.5C_3H_8O$ (**2d**·HCl·0.5H$_2$O·0.5C$_3$H$_8$O): C, 66.19; H, 6.83; N, 2.77; found: C, 66.17; H, 6.92; N, 2.91%. $[\alpha]_D^{20}$ −136.5 (c 0.68, MeOH, HCl·0.5H$_2$O·0.5i-PrOH).

(7aR,12bS)-9-Hydroxy-3-(4-fluorophenethyl)-2,3,4,4a,5,6-hexahydro-1H-4,12-methanobenzofuro[3,2-e]-isoquinolin-7(7aH)-one (**2e**): The general procedure with **S10** (0.406 g, 1.5 mmol), 1-(2-bromoethyl)-4-fluorobenzene (0.460 mL, 3.3 mmol), NaHCO$_3$ (0.504 g, 6 mmol), and DMF (10 mL). Purification by column chromatography afforded **2e** free base (0.290 g, 50%) as a colorless oil. ^{1}H-NMR (CD$_3$OD): δ 7.24 (dd, J = 8.2 Hz, 5.4 Hz, 2H), 6.99 (t, J = 8.8 Hz, 2H), 6.60 (d, J = 8.0 Hz, 1H), 6.56 (d, J = 8.4 Hz, 1H), 4.77 (s, 1H), 3.30 (s, 1H), 2.97 (d, J = 18.4 Hz, 1H), 2.83–2.66 (m, 5H), 2.61 (dt, J = 12.8 Hz, 3.4 Hz, 1H), 2.52 (td, J = 14.2 Hz, 4.6 Hz, 1H), 2.37 (dd, J = 18.6 Hz, 5.8 Hz, 1H), 2.29 (dt, J = 14.0 Hz, 2.8 Hz, 1H), 2.22 (td, J = 12.0 Hz, 3.0 Hz, 1H), 2.12 (td, J = 12.0 Hz, 4.4 Hz, 1H), 1.88–1.82 (m, 1H), 1.69 (d, J = 12.4 Hz, 1H), 1.15 (ddd, J = 27.2 Hz, 13.2 Hz, 2.4 Hz, 1H); ^{13}C-NMR (CD$_3$OD): δ 210.3, 162.7, 160.2, 144.1, 139.2, 136.0(2), 130.0(2), 127.0, 124.9, 119.6, 117.3, 114.6, 114.4, 91.0, 57.2, 56.6, 47.2, 45.0, 41.5, 39.4, 34.7, 32.8, 25.4, 20.4; HRMS (TOF MS ES+) calcd for $C_{24}H_{25}FNO_3$ (M + H+) 394.1818, found 394.1825. An HCl salt was prepared by dissolving **2e** free base in hot *i*-PrOH (5.0 mL) followed by the addition of concentrated aq HCl (0.10 mL, 3 equiv) and cooling to 5 °C. The crystals were filtered and air-dried to give **2e** as its HCl salt. Anal. Calcd for $C_{24}H_{24}FNO_3 \cdot HCl \cdot 1.5H_2O$ (**2e**·HCl·1.5H$_2$O): C, 63.14; H, 6.03; N, 2.98; found: C, 63.09; H, 6.18; N, 3.07%. $[\alpha]_D^{20}$ − 137.8 (*c* 0.65, MeOH, HCl·1.5H$_2$O).

(7aR,12bS)-9-Hydroxy-3-(3-fluorophenethyl)-2,3,4,4a,5,6-hexahydro-1H-4,12-methanobenzofuro[3,2-e]-isoquinolin-7(7aH)-one (**2f**): The general procedure with **10** (0.406 g, 1.5 mmol), 1-(2-bromoethyl)-3-fluorobenzene (0.460 mL, 3.3 mmol), NaHCO$_3$ (0.504 g, 6 mmol), and DMF (10 mL). Purification by column chromatography afforded **2f** free base (0.270 g, 46%) as colorless oil. ^{1}H-NMR (CD$_3$OD): δ 7.27 (dd, J = 14.0 Hz, 8.0 Hz, 1H), 7.05 (d, J = 7.6 Hz, 1H), 6.99 (d, J = 10.4 Hz, 1H), 6.90 (td, J = 8.6 Hz, 2.4 Hz, 1H), 6.61 (d, J = 8.4 Hz, 1H), 6.56 (d, J = 8.0 Hz, 1H), 4.76 (s, 1H), 3.34–3.32 (m, 1H), 2.96 (d, J = 18.4 Hz, 1H), 2.85–2.68 (m, 5H), 2.60 (dt, J = 12.6 Hz, 3.4 Hz, 1H), 2.52 (td, J = 14.0 Hz, 4.6 Hz, 1H), 2.36 (dd, J = 18.4 Hz, 5.6 Hz, 1H), 2.28 (dt, J = 13.8 Hz, 2.1 Hz, 1H), 2.21 (td, J = 12.4 Hz, 3.2 Hz, 1H), 2.11 (td, J = 12.2 Hz, 4.4 Hz, 1H), 1.87–1.81 (m, 1H), 1.67 (d, J = 12.4 Hz, 1H), 1.14 (ddd, J = 26.8 Hz, 13.4 Hz, 2.4 Hz, 1H); ^{13}C-NMR (CD$_3$OD): δ 210.4, 164.1, 161.7, 144.1, 143.1, 143.0, 139.2, 129.7, 129.6, 127.0, 124.9, 124.3, 124.2, 119.7, 117.4, 115.1, 114.9, 112.5, 112.2, 91.0, 57.2, 56.1, 47.2, 44.9, 41.5, 39.4, 34.7, 33.3, 25.3, 20.4; HRMS (TOF MS ES+) calcd for $C_{24}H_{25}FNO_3$ [M + H]+ 394.1818, found 394.1821. An HCl salt was prepared by dissolving **2f** free base in hot *i*-PrOH (5.0 mL) followed by the addition of concentrated aqueous HCl (0.10 mL, 3 equiv) and cooling to 5 °C. The crystals were filtered and air-dried to give **2f** as its HCl salt. Anal. Calcd for $C_{24}H_{24}FNO_3 \cdot HCl \cdot 1.25H_2O$ (**2f**·HCl·1.25H$_2$O): C, 63.71; H, 6.13; N, 3.10; found: C, 63.71; H, 6.11; N, 3.11%. $[\alpha]_D^{20}$ −149.2 (*c* 0.48, MeOH, HCl·1.25H$_2$O).

(7aR,12bS)-9-Hydroxy-3-(2-fluorophenethyl)-2,3,4,4a,5,6-hexahydro-1H-4,12-methanobenzofuro[3,2-e]-isoquinolin-7(7aH)-one (**2g**): The general procedure with **S10** (0.406 g, 1.5 mmol), 1-(2-bromoethyl)-2-fluorobenzene (0.460 mL, 3.3 mmol), NaHCO$_3$ (0.504 g, 6 mmol), and DMF (10 mL). Purification by column chromatography afforded **2g** free base (0.260 g, 45%) as a colorless oil. ^{1}H-NMR (CD$_3$OD): δ 7.31–7.27 (m, 1H), 7.24–7.19 (m, 1H), 7.11–7.01 (m, 2H), 6.61 (d, J = 8.4 Hz, 1H), 6.56 (d, J = 8.0 Hz, 1H), 4.77 (s, 1H), 3.36 (dd, J = 5.2 Hz, 2.8 Hz, 1H), 2.96 (d, J = 18.4 Hz, 1H), 2.94–2.66 (m, 5H), 2.61 (dt, J = 12.8 Hz, 3.4 Hz, 1H), 2.40 (td, J = 14.0 Hz, 4.6 Hz, 1H), 2.38 (dd, J = 18.6 Hz, 5.8 Hz, 1H), 2.29 (dt, J = 14.0 Hz, 3.0 Hz, 1H), 2.23 (td, J = 12.4 Hz, 3.2 Hz, 1H), 2.12 (td, J = 12.2 Hz, 4.6 Hz, 1H), 1.89–1.82 (m, 1H), 1.70–1.67 (m, 1H), 1.15 (ddd, J = 27.2 Hz, 13.4 Hz, 2.4 Hz, 1H); ^{13}C-NMR (CD$_3$OD): δ 210.4, 162.4, 160.0, 144.0, 139.2, 130.9, 130.8, 127.8, 127.7, 127.0, 126.8, 126.6, 124.9, 123.9(2), 119.6, 117.3, 114.7, 114.5, 91.0, 57.2, 55.0, 47.2, 45.0, 41.5, 39.4, 34.7, 26.9(2), 25.4, 20.4; HRMS (TOF MS ES+) calcd for $C_{24}H_{25}FNO_3$ [M + H]+ 394.1818, found 394.1822. An HCl salt was prepared by dissolving **2g** free base in hot *i*-PrOH (5.0 mL) followed by the addition of concentrated aq HCl (0.10 mL, 3 equiv)

and cooling to 5 °C. The crystals were filtered and air-dried to give **2g** as its HCl salt. Anal. Calcd for $C_{24}H_{24}FNO_3 \cdot HCl \cdot 1.5H_2O$ (**2g**·HCl·1.5H$_2$O): C, 63.51; H, 5.74; N, 3.05; found: C, 63.09; H, 6.18; N, 3.07%. $[\alpha]_D^{20}$ −135.7 (c 1.25, MeOH, HCl·1.5H$_2$O).

(7aR,12bS)-9-Hydroxy-3-(4-(trifluoromethyl)phenethyl)-2,3,4,4a,5,6-hexahydro-1H-4,12-methanobenzo furo-[3,2-e]isoquinolin-7(7aH)-one (**2h**): The general procedure with **S10** (0.406 g, 1.5 mmol), 1-(2-bromoethyl)-4-(trifluoromethyl)benzene (0.554 mL, 3.3 mmol), NaHCO$_3$ (0.504 g, 6 mmol), and DMF (10 mL). Purification by column chromatography afforded **2h** free base (0.145 g, 25%) as a colorless oil. ^{1}H-NMR (CD$_3$OD): δ 7.58 (d, J = 8.0 Hz, 2H), 7.45 (d, J = 8.0 Hz, 2H), 6.61 (d, J = 8.4 Hz, 1H), 6.56 (d, J = 8.4 Hz, 1H), 4.77 (s, 1H), 3.34–3.32 (m, 1H), 2.97 (d, J = 18.4 Hz, 1H), 2.93–2.72 (m, 5H), 2.60 (dt, J = 12.8 Hz, 3.4 Hz, 1H), 2.54 (td, J = 14.0 Hz, 4.8 Hz, 1H), 2.38 (dd, J = 18.6 Hz, 5.8 Hz, 1H), 2.29 (dt, J = 14.0 Hz, 3.0 Hz, 1H), 2.23 (td, J = 12.2 Hz, 3.4 Hz, 1H), 2.12 (td, J = 12.2 Hz, 4.2 Hz, 1H), 1.88–1.82 (m, 1H), 1.69 (d, J = 11.6 Hz, 1H), 1.15 (ddd, J = 27.2 Hz, 13.2 Hz, 2.4 Hz, 1H); ^{13}C-NMR (CD$_3$OD): δ 210.4, 144.1, 139.2, 129.0, 128.5, 128.1, 127.8, 127.5, 127.0, 124.9, 124.8(2), 124.7(2), 119.6, 117.3, 91.0, 57.3, 56.0, 47.2, 44.8, 41.6, 39.4, 34.7, 33.4, 25.3, 20.5; HRMS (TOF MS ES$^+$) calcd for $C_{25}H_{25}F_3NO_3$ [M + H]$^+$ 444.1787, found 444.1788. An HCl salt was prepared by dissolving **2h** free base in hot i-PrOH (5.0 mL) followed by the addition of concentrated aq HCl (0.10 mL, 3 equiv) and cooling to 5 °C. The crystals were filtered and air-dried to give **2h** as its HCl salt. Anal. Calcd for $C_{25}H_{24}F_3NO_3 \cdot HCl \cdot 0.5H_2O \cdot 0.5C_3H_8O$ (**2h**·HCl·0.5H$_2$O·0.5C$_3$H$_8$O): C, 61.31; H, 5.73; N, 2.60; found: C, 61.33; H, 5.83; N, 2.70%. $[\alpha]_D^{20}$ − 122.0 (c 0.4, MeOH, HCl·0.5H$_2$O·0.5i-PrOH).

(7aR,12bS)-3-(4-Chlorophenethyl)-9-hydroxy-2,3,4,4a,5,6-hexahydro-1H-4,12-methanobenzofuro[3,2-e]-isoquinolin-7(7aH)-one (**2i**): See the General Procedure in 3.2.

(4R,7aR,12bS)-3-(4-Bromophenethyl)-9-hydroxy-2,3,4,4a,5,6-hexahydro-1H-4,12-methanobenzofuro[3,2-e]-isoquinolin-7(7aH)-one oxalate (**2j**): The general procedure with **S10** (0.3 g, 1.11 mmol), 4-bromophenethyl bromide (0.586 g, 2.22 mmol), NaHCO$_3$ (0.50 g, 5.95 mmol), and DMF (10 mL) at room temperature. The reaction was heated to 60 °C for 20 h cooled to room temperature, and filtered through a pad of Celite. The DMF was removed via azeotrope with toluene (3 × 20 mL), then purification by SiO$_2$ column chromatography with 10% NH$_4$OH in MeOH/CHCl$_3$ (0% → 5% of 10% NH$_4$OH) gave the base **2j** ree base (0.212 g isolated, 41% yield) as a light brown oil. An oxalate salt was prepared by dissolving **2j** in a minimal amount of hot i-PrOH followed by addition of a concentrated solution of oxalic acid in isopropanol. Cooling at 5 °C overnight gave **2j·oxalate** as a precipitate (0.131 g, 44/%), mp 201–204 °C. ^{1}H-NMR (CD$_3$OD): δ 7.39 (d, J = 8.1 Hz, 2H), 7.07 (d, J = 8.1 Hz, 2H), 6.71 (d, J = 8.1 Hz, 1H), 6.58 (d, J = 8.1 Hz, 1H), 4.65 (s, 1H), 3.34 (d, J = 0.4 Hz, 1H), 2.96 (t, J = 15.8 Hz, 1H), 2.78–2.69 (m, 5H), 2.65–2.61 (m, 1H), 2.38–2.32 (m, 3H), 2.27–2.21 (m, 1H), 2.16–2.07 (m, 1H), 1.84–1.76 (m, 2H), 1.27–1.18 (m, 2H). ^{13}C-NMR (CD$_3$OD): δ 209.12, 144.04, 139.08, 138.89, 131.39, 130.47, 126.78, 125.05, 120.26, 119.89, 118.00, 91.35, 57.67, 56.64, 47.40, 45.03, 42.11, 40.13, 35.16, 33.63, 25.41, 20.98; HRMS (TOF MS ES$^+$) $C_{24}H_{24}BrNO_3$ (M+H$^+$) 454.1018, found 454.1021. Anal. Calcd for $C_{24}H_{24}BrNO_3 \cdot C_2H_2O_4 \cdot 2H_2O$ (**2j**·C$_2$H$_2$O$_4$·2H$_2$O) C, 54.31%; H, 5.15%; N, 2.44%; found: C, 54.09%; H, 5.04%; N, 2.71%. $[\alpha]_D^{20}$ −87.0 (c 1.2, MeOH, C$_{24}$H$_{24}$BrNO$_3$·C$_2$H$_2$O$_4$·2H$_2$O).

(7aR,12bS)-3-(2,6-Dichlorophenethyl)-9-hydroxy-2,3,4,4a,5,6-hexahydro-1H-4,12-methanobenzofuro[3,2-e] isoquinolin-7(7aH)-one (**2k**): The general procedure with **S10** (0.56 g, 2 mmol), 2,6-dichlorophenethyl bromide (1.0 g, 4 mmol), NaHCO$_3$ (0.70 g, 8.3 mmol), and DMF (10 mL). Purification by column chromatography afforded **2k** free base (0.012 g, 0.02 mmol, 2%) as a yellow oil. The oil was taken up in acetone (2 mL) and oxalic acid (0.002 g) added to give pure **2k·oxalate** (0.014 g) as a white powder. ^{1}H-NMR (DMSO-d$_6$): δ 7.49 (d, J = 8.0 Hz, 2H), 7.32 (t, J = 8.0 Hz, 1H), 6.58 (q, J = 7.5 Hz, 2H), 4.91 (s, 1H), 3.72–3.70 (m, 1H), 3.24–3.13 (m, 2H), 3.10–2.93 (m, 3H), 2.91–2.81 (m, 1H), 2.76–2.66 (m, 1H), 2.63–2.54 (m, 2H), 2.39–2.32 (m, 1H), 2.20–2.16 (m, 2H), 1.86–1.83 (m, 1H), 1.65–1.62 (m, 1H), 1.06–0.95 (m, 1H); ^{13}C-NMR (DMSO-d$_6$): δ 208.6, 163.2, 144.4, 140.0, 135.2, 129.9, 129.0, 120.0, 117.7, 90.4, 57.9, 46.2, 31.1, 25.0; m.p. 204-206 °C (decomp); HRMS (ESI): Calcd for $C_{26}H_{26}Cl_2NO_7$ [M + H]$^+$ 444.1133, found: 444.1129; Anal. Calcd for $C_{26}H_{25}Cl_2NO_7 \cdot 2.25 H_2O$: C, 54.32; H, 5.17; N, 2.44; found: C, 54.22; H, 4.86; N, 2.59.

3.3. In Vitro Pharmacology.

3.3.1. Opioid Receptor Binding Affinity

Frozen whole rat brains excluding cerebellum were thawed on ice, homogenized in 50 mM Tris HCl, pH 7.5 using a Polytron (Brinkman Instruments, Westbury, NY, USA), setting 6 for 20 s), and centrifuged at 30,000× g for 10 min at 4 °C. The supernatant was discarded and the pellet was re-suspended in fresh buffer and spun at 30,000× g for 10 min. The supernatant was discarded and the pellet was re-suspended to give 100 mg/mL original wet weight. Ligand binding experiments were conducted in polypropylene assay tubes containing 0.5 mL Tris HCl buffer for 60 min at room temperature. [^{3}H]DADLE (final concentration 1 nM, PolyPeptide Laboratories, San Diego, CA, USA), [^{3}H]DAMGO (final concentration 1 nM, PolyPeptide Laboratories, San Diego, CA, USA) or [^{3}H]U69,593 (final concentration 1 nM, Perkin Elmer Life Sciences, Waltham, MA, USA) were used to determine binding at δ-, μ- and κ-opioid receptor sites, respectively. Unlabeled DAMGO (final concentration, 30 nM) was added to the delta assay tubes to block μ-receptor binding. All assay tubes contained 100 μL homogenate suspension. Nonspecific binding was determined in all assays using 0.01 mM naloxone. Incubations were terminated by rapid filtration through Whatman GF/B filters, presoaked in 0.1% polyethyleneimine, using a Brandel R48 filtering manifold (Brandel Instruments Gaithersburg, Maryland). The filters were washed twice with 5 mL cold buffer and transferred to scintillation vials. Cytoscint (MP BioMedicals, Santa Ana, CA, USA) 3.0 mL) was added and the vials were counted the next day using a Perkin Elmer TriCarb liquid scintillation counter. Data were analyzed with GraphPad Prism software (GraphPad Inc., San Diego, CA, USA).

3.3.2. Stimulation of [^{35}S]GTPγS Binding

All tissue culture reagents were purchased from Gibco Life Sciences (Grand Island, NY, USA). C6-rat glioma cells stably transfected with a rat MOR or rat DOR [38] and Chinese hamster ovary (CHO) cells stably expressing a human KOR [39] were used for all in vitro assays. Cells were grown to confluence at 37 °C in 5% CO_2 in Dulbecco's Modified Eagle Medium (DMEM) containing 10% fetal bovine serum and 5% penicillin/ streptomycin. Membranes were prepared by washing confluent cells three times with ice-cold phosphate buffered saline (0.9% NaCl, 0.61 mM Na_2HPO_4, 0.38 mM KH_2PO_4, pH 7.4). Cells were detached from the plates by incubation in warm harvesting buffer (20 mM HEPES, 150 mM NaCl, 0.68 mM EDTA, pH 7.4) and pelleted by centrifugation at 1600 rpm for 3 min. The cell pellet was suspended in ice-cold 50 mM Tris-HCl buffer, pH 7.4, and homogenized with a Tissue Tearor (Biospec Products, Inc., Bartlesville, OK, USA) for 20 s. The homogenate was centrifuged at 15,000 rpm for 20 min at 4 °C. The pellet was re-homogenized in 50 mM Tris-HCl with a Tissue Tearor for 10 s, followed by re-centrifugation. The final pellet was re-suspended in 50 mM Tris-HCl and frozen in aliquots at 80 °C. Protein concentration was determined via a BCA protein assay (Thermo Scientific Pierce, Waltham, MA, USA) using bovine serum albumin as the standard.

Agonist stimulation of [^{35}S]guanosine 5'-O-[γ-thio]triphosphate ([^{35}S]GTPγS, 1250 Ci, 46.2 TBq/mmol) binding to G-protein was measured as described previously [40]. Briefly, membranes (10–20 μg of protein/tube) were incubated 1 h at 25 °C in GTPγS buffer (50 mM Tris-HCl, 100 mM NaCl, 5 mM $MgCl_2$, pH 7.4) containing 0.1 nM [35S]GTPγS, 30 μM guanosine diphosphate (GDP), and varying concentrations of test compound. G-Protein activation following receptor stimulation of [^{35}S]GTPγS (% stimulation) with test compound was compared with 10 μM of the standard compounds [D-Ala2,N-MePhe4,Gly-ol]- enkephalin (DAMGO) at MOR, D-Pen2,5-enkephalin (DPDPE) at DOR, or U69,593 at KOR. The reaction was terminated by vacuum filtration of GF/C filters that were washed 10 times with GTPγS buffer. Bound radioactivity on dried filters was determined by liquid scintillation counting, after saturation with EcoLume liquid scintillation cocktail, in a Wallac 1450 MicroBeta (PerkinElmer, Waltham, MA, USA). The results are presented as the mean ± standard error (SEM) from at least three separate assays performed in duplicate; potency (EC50 (nM)) and % stimulation were determined using nonlinear regression analysis with GraphPad Prism.

3.3.3. Forskolin-Induced cAMP Accumulation Assays

Cell Lines and Cell Culture

HitHunter Chinese hamster ovary cells (CHO-K1) that express human µ-opioid receptor (OPRM1), human κ-opioid receptor (OPRMK1), and human δ-receptor (OPRMD1) were used for the forskolin-induced cAMP accumulation assay. PathHunter CHO cells expressing human µ-opioid receptor β-arrestin-2 EFC cells were used for the β-arrestin-2 EFC recruitment assay. Both cell lines were purchased from Eurofins DiscoverX (Fremont, CA, USA). Cell culture was performed as previously described [41].

Assays

These were performed as previously described using HitHunter CHO-K1 cells expressing either human OPRM1, OPRK1, or OPRMD1 cells. Briefly, cells were dissociated from culture plates and plated at 10,000 cells/well in a 384-well tissue culture plate and incubated overnight at 37 °C in 5% CO_2. Stock solutions of compound were made in 100% DMSO at a 5 mM concentration. A serial dilution of 10 concentrations was made using 100% DMSO, creating 100× solutions of the compound for treatment. The 100× solutions were then diluted to 5× solutions using assay buffer consisting of Hank's Buffered Salt Solution, HEPES, and forskolin. The HitHunter cAMP Assay for Small Molecules by DiscoverX was then used according to manufacturer's directions, utilizing the 5× solutions containing the compound studied. Cells were incubated with compound for 30 min at a 1× concentration. The following day, the Cytation 5 plate reader and Gen5 Software were used to quantify luminescence (BioTek, Winooski, VT, USA) [41].

3.3.4. β-Arrestin-2 EFC Recruitment Assay

Assays were performed as previously described [41] using PathHunter human µ-opioid receptor β-arrestin-2 EFC cells. Briefly, cells were dissociated from culture plates and plated at 5000 cells/well in a 384-well tissue culture plate and incubated overnight at 37 °C in 5% CO_2. Stock solutions of compound were made in 100% DMSO for a final concentration of 5 mM. A serial dilution of 11 concentrations was made using 100% DMSO to create 100× solutions of the compound. Assay buffer containing Hank's Buffered Salt Solution and HEPES was used to dilute the 100× solutions to 5× solutions. The DiscoverX PathHunter assay was used according to manufacturer's instructions. Cells were treated with the compounds for a final 1× concentration for 90 min. at 37 °C and 5% CO_2. Reagents from the assay kit were used accordingly and the cell culture plate was protected from light for 1 h. Cytation 5 plate reader and Gen5 Software were used to quantify luminescence (BioTek).

3.3.5. Data Analysis

Data were analyzed as previously described [42] using GraphPad Prism 6.0 software (GraphPad, San Diego, CA, USA different address given before). Briefly, sigmoidal dose-response curves in the forskolin-induced cAMP accumulation assay and the β-arrestin2 EFC recruitment assay were generated using nonlinear regression analysis. Compounds were evaluated in triplicate in individual experiments with $n \geq 2$. All values in the cAMP accumulation assay and β-arrestin2 recruitment assay are reported as the mean ± SEM. Bias factors were calculated using Equation (1) shown below.

$$Log\ (bias\ factor) = \left(Log\left(\frac{EC50\ test \times Emax\ DAMGO}{Emax\ test \times EC50\ DAMGO}\right)\right)_{cAMP} - \left(Log\left(\frac{EC50\ test \times Emax\ DAMGO}{Emax\ test \times EC50\ DAMGO}\right)\right)_{\beta-arrestin} \quad (1)$$

3.4. In Vivo Pharmacolog

3.4.1. Measurement of Respiration Rate and Arterial Oxygen Saturation in Mice

Male Swiss Webster mice (Taconic Biosciences, Germantown, NY, USA) weighing 30–35 g were used. Mice were housed in a temperature- and humidity-controlled environment with a 12-h light-dark cycle in the Temple University Animal Care Facility. They were supplied with food and water ad libitum. Before any procedure was applied, the mice were acclimated for 1 week in the animal facility. Behavioral testing was performed between 11:00 a.m. and 5:00 p.m. On the day of the experiment, mice were brought to the room and acclimated for 45–60 min in the observation boxes All animal care and experimental procedures were approved by the Institutional Animal Care and Use Committee of Temple University (Protocol #4793 Respiration Measurement in Mice; Approval Date: 1 June 2018), and conducted according to the NIH Guide for the Care and Use of Laboratory Animals.

Respiration and oxygen saturation (SpO_2) were measured using MouseOx Plus Rat and Mouse Pulse Oximeter (Starr Life Sciences Corp, Oakmont, PA, USA) in conscious, freely moving animals. Animals were exposed to 4% isoflurane for 30 s to connect throat collar sensor and to inject (s.c.) either saline, morphine 10 mg/kg, or **2i** (0.01–0.1 mg/kg, n = 6–8). Mice were then placed into observation boxes and recording was started 5 min later to eliminate any anesthesia effect. Respiration and SpO_2 were recorded every second and averaged over 1-min periods for 40 min. Morphine, 10 mg/kg, was used as a positive control [43].

3.4.2. Statistical Analysis

Area under the curve (AUC) was calculated from 6 min to 45 min and analyzed using one-way analysis of variance (ANOVA) followed by Dunnett's multiple comparison test. Data are expressed as mean ± standard error of the mean (S.E.M.), and $p < 0.05$ was accepted as statistically significant. GraphPad Prism, version 7, was used for data analysis.

3.5. Warm-Water Squirrel Tail-Withdrawal and Operant Responding

Male squirrel monkeys (Saimiri sciureus) were housed in a climate-controlled vivarium with a 12-h light/dark cycle (7 AM–7 PM) in the McLean Hospital Animal Care Facility (licensed by the U.S. Department of Agriculture and compliant with guidelines provided by the Committee on Care and Use of Laboratory Animals of the Institute of Laboratory Animals Resources, Commission on Life Sciences, National Research Council; 2011). Tail withdrawal latencies and food-maintained behavior were assessed as described previously [44]. Briefly, monkeys were seated in customized Plexiglas chairs that allowed their tails to hang freely behind the chair and were equipped with colored stimulus lights, a response lever, and a receptacle into which 0.15 mL of 30% sweetened condensed milk could be delivered. Animals were trained to respond under a fixed-ratio 10-response (FR10) schedule of food reinforcement in the presence of red stimulus lights. Completion of 10 responses in less than 20 s resulted in milk delivery, and initiated a timeout (TO) period of 30 s during which all stimulus lights remained off. Failure to complete 10 responses within 20 s initiated the 30 s TO. Tail withdrawal latencies were measured during the 30 s TO periods by immersing the subject's tail in water held at 35 °C, 50 °C, 52 °C, or 55 °C (each temperature of water was presented in a randomized order). Experimental sessions were 4 or 5 sequential cycles, each composed of a 10 min TO during which no lights were on and responding had no programmed consequences followed by a 5 min response component during which the FR10 schedule of food reinforcement and interspersed determinations of tail withdrawal latencies was in effect. Cumulative doses of **2i** or morphine were administered shortly after the onset of the 10 min TO.

3.6. Squirrel Monkey Ventilation

Male squirrel monkeys were acclimated to a customized round acrylic chamber (13.75″ day × 15″ h) that served as a whole-body plethysmograph (EMKA Technologies, Montreal, PQ, Canada). Gas (either air or a 5% CO_2 in air mixture) was introduced to and extracted from the chamber at a constant flow rate of 5 L/min. Experimental sessions consisted of 4–6 consecutive 30 min cycles, each comprising a 15 min exposure to air followed by a 15 min exposure to 5% CO_2. Drug effects were determined using cumulative dosing procedures, and injections were administered following each exposure to 5% CO_2. Respiratory rate and tidal volume (mL/breath) were recorded over 1 min periods and were multiplied to provide minute volumes. Data from the last three minutes of each exposure to air or CO2 were averaged and used for analysis of drug effects on ventilation.

4. Computational Methods

All the ligands considered in this study and their conformers (see Table S1 and Figure S2A in SI) in their protonated form were geometry optimized via quantum chemical (QM) calculations at the B3LYP/6-31G* level in the gaseous phase as implemented in Gaussian 09 software [45]. The atomic polar tensor derived charges from these calculations were used to assign a partial charge on each atom for the ligands. All other parameters were determined by chemical analogy with the topology and the parameters files of the all-atom CHARMM force field (version c42b2) [46]. The structures of the inactive forms of MOR (PDB # 4DKL) and DOR (4EJ4) were taken as the starting configurations. After removing the cocrystallized ligands and crystal water/ions, the intracellular loop (ICL3) connecting TM5 and TM6 was first modeled in each receptor using MM (ab initio) methods [8,47,48]. The modeled receptors were then embedded in a membrane composed of zwitterionic 1-palmitoyl-2-oleoyl-phosphatidylcholine lipid molecules with initial concentrations of Na^+, K^+, and Cl^- ions in the extracellular (EC) and intracellular (IC) regions. All the amino acids were assumed to be neutral at physiological pH except Asp^-, Glu^-, Lys^+ and Arg^+; additional ions were used to neutralize the systems. The initial orientation and relative position of the receptor with respect to the membrane were obtained from the OPM database [49]. The receptor and the membrane were then solvated in TIP3P water, and a single Na^+ ion was introduced in the binding pocket and coordinated as in the DOR (4N6H) [50]. The system was then energy minimized and thermally equilibrated according to the following protocol: first, the conformation of the receptor and Na^+ were kept fixed, and the membrane and water were gradually heated to the target temperature (37 °C) at constant pressure (1 atm); the system was then equilibrated for 5 ns; the constraints on the side chains and ion were then removed, and the system equilibrated for another 5 ns; finally, all the constraints were removed, and the system equilibrated for another 5 ns. Throughout the entire equilibration process, the ion remained coordinated with the anchoring aspartic acid D147 (MOR) and D128 (DOR) (sequence numbering follows the corresponding crystal structures). A conformation (snapshot) of each system at the end of the final equilibration phase was used to dock the ligands. These are the basal conformations that all the ligands "see" before entering the binding pocket, and were used for all the comparative analyses, regardless of the experimentally determined activity or pharmacological outcome. After removing the Na^+ ion, the ligands (and their conformers) were rigidly docked into the binding pocket based on two criteria: the close contact between the charged amine and the anchoring Asp^- and the binding mode of the antagonists β-FNA and naltrindole co-crystallized with the MOR and the DOR, respectively. Several conformers (cf. Figure S2) could be eliminated by steric considerations alone. Others (especially those involving rotations of ϕ_1; cf. Figure S2) could still dock without apparent steric clashes upon small relaxations of the pocket side chains, but they tended to lose the critical interaction with Asp^- in the course of equilibration or early production; when this occurred in repeated simulations, the conformer was discarded. Overall, between one and four stable conformers were left for each ligand (see Table S2). The three-stage equilibration protocol described above for Na^+ was repeated for each ligand/conformer after docking. Steric relaxation of the ligand and residues in the pocket set in during the early stages of equilibration. Five independent 50 ns molecular dynamics simulations were conducted for each system at 37 °C and 1 atm, using periodic boundary conditions and particle mesh Ewald summations. This simulation time was sufficient to ensure convergence and statistical analysis of the quantities of interest (hydrophobic contacts, H-bonds, electrostatic interactions), which were computed after structural relaxation set in (estimated from Cα-RMSD vs. time), typically during the last half of the dynamic trajectory (production run). The results combine data from all the independent simulations for each ligand conformer/OR.

5. Conclusions

We hypothesized that substituents at the tail end of the body of a large molecule might modify the in vitro activity and/or potency of the compound and possibly modify a G-protein biased compound that acted primarily through MOR to a bifunctional ligand. We found that a substituent, a chlorine atom, modified the activity of N-phenethylnorhydromorphone (**S11**), a potent full agonist with a DOR-MOR δ/μ potency ratio of 38.5, to a compound with a δ/μ potency ratio of 1.2, N-p-chloro phenethylnorhydromorphone (**2i**). It exhibited potent partial MOR agonist and potent full DOR agonist activity. In fact, the introduction of a p-Cl substituent (**2i**) in the N-phenethyl moiety did not particularly reduce the MOR potency of **S11** but instead increased its DOR potency; it induced a change from a molecule that acted primarily as a MOR ligand to a bifunctional compound with the ability to interact potently with MOR and DOR. This change was due to a simple substituent at the tail end of the compound. Molecular modeling and simulations found that the substituent on the aromatic ring of the N-phenethyl moiety is located in an area where relatively small changes in the N-phenylethyl ring via substitution perturb residues located in quite different regions of the opioid receptors and engage different TMHs. In theory, the combination of MOR and DOR properties found in **2i** might have made the compound less likely than other potent analgesics to cause respiratory depression [17]. Indeed, that was found to be the case in mice using normal air, where a clear difference was found between the effects of **2i** and morphine on respiration. Both **2i** and morphine are partial agonists; if the lack of effect on respiration was due to the partial agonist character of **2i**, the same effect would be expected with morphine. The ability of **2i** to recruit β-arrestin2 at least as well as morphine (Table 2) would predict that it should exhibit all of the side-effects known to occur with morphine. The inability of **2i** to depress respiration in mice might indicate that the recruitment of β-arrestin2 may not be the cause of all of the side-effects seen with opioids [4]. However, with squirrel monkeys under more stringent conditions, in an assay using 5% CO_2 mixed in air, **2i** was found to be as effective as morphine in depressing respiration. Further work is necessary to determine whether **2i** will produce the gastrointestinal effects, tolerance, and dependence that occur with other G-protein biased opioids.

6. Patents

K. C. Rice, A. E. Jacobson, F. Li, E. Gutman, E. W. Bow: Biased Potent Opioid-Like Agonists as Improved Medications to Treat Chronic and Acute Pain and Methods of Using the Same. International Application PCT/US19/22701, 18 March 2019 (PCT Application Serial No.: PCT/US2019/022701, filed 18 March 2019). Patent No. WO 2019182950.

Supplementary Materials: ^{1}H and ^{13}C-NMR spectra of novel compounds, molecular modeling, and dynamics simulations, and Scheme S1, the Synthesis of hydromorphone (**S5**). N-norhydromorphone (**S10**) and N-phenethy lnorhydromorphone (**S11**).

Author Contributions: Conceptualization, A.E.J.; Data curation, C.A.H., R.D.H., S.A.H., Y.-S.L., S.K., R.S.C., E.B.G., T.A.K., J.L.K., A.M.C. and J.R.T.; Formal analysis, S.A.H., Y.-S.L., S.K., R.S.C., T.E.P., S.L.W., C.A.P., J.B., S.I., E.B.G., M.W.A., T.A.K. and J.L.K.; Funding acquisition, C.A.P., J.B., M.W.A. and J.R.T.; Investigation, T.C.I., C.A.H., R.D.H., S.A.H., Y.-S.L., S.K., R.S.C., T.E.P., S.L.W., S.I., T.A.K. and A.M.C.; Methodology, M.W., S.A.H., Y.-S.L., S.K., R.S.C., T.E.P., S.L.W., C.A.P., J.B., J.R.T., A.E.J. and K.C.R.; Project administration, K.C.R.; Resources, K.C.R.; Supervision, T.E.P., C.A.P., J.B., M.W.A., J.L.K., J.R.T., A.E.J. and K.C.R.; Validation, T.C.I.; Writing—original draft, A.E.J.; Writing—review & editing, S.A.H., Y.-S.L., S.K., T.E.P., C.A.P., J.B., S.I., E.B.G., M.W.A., J.L.K., J.R.T. and K.C.R. All authors have read and agreed to the published version of the manuscript.

Funding: The work of SI: EBG, ad MWA was supported by NIDA grant P30 DA13429. The work of JRT was supported by NIDA grant DA039997. The work of SK, RSC and TEP was supported by NIDA grant DA018151. The work of SLW, CAP, and JB was supported by NIDA grants DA035857 and DA047574.The work of MW, TCI, CAH, AEJ and KCR was supported by the NIH Intramural Research Programs of the National Institute on Drug Abuse and the National Institute of Alcohol Abuse and Alcoholism. The work of TAK and JLK was supported by the NIH Intramural Research Programs of the National Institute on Drug Abuse. The work of SAH and YSL was supported by the NIH Intramural Research Program through the Center for Information Technology. The computational studies utilized PC/LINUX clusters at the Center for Molecular Modeling of the NIH (http://cmm.cit.nih.gov) and *the computational resources of the NIH HPC Biowulf cluster* (http://hpc.nih.gov). The work of TAK and JLK was supported by the NIH Intramural Research Programs of the National Institute on Drug Abuse. We thank the NIDA Drug Supply for providing compounds used in the forskolin-induced cAMP assays. We also thank John Lloyd and Noel Whittaker (Mass Spectrometry Facility, NIDDK) for the mass spectral data, and S. Steven Negus (Dept. of Pharmacology and Toxicology. Virginia Commonwealth University, Richmond VA) for helpful discussions about the possible pharmacological effects of compounds with MOR and DOR agonist activity.

Conflicts of Interest: The authors declare no conflict of interest.

References

1. Bohn, L.M.; Aubé, J. Seeking (and Finding) Biased Ligands of the Kappa Opioid Receptor. *ACS Med. Chem. Lett.* **2017**, *8*, 694–700. [CrossRef] [PubMed]
2. Bond, R.A.; Lucero Garcia-Rojas, E.Y.; Hegde, A.; Walker, J.K.L. Therapeutic Potential of Targeting ß-Arrestin. *Front. Pharmacol.* **2019**, *10*, 124. [CrossRef] [PubMed]
3. Whalen, E.J.; Rajagopal, S.; Lefkowitz, R.J. Therapeutic potential of β-arrestin- and G protein-biased agonists. *Trends Mol. Med.* **2011**, *17*, 126–139. [CrossRef] [PubMed]
4. Kliewer, A.; Gillis, A.; Hill, R.; Schmidel, F.; Bailey, C.; Kelly, E.; Henderson, G.; Christie, M.J.; Schulz, S. Morphine-induced respiratory depression is independent of β-arrestin2 signalling. *Br. J. Pharmacol.* **2020**. [CrossRef]
5. Ben Haddou, T.; Béni, S.; Hosztafi, S.; Malfacini, D.; Calo, G.; Schmidhammer, H.; Spetea, M. Pharmacological investigations of N-substituent variation in morphine and oxymorphone: Opioid receptor binding, signaling and antinociceptive activity. *PLoS ONE* **2014**, *9*, e99231. [CrossRef]
6. May, E.L.; Eddy, N.B. Structures Related to Morphine. XII.1 (±) 2′ Hydroxy-5,9-dimethyl-2-phenethyl-6,7-benzomorphan (NIH 7519) and Its Optical Forms. *J. Org. Chem.* **1959**, *24*, 1435–1437. [CrossRef]
7. Hashimoto, A.; Jacobson, A.E.; Rothman, R.B.; Dersch, C.M.; George, C.; Flippen-Anderson, J.L.; Rice, K.C. Probes for narcotic receptor mediated phenomena. Part 28: New opioid antagonists from enantiomeric analogues of 5-(3-hydroxyphenyl)-N-phenylethylmorphan. *Bioorg. Med. Chem.* **2002**, *10*, 3319–3329. [CrossRef]
8. Truong, P.M.; Hassan, S.A.; Lee, Y.-S.; Kopajtic, T.A.; Katz, J.L.; Chadderdon, A.M.; Traynor, J.R.; Deschamps, J.R.; Jacobson, A.E.; Rice, K.C. Modulation of opioid receptor affinity and efficacy via N-substitution of 9β-hydroxy-5-(3-hydroxyphenyl)morphan: Synthesis and computer simulation study. *Bioorg. Med. Chem.* **2017**, *25*, 2406–2422. [CrossRef]
9. Lo, K. Synthesis of *N*-phenethylnorhydromorphone: A Hydromorphone Analogue. Ph.D. Thesis, University of British Columbia, Vancouver, BC, Canada, 2001. Available online: http://hdl.handle.net/2429/11862 (accessed on 26 March 2020).
10. Portoghese, P.S.; Sultana, M.; Nagase, H.; Takemori, A.E. Application of the message-address concept in the design of highly potent and selective non-peptide delta opioid receptor antagonists. *J. Med. Chem.* **1988**, *31*, 281–282. [CrossRef]
11. Bender, A.M.; Clark, M.J.; Agius, M.P.; Traynor, J.R.; Mosberg, H.I. Synthesis and evaluation of 4-substituted piperidines and piperazines as balanced affinity μ opioid receptor (MOR) agonist/δ opioid receptor (DOR) antagonist ligands. *Bioorg. Med. Chem. Lett.* **2014**, *24*, 548–551. [CrossRef]
12. Wade, P.R.; Palmer, J.M.; McKenney, S.; Kenigs, V.; Chevalier, K.; Moore, B.A.; Mabus, J.R.; Saunders, P.R.; Wallace, N.H.; Schneider, C.R.; et al. Modulation of gastrointestinal function by MuDelta, a mixed μ opioid receptor agonist/ μ opioid receptor antagonist. *Br. J. Pharmacol.* **2012**, *167*, 1111–1125. [CrossRef] [PubMed]
13. Olson, K.M.; Keresztes, A.; Tashiro, J.K.; Daconta, L.V.; Hruby, V.J.; Streicher, J.M. Synthesis and Evaluation of a Novel Bivalent Selective Antagonist for the Mu-Delta Opioid Receptor Heterodimer that Reduces Morphine Withdrawal in Mice. *J. Med. Chem.* **2018**, *61*, 6075–6086. [CrossRef] [PubMed]
14. Qi, J.; Mosberg, H.I.; Porreca, F. Modulation of the Potency and Efficacy of Mu-Mediated Antinociception by Delta-Agonists in the Mouse. *J. Pharmacol. Exp. Ther.* **1990**, *254*, 683–689. [PubMed]
15. Ananthan, S. Opioid Ligands with mixed mu/delta opioid receptor interactions: An emerging approach to novel analgesics. *AAPS J.* **2006**, *8*, E118–E125. [CrossRef] [PubMed]

16. Lowery, J.J.; Raymond, T.J.; Giuvelis, D.; Bidlack, J.M.; Polt, R.; Bilsky, E.J. In vivo characterization of MMP-2200, a mixed δ/μ opioid agonist, in mice. *J. Pharmacol. Exp. Ther.* **2011**, *336*, 767–778. [CrossRef]
17. Su, Y.-F.; McNutt, R.W.; Chang, K.-J. Delta-Opioid Ligands Reverse Alfentanil-Induced Respiratory Depression but Not Antinociception. *J. Pharmacol. Exp. Ther.* **1998**, *287*, 815–823.
18. Montandon, G.; Slutsky, A.S. Solving the Opioid Crisis: Respiratory Depression by Opioids as Critical End Point. *CHEST* **2019**, *156*, 653–658. [CrossRef]
19. Bertha, C.M.; Flippen-Anderson, J.L.; Rothman, R.B.; Porreca, F.; Davis, P.; Xu, H.; Becketts, K.; Cha, X.-Y.; Rice, K.C. Probes for Narcotic Receptor-Mediated Phenomena. 20. Alteration of Opioid Receptor Subtype Selectivity of the 5-(3-Hydroxyphenyl)morphans by Application of the Message-Address Concept: Preparation of delta.-Opioid Receptor Ligands. *J. Med. Chem.* **1995**, *38*, 1523–1537. [CrossRef]
20. Bertha, C.M.; Ellis, M.; Flippen-Anderson, J.L.; Porreca, F.; Rothman, R.B.; Davis, P.; Xu, H.; Becketts, K.; Rice, K.C. Probes for Narcotic Receptor-Mediated Phenomena. 21. Novel Derivatives of 3-(1,2,3,4,5,11-Hexahydro-3-methyl-2,6-methano-6H-azocino[4¨CC5-b]indol-6-yl)-phenols with Improved Œ¥ Opioid Receptor Selectivity. *J. Med. Chem.* **1996**, *39*, 2081–2086. [CrossRef]
21. Breslin, H.J.; Miskowski, T.A.; Rafferty, B.M.; Coutinho, S.V.; Palmer, J.M.; Wallace, N.H.; Schneider, C.R.; Kimball, E.S.; Zhang, S.P.; Li, J.; et al. Rationale, design, and synthesis of novel phenyl imidazoles as opioid receptor agonists for gastrointestinal disorders. *J. Med. Chem.* **2004**, *47*, 5009–5020. [CrossRef]
22. Zhang, Q.; Keenan, S.M.; Peng, Y.Y.; Nair, A.C.; Yu, S.J.; Howells, R.D.; Welsh, W.J. Discovery of novel triazole-based opioid receptor antagonists. *J. Med. Chem.* **2006**, *49*, 4044–4047. [CrossRef] [PubMed]
23. Ananthan, S.; Saini, S.; Dersch, C.; Xu, H.; McGlinchey, N.; Giuvelis, D.; Bilsky, E.J.; Rothman, R.B. 14-Alkoxy- and 14-acyloxypyridomorphinans: Mu agonist/delta antagonist opioid analgesics with diminished tolerance and dependence side effects. *J. Med. Chem.* **2012**, *55*, 8350–8363. [CrossRef] [PubMed]
24. Breslin, H.; Diamond, C.; Kavash, R.; Cai, C.; Dyatkin, A. Identification of a dual delta OR antagonist/mu OR agonist as a potential therapeutic for diarrhea-predominant Irritable Bowel Syndrome (IBS-d). *Bioorg. Med. Chem. Lett.* **2012**, *22*, 4869–4872. [CrossRef] [PubMed]
25. Healy, J.R.; Bezawada, P.; Shim, J.; Jones, J.W.; Kane, M.A.; MacKerell, A.D.; Coop, A.; Matsumoto, R.R. Synthesis, Modeling, and Pharmacological Evaluation of UMB 425, a Mixed μ Agonist/δ Antagonist Opioid Analgesic with Reduced Tolerance Liabilities. *ACS Chem. Neurosci.* **2013**, *4*, 1256–1266. [CrossRef]
26. Yadlapalli, J.S.K.; Ford, B.M.; Ketkar, A.; Wan, A.; Penthala, N.R.; Eoff, R.L.; Prather, P.L.; Dobretsov, M.; Crooks, P.A. Antinociceptive effects of the 6-O-sulfate ester of morphine in normal and diabetic rats: Comparative role of mu- and delta-opioid receptors. *Pharmacol. Res.* **2016**, *113 Pt A*, 335–347. [CrossRef]
27. Stevenson, G.W.; Luginbuhl, A.; Dunbar, C.; LaVigne, J.; Dutra, J.; Atherton, P.; Bell, B.; Cone, K.; Giuvelis, D.; Polt, R.; et al. The mixed-action delta/mu opioid agonist MMP-2200 does not produce conditioned place preference but does maintain drug self-administration in rats, and induces in vitro markers of tolerance and dependence. *Pharmacol. Biochem. Behav.* **2015**, *132*, 49–55. [CrossRef]
28. Przybyl, A.K.; Flippen-Anderson, J.L.; Jacobson, A.E.; Rice, K.C. Practical and High-Yield Syntheses of Dihydromorphine from Tetrahydrothebaine and Efficient Syntheses of (8S)-8-Bromomorphide. *J. Org. Chem.* **2003**, *68*, 2010–2013. [CrossRef]
29. Csuk, R.; Vasileva, G.; Barthel, A. Towards an Efficient Preparation of Hydromorphone. *Synthesis* **2012**, *44*, 2840–2842. [CrossRef]
30. Iijima, I.; Minamikawa, J.; Jacobson, A.E.; Brossi, A.; Rice, K.C. Studies in the (+)-morphinan series. 5. Synthesis and biological properties of (+)-naloxone. *J. Med. Chem.* **1978**, *21*, 398–400. [CrossRef]
31. Purington, L.C.; Sobczyk-Kojiro, K.; Pogozheva, I.D.; Traynor, J.R.; Mosberg, H.I. Development and in vitro characterization of a novel bifunctional μ-agonist/δ-antagonist opioid tetrapeptide. *ACS Chem. Biol.* **2011**, *6*, 1375–1381. [CrossRef]
32. Beck, T.C.; Hapstack, M.A.; Beck, K.R.; Dix, T.A. Therapeutic Potential of Kappa Opioid Agonists. *Pharmaceuticals* **2019**, *12*, 95. [CrossRef] [PubMed]
33. Dumitrascuta, M.; Bermudez, M.; Ben Haddou, T.; Guerrieri, E.; Schläfer, L.; Ritsch, A.; Hosztafi, S.; Lantero, A.; Kreutz, C.; Massotte, D.; et al. N-Phenethyl Substitution in 14-Methoxy-N-methylmorphinan-6-ones Turns Selective μ Opioid Receptor Ligands into Dual μ/δ Opioid Receptor Agonists. *Sci. Rep.* **2020**, *10*, 5653. [CrossRef] [PubMed]
34. Metrangolo, P.; Murray, J.S.; Pilati, T.; Politzer, P.; Resnati, G.; Terraneo, G. Fluorine-Centered Halogen Bonding: A Factor in Recognition Phenomena and Reactivity. *Cryst. Growth Des.* **2011**, *11*, 4238–4246. [CrossRef]

35. Kolář, M.H.; Hobza, P. Computer Modeling of Halogen Bonds and Other σ-Hole Interactions. *Chem. Rev.* **2016**, *116*, 5155–5187. [CrossRef]
36. Matter, H.; Nazaré, M.; Güssregen, S.; Will, D.W.; Schreuder, H.; Bauer, A.; Urmann, M.; Ritter, K.; Wagner, M.; Wehner, V. Evidence for C-Cl/C-Br⋯π Interactions as an Important Contribution to Protein–Ligand Binding Affinity. *Angew. Chem. Int. Ed. Engl.* **2009**, *48*, 2911–2916. [CrossRef]
37. Chan, H.C.S.; Wang, J.; Palczewski, K.; Filipek, S.; Vogel, H.; Liu, Z.-J.; Yuan, S. Exploring a new ligand binding site of G protein-coupled receptors. *Chem. Sci.* **2018**, *9*, 6480–6489. [CrossRef]
38. Lee, K.O.; Akil, H.; Woods, J.H.; Traynor, J.R. Differential binding properties of oripavines at cloned mu- and delta-opioid receptors. *Eur. J. Pharmacol.* **1999**, *378*, 323–330. [CrossRef]
39. Husbands, S.M.; Neilan, C.L.; Broadbear, J.; Grundt, P.; Breeden, S.; Aceto, M.D.; Woods, J.H.; Lewis, J.W.; Traynor, J.R. BU74, a complex oripavine derivative with potent kappa opioid receptor agonism and delayed opioid antagonism. *Eur. J. Pharmacol.* **2005**, *509*, 117–125. [CrossRef]
40. Traynor, J.R.; Nahorski, S.R. Modulation of mu-opioid agonists of guanisine-5'-O-(3-[^{35}S]thio)triphosphate binding to membranes from human neurobastoma SH-SY5Y cells. *J. Mol. Pharmacol.* **1995**, *47*, 848–854.
41. Crowley, R.S.; Riley, A.P.; Sherwood, A.M.; Groer, C.E.; Shivaperumal, N.; Biscaia, M.; Paton, K.; Schneider, S.; Provasi, D.; Kivell, B.M.; et al. Synthetic Studies of Neoclerodane Diterpenes from Salvia divinorum: Identification of a Potent and Centrally Acting μ Opioid Analgesic with Reduced Abuse Liability. *J. Med. Chem.* **2016**, *59*, 11027–11038. [CrossRef]
42. Riley, A.P.; Groer, C.E.; Young, D.; Ewald, A.W.; Kivell, B.M.; Prisinzano, T.E. Synthesis and κ-opioid receptor activity of furan-substituted salvinorin A analogues. *J. Med. Chem.* **2014**, *57*, 10464–10475. [CrossRef] [PubMed]
43. Hill, R.; Disney, A.; Conibear, A.; Sutcliffe, K.; Dewey, W.; Husbands, S.; Bailey, C.; Kelly, E.; Henderson, G. The novel μ-opioid receptor agonist PZM21 depresses respiration and induces tolerance to antinociception. *Br. J. Pharmacol.* **2018**, *175*, 2653–2661. [CrossRef] [PubMed]
44. Withey, S.L.; Paronis, C.A.; Bergman, J. Concurrent Assessment of the Antinociceptive and Behaviorally Disruptive Effects of Opioids in Squirrel Monkeys. *J. Pain* **2018**, *19*, 728–740. [CrossRef]
45. Frisch, M.J.; Trucks, G.W.; Schlegel, H.B.; Scuseria, G.E.; Robb, M.A.; Cheeseman, J.R.; Scalmani, G.; Barone, V.; Mennucci, B.; Petersson, G.A.; et al. *Gaussian 09, Revision A.02*; Gaussian Inc.: Wallingford, CT, USA, 2009.
46. Brooks, B.R.; Brooks, C.L., 3rd; Mackerell, A.D., Jr.; Nilsson, L.; Petrella, R.J.; Roux, B.; Won, Y.; Archontis, G.; Bartels, C.; Boresch, S.; et al. CHARMM: The Biomolecular Simulation Program. *J. Comput. Chem.* **2009**, *30*, 1545–1614. [CrossRef]
47. Mehler, E.L.; Hassan, S.A.; Kortagere, S.; Weinstein, H. Ab initio computational modeling of loops in G-protein-coupled receptors: Lessons from the crystal structure of rhodopsin. *Proteins* **2006**, *64*, 673–690. [CrossRef] [PubMed]
48. Mehler, E.L.; Periole, X.; Hassan, S.A.; Weinstein, H. Key issues in the computational simulation of GPCR function: Representation of loop domains. *J. Comput. Aided Mol. Des.* **2002**, *16*, 841–853. [CrossRef]
49. Lomize, M.A.; Lomize, A.L.; Pogozheva, I.D.; Mosberg, H.I. OPM: Orientations of proteins in membranes database. *Bioinformatics* **2006**, *22*, 623–625. [CrossRef]
50. Fenalti, G.; Giguere, P.M.; Katritch, V.; Huang, X.P.; Thompson, A.A.; Cherezov, V.; Roth, B.L.; Stevens, R.C. Molecular control of δ-opioid receptor signalling. *Nature* **2014**, *506*, 191–196. [CrossRef]

Sample Availability: Not available.

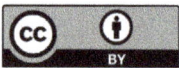

© 2020 by the authors. Licensee MDPI, Basel, Switzerland. This article is an open access article distributed under the terms and conditions of the Creative Commons Attribution (CC BY) license (http://creativecommons.org/licenses/by/4.0/).

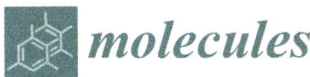

Communication

Structure-Activity Relationship between Thiol Group-Trapping Ability of Morphinan Compounds with a Michael Acceptor and Anti-*Plasmodium falciparum* Activities

Noriki Kutsumura [1,2], Yasuaki Koyama [2], Tsuyoshi Saitoh [1], Naoshi Yamamoto [1], Yasuyuki Nagumo [1], Yoshiyuki Miyata [3], Rei Hokari [4], Aki Ishiyama [4], Masato Iwatsuki [4], Kazuhiko Otoguro [4], Satoshi Ōmura [4] and Hiroshi Nagase [1,2,*]

1. International Institute for Integrative Sleep Medicine (WPI-IIIS), University of Tsukuba, 1-1-1 Tennodai, Tsukuba, Ibaraki 305-8575, Japan; kutsumura.noriki.gn@u.tsukuba.ac.jp (N.K.); tsuyoshi-saito.gf@u.tsukuba.ac.jp (T.S.); yamamoto.naoshi.gu@u.tsukuba.ac.jp (N.Y.); nagumo.yasuyuki.fu@u.tsukuba.ac.jp (Y.N.)
2. Graduate School of Pure and Applied Sciences, University of Tsukuba, 1-1-1 Tennodai, Tsukuba, Ibaraki 305-8571, Japan; kykoyamayasuaki@gmail.com
3. School of Medicine, Keio University, 35, Shinanomachi, Shinjuku, Tokyo 160-8582, Japan; yomiyat@keio.jp
4. Kitasato Institute for Life Sciences, Kitasato University, 5-9-1 Shirokane, Minato-ku, Tokyo 108-8641, Japan; hokari@lisci.kitasato-u.ac.jp (R.H.); ishiyama@lisci.kitasato-u.ac.jp (A.I.); iwatuki@lisci.kitasato-u.ac.jp (M.I.); tsuchikurekai@gmail.com (K.O.); omuras@insti.kitasato-u.ac.jp (S.Ō.)
* Correspondence: nagase.hiroshi.gt@u.tsukuba.ac.jp; Tel.: +81-29-853-6437

Academic Editors: Mariana Spetea and Helmut Schmidhammer
Received: 24 January 2020; Accepted: 28 February 2020; Published: 2 March 2020

Abstract: 7-Benzylidenenaltrexone (BNTX) and most of its derivatives showed in vitro antimalarial activities against chloroquine-resistant and -sensitive *Plasmodium falciparum* strains (K1 and FCR3, respectively). In addition, the time-dependent changes of the addition reactions of the BNTX derivatives with 1-propanethiol were examined by ^{1}H-NMR experiments to estimate their thiol group-trapping ability. The relative chemical reactivity of the BNTX derivatives to trap the thiol group of 1-propanethiol was correlated highly with the antimalarial activity. Therefore, the measurements of the thiol group-trapping ability of the BNTX derivatives with a Michael acceptor is expected to become an alternative method for in vitro malarial activity and related assays.

Keywords: morphinan; BNTX; δ opioid receptor antagonist; ^{1}H-NMR experiments; mechanism elucidation

---

1. Introduction

Malaria is one of the world's deadliest infectious diseases and it is widespread in the tropical and subtropical regions located in a broad band around the equator, including Africa, Southeast Asia, Middle East, and Latin America. In 2017, an estimated 219 million malaria infections were reported in 87 countries, including about 435,000 deaths from malaria [1]. Malaria also causes serious complications, such as cerebral malaria involving encephalopathy [2], blackwater fever [3], and acute respiratory distress syndrome (ARDS) [4]. Since 2001, the World Health Organization (WHO) has recommended Artemisinin-based combination therapy (ACT) for antimalarial medication. However, not only general drug-resistant type of malaria, such as chloroquine-resistance (CQ-resistance), but also artemisinin-resistant malaria has been identified, creating a critical social situation [5,6].

Against such a background, we first reported that a δ opioid receptor (DOR) antagonist 7-benzylidenenaltrexone (BNTX, **1**, Figure 1) had a potent CQ-resistance reversing effect on *Plasmodium* *chabaudi*, that is, the combined administration of **1** (perorally) and CQ (intravenously) decreased the number of parasitized red blood cells in mice infected with CQ-resistant malaria [7]. These research results revealed that DOR antagonism was particularly important for the CQ-resistance reversing effect. Further studies suggested that the CQ-resistance reversing effect of **1** was closely related to not only the DOR antagonism but also to the presence of a Michael acceptor moiety in morphinan compound **1**. Although a correlation between the DOR antagonism and its CQ-resistance reversing effect on malaria parasites has not yet been clearly elucidated, the Michael acceptor structure could be involved in the effect by reacting with the thiol group of the glutathione-system to increase oxidative stress in the host [8]. In addition, Asahi and co-workers also reported that the morphinan **1** effectively inhibited the successive ring–trophozoite–schizont progression of *P. falciparum* during early developmental stages, which are associated with the development of pyknosis in ring forms, as compared to another antimalarial drug dihydroartemisinin [9]. In another study of **1** in protozoal infections, **1** and its derivatives exhibited in vitro antitrichomonal activity against *Trichomonas vaginalis* and the activity was also related to the presence of a Michael acceptor moiety in the morphinan derivatives [10,11]. Thus, "thiol group-trapping action by Michael acceptors such as an α,β-unsaturated ketone moiety" in morphinan compounds could be considered as a common factor for both the CQ-resistance reversing effect in malaria and the antitrichomonal effects. Therefore, we hypothesized that chemical enhancement of the ability to trap thiol groups (for example: glutathione et al. in malaria [12–14]; cysteine et al. in trichomonads [15–19]) would affect the inhibition of each antioxidant system, leading to the direct improvement of antiprotozoal activity (Figure 1). Morphinan compounds such as **1** have been recognized as structurally typical drug-like compounds, such as some compounds (morphine, codeine, and nalfurafine [20], etc.) have been used in clinical practice. In fact, we have already confirmed in vivo experiments that the morphinan compound **1** is effective against CQ-resistant malaria [7,8]. However, there have been no applications of morphinan compounds to protozoal infections, and this study is quite significant in the search for new lead compounds for protozoal infections. In this paper, we investigated the correlation between the thiol group-trapping ability of **1** and its derivatives and in vitro antimalarial activity.

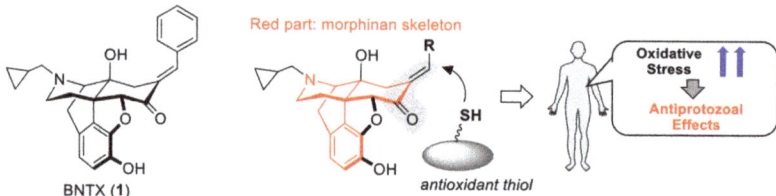

Figure 1. Structure of BNTX (**1**) and a plausible explication of antiprotozoal effects by the morphinan compounds.

2. Results and Discussion

First, BNTX (**1**) and the related derivatives **2–20** (see Table 1), which were prepared by the previously reported synthetic methods [10,11], were evaluated for in vitro antimalarial activities against CQ-resistant and -sensitive *Plasmodium falciparum* strains (K1 and FCR3, respectively) (Table 1) [21]. All compounds **1–20** exhibited moderate antimalarial activity against the CQ-resistant K1 strain (IC$_{50}$ = 2.08–19.8 μM), except for the dimethylamino-substituted derivative **17**. These compounds also exhibited similar activity against the CQ-sensitive FCR3 strain (IC$_{50}$ = 1.94–15.0 μM), with the exception of **17** and the reduced derivative **20**. Notably, the morphinan derivatives bearing an electron-withdrawing substituted benzylidene group such as the compounds **6**, **8**, **9**, and **11** tended to exhibit relatively high antimalarial activities. On the contrary, the electron-donating substituted derivatives **16** and **17** tended to exhibit weak activities. These results thus suggested that inductive effects caused by introducing substituents into the benzylidene site affected antimalarial activity to some extent. For the compounds with alkylidene groups (**14**, **15**, and **18**), the antimalarial activity increased as the ring size increased.

Of particular importance is the result that the antimalarial activity of the saturated derivative **20** lacking a Michael acceptor was significantly deactivated, as in our previous studies [8,11]. In the first in vitro antimalarial activity evaluation of a variety of BNTX derivatives, almost all derivatives were found to exhibit moderate antimalarial activity, although none of them were as potent as the clinical drugs artemisinin and chloroquine. Furthermore, the antimalarial activity correlated with electron density of the Michael acceptor, as we predicted.

Table 1. In vitro antimalarial activity of the morphinan derivatives **1–20**.

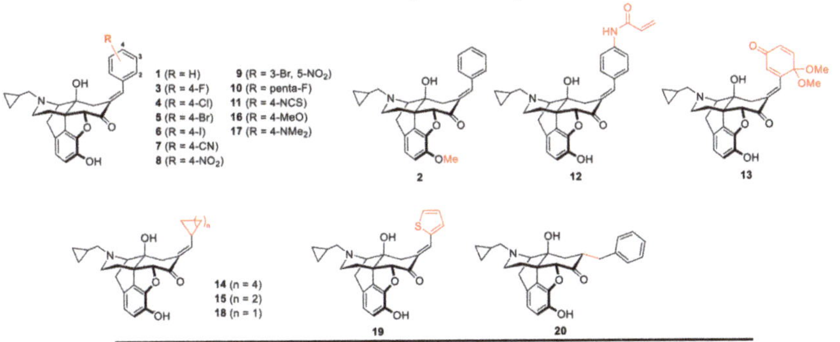

Compound	IC$_{50}$ (μM)		Compound	IC$_{50}$ (μM)	
	K1 [a]	FCR3 [b]		K1 [a]	FCR3 [b]
Artemisinin	0.03	0.04	10 [d]	7.33	6.38
Chloroquine	0.57	0.07	11 [c]	2.60	2.50
BNTX (1) [c]	4.08	3.26	12 [d]	0.93	1.66
2 [d]	4.31	3.94	13 [d]	7.89	9.43
3 [d]	3.60	2.86	14 [d]	2.08	1.95
4 [d]	2.82	2.67	15 [d]	7.37	7.16
5 [d]	3.07	2.76	16 [d]	7.58	6.61
6 [d]	2.78	2.24	17 [d]	>20.1	N/A
7 [d]	3.16	2.38	18 [d]	18.3	15.0
8 [d]	3.04	2.24	19 [d]	15.6	10.3
9 [d]	2.99	2.13	20 [d]	19.8	>21.5

[a] chloroquine-resistant *P. falciparum* strain. [b] chloroquine-sensitive *P. falciparum* strain. [c] hydrochloride. [d] tartrate.

Next, to easily evaluate the thiol group-trapping ability of BNTX (**1**) and the various derivatives **2–20**, we examined the time-dependent changes of the addition reactions of the compounds **1–20** with 1-propanethiol (as a simple model compound with a thiol group) by utilizing ^{1}H-NMR. A typical experimental example is as follows (Scheme 1). 1-Propanethiol was added to a solution of **1** in DMSO-d_6 (4 mM) at 37 ^{0}C, and the reaction system was kept at the same temperature. Then, the residual rate of **1** was calculated by measuring the integral value of the vinyl proton at constant time intervals. In addition, the time-dependent change of each reaction of **1** with the addition of increasing amounts of 1-propanethiol was performed (1, 3, 10, and 30 equiv.) as shown in Figure 2.

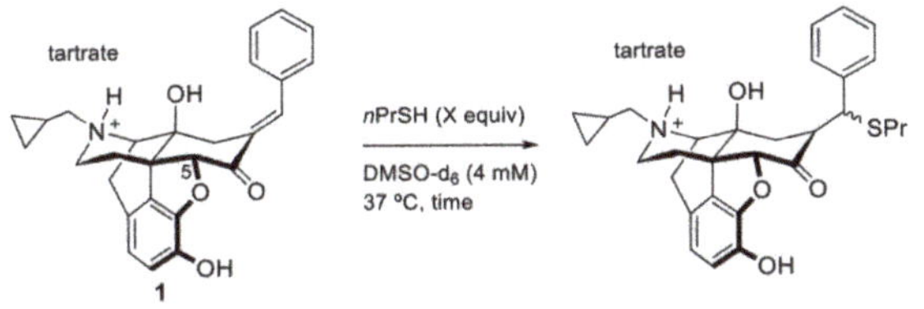

Scheme 1. Reactions of **1** with 1-propanethiol.

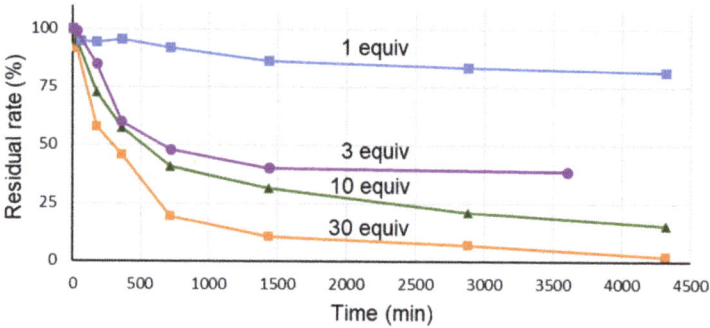

Figure 2. Temporal change of the addition reaction and the residual rate of **1**.

The correlation chart between the elapsed time of the reaction and the residual rate of **1** showed that the addition reaction of 1-propanethiol achieved equilibrium and the residual rate of substrate **1** converged to a steady-state. General glutathione levels in healthy human erythrocytes cover a wide range (0.4 to 3.0 mM [22] or 0.1 to 10 mM [23]). Therefore, we decided to evaluate the thiol group-trapping ability of **1–20** with 3 equivalents of 1-propanethiol (12 mM), because the addition reaction proceeded very slowly when the concentration of 1-propanethiol was 4.0 mM (1.0 equivalent) as shown in Figure 2. Table 2 shows the residual rate (%) of the starting materials **1–20** after 1 day or 2 days (also see the Supplementary Materials). The residual rate of starting morphinan derivatives was calculated by measuring the integral value of the proton at the C5-posidion because of ease of comparison of integral values before and after addition reaction.

Table 2. The residual rate of the derivatives **1–20** after 1 or 2 days.

Compound	Residual Rate (%)		Compound	Residual Rate (%)	
	1 day	2 days		1 day	2 days
1[c]	40.2	38.7 [b]	**11**[a]	35.1	14.0
2[c]	36.0	34.1 [b]	**12**[c]	54.9	53.2
3[c]	70.0	56.0	**13**[c]	45.8	38.6
4[c]	46.4	36.3	**14**[c]	25.3	16.2
5[c]	41.8	31.2	**15**[c]	6.8	6.0
6[c]	51.3	40.1	**16**[c]	79.0	66.8
7[c]	24.6	17.7	**17**[c]	90.0	88.3
8[c]	15.6	10.3	**18**[c]	82.6	80.2
9[c]	6.7	6.3	**19**[c]	90.9	83.8
10[c]	36.6	24.8	**20**[c]	97.9	89.8

[a] hydrochloride. [b] 2.5 days later. [c] tartrate.

Furthermore, we created a correlation diagram in which the antimalarial activities (IC$_{50}$ values) of the BNTX derivatives shown in Table 1 were on the vertical axis, and the residual rate (%) of the individual derivatives shown in Table 2 was on the horizontal axis, with the exception of compounds **17** and **20** (Figure 3). The data showed a clear tendency for the morphinan derivatives with higher thiol group-trapping ability to have higher antimalarial activity (shown enclosed in the red circle in Figure 3). In contrast, the correlation diagram also showed that a lower ability to capture thiol groups was associated with a lower antimalarial activity of the derivatives. These experimental results partly support the recent research reports on thiol group-trapping effects by other laboratories [24–29]. Thus, as we initially described our hypothesis, the antiprotozoal activity (antimalarial or antitrichomonal activity) of the BNTX (**1**) and its derivatives with a Michael acceptor may be expressed by inhibiting the respective antioxidant system of infectious protozoa. In the near future, we aim to further elucidate the mechanism of antimalarial activity of the morphinan compounds by applying these results to in vivo assays, which we have performed in previous studies. When evaluating antimalarial activity of the morphinan derivatives, the examination of the thiol group-trapping ability through an organic chemistry approach might become a reliable primary screening tool.

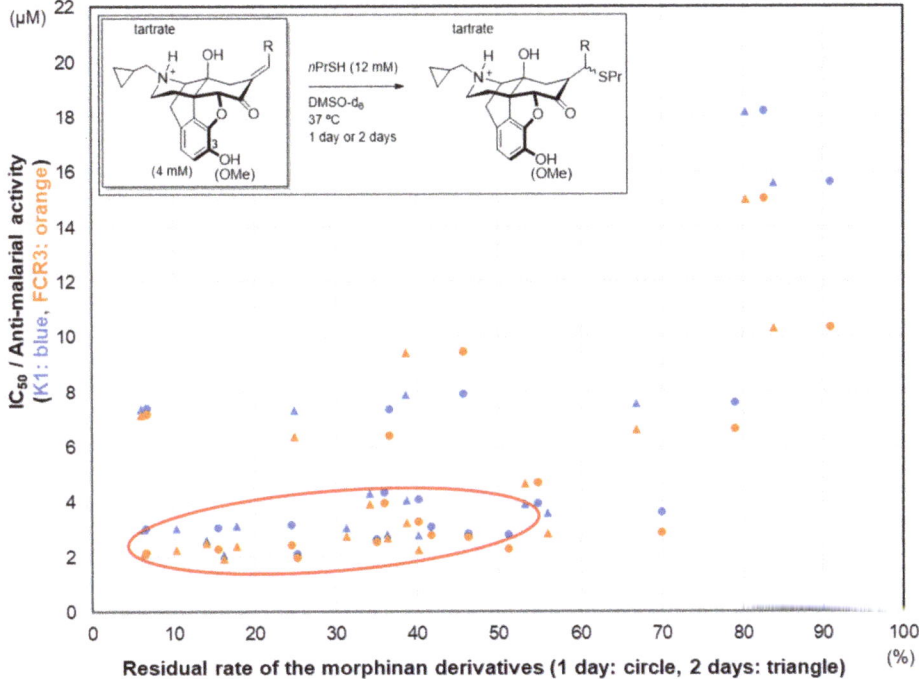

Figure 3. Relationship between antimalarial activities of the BNTX derivatives and the thiol group-trapping ability. Blue symbols represent K1, the CQ-resistant strain, while the orange symbols represent the CQ-sensitive strain, FCR-3. The filled circles (●) indicate the residual rates at day 1 and the filled triangles (▲) represent the day 2 values. [a] The residual rates of **1** and **2** after 2.5 days were adopted.

3. Materials and Methods

All melting points were determined on a Yanaco MP-500P melting point (Mp) apparatus (Tokyo, Japan) and were uncorrected. Infrared spectra (IR) were recorded with a JASCO FT/IR 4100 spectrophotometer (Tokyo, Japan). ^{1}H and ^{13}C NMR spectra data were obtained with JEOL JNM-ECS 400 instruments (Tokyo, Japan). Chemical shifts are quoted in ppm using tetramethylsilane (δ = 0 ppm) as the reference for ^{1}H NMR spectroscopy (JEOL RESONANCE, Tokyo, Japan), CDCl$_3$ (δ = 77.0 ppm) for ^{13}C NMR spectroscopy. Mass spectra were measured with a JEOL JMS-T100LP spectrometer. Elemental analysis was performed with a J-SCIENCE MICRO CORDER JM-10 model analyzer. Column chromatography was carried out on silica gel (Fuji Silysia, CHROMATOREX PSQ60B, Aichi, Japan). Thin layer chromatography (TLC) and preparative TLC were performed on Merck Kieselgel 60 F$_{254}$ (0.25 mm and 0.50 mm) plates (Darmstadt, Germany). All reactions were performed under an argon atmosphere. Synthetic procedures and analytical data for the compounds **1–7**, **16**, **17**, **19**, and **20** were reported in our previous paper [11]. Additionally, the analytical data of compound **8** have been reported [30].

3.1. Experimental Data

(12b*S*)-6-((*E*)-3-Bromo-5-nitrobenzylidene)-3-(cyclopropylmethyl)-4a,9-dihydroxy-2,3,4,4a,5,6-hexahydro-1*H*-4,12-methanobenzofuro[3,2-*e*]isoquinolin-7(7a*H*)-one (**9**): IR (neat) cm^{-1}: 3348, 2925,

2831, 1695, 1533, 1347, 1051. ^{1}H NMR (400 MHz, CDCl$_3$): δ (ppm) 0.12–0.17 (m, 2H), 0.54–0.58 (m, 2H), 0.83–0.89 (m, 1H), 1.67 (d, J = 13.3 Hz, 1H), 2.30–2.43 (m, 5H), 2.66–2.76 (m, 2H), 2.85 (d, J = 15.1 Hz, 1H), 3.13–3.24 (m, 2H), 4.71 (s, 1H), 6.66 (d, J = 8.2 Hz, 1H), 6.76 (d, J = 8.2 Hz, 1H), 7.46 (d, J = 2.3 Hz, 1H), 7.79 (dd, J = 1.8, 1.8 Hz, 1H), 8.15 (dd, J = 1.8, 1.8 Hz, 1H), 8.31 (dd, J = 1.8, 1.8 Hz, 1H). The OH peaks were not observed. ^{13}C NMR (100 MHz, CDCl$_3$): δ (ppm) 3.7, 4.2, 9.2, 22.8, 31.6, 33.5, 43.3, 48.1, 59.3, 61.6, 70.6, 89.9, 117.8, 120.4, 123.0 (× 2), 124.4, 126.3, 129.4, 135.1, 136.5, 138.3, 138.4 (× 2), 143.7, 148.7, 198.7. HR-MS (ESI): m/z [M + H]$^+$ calcd for C$_{27}$H$_{26}$BrN$_2$O$_6$: 553.09742, found: 553.09566.

9·*tartrate*: Mp (dec) 166.0–168.0 °C. Anal. Calcd for C$_{27}$H$_{25}$BrN$_2$O$_6$·C$_4$H$_6$O$_6$·1.9H$_2$O: C, 50.47; H, 4.75; N, 3.80, found: C, 50.34; H, 4.91; N, 3.65.

(4R,4aS,7aR,12bS,E)-3-(Cyclopropylmethyl)-4a,9-dihydroxy-6-((perfluorophenyl)methylene)-2,3,4,4a,5,6-hexahydro-1H-4,12-methanobenzofuro[3,2-e]isoquinolin-7(7aH)-one (**10**): IR (KBr) cm^{-1}: 3377, 2927, 1698, 1521, 1496. ^{1}H NMR (400 MHz, CDCl$_3$): δ (ppm) 0.11–0.15 (m, 2H), 0.52–0.55 (m, 2H), 0.81–0.84 (m, 1H), 1.63–1.66 (m, 1H), 2.24–2.50 (m, 6H), 2.64–2.74 (m, 2H), 3.13 (d, J = 18.8 Hz, 1H), 3.19 (d, J = 6.0 Hz, 1H), 4.72 (s, 1H), 6.66 (d, J = 8.2 Hz, 1H), 6.75 (d, J = 8.2 Hz, 1H), 7.21 (s, 1H). The OH peaks were not observed. ^{13}C NMR (100 MHz, CDCl$_3$): δ (ppm) 3.6, 4.2, 9.2, 22.7, 31.6, 35.1, 43.4, 48.1, 59.3, 61.4, 70.2, 89.7, 117.8, 120.4, 123.5, 124.4, 129.3, 138.3, 139.7, 143.5, 197.9. Some aromatic carbons were not observed. HR-MS (ESI): m/z [M + H]$^+$ calcd for C$_{27}$H$_{23}$F$_5$NO$_4$: 520.15472, found: 520.15331.

10·*tartrate*: Mp (dec) 178.2–179.9 °C. Anal. Calcd for C$_{27}$H$_{22}$F$_5$NO$_4$·C$_4$H$_6$O$_6$·2H$_2$O: C, 52.77; H, 4.57; N, 1.99, found: C, 52.82; H, 4.68; N, 2.23.

(12bS)-3-(Cyclopropylmethyl)-4a,9-dihydroxy-6-((E)-4-isothiocyanatobenzylidene)-2,3,4,4a,5,6-hexahydro-1H-4,12-methanobenzofuro[3,2-e]isoquinolin-7(7aH)-one (**11**): IR (KBr) cm^{-1}: 3409, 2924, 2096, 1685, 1596.

^{1}H NMR (400 MHz, CDCl$_3$): δ (ppm) 0.13–0.15 (m, 2H), 0.54–0.56 (m, 2H), 0.83–0.88 (m, 1H), 1.66–1.68 (m, 1H), 2.26–2.48 (m, 5H), 2.64–2.74 (m, 2H), 2.92 (d, J = 15.6 Hz, 1H), 3.15 (d, J = 18.8 Hz, 1H), 3.21 (d, J = 6.0 Hz, 1H), 4.69 (s, 1H), 6.65 (d, J = 8.0 Hz, 1H), 6.75 (d, J = 8.0 Hz, 1H), 7.21 (d, J = 8.2 Hz, 2H), 7.34 (d, J = 8.2 Hz, 2H), 7.58 (d, J = 8.3 Hz, 1H). The OH peaks were not observed. ^{13}C NMR (100 MHz, CDCl$_3$): δ (ppm) 3.7, 4.1, 9.3, 22.8, 31.7, 33.7, 43.3, 47.8, 59.4, 61.6, 70.2, 89.9, 117.7, 120.2, 124.5, 125.8 (× 2), 129.7, 131.4 (× 2), 131.5, 133.3, 134.1, 136.4, 138.3, 138.6, 143.7, 198.6. HR-MS (ESI): m/z [M + H]$^+$ calcd for C$_{28}$H$_{27}$N$_2$O$_4$S: 487.16915, found: 487.16863.

11·*hydrochloride*: Mp (dec) 189.6–191.3 °C. Anal. Calcd for C$_{28}$H$_{26}$N$_2$O$_4$S·HCl·2.3H$_2$O: C, 59.58; H, 5.64; N, 4.96, found: C, 59.42; H, 5.55; N, 4.82.

N-(4-((E)-((4R,4aS,7aR,12bS)-3-(Cyclopropylmethyl)-4a,9-dihydroxy-7-oxo-1,2,3,4,4a,5,7,7a-octahydro-6H-4,12-methanobenzofuro[3,2-e]isoquinolin-6-ylidene)methyl)phenyl)acrylamide (**12**): IR (KBr) cm^{-1}: 3435, 2925, 1672, 1592. ^{1}H NMR (400 MHz, CDCl$_3$): δ (ppm) 0.13–0.16 (m, 2H), 0.52–0.57 (m, 2H), 0.83–0.86 (m, 1H), 1.64–1.66 (m, 1H), 2.26–2.47 (m, 5H), 2.66–2.72 (m, 2H), 3.00 (d, J = 15.6 Hz, 1H), 3.15 (d, J = 18.8 Hz, 1H), 3.24 (d, J = 6.4 Hz, 1H), 4.68 (s, 1H), 5.78 (dd, J = 10.1, 1.1 Hz, 1H), 6.26 (dd, J = 16.7, 10.7 Hz, 1H), 6.44 (dd, J = 16.7, 1.1 Hz, 1H), 6.64 (d, J = 8.2 Hz, 1H), 6.74 (d, J = 8.2 Hz, 1H), 7.28 (d, J = 8.2 Hz, 2H), 7.57–7.63 (m, 4H). The OH peaks were not observed. ^{13}C NMR (100 MHz, CDCl$_3$): δ (ppm) 3.6, 4.2, 9.3, 22.9, 31.8, 33.8, 43.4, 47.7, 59.4, 61.5, 70.2, 90.0, 117.7, 119.5 (× 2), 120.1, 124.6, 128.4, 129.8, 130.9, 131.1, 131.4 (× 2), 131.5, 138.4, 138.5, 140.1, 143.8, 163.6, 198.4. HR-MS (ESI): m/z [M + H]$^+$ calcd for C$_{30}$H$_{31}$N$_2$O$_5$: 499.22330, found: 499.22469.

12·*tartrate*: Mp (dec) 202.0–203.9 °C. Anal. Calcd for C$_{30}$H$_{30}$N$_2$O$_5$·C$_4$H$_6$O$_6$·2.8H$_2$O: C, 58.41; H, 6.00; N, 4.01, found: C, 58.46; H, 5.81; N, 4.11.

(4R,4aS,7aR,12bS,E)-3-(Cyclopropylmethyl)-6-((6,6-dimethoxy-3-oxocyclohexa-1,4-dien-1-yl)methylene)-4a,9-dihydroxy-2,3,4,4a,5,6-hexahydro-1H-4,12-methanobenzofuro[3,2-e]isoquinolin-7(7aH)-one (**13**): IR (KBr) cm^{-1}: 3417, 2937, 1671, 1632. ^{1}H NMR (400 MHz, CDCl$_3$): δ (ppm) 0.14–0.15 (m, 2H),

0.54–0.59 (m, 2H), 0.83–0.86 (m, 1H), 1.63–1.66 (m, 1H), 2.23–2.40 (m, 4H), 2.46 (dd, J = 12.0, 6.2 Hz, 1H), 2.65 (dd, J = 18.5, 6.4 Hz, 1H), 2.73 (dd, J = 12.0, 4.1 Hz, 1H), 2.93 (d, J = 15.1 Hz, 1H), 3.13 (d, J = 18.5 Hz, 1H), 3.21 (d, J = 6.4 Hz, 1H), 3.25 (s, 6H), 4.69 (s, 1H), 6.29 (s, 1H), 6.44 (dd, J = 10.4, 2.1 Hz, 1H), 6.64 (d, J = 8.2 Hz, 1H), 6.74 (d, J = 8.2 Hz, 1H), 6.81 (d, J = 10.4 Hz, 1H), 7.27 (s, 1H). The OH peaks were not observed. ^{13}C NMR (100 MHz, CDCl$_3$): δ (ppm) 3.7, 4.1, 9.3, 22.7, 31.5, 34.6, 43.3, 48.0, 51.2, 51.3, 59.4, 61.6, 70.4, 89.9, 94.9, 117.6, 120.2, 124.6, 129.5, 131.1, 131.7, 132.9, 138.2, 138.4, 143.6, 144.4, 151.4, 185.0, 198.5. HR-MS (ESI): m/z [M + H]$^+$ calcd for C$_{29}$H$_{32}$NO$_7$: 506.21788, found: 506.21626.

13·tartrate: Mp (dec) 218.6–220.5 °C. Anal. Calcd for C$_{29}$H$_{31}$NO$_7$·C$_4$H$_6$O$_6$·3.5H$_2$O: C, 55.15; H, 6.17; N, 1.95, found: C, 55.17; H, 5.79; N, 1.92.

(4R,4aS,7aR,12bS,E)-6-(Cyclohexylmethylene)-3-(cyclopropylmethyl)-4a,9-dihydroxy-2,3,4,4a,5,6-hexahydro-1H-4,12-methanobenzofuro[3,2-e]isoquinolin-7(7aH)-one (**14**): IR (KBr) cm^{-1}: 3422, 2925, 1686. ^{1}H NMR (400 MHz, CDCl$_3$): δ (ppm) 0.14–0.15 (m, 2H), 0.52–0.60 (m, 2H), 0.86–0.87 (m, 1H), 1.06–1.29 (m, 5H), 1.44 (d, J = 12.8 Hz, 1H), 1.59–1.73 (m, 5H), 2.09 (dd, J = 15.1, 2.8 Hz, 1H), 2.21–2.46 (m, 5H), 2.60–2.73 (m, 3H), 3.10 (d, J = 18.3 Hz, 1H), 3.24 (s, 1H), 4.59 (s, 1H), 6.55–6.60 (m, 2H), 6.70 (d, J = 8.2 Hz, 1H). The OH peaks were not observed. ^{13}C NMR (100 MHz, CDCl$_3$): δ (ppm) 3.8, 4.1, 9.3, 22.9, 25.4, 25.5, 25.7, 31.4 (× 2), 31.9, 32.5, 37.2, 43.4, 47.9, 59.4, 61.8, 70.1, 90.1, 117.5, 119.9, 124.4, 129.8, 130.5, 138.3, 143.6, 149.4, 198.7. HR-MS (ESI): m/z [M + H]$^+$ calcd for C$_{27}$H$_{34}$NO$_4$: 436.24878, found: 436.24706. **14**·tartrate: Mp (dec) 176.8–178.8 °C. Anal. Calcd for C$_{27}$H$_{33}$NO$_4$·C$_4$H$_6$O$_6$·1.8H$_2$O: C, 60.24; H, 6.95; N, 2.27, found: C, 60.39; H, 6.92; N, 2.14.

(4R,4aS,7aR,12bS,E)-6-(Cyclobutylmethylene)-3-(cyclopropylmethyl)-4a,9-dihydroxy-2,3,4,4a,5,6-hexahydro-1H-4,12-methanobenzofuro[3,2-e]isoquinolin-7(7aH)-one (**15**): IR (KBr) cm^{-1}: 3419, 2936, 1685, 1612. ^{1}H NMR (400 MHz, CDCl$_3$): δ (ppm) 0.15–0.16 (m, 2H), 0.56–0.57 (m, 2H), 0.86–0.89 (m, 1H), 1.60–1.63 (m, 1H), 1.85–2.12 (m, 6H), 2.21–2.39 (m, 4H), 2.46 (dd, J = 12.6, 6.2 Hz, 1H), 2.56–2.65 (m, 2H), 2.70–2.74 (m, 1H), 3.09–3.24 (m, 3H), 4.60 (s, 1H), 6.60 (d, J = 8.2 Hz, 1H), 6.71 (d, J = 8.2 Hz, 1H), 6.88 (dd, J = 8.7, 2.3 Hz, 1H). The OH peaks were not observed. ^{13}C NMR (100 MHz, CDCl$_3$): δ (ppm) 3.7, 4.1, 9.3, 19.1, 22.8, 28.65, 28.67, 31.7, 32.5, 34.3, 43.3, 47.9, 59.4, 61.7, 70.0, 90.1, 117.3, 119.9, 124.6, 129.9, 130.3, 138.2, 143.6, 148.9, 197.9. HR-MS (ESI): m/z [M + H]$^+$ calcd for C$_{25}$H$_{30}$NO$_4$: 408.21748, found: 408.21657.

15·tartrate: Mp (dec) 166.9–168.9 °C. Anal. Calcd for C$_{25}$H$_{29}$NO$_4$·C$_4$H$_6$O$_6$·1.4H$_2$O: C, 59.76; H, 6.54; N, 2.40, found: C, 59.73; H, 6.72; N, 2.48.

(4R,4aS,7aR,12bS,E)-3-(Cyclopropylmethyl)-6-(cyclopropylmethylene)-4a,9-dihydroxy-2,3,4,4a,5,6-hexahydro-1H-4,12-methanobenzofuro[3,2-e]isoquinolin-7(7aH)-one (**18**): Mp (dec) 222.0–223.8 °C. IR (KBr) cm^{-1}: 3399, 2924, 2821, 1678, 1328. ^{1}H NMR (400 MHz, CDCl$_3$): δ (ppm) 0.14–0.18 (m, 2H), 0.54–0.59 (m, 2H), 0.63–0.75 (m, 2H), 0.87–1.01 (m, 3H), 1.51–1.55 (m, 1H), 1.62–1.65 (m, 1H), 2.23–2.50 (m, 5H), 2.61–2.73 (m, 2H), 2.80 (d, J = 15.6 Hz, 1H), 3.14 (d, J = 18.8 Hz, 1H), 3.27 (d, J = 6.0 Hz, 1H), 4.61 (s, 1H), 5.28 (brs, 1H), 6.21 (dd, J = 11.2, 2.1 Hz, 1H), 6.60 (d, J = 8.2 Hz, 1H), 6.71 (d, J = 8.2 Hz, 1H). The OH peak was not observed. ^{13}C NMR (100 MHz, CDCl$_3$): δ (ppm) 3.6, 4.1, 9.35, 9.38, 9.8, 12.2, 22.9, 31.8, 32.4, 43.4, 47.7, 59.4, 61.6, 69.9, 90.0, 117.3, 119.8, 124.6, 129.3, 130.0, 138.2, 143.7, 150.9, 196.1. HR-MS (ESI): m/z [M + H]$^+$ calcd for C$_{24}$H$_{28}$NO$_4$: 394.20183, found: 394.20102.

18·tartrate: Mp (dec) 173.0–175.0 °C. Anal. Calcd for C$_{24}$H$_{27}$NO$_4$·C$_4$H$_6$O$_6$·1.2H$_2$O: C, 59.50; H, 6.31; N, 2.48, found: C, 59.67; H, 6.33; N, 2.22.

3.2. Antimalarial Assay

The evaluation of antimalarial activity was conducted as previously reported [21]. Briefly, cultured *P. falciparum* (chloroquine sensitive FCR3 strain and chloroquine resistant K1 strain) in Type A$^+$ blood was seeded in 96-well culture plates (parasitemia 0.5%–1%, hematocrit 2.0%) and incubated with test drugs for 72 h in RPMI medium supplemented with 10% human plasma at 37 °C, under 93%

N₂, 4% CO_2, and 3% O_2. After incubation, parasite lactate dehydrogenase activity was assayed to determine parasite growth and calculate the antimalarial activity in comparison with the controls that had received no drugs. This study was approved by "Kitasato Institute Hospital Research Ethics Committee (No12102)" on donated human blood from volunteers.

4. Conclusions

In conclusion, the antimalarial activities of the BNTX derivatives with a Michael acceptor were evaluated using CQ-resistant K1 and -sensitive FCR3 strains. Moreover, the thiol group-trapping abilities of the derivatives were also investigated relatively, using ^{1}H-NMR experiments. The experimental results strongly supported a correlation between the antimalarial activity and the chemical reactivity of the BNTX derivatives with 1-propanethiol. Thus, the measurement of the thiol group-trapping ability of the derivatives with a Michael acceptor could become a reliable and valid screening technique for antimalarial or related activities.

Supplementary Materials: The addition reactions of 1-propanethiol (Table 2) in detail are available online.

Author Contributions: Conceptualization, N.K. and H.N.; Methodology, N.K.; Supervision, H.N.; Synthetic experiments, Y.K.; Evaluation of compounds, R.H., A.I., and M.I.; Analysis and Data Curation, N.K. and Y.K.; Investigation, T.S., N.Y., Y.N., Y.M., K.O., and S.Ō.; Writing, N.K.; Funding Acquisition, N.K. All authors have read and agreed to the published version of the manuscript.

Funding: This work was partly supported by JSPS KAKANHI Grant Number JP19K05710 (N.K.), and TORAY Industries, Inc.

Conflicts of Interest: The authors declare no conflict of interest.

References

1. World Health Organization. Malaria. Available online: https://www.who.int/news-room/fact-sheets/detail/malaria (accessed on 4 October 2019).
2. Beare, N.A.V.; Lewallen, S.; Taylor, T.E.; Molyneux, M.E. Redefining cerebral malaria by including malaria retinopathy. *Future Microbiol.* **2011**, *6*, 349–355. [CrossRef] [PubMed]
3. Bartoloni, A.; Zammarchi, L. Clinical aspects of uncomplicated and severe malaria. *Mediterr. J. Hematol. Infect. Dis.* **2012**, *4*, e2012026. [CrossRef] [PubMed]
4. Taylor, W.R.J.; Hanson, J.; Turner, G.D.H.; White, N.J.; Dondorp, A.M. Respiratory manifestations of malaria. *Chest* **2012**, *142*, 492–505. [CrossRef] [PubMed]
5. Wongsrichanalai, C.; Meshnick, S.R. Declining artesunate-mefloquine efficacy against falciparum malaria on the Cambodia-Thailand border. *Emerg. Infect. Dis.* **2008**, *14*, 716–719. [CrossRef] [PubMed]
6. Ashley, E.A.; Dhorda, M.; Fairhurst, R.M.; Amaratunga, C.; Lim, P.; Suon, S.; Sreng, S.; Anderson, J.M.; Mao, S.; Sam, B.; et al. Spread of artemisinin resistance in *Plasmodium falciparum* malaria. *N. Engl. J. Med.* **2014**, *371*, 411–423. [CrossRef]
7. Miyata, Y.; Fujii, H.; Osa, Y.; Kobayashi, S.; Takeuchi, T.; Nagase, H. Opioid δ₁ receptor antagonist 7-benzylidenenaltrexone as an effective resistance reverser for chloroquine-resistant *Plasmodium chabaudi*. *Bioorg. Med. Chem. Lett.* **2011**, *21*, 4710–4712. [CrossRef]
8. Miyata, Y.; Fujii, H.; Uenohara, Y.; Kobayashi, S.; Takenouchi, T.; Nagase, H. Investigation of 7-benzylidenenaltrexone derivatives as resistance reverser for chloroquine-resistant *Plasmodium chabaudi*. *Bioorg. Med. Chem. Lett.* **2012**, *22*, 5174–5176. [CrossRef]
9. Asahi, H.; Inoue, S.-I.; Niikura, M.; Kunigo, K.; Suzuki, Y.; Kobayashi, F.; Sendo, F. Profiling molecular factors associated with pyknosis and developmental arrest induced by an opioid receptor antagonist and dihydroarthemisinin in *Plasmodium falciparum*. *PLoS ONE* **2017**, *12*, e0184874. [CrossRef]
10. Kutsumura, N.; Nakajima, R.; Koyama, Y.; Miyata, Y.; Saitoh, T.; Yamamoto, N.; Iwata, S.; Fujii, H.; Nagase, H. Investigation of 7-benzylidenenaltrexone derivatives as a novel structural antitrichomonal lead compound. *Bioorg. Med. Chem. Lett.* **2015**, *25*, 4890–4892. [CrossRef]
11. Kutsumura, N.; Koyama, Y.; Nagumo, Y.; Nakajima, R.; Miyata, Y.; Yamamoto, N.; Saitoh, T.; Yoshida, N.; Iwata, S.; Nagase, H. Antitrichomonal activity of δ opioid receptor antagonists, 7-benzylidenenaltrexone derivatives. *Bioorg. Med. Chem.* **2017**, *25*, 4375–4383. [CrossRef]

12. Dubois, V.L.; Platel, D.F.N.; Pauly, G.; Tribouleyduret, J. *Plasmodium berghei*: Implication of intracellular glutathione and its related enzyme in chloroquine resistance in vivo. *Exp. Parasitol.* **1995**, *81*, 117–124. [CrossRef] [PubMed]
13. Ginsburg, H.; Famin, O.; Zhang, J.; Krugliak, M. Inhibition of glutathione-dependent degradation of heme by chloroquine and amodiaquine as a possible basis for their antimalarial mode of action. *Biochem. Pharmacol.* **1998**, *56*, 1305–1313. [CrossRef]
14. Famin, O.; Krugliak, M.; Ginsburg, H. Kinetics of inhibition of glutathione-mediated degradation of ferriprotoporphyrin IX by antimalarial drugs. *Biochem. Pharmacol.* **1999**, *58*, 59–68. [CrossRef]
15. Ellis, J.E.; Yarlett, N.; Cole, D.; Humphreys, M.J.; Lloyd, D. Antioxidant defences in the microaerophilic protozoan *Trichomonas vaginalis*: Comparison of metronidazole-resistant and sensitive strains. *Microbiology* **1994**, *140*, 2489–2494. [CrossRef]
16. Coombs, G.H.; Westrop, G.D.; Suchan, P.; Puzova, G.; Hirt, R.P.; Embley, T.M.; Mottram, J.C.; Müller, S. The amitochondriate eukaryote Trichomonas vaginalis contains a divergent thioredoxin-linked peroxiredoxin antioxidant system. *J. Biol. Chem.* **2004**, *279*, 5249–5256. [CrossRef]
17. Pal, C.; Bandyopadhyay, U. Redox-active antiparasitic drugs. *Antiox. Redox Signal.* **2012**, *17*, 555–587. [CrossRef]
18. Beltrán, N.C.; Horváthová, L.; Jedelský, P.L.; Šedinová, M.; Rada, P.; Marcinčiková, M.; Hrdý, I.; Tachezy, J. Iron-induced changes in the proteome of *Trichomonas vaginalis* hydrogenosomes. *PLoS ONE* **2013**, *8*, e65148. [CrossRef]
19. Puente-Rivera, J.; Ramón-Luing, L.Á.; Figueroa-Angulo, E.E.; Ortega-López, J.; Arroyo, R. Trichocystatin-2(TC-2): An endogenous inhibitor of cysteine proteinases in *Trichomonas vaginalis* is associated with TvCP39. *Int. J. Biochem. Cell Biol.* **2014**, *54*, 255–265. [CrossRef]
20. Nagase, H.; Hayakawa, J.; Kawamura, K.; Kawai, K.; Takezawa, Y.; Matsuura, H.; Tajima, C.; Endo, T. Discovery of a structurally novel opioid κ-agonist derived from 4,5-epoxymorphinan. *Chem. Pharm. Bull.* **1998**, *46*, 366–369. [CrossRef]
21. Otoguro, K.; Kohana, A.; Manabe, C.; Ishiyama, A.; Ui, H.; Shiomi, K.; Yamada, H.; Omura, S. Potent antimalarial activities of polyether antibiotic, X-206. *J. Antibiot.* **2001**, *54*, 658–663. [CrossRef]
22. Van't Erve, T.J.; Wagner, B.A.; Ryckman, K.K.; Raife, T.J.; Buettner, G.R. The concentration of glutathione in human erythrocytes is a heritable trait. *Free Radic. Biol. Med.* **2013**, *65*, 742–749. [CrossRef] [PubMed]
23. Atamna, H.; Ginsburg, H. The malaria parasite supplies glutathione to its host cell–Investigation of glutathione transport and metabolism in human erythrocytes infected with *Plasmodium falciparum*. *Eur. J. Biochem.* **1997**, *250*, 670–679. [CrossRef] [PubMed]
24. Müller, T.; Johann, L.; Jannack, B.; Brückner, M.; Lanfranchi, D.A.; Bauer, H.; Sanchez, C.; Yardley, V.; Deregnaucourt, C.; Schrével, J.; et al. Glutathione reductase-catalyzed cascade of redox reactions to bioactive potent antimalarial 1,4-naphthoquinones–A new strategy to combat malarial parasites. *J. Am. Chem. Soc.* **2011**, *133*, 11557–11571. [CrossRef] [PubMed]
25. Liu, Q.; Sabnis, Y.; Zhao, Z.; Zhang, T.; Buhrlage, S.J.; Jones, L.H.; Gray, N.S. Developing irreversible inhibitors of the protein kinase cysteinome. *Chem. Biol.* **2013**, *20*, 146–159. [CrossRef] [PubMed]
26. Lanning, B.R.; Whitby, L.R.; Dix, M.M.; Douhan, J.; Gilbert, A.M.; Hett, E.C.; Johnson, T.O.; Joslyn, C.; Kath, J.C.; Niessen, S.; et al. A road map to evaluate the proteome-wide selectivity of covalent kinase inhibitors. *Nat. Chem. Biol.* **2014**, *10*, 760–767. [CrossRef] [PubMed]
27. Goedken, E.R.; Argiriadi, M.A.; Banach, D.L.; Fiamengo, B.A.; Foley, S.E.; Frank, K.E.; George, J.S.; Harris, C.M.; Hobson, A.D.; Ihle, D.C.; et al. Tricyclic covalent inhibitors selectively target Jak3 through an active site thiol. *J. Biol. Chem.* **2015**, *290*, 4573–4589. [CrossRef]
28. Jackson, P.A.; Widen, J.C.; Harki, D.A.; Brummond, K.M. Covalent modifiers: A chemical perspective on the reactivity of α,β-unsaturated carbonyls with thiols via hetero-Michael addition reactions. *J. Med. Chem.* **2017**, *60*, 839–885. [CrossRef]

29. Shindo, N.; Fuchida, H.; Sato, M.; Watari, K.; Shibata, T.; Kuwata, K.; Miura, C.; Okamoto, K.; Hatsuyama, Y.; Tokunaga, K.; et al. Selective and reversible modification of kinase cysteines with chlorofluoroacetamides. *Nat. Chem. Biol.* **2019**, *15*, 250–258. [CrossRef]
30. Ohkawa, S.; Portoghese, P.S. 7-Arylidenenaltrexones as selective δ_1 opioid receptor antagonists. *J. Med. Chem.* **1998**, *41*, 4177–4180. [CrossRef]

Sample Availability: Samples of the compounds are available from the authors.

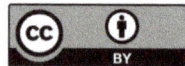

© 2020 by the authors. Licensee MDPI, Basel, Switzerland. This article is an open access article distributed under the terms and conditions of the Creative Commons Attribution (CC BY) license (http://creativecommons.org/licenses/by/4.0/).

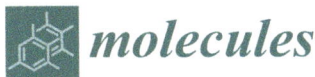 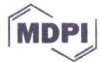

Article

Effects of *N*-Substituents on the Functional Activities of Naltrindole Derivatives for the δ Opioid Receptor: Synthesis and Evaluation of Sulfonamide Derivatives

Chiharu Iwamatsu [1], Daichi Hayakawa [2], Tomomi Kono [1], Ayaka Honjo [1], Saki Ishizaki [1], Shigeto Hirayama [1,3], Hiroaki Gouda [2] and Hideaki Fujii [1,3,*]

[1] Laboratory of Medicinal Chemistry, School of Pharmacy, Kitasato University, 5-9-1, Shirokane, Minato-ku, Tokyo 108-8641, Japan; ml18101@st.kitasato-u.ac.jp (C.I.); r.tymo-hone@i.softbank.jp (T.K.); ml17117@st.kitasato-u.ac.jp (A.H.); pl17007@st.kitasato-u.ac.jp (S.I.); hirayamas@pharm.kitasato-u.ac.jp (S.H.)

[2] Division of Biophysical Chemistry, Department of Pharmaceutical Sciences, School of Pharmacy, Showa University, 1-5-8 Hatanodai, Shinagawa-ku, Tokyo 142-8555, Japan; d-hayakawa@pharm.showa-u.ac.jp (D.H.); godah@pharm.showa-u.ac.jp (H.G.)

[3] Medicinal Research Laboratories, School of Pharmacy, Kitasato University, 5-9-1, Shirokane, Minato-ku, Tokyo 108-8641, Japan

* Correspondence: fujiih@pharm.kitasato-u.ac.jp; Tel.: +81-3-5791-6372

Academic Editors: Helmut Schmidhammera and Mariana Spetea
Received: 31 July 2020; Accepted: 19 August 2020; Published: 20 August 2020

Abstract: We have recently reported that *N*-alkyl and *N*-acyl naltrindole (NTI) derivatives showed activities for the δ opioid receptor (DOR) ranging widely from full inverse agonists to full agonists. We newly designed sulfonamide-type NTI derivatives in order to investigate the effects of the *N*-substituent on the functional activities because the side chain and S=O part in the sulfonamide moiety located in spatially different positions compared with those in the alkylamine and amide moieties. Among the tested compounds, cyclopropylsulfonamide **9f** (SYK-839) was the most potent full inverse agonist for the DOR, whereas phenethylsulfonamide **9e** (SYK-901) showed full DOR agonist activity with moderate potency. These NTI derivatives are expected to be useful compounds for investigation of the molecular mechanism inducing these functional activities.

Keywords: δ opioid receptor; NTI derivative; sulfonamide; inverse agonist; neutral antagonist; agonist

---

1. Introduction

The ligands interacting with receptors have long been classified into agonists and antagonists. However, it is now widely accepted that there are agonists, neutral antagonists, and inverse agonists. Agonists interact with receptors in the active state to induce physiological activities, whereas inverse agonists, which bind to receptors in the inactive state, can suppress the constitutive activities of receptors. The constitutive activity is characterized as activities induced by receptors in the absence of agonists [1–3]. Neutral antagonists themselves do not exhibit any activities and can block the functions of both agonists and inverse agonists. Recently, the relationship between some disease states and the constitutive activity of receptors, and developments of inverse agonists have been reported [4–20]. In the opioid field, since Costa and Herz firstly reported that peptidic ICI-174,864 showed δ opioid receptor (DOR) inverse agonist activity [21], several peptidic and non-peptidic DOR inverse agonists have been developed [4]. Possible pharmacological effects resulting from DOR inverse agonism include anorexia [22,23], short-term memory improvement [24], and antitussive effects [25]. We also recently reported several DOR inverse agonists with the skeleton of naltrindole (NTI) [24–26], which was developed as a selective DOR antagonist by Portoghese et al. [27,28].

Interestingly, a series of compounds we reported induced activities from full inverse agonists to full agonists depending on their substituents on the 17-nitrogen atom (Figure 1) [24–26,29]. Amide-type compound SKY-623 bearing 17-cyclopropanecarbonyl group was a DOR full inverse agonist with high potency [25]. Well-known NTI with the 17-cyclopropylmethyl substituent was a neutral antagonist [27,28]. In contrast, SYK-754 possessing the phenylacetyl group as a 17-substituent was a DOR full agonist with moderate potency [29]. The 17-substituent of the morphinan skeleton, which is a representatively fundamental core of opioid ligands and is shared among NTI and many clinically used opioids like morphine, oxymorphone, and naloxone, is a determinant of the activities of ligands, either agonist or antagonist [30]. Especially, this tendency is observed in the ligands showing selectivity for the μ opioid receptor (MOR), which is one of the known opioid receptor types, encompassing MOR, DOR, and κ opioid receptor (KOR). For example, naltrexone and naloxone with a bulky 17-substituent like cyclopropylmethyl and allyl, respectively, are antagonists, while morphine and oxymorphone, having a small methyl group at the 17-nitrogen, are agonists. However, to the best of our knowledge, this is the first example of opioid ligands with common structures, but possessing different 17-substituents, whose activities range from full inverse agonists to full agonists. It is also worth noting that amide-type compounds SYK-623 and SYK-754 showed opioid functionality even though they lack a basic nitrogen. The basic nitrogen in opioid ligands, which is protonated under the physiological environment, is well-known to be an essential pharmacophore. Indeed, co-crystals of opioid receptors with specific antagonists or agonists have been resolved to reveal the interaction between the protonated nitrogen atom in the ligands and the aspartic acid residue in the receptor [31–35]. Moreover, such interaction between a ligand and the receptor has also been recently elucidated by cryo-electron microscopic analysis of the ligand-receptor complex [36,37]. The neoclerodane diterpene salvinolin A is known to be a non-nitrogenous KOR agonist [38]. However, salvinolin A has been reported to bind to the KOR in a different fashion from that of morphinan derivatives [39]. Taken together, several NTI derivatives that we have reported (Figure 1) are expected to be useful compounds to elucidate the binding modes of these structures and to investigate the effects of the N-substituents on the conformational changes of the DOR that induce functional activities from inverse agonists to agonists. We were therefore interested in sulfonamide-type NTI derivatives, because not only the orientation of the sidechain, but also the chemical property of the nitrogen atom in the sulfonamide moiety differs from those of tertiary alkyl or amide-type compounds. Herein, we will report the synthesis of sulfonamide-type NTI derivatives and the evaluation of their opioid activities. We also compared activities among the NTI derivatives having corresponding tertiary alkyl amine, amide, and sulfonamide moieties.

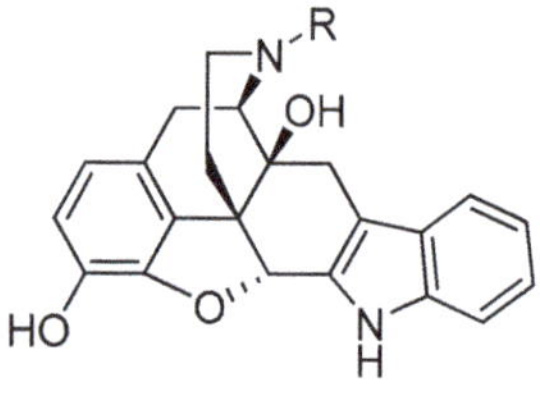

SYK-623: R = (C=O)c-Pr: DOR full inverse agonist
NTI: R = CH$_2$c-Pr: DOR neutral antagonist
SYK-754: R = (C=O)CH$_2$Ph: DOR full agonists

Figure 1. Structures of SYK-623 (DOR full inverse agonist), NTI (DOR neutral antagonist), and SYK-882 (DOR full agonist).

2. Results and Discussion

2.1. The Most Stable Conformations of the Corresponding Alkyl-, Amide-, and Sulfonamide-Type Compounds and the Comparison of the Basicities of Their Nitrogen Atoms

In order to clarify the structural differences among alkylamines, amides, and sulfonamides, we calculated the most stable conformations of 1-(2,2,2-trifluoroethyl)piperidine (**A**), 1-(trifluoroacetyl)piperidine (**B**), and 1-(trifluoromethylsulfonyl)piperidine (**C**) as model compounds at the ωB97XD/6-31G(d,p) level (Figure 2). The orientations of trifluoromethyl parts in the three model compounds differed from each other. The C=O or S=O moieties in piperidines **B** or **C**, which were possible functionalities to interact with the receptor, were also oriented toward distinct directions. The active conformers, which interact with the target proteins, do not necessarily correspond to the most stable conformations. However, it is obvious that the relative relationship among the spatial locations of the piperidine ring, side chain, and the C=O or S=O moieties varied among the three piperidines. As the nitrogens of piperidines **A** and **B** are sp^3 and sp^2 hybridized, respectively, the structures of these nitrogens were trigonal pyramid and the trigonal plannar, respectively. Meanwhile, the nitrogen of piperidine **C** was observed to be slightly pyramidalized. According to the calculations by Advanced Chemistry Development (ACD/Labs) Software V11.02, the nitrogen of piperidine **A** is basic, whereas piperidines **B** and **C** have no basic nitrogens: the predicted pKa values were 6.79 ± 0.10 for **A**, −1 ± 0.20 for **B**, and −7.81 ± 0.20 for **C**. The amide-type NTI derivative SYK-623 (Figure 1) was a DOR full inverse agonist, even though it lacked a basic nitrogen, a known important pharmacophore. This observation evoked the idea that the C=O moiety might compensate for the interaction between the protonated nitrogen and the receptor. It is interesting to consider whether the S=O moieties in sulfonamide-type NTI derivatives, which were oriented differently from the C=O part in amide-type NTI derivatives, can function as a surrogate for the amide carbonyl moiety.

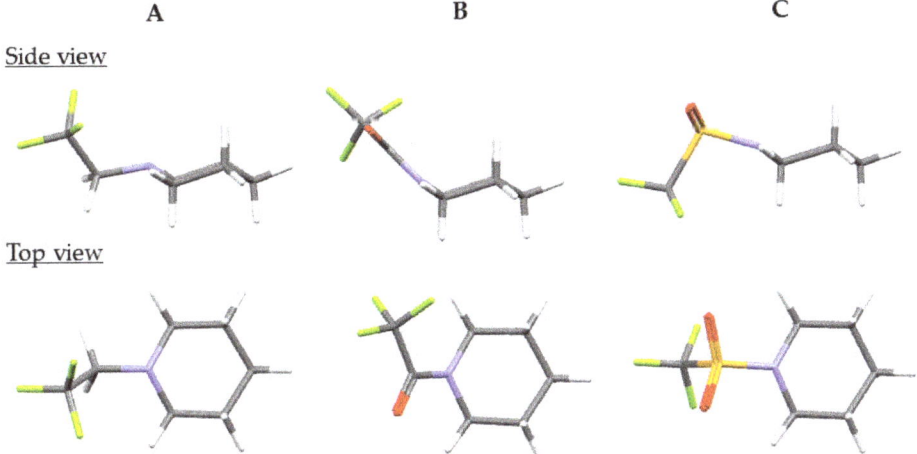

Figure 2. The most stable conformations of 1-(2,2,2-trifluoroethyl)piperidine (**A**), 1-(trifluoroacetyl)piperidine (**B**), and 1-(trifluoromethylsulfonyl)piperidine (**C**). The conformers were obtained by the ωB97XD/6-31G(d,p) level calculation.

2.2. Chemical Synthesis

Compound **7** [24,25], which is the key intermediate for the synthesis of the target sulfonamide-type NTI derivatives, was synthesized from naltrexone hydrochloride (**1**) (Scheme 1). Fischer indolization of **1** with phenylhydrazine hydrochloride gave NTI (**2**) [27,28] in 99% yield, which was treated with acetic anhydride to afford diacetate **3** in 95% yield. The reaction of **3** with Troc-Cl provided a mixture of compounds **4** and **4'**. Although the dealkylation with chloroformates is the usual method [40–42], the application of the methodology to 14-hydroxymorphinan derivatives requires the protection of the 14-hydroxy group because the cleavage reaction of the D-ring (piperidine ring) reportedly proceeded when applying the methodology to 14-hydroxy free morphinan derivatives [43]. Although the treatment with zinc and acetic acid is the usual deprotection procedure for the *N*-Troc group [44], the application of the deprotection conditions to the 14-acetoxy morphinan derivatives like **4** and

4′ sometimes facilitated the migration of the acetyl group from the 14-O-position to the 17-nitrogen. Therefore, we attempted to hydrolyze the 14-acetate under basic conditions using methanol as a solvent to afford compounds **5** and **6** in 60% and 21% yields, respectively. As compound **5** was unexpectedly obtained, we explored the optimal conditions of hydrolysis (see the Supporting Information for details). The treatment of a mixture of **4** and **4′** with 4 M NaOH aqueous solution using THF as a solvent selectively furnished compound **5** and methyl carbamate **6** was almost not detected. Finally, the key intermediate **7** was prepared by introduction of TBS group at the phenolic hydroxy group of **5**. Although we previously reported the synthesis of **7** from **1** [24], the synthetic method shown in Scheme 1 was four steps shorter and provided the key intermediate **7** in higher total yield than the previous method (see the Supporting Information for details). Portoghese et al. and Rice et al. independently reported the synthesis of the **5** hydrochloride from noroxymorphone in one step (see the Supporting Information for details) [45,46]. However, noroxymorphone is difficult to obtain and very expensive compared with naltrexone hydrochloride (**1**).

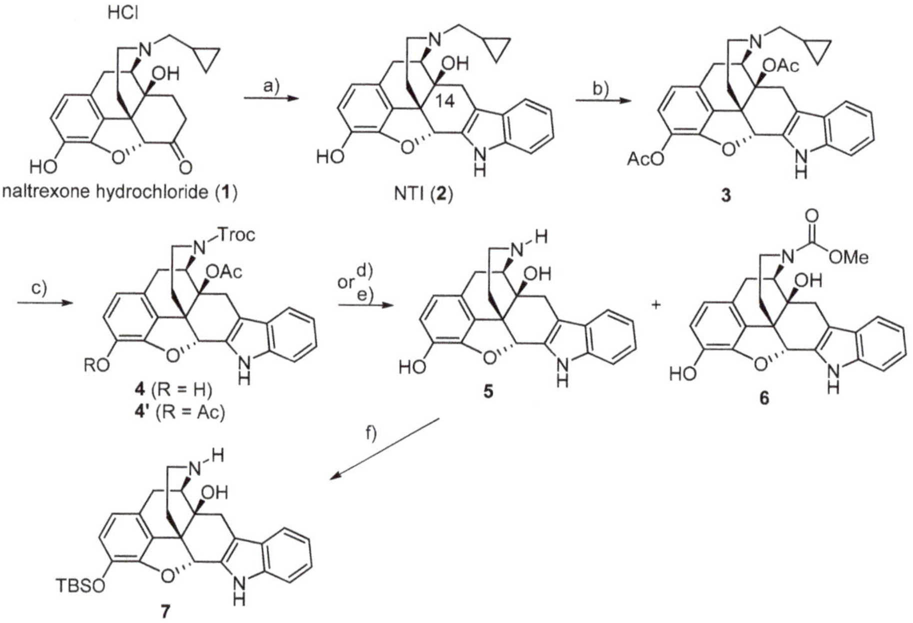

Scheme 1. Synthesis of the key intermediate **7**. Reagents and conditions: (**a**) PhNHNH$_2$·HCl, MeSO$_3$H, EtOH, reflux, 99%; (**b**) Ac$_2$O, 85 °C, 95%; (**c**) Troc-Cl, K$_2$CO$_3$, 1,1,2,2-tetrachloroethane, reflux, 92%; (**d**) 4 M NaOH aq, MeOH, reflux, **5**: 60% from **3**, **6**: 21% from **3**; (**e**) 4 M NaOH aq, THF, reflux, **5**: 72% from **3**, **6**: trace from **3**; (**f**) TBSCl, imidazole, DMF, rt, 70%.

Designed sulfonamide-type NTI derivatives **9** were synthesized from the key intermediate **7** (Scheme 2). Sulfonylation of **7** and the followed deprotection of TBS group gave compounds **9a–g**. For the synthesis of vinyl sulfonamide derivatives **8g**, 2-chloroethylsulfonyl chloride was used in the presence of NaOH instead of triethylamine. The change from triethylamine to more basic NaOH effectively expedited E2 elimination to provide the vinylsulfonyl moiety.

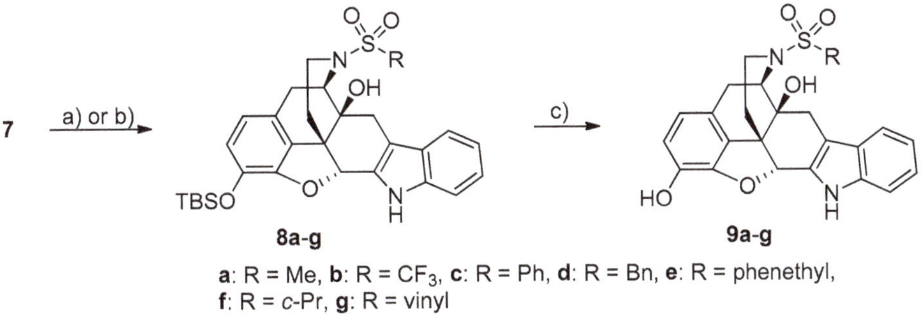

Scheme 2. Synthesis of sulfonamide-type NTI derivatives **9**. Reagents and conditions: (**a**) RSO$_2$Cl, Et$_3$N, CH$_2$Cl$_2$, 0 °C, 46–98%; (**b**) ClCH$_2$CH$_2$SO$_2$Cl, 0.5 M NaOH aq, CH$_2$Cl$_2$, 0 °C, 56% (**8g**); (**c**) 1.0 M TBAF, THF, rt, 71–96%.

2.3. Binding Affinity and Functional Activity

The binding affinities of the synthesized compounds **9** for the opiod receptors were evaluated by competitive binding assays according to the previously reported methods [47] (Table 1). Although the binding affinity of compound **9d** for the DOR was low, the other tested compounds **9** bound to the DOR with strong to moderate affinities. Among them, compound **9f** with a cyclopropylsulfonyl group was the strongest binder to the DOR with a K$_i$ value of 7.44 nM. However, its affinity for the DOR was over 10-fold lower than that of the mother compound NTI. Compounds **9c** and **9f**, which had relatively high affinities for the DOR, showed binding affinities for the KOR, but their affinities for the KOR were lower than those for the DOR. All the tested compounds exhibited almost no affinities for the MOR. The DOR selectivities displayed by the tested compounds tended to also be observed in the series of alkyl- and amide-type NTI derivatives.

As all the tested compounds **9** showed DOR selectivities, we evaluated the functional activities of **9** for the DOR by [^{35}S]GTPγS binding assays according to the previously reported methods [47] (Table 1). Compounds **9a**, **9b**, **9f**, and **9g** showed inverse agonist activities. Among them, compounds **9f** and **9g** showing high efficacies were almost full inverse agonists. The activity of **9f** was comparable to that to SYK-623 (EC$_{50}$ = 0.969 nM, E$_{max}$ = −91.2%) [25]. Interestingly, both compounds possessing the cyclopropyl moiety together with either a C=O or a S=O functionality were inverse agonists, while the NTI-bearing cyclopropylmethyl group, with neither the C=O nor S=O moiety, was a neutral antagonist. Benzylsulfonamide **9d** and phenethylsulfonamide **9e** were DOR agonists. Morphine derivatives with large and small N-substituents are known to show antagonist and agonist activities, respectively, while the N-phenethyl derivative bearing a larger N-substituent was an agonist [30]. Although it is not fully clear why such outcomes were observed, the observations for compounds **9d** and **9e** may result from a similar cause. As no [^{35}S]GTPγS binding was measured for compound **9c**, **9c** was a neutral DOR antagonist.

We summarized the binding affinities and functional acitvities of the corresponding alkyl-, amide-, and sulfonamide-type NTI derivatives for the DOR in Table 2. Full agonists, partial agonists, neutral antagonists, partial inverse agonists, and full inverse agonists were categorized based on the following criteria: E$_{max}$ ≥ 80% for full agonists, 80% > E$_{max}$ ≥ 10% for partial agonists, 10% > E$_{max}$ > −10% for neutral antagonists, −10% ≥ E$_{max}$ > −80% for partial inverse agonists, and −80% ≥ E$_{max}$ for full inverse agonists. In the case that the substituent R was methyl, trifluoromethyl, phenyl, or cyclopropyl group, NTI derivatives were neutral antagonsts or inverse agonists. However, no clear trend dependent on the moiety X was observed. On the other hand, the derivatives bearing benzyl or phenethyl substituent as the R group exhibited agonist activities regardless of the moiety X. Although all the derivatives with the phenyl, benzyl, or phenethyl substituent as the R group possessed the phenyl ring in their N-substituents, regardless of the moiety X, the derivatives with benzyl-X- or phenethyl-X-group showed positive intrinsic activities whereas N-(phenyl-X)- derivatives displayed no positive intrinsic activities. It is not clear why such results were obtained, but the length between the phenyl ring and morphinan core structure may play a key role. When the substituent R is a vinyl group, the X moiety seemed to control the functional activities: an alkyl-type derivative (X = CH$_2$) was an agonist while amide-type (X = CO) or sulfonamide-type (X = SO$_2$) derivatives were inverse agonists. The outcomes shown in Table 2 critically suggest that the N-substituent (R-X- group) would affect the functional activity. This observation is consistent with the idea that binding of these different structures would selectively alter the conformation of the DOR to induce an agonistic, inverse agonistic activity, or no activity at all. However, it is not yet known which functional group or which interaction would control the conformational changes of the receptor based on the classical structure-activity relationship study carried out in this research. Further investigations using computational simulation, X-ray crystallographic or cryo-electron microscopic studies of the complex of these ligands with the DOR are expected to reveal key insights.

Table 1. Binding affinities of compounds **9** for the opioid receptors [a] and functional activities of compounds **9** for the DOR [b].

Compd	R	Binding Affinity, nM (95% CI)			Functional Activity for DOR	
		K_i (DOR)	K_i (MOR)	K_i (KOR)	EC$_{50}$, nM (95% CI)	E$_{max}$, % (95% CI)
DPDPE [c]	—	NT [d]	NT [d]	NT [d]	4.66 (2.08–10.4)	100 [e]
ICI-174,864 [c]	—	422 (215–829)	NT [d]	NT [d]	114 (67.9–192)	−100 [f]
NTI [c]	—	0.457 (0.192–1.09)	30.7 (12.5–75.4)	14.7 (3.16–68.5)	ND [g]	7.50 [h]
9a	Me	284 (151–535)	10,100 (1920–16,600)	ND [g]	0.468 (0.0816–2.68)	−48.8 (−58.2—39.5)
9b	CF$_3$	365 (193–692)	11,800 (1740–80,300)	675 (210–2170)	ND [g]	−36.1 [h]
9c	Ph	49.6 (26.2–93.9)	20,500 (1560–269,000)	95.6 (41.4–220)	ND [g]	ND [g]
9d	Bn	734 (326–1660)	5180 (1930–13,900)	18,800 (6010–58,800)	310 (82.1–177)	47.1 (36.9–57.3)
9e	Phenethyl	132 (57.0–304)	1400 (261–7440)	17,800 (6840–46,300)	75.8 (39.5–146)	88.1 (79.2–97.0)
9f	c-Pr	7.44 (3.53–15.7)	3900 (1450–10,500)	13.6 (5.45–33.7)	1.59 (0.825–3.05)	−80.5 (−87.7—73.4)
9g	vinyl	196 (87.5–440)	3570 (1420–8970)	59,100 (2190–160,000)	7.80 (1.58–38.4)	−80.2 (−97.8—62.6)

[a] Evaluated by the ability of each compound to displace [^{3}H]DAMGO (MOR), [^{3}H]DPDPE (DOR), or [^{3}H]U-69,593 (KOR) binding to the CHO cells expressing human MOR, DOR, or KOR. The data represent means of three samples. [b] Membranes were incubated with [^{35}S]GTPγS and GDP in the presence of the test compound. The human DOR recombinant cell membrane (CHO) was used in this assay. The data represent means of three samples. [c] From ref. [24]. [d] NT: Not tested. [e] DPDPE (1 μM) was used as the standard DOR agonist. [f] ICI-174,864 (10 μM) was used as the standard DOR inverse agonist. [g] ND: Not determined. [h] Percent stimulation at 10 μM of the tested compound. 95% CI: 95% confidence interval.

Table 2. Comparison of binding affinity and functional activity for the DOR among the corresponding alkyl-, amide-, and sulfonamide-type NTI derivatives.

R	Alkyl-Type, X = CH$_2$ (95% CI)	Amide-Type, X = CO (95% CI)	Sulfonamide-Type, X = SO$_2$ (95% CI)
Me	SYK-323 [a] K_i = 2.71 nM (1.93–3.82) EC$_{50}$: ND [c] E$_{max}$: ND [c]	SYK-747 [b] K_i = 977 nM (332–2,880) EC$_{50}$: ND [c] E$_{max}$ = −4.86% [d]	9a (SYK-884) K_i = 284 nM (151–535) EC$_{50}$ = 0.468 nM (0.0816–2.68) E$_{max}$ = −48.8% (−58.2−−39.5)
CF$_3$	SYK-165 [a] K_i = 134 nM (75.4–239) EC$_{50}$ = 45.5 nM (17.5–118) E$_{max}$ = −44.8% (−51.9−−37.7)	SYK-752 [b] K_i = 7.84 nM (4.30–14.3) EC$_{50}$: ND [c] E$_{max}$ = −1.10% [d]	9b (SYK-837) K_i = 365 nM (193–692) EC$_{50}$: ND [c] E$_{max}$ = −36.1% [d]
Ph	SYK-619 [e] K_i = 15.8 nM (7.23–34.7) EC$_{50}$ = 16.1 nM (7.31–35.4) E$_{max}$ = −56.5% (−63.3−−49.8)	SYK-736 [b] K_i = 290 nM (177–476) EC$_{50}$ = 322 nM (51.5–2,010) E$_{max}$ = −92.7% (−122−−62.6)	9c (SYK-838) K_i = 49.6 nM (26.2–93.9) EC$_{50}$: ND [c] E$_{max}$: ND [c]
Bn	SYK-707 [e] K_i = 1.94 nM (1.50–2.50) EC$_{50}$ = 15.1 nM (2.67–85.0) E$_{max}$ = 40.3% (30.4–50.2)	SYK-754 [f] K_i = 89.0 nM (66.6–119) EC$_{50}$ = 127 nM (80.1–201) E$_{max}$ = 88.5% (81.6–95.3)	9d (SYK-887) K_i = 734 nM (326–1,660) EC$_{50}$ = 310 nM (82.1–117) E$_{max}$ = 47.1% (36.9–57.3)
Phenethyl	SYK-903 [g] K_i = 166 nM (65.5–419) EC$_{50}$ = 7.37 nM (3.80–14.3) E$_{max}$ = 105% (96.2–114)	SYK-753 [f] K_i = 41.5 nM (28.5–60.6) EC$_{50}$ = 132 nM (51.5–336) E$_{max}$ = 97.5% (82.6–112)	9e (SYK-901) K_i = 132 nM (57.0–304) EC$_{50}$ = 75.8 nM (39.5–146) E$_{max}$ = 88.1% (79.2–97.0)
c-Pr	NTI [e] K_i = 0.46 nM (0.192–1.09) EC$_{50}$: ND [c] E$_{max}$ = 7.50% [d]	SYK-623 [b] K_i = 17.3 nM (10.3–28.9) EC$_{50}$ = 0.969 nM (0.406–2.93) E$_{max}$ = −91.2% (−99.8−−82.7)	9f (SYK-839) K_i = 7.44 nM (3.53–15.7) EC$_{50}$ = 1.59 nM (0.825–3.05) E$_{max}$ = −80.5% (−87.7−−73.4)
vinyl	SYK-706 [e] K_i = 0.609 nM (0.407–0.913) EC$_{50}$ = 101 nM (4.46–2,280) E$_{max}$ = 16.2% (8.14–24.3)	SYK-836 [b] K_i = 1.16 nM (0.508–2.63) EC$_{50}$ = 1.43 nM (0.819–2.59) E$_{max}$ = −86.2% (−92.2−−80.2)	9g (SYK-886) K_i = 196 nM (87.5–440) EC$_{50}$ = 7.80 nM (1.58–38.4) E$_{max}$ = −80.2% (−97.8−−62.6)

: Full agonist (E$_{max}$ ≥ 80%), : partial agonist (80% > E$_{max}$ ≥ 10%), : neutral antagonist (10% > E$_{max}$ > −10%), : partial inverse agonist (−10% ≥ E$_{max}$ > −80%), : full inverse agonist (−80% ≥ E$_{max}$). [a] From ref. [26]. [b] From ref. [25]. [c] ND: Not determined. [d] Percent stimulation at 10 μM of the tested compound. [e] From ref. [24]. [f] From ref. [29]. [g] SYK-903 was newly synthesized and evaluated in comparison with SYK-836 and SYK-886. The synthetic method and its spectral data are described in the Supporting Information. The data represent means of three or four samples. 95% CI: 95% confidence interval.

3. Materials and Methods

3.1. General Information

All reagents and solvents were obtained from commercial suppliers and were used without further purification. Melting points were determined on a Yanako MP-500P melting point apparatus and were uncorrected. IR spectra were recorded on a JASCO FT/IR-460Plus. NMR spectra were recorded on an Agilent Technologies VXR-400NMR for ^{1}H- and ^{13}C-NMR. Chemical shifts were reported as δ values (ppm) referenced to tetramethylsilane, acetone-d_6, methanol-d_4, or dimethyl sulfoxide-d_6. MS were obtained on a JMS-AX505HA, JMS-700 MStation, or JMS-100LP instrument by applying an electrospray ionization (ESI) method. Elemental analyses were determined with a Yanako MT-5 and JM10 for carbon, hydrogen, and nitrogen. The progress of the reaction was determined on Merck Silica Gel Art. 5715 (TLC) visualized by exposure to UV light or with sodium phosphomolybdate solution (sodium phosphomolybdate (9.68 g) in distilled water (400 mL), sulfuric acid (20 mL), and 85% phosphoric acid (6 mL)). Column chromatographies were carried out using Fuji Silysia CHROMATOREX® PSQ 60B (60 µm) or Fuji Silysia CHROMATOREX® NH-DM2035 (60 µm). The reactions were performed under an argon atmosphere unless otherwise noted.

3.2. Procedures for the Synthesis All the New Compounds and Their Spectroscopic Data

3.2.1. 17-Cyclopropyl-6,7-didehydro-4,5α-epoxyindolo[2′,3′:6,7]morphinan-3,14β-diyl Diacetate (3)

A solution of NTI (220 mg, 0.53 mmol) in acetic anhydride (5 mL) was stirred at 83 °C for 2 h. After cooling to room temperature, the reaction mixture was poured into saturated sodium bicarbonate aqueous solution and extracted with chloroform. The combined organic layers were washed with brine and dried over anhydrous sodium sulfate. After removing the solvent *in vacuo*, the residue was purified by silica gel column chromatography to give the title compound 3 (252 mg, 95%) as a yellow amorphous material; IR (film) cm^{-1}: 3375, 1730, 1450, 1367, 1255, 1231, 1190, 1155, 1046, 1016, 744. ^{1}H NMR (400 MHz, CDCl$_3$): δ 0.05–0.17 (m, 2H), 0.46–0.57 (m, 2H), 0.77–0.88 (m, 1H), 1.78 (dd, J = 2.0, 12.2 Hz, 1H), 1.96 (s, 3H), 2.24 (s, 3 H), 2.25–2.32 (m, 1H), 2.28 (dd, J = 6.9, 12.5 Hz, 1H), 2.42 (dd, J = 6.1, 12.5 Hz, 1H), 2.53 (ddd, J = 5.3, 12.3, 12.3 Hz, 1H), 2.55 (dd, J = 1.3, 16.9 Hz, 1H), 2.72-2.80 (m, 2H), 3.18 (d, J = 18.8 Hz, 1H), 3.82 (d, J = 16.9 Hz, 1H), 4.70 (d, J = 6.2 Hz, 1H), 5.69 (s, 1H), 6.64 (d, J = 8.2 Hz, 1H), 6.76 (d, J = 8.2 Hz, 1H), 7.03–7.08 (m, 1H), 7.15–7.21 (m, 1H), 7.34 (br d, J = 8.2 Hz, 1H), 7.42 (br d, J = 7.8 Hz, 1H), 8.09 (s, 1H). ^{13}C NMR (100 MHz, CDCl$_3$): δ 3.7, 3.8, 9.5, 20.5, 22.3, 24.0, 24.5, 30.9, 43.7, 48.2, 55.7, 59.5, 83.8, 85.7, 110.9, 111.3, 118.7, 119.1, 119.4, 122.4, 122.9, 126.6, 128.6, 130.8, 132.0, 132.8, 137.0, 146.9, 168.5, 170.6. HR-MS (ESI): Calcd for C$_{30}$H$_{31}$N$_2$O$_5$ [M + H]$^+$: 499.2233. Found: 499.2246.

3.2.2. 6,7-Didehydro-4,5α-epoxyindolo[2′,3′:6,7]morphinan-3,14β-diol (nor-NTI) (5)

To a solution of compound 3 (1.6 g, 3.22 mmol) in 1,1,2,2-tetrachloroethane (10 mL) were added potassium carbonate (2.2 g, 16.1 mmol) and 2,2,2-trichloroethyl chloroformate (2.22 mL, 16.1 mmol), and the mixture was refluxed for 20 h with stirring. After cooling to room temperature, the reaction mixture was poured into saturated sodium bicarbonate aqueous solution and extracted with chloroform. The combined organic layers were washed with brine and dried over anhydrous sodium sulfate. After removing the solvent in vacuo, the obtained crude product was used in the next reaction without any purification.

To a solution of the crude product in THF (15 mL) was added 4 M sodium hydroxide aqueous solution and the mixture was refluxed for 24 h with stirring. After cooling to room temperature, the reaction mixture was poured into saturated sodium bicarbonate aqueous solution and adjusted to pH 7–8 by addition of 2 M hydrochloric acid, then extracted with a mixed solvent (chloroform:ethanol = 3:1). The combined organic layers were washed with brine and dried over anhydrous sodium sulfate. After removing the solvent in vacuo, the residue was purified by silica gel column chromatography to give the title compound 5 (834 mg, 72% from 3) as a yellow amorphous material; IR (film) cm^{-1}: 3292, 1617, 1501, 1457, 1325, 1240, 1164, 1072, 868. ^{1}H NMR (400 MHz, methanol-d_4): δ 1.90 (dd, J = 3.8, 13.2 Hz, 1H), 2.65 (dd, J = 1.2, 16.0 Hz, 1H), 2.66 (ddd, J = 5.2, 13.4, 13.4 Hz, 1H), 2.92 (d, J = 16.0 Hz, 1H), 2.99 (ddd, J = 4.1, 13.2, 13.2 Hz, 1H), 3.12–3.18 (m, 1H), 3.21 (d, J = 19.2 Hz, 1H), 3.46 (dd, J = 6.8, 19.2 Hz, 1H), 3.80 (d, J = 6.8 Hz, 1H), 5.68 (s, 1H), 6.639 (d, J = 8.2 Hz, 1H), 6.648 (d, J = 8.2 Hz, 1H), 6.97 (ddd, J = 0.9, 7.1, 8.0 Hz, 1H), 7.11 (ddd, J = 1.1, 7.1, 8.2 Hz, 1H), 7.33 (d, J = 8.2 Hz, 1H), 7.38 (d, J = 8.0 Hz, 1H), 7.89 (s, 1H), three protons (OH × 2 and NH) were not observed. ^{13}C NMR (100 MHz, DMSO-d_6): δ 47.1, 54.3, 56.1, 67.0, 71.7, 72.1, 79.2, 84.3, 109.6, 111.4, 114.6, 118.3, 118.5, 121.8, 125.0, 126.3, 129.4, 130.2, 136.8, 141.9, 143.9, 170.6. HR-MS (ESI): Calcd for C$_{22}$H$_{21}$N$_2$O$_3$ [M + H]$^+$: 361.1552. Found: 361.1563.

3.2.3. Methyl 6,7-Didehydro-4,5α-epoxy-3,14β-dihydorxyindolo[2′,3′:6,7]morphinan-17-ylcarboxylate (6)

The hydrolysis of the crude compound, which was obtained by the reaction of compound **3** with 2,2,2-trichloroethyl chloroformate, was carried out using methanol instead of THF as a solvent, provided compound **5** (60%) and the title compound **6** (21%) as off-white amorphous material; IR (film) cm^{-1}: 3400, 1673, 1454, 1325, 909, 735. ^{1}H NMR (400 MHz, methanol-d_4): δ 1.58–1.68 (m, 1H), 2.39–2.50 (m, 1H), 2.60 (d, J = 15.7 Hz, 0.5H), 2.62 (d, J = 15.7 Hz, 0.5H), 2.82-2.99 (m, 3H), 3.32 (d, J = 18.2 Hz, 0.5H), 3.33 (d, J = 18.2 Hz, 0.5H), 3.71 (s, 1.5H), 3.73 (s, 1.5H), 4.00 (dd, J = 5.0, 13.7 Hz, 0.5H), 4.06 (dd, J = 5.0, 13.7 Hz, 0.5H), 4.59 (d, J = 6.5 Hz, 0.5H), 4.65 (d, J = 6.4 Hz, 0.5H), 5.59 (s, 1H), 6.54 (d, J = 8.1 Hz, 1H), 6.59 (d, J = 8.1 Hz, 1H), 6.94 (ddd, J = 0.9, 7.1, 7.9 Hz, 1H), 7.07 (ddd, J = 1.0, 7.1, 8.1 Hz, 1H), 7.30 (d, J = 8.1 Hz, 1H), 7.37 (d, J = 7.9 Hz, 1H), 7.87 (s, 1H), two protons (OH × 2) were not observed. ^{13}C NMR (100 MHz, methanol-d_4): δ 30.2, 30.4, 33.6, 38.2, 38.5, 48.8, 53.3, 58.0, 58.3, 74.4, 79.5, 85.99, 86.03, 110.8, 110.9, 112.2, 118.7, 119.4, 119.5, 119.8, 120.1, 123.3, 125.3, 128.1, 130.6, 130.7, 131.6, 138.8, 141.3, 144.9, 158.6. HR-MS (ESI): Calcd for $C_{24}H_{22}N_2NaO_5$ [M + Na]$^+$: 441.1426. Found: 441.1412.

3.2.4. General Synthesis of Sulfonamides 8

To a solution of compound **7** in dichloromethane were added sulfonyl chloride (RSO$_2$Cl) or trifluoromethylsulfonyl anhydride (2–4 eq) and triethylamine (2–4 eq), and the mixture was stirred at 0 °C. The progress of the reaction was monitored by TLC analysis. After completion of the reaction, the reaction mixture was poured into saturated sodium bicarbonate aqueous solution and extracted with chloroform. The combined organic layers were washed with brine and dried over anhydrous sodium sulfate. After removing the solvent *in vacuo*, the residue was purified by silica gel column chromatography.

3-((tert-Butyldimethylsilyl)oxy)-6,7-didehydro-4,5α-epoxy-17-(methylsulfonyl)indolo[2′,3′:6,7]morphinan-14β-ol (**8a**)

Yield: 78%, white oil, IR (neat) cm^{-1}: 3583, 2927, 1497, 1443, 1323, 1274, 1147, 1044, 955, 906, 842. ^{1}H NMR (400 MHz, CDCl$_3$): δ 0.02 (s, 3H), 0.04 (s, 3H), 0.89 (s, 9H), 1.82 (dd, J = 2.2, 12.8 Hz, 1H), 2.50 (ddd, J = 5.4, 12.8, 12.8 Hz, 1H), 2.69 (d, J = 15.9 Hz, 1H), 2.91 (d, J = 15.9 Hz, 1H), 3.03 (s, 3H), 3.15 (ddd, J = 3.5, 13.3, 13.3 Hz, 1H), 3.17 (d, J = 18.8 Hz, 1H), 3.39 (dd, J = 6.6, 18.8 Hz, 1H), 3.74 (dd, J = 5.3, 13.7 Hz, 1H), 4.41 (d, J = 6.6 Hz, 1H), 5.58 (s, 1H), 6.56 (d, J = 8.2 Hz, 1H), 6.61 (d, J = 8.2 Hz, 1H), 7.07 (ddd, J = 0.9, 7.1, 7.9 Hz, 1H), 7.19 (ddd, J = 1.1, 7.1, 8.1 Hz, 1H), 7.34 (br d, J = 8.2 Hz, 1H), 7.41 (br d, J = 8.0 Hz, 1H), 8.11 (s, 1H), a proton (OH) was not observed. ^{13}C NMR (100 MHz, CDCl$_3$): δ −4.8, −4.7, 18.2, 25.5, 29.7, 29.8, 33.9 , 38.9, 45.9, 47.9, 58.4, 73.3, 83.7, 109.7, 111.3, 118.8, 119.3, 119.8, 122.6, 123.4, 125.1, 126.5, 128.8, 129.3, 137.1, 138.9, 146.6. HR-MS (ESI): Calcd for $C_{29}H_{36}N_2NaO_5SSi$ [M + Na]$^+$: 575.2012. Found: 575.2029.

3-((tert-Butyldimethylsilyl)oxy)-6,7-didehydro-4,5α-epoxy-17-(1,1,1-trifluoromethylsulfonyl)indolo[2′,3′:6,7]morphinan-14β-ol (**8b**)

Yield: 74%, white amorphous material, IR (film) cm^{-1}: 3417, 2930, 2857, 1605, 1498, 1382, 1195, 1115, 1044, 842. ^{1}H NMR (400 MHz, CDCl$_3$): δ 0.02 (s, 3H), 0.04 (s, 3H), 0.88 (s, 9H), 1.75 (br d, J = 12.8 Hz, 1H), 2.53–2.81 (m, 3 H), 3.09 (d, J = 18.9 Hz, 1H), 3.24 (ddd, J = 2.9, 13.5, 13.5 Hz, 1H), 3.40 (dd, J = 6.6, 18.9 Hz, 1H), 3.86 (dd, J = 4.6, 13.9 Hz, 1H), 4.34 (d, J = 6.6 Hz, 1H), 5.57 (s, 1H), 6.57 (d, J = 8.2 Hz, 1H), 6.63 (d, J = 8.2 Hz, 1H), 7.05–7.10 (m, 1H), 7.20 (ddd, J = 1.1, 7.1, 8.2 Hz, 1H), 7.33 (dd, J = 0.7, 8.2 Hz, 1H), 7.37 (br d, J = 7.8 Hz, 1H), 8.15 (s, 1H), a proton (OH) was not observed. ^{13}C NMR (100 MHz, CDCl$_3$): δ −4.8, −4.7, 18.2, 25.5, 29.68, 29.71, 29.9, 40.5, 47.5, 60.0, 72.4, 83.6, 109.7, 111.3, 118.8, 119.2, 119.8, 122.8, 123.3, 124.0, 126.4, 128.6, 129.3, 137.1, 139.2, 146.6, the carbon binding to fluorines was not determined. HR-MS (ESI): Calcd for $C_{29}H_{34}F_3N_2O_5SSi$ [M + H]$^+$: 607.1910. Found: 607.1898.

3-((tert-Butyldimethylsilyl)oxy)-6,7-didehydro-4,5α-epoxy-
17-(phenylsulfonyl)indolo[2′,3′:6,7]morphinan-14β-ol (8c)

Yield: 90%, white oil, IR (neat) cm^{-1}: 3399, 3059, 3023, 2928, 2857, 1714, 1631, 1604, 1496, 1455. ^{1}H NMR (400 MHz, CDCl$_3$): δ −0.02 (s, 3H), 0.01 (s, 3H), 0.87 (s, 9H), 1.82 (dd, J = 1.0, 13.0 Hz, 1H), 2.45 (ddd, J = 5.4, 12.8, 12.8 Hz, 1H), 2.606 (d, J = 15.8 Hz, 1H), 2.609 (d, J = 18.8 Hz, 1H), 2.82 (s, 1H), 2.922 (d, J = 15.8 Hz, 1H), 2.924 (ddd, J = 3.6, 12.6, 12.6 Hz, 1H), 3.10 (dd, J = 6.6, 18.8 Hz, 1H), 3.80 (dd, J = 5.2, 12.7 Hz, 1H), 4.42 (d, J = 6.6 Hz, 1H), 5.58 (s, 1H), 6.36 (d, J = 8.2 Hz, 1H), 6.52 (d, J = 8.2 Hz, 1H), 7.04 (ddd, J = 0.9, 7.0, 7.9 Hz, 1H), 7.16 (ddd, J = 1.1, 7.0, 8.2 Hz, 1H), 7.30 (br d, J = 8.2 Hz, 1H), 7.39(br d, J = 7.8 Hz, 1H), 7.53–7.60 (m, 2H), 7.61–7.66 (m, 1H), 7.87–7.92 (m, 2H), 8.06 (s, 1H). ^{13}C NMR (100 MHz, CDCl$_3$): δ −4.8, −4.7, 18.2, 25.5, 29.1, 30.1, 30.5, 38.7, 47.7, 58.7, 72.8, 84.1, 110.7, 111.1, 118.9, 119.5, 122.4, 123.1, 124.7, 126.5, 127.2, 128.4, 129.4, 129.8, 132.9, 137.1, 138.9, 139.8, 146.5, two signals in the aromatic region would be overlapped. HR-MS (ESI): Calcd for C$_{34}$H$_{39}$N$_2$O$_5$SSi [M + H]$^+$: 615.2349. Found: 615.2359.

17-(Benzylsulfonyl)-3-((tert-butyldimethylsilyl)oxy)-6,7-didehydro-
4,5α-epoxyindolo[2′,3′:6,7]morphinan-14β-ol (8d)

Yield: 98%, white amorphous material, IR (film) cm^{-1}: 3397, 3061, 2953, 2928, 2856, 1497, 1324, 1274, 1043, 852. ^{1}H NMR (400 MHz, CDCl$_3$): δ 0.00 (s, 3H), 0.02 (s, 3H), 0.88 (s, 9H), 1.68 (dd, J = 2.0, 12.9 Hz, 1H), 2.33 (ddd, J = 5.4, 12.9, 12.9 Hz, 1H), 2.61 (d, J = 15.6 Hz, 1H), 2.84 (d, J = 15.6 Hz, 1H), 2.94 (d, J = 19.0 Hz, 1H), 3.02 (ddd, J = 3.5, 13.2, 13.2 Hz, 1H), 3.24 (dd, J = 6.6, 19.0 Hz, 1H), 3.38 (dd, J = 5.3, 13.6 Hz, 1H), 4.23 (d, J = 6.6 Hz, 1H), 4.32 (d, J = 14.0 Hz, 1H), 4.42 (d, J = 14.0 Hz, 1H), 5.54 (s, 1H), 6.49 (d, J = 8.2 Hz, 1H), 6.57 (d, J = 8.2 Hz, 1H), 7.04 (ddd, J = 0.9, 7.1, 7.9 Hz, 1H), 7.17 (ddd, J = 1.0, 7.1, 8.2 Hz, 1H), 7.32 (d, J = 8.2 Hz, 1H), 7.38 (d, J = 7.9 Hz, 1H), 7.37–7.50 (m, 5H), 8.07 (s,1H), a proton (OH) was not observed. ^{13}C NMR (100 MHz, CDCl$_3$): δ −4.8, −4.7, 18.2, 25.5, 29.5, 29.6, 33.2, 39.5, 47.7, 58.7, 58.9, 73.0, 83.9, 110.4, 111.2, 118.8, 119.0, 119.6, 122.4, 123.1, 125.1, 126.6, 128.6, 128.8, 128.9, 129.4, 129.7, 130.6, 137.1, 138.8, 146.4. HR-MS (ESI): Calcd for C$_{35}$H$_{41}$N$_2$O$_5$SSi [M + H]$^+$: 629.2505. Found: 629.2492.

3-((tert-Butyldimethylsilyl)oxy)-6,7-didehydro-4,5α-epoxy-
17-((2-phenyethyl)sulfonyl)indolo[2′,3′:6,7]morphinan-14β-ol (8e)

Yield: 46%, pale yellow oil, IR (neat) cm^{-1}: 2928, 1497, 1443, 1275, 1147, 1044, 907, 853, 741, 423. ^{1}H NMR (400 MHz, CDCl$_3$): δ 0.01 (s, 3H), 0.04 (s, 3H), 0.88 (s, 9H), 1.78 (br d, J = 12.7 Hz, 1H), 2.47 (ddd, J = 5.3, 12.7, 12.7 Hz, 1 H), 2.68 (d, J = 15.8 Hz, 1H), 2.87 (d, J = 15.8 Hz, 1H), 3.11-3.23 (m , 4H), 3.32-3.43 (m, 3 H), 3.75 (dd, J = 5.1, 13.6 Hz, 1H), 4.33 (d, J = 6.4 Hz, 1H), 5.55 (s, 1H), 6.54 (d, J = 8.2 Hz, 1H), 6.60 (d, J = 8.2 Hz, 1H), 7.04–7.09 (m, 1H), 7.16-7.35 (m, 7H), 7.40 (br d, J = 7.9 Hz, 1H), 8.13 (br s, 1H), a proton (OH) was not observed. ^{13}C NMR (100 MHz, CDCl$_3$): δ −4.8, −4.7, 18.2, 25.5, 28.4, 29.7, 29.8, 33.6, 38.9, 47.9, 54.4, 58.4, 73.1, 83.9, 110.1, 111.2, 118.8, 119.1, 119.7, 122.5, 123.2, 125.1, 126.6, 126.8, 128.4, 128.7, 128.8, 129.6, 137.1, 138.2, 138.8, 146.5. HR-MS (ESI): Calcd for C$_{36}$H$_{42}$N$_2$NaO$_5$SSi [M + Na]$^+$: 665.2481. Found: 665.2468.

3-((tert-Butyldimethylsilyl)oxy)-17-(cyclopropylsulfonyl)-6,7-didehydro-
4,5α-epoxyindolo[2′,3′:6,7]morphinan-14β-ol (8f)

Yield: 98%, white amorphous material, IR (film) cm^{-1}: 3397, 2928, 1604, 1497, 1444, 1325, 1274, 1147, 1046, 937, 906, 852. ^{1}H NMR (400 MHz, CDCl$_3$): δ 0.01 (s, 3H), 0.04 (s, 3H), 0.89 (s, 9H), 1.00–1.10 (m, 2H), 1.20–1.28 (m, 2H), 1.83 (br d, J = 11.2 Hz, 1H), 2.44–2.55 (m, 2H), 2.67 (d, J = 15.8 Hz, 1H), 2.83 (s, 1H), 2.93 (d, J = 15.8 Hz, 1H), 3.13 (ddd, J = 3.4, 12.9, 12.9 Hz, 1H), 3.32 (d, J = 18.7 Hz, 1H), 3.37 (dd, J = 6.2, 18.7 Hz, 1H), 3.73 (dd, J = 5.0, 13.0 Hz, 1H), 4.35 (d, J = 6.2 Hz, 1H), 5.60 (s, 1H), 6.55 (d, J = 8.2 Hz, 1H), 6.60 (d, J = 8.2 Hz, 1H), 7.05 (br dd, J = 7.5, 7.5 Hz, 1H), 7.18 (br dd, J = 7.6, 7.6 Hz, 1H), 7.32 (d, J = 8.2 Hz, 1H), 7.40 (d, J = 7.9 Hz, 1H), 8.09 (s, 1H). ^{13}C NMR (100 MHz, CDCl$_3$): δ −4.8, −4.7, 5.3, 5.7, 18.2, 25.5, 29.2, 29.7, 30.0, 32.4, 38.9, 47.7, 58.8, 72.8, 84.1, 110.5, 111.2, 118.8, 118.9, 119.5, 122.4,

123.0, 124.9, 126.5, 128.6, 129.9, 137.1, 138.9, 146.5. HR-MS (ESI): Calcd for $C_{31}H_{39}N_2O_5SSi$ [M + H]$^+$: 579.2349. Found: 579.2367.

3.2.5. 3-((tert-Butyldimethylsilyl)oxy)-6,7-didehydro-4,5α-epoxy-17-(ethenylsulfonyl)indolo[2',3':6,7]morphinan-14β-ol (8g)

To a solution of compound 7 (29.9 mg, 0.063 mmol) in dichloromethane (3 mL) were added 2-chloroethanesulfonyl chloride (22.0 μL, 0.20 mmol) and 0.5 M sodium hydroxide aqueous solution (15 μL), and the mixture was stirred at 0 °C for 20 h. The reaction mixture was poured into saturated sodium bicarbonate aqueous solution and extracted with chloroform. The combined organic layers were washed with brine and dried over anhydrous sodium sulfate. After removing the solvent *in vacuo*, the residue was purified by silica gel column chromatography to give the title compound 8f (19.8 mg, 56%) as a white amorphous material; IR (film) cm^{-1}: 3397, 2928, 2857, 1497, 1444, 1325, 1148, 1043, 852, 744. ^{1}H NMR (400 MHz, CDCl$_3$): δ 0.01 (s, 3H), 0.04 (s, 3H), 0.88 (s, 9H), 1.80 (dd, *J* = 2.1, 13.0 Hz, 1H), 2.46 (ddd, *J* = 5.4, 12.8, 12.8 Hz, 1H), 2.67 (dd, *J* = 0.9, 15.9 Hz, 1H), 2.91 (d, *J* = 15.9 Hz, 1H), 3.06 (ddd, *J* = 3.5, 13.1, 13.1 Hz, 1H), 3.17 (d, *J* = 18.8 Hz, 1H), 3.34 (dd, *J* = 6.5, 18.8 Hz, 1H), 3.63 (dd, *J* = 5.3, 13.3 Hz, 1H), 4.37 (d, *J* = 6.5 Hz, 1H), 5.58 (s, 1H), 5.99 (d, *J* = 10.0 Hz, 1H), 6.31 (d, *J* = 16.6 Hz, 1H), 6.54 (d, *J* = 8.2 Hz, 1H), 6.60 (d, *J* = 8.2 Hz, 1H), 6.65 (dd, *J* = 10.0, 16.6 Hz, 1H), 7.06 (ddd, *J* = 0.8, 7.0, 7.9 Hz, 1H), 7.18 (ddd, *J* = 1.1, 7.0, 8.2 Hz, 1H), 7.33 (br d, *J* = 8.2 Hz, 1H), 7.40 (br d, *J* = 7.8 Hz, 1H), 8.10 (s, 1H), a proton (OH) was not observed. ^{13}C NMR (100 MHz, CDCl$_3$): δ −4.8, −4.7, 18.2, 25.5, 29.4, 29.6, 32.6, 38.3, 47.8, 58.4, 72.9, 84.0, 110.4, 111.2, 118.9, 119.1, 119.6, 122.5, 123.2, 124.9, 126.6, 127.1, 128.6, 129.7, 135.7, 137.1, 138.9, 146.5. HR-MS (ESI): Calcd for $C_{30}H_{37}N_2O_5SSi$ [M + H]$^+$: 565.2192. Found: 565.2195.

3.2.6. General Synthesis of Test Compounds 9

To a solution of compound 8 in THF was added 1.0 M solution of tetrabutylammonium fluoride in THF (excess), and the mixture was stirred at room temperature. The progress of the reaction was monitored by TLC analysis. After completion of the reaction, the reaction mixture was poured into saturated sodium bicarbonate aqueous solution and extracted with a mixed solvent (chloroform: ethanol = 3:1). The combined organic layers were washed with brine and dried over anhydrous sodium sulfate. After removing the solvent *in vacuo*, the residue was purified by silica gel column chromatography.

6,7-Didehydro-4,5α-epoxy-17-(methylsulfonyl)indolo[2',3':6,7]morphinan-3,14β-diol (9a)

Yield: 87%, white amorphous material, IR (film) cm^{-1}: 3855, 3823, 3364, 1691, 1314, 1149, 899, 803, 752, 467. ^{1}H NMR (400 MHz, CDCl$_3$): δ 1.80 (dd, *J* = 2.2, 12.9 Hz, 1H), 2.49 (ddd, *J* = 5.4, 12.8, 12.8 Hz, 1H), 2.61 (dd, *J* = 0.9, 15.9 Hz, 1H), 2.67 (s, 1H), 2.91 (d, *J* = 15.9 Hz, 1H), 3.22 (s, 3H), 3.14 (ddd, *J* = 3.5, 13.3, 13.3 Hz, 1H), 3.16 (d, *J* = 18.7 Hz, 1H), 3.36 (dd, *J* = 6.5, 18.7 Hz, 1H), 3.74 (dd, *J* = 5.3, 13.6 Hz, 1H), 4.40 (d, *J* = 6.5 Hz, 1H), 5.02 (br s, 1H), 5.61 (s, 1H), 6.58 (d, *J* = 8.2 Hz, 1H), 6.65 (d, *J* = 8.2 Hz, 1H), 7.07 (ddd, *J* = 0.9, 7.0, 7.9 Hz, 1H), 7.18 (ddd, *J* = 1.1, 7.0, 8.2 Hz, 1H), 7.28 (d, *J* = 8.2 Hz, 1H), 7.40 (d, *J* = 7.9 Hz, 1H), 8.29 (s, 1H). ^{13}C NMR (100 MHz, CDCl$_3$): δ 29.5, 30.9, 32.9, 38.6, 40.0, 48.0, 58.4, 73.2, 85.0, 110.5, 111.4, 117.8, 118.9, 119.6, 119.8, 123.4, 124.1, 126.5, 128.4, 129.2, 137.1, 139.3, 143.0. HR-MS (ESI): Calcd for $C_{23}H_{23}N_2O_5S$ [M + H]$^+$: 439.1328. Found: 439.1336. Anal. Calcd for $C_{23}H_{22}N_2O_5S\cdot1.1EtOH$: C, 61.87; H, 5.89; N, 5.73. Found C, 61.47; H, 5.53; N, 5.36.

6,7-Didehydro-4,5α-epoxy-17-(1,1,1-trifluoromethylsulfonyl)indolo[2',3':6,7]morphinan-3,14β-diol (9b)

Yield: 74%, white amorphous material, IR (film) cm^{-1}: 3410, 2924, 1707, 1638, 1618, 1508, 1456, 1380, 1195, 1113. ^{1}H NMR (400 MHz, CDCl$_3$): δ 1.77 (br d, *J* = 12.6 Hz, 1H), 2.63 (ddd, *J* = 5.3, 12.8, 12.8 Hz, 1H), 2.65 (d, *J* = 15.9 Hz, 1H), 2.82 (d, *J* = 15.9 Hz, 1H), 3.16 (d, *J* = 18.9 Hz, 1H), 3.25 (ddd, *J* = 2.8, 13.3, 13.3 Hz, 1H), 3.44 (dd, *J* = 6.7, 18.9 Hz, 1H), 3.88 (dd, *J* = 4.9, 13.8 Hz, 1H), 4.38 (d, *J* = 6.7 Hz, 1H), 4.92 (br s, 1H), 5.65 (s, 1H), 6.61 (d, *J* = 8.2 Hz, 1H), 6.68 (d, *J* = 8.2 Hz, 1H), 7.08 (dd, *J* = 7.4, 7.4 Hz, 1H), 7.13-7.28 (m, 1H), 7.32 (br d, *J* = 8.2 Hz, 1H), 7.37 (br d, *J* = 7.9 Hz, 1H), 8.25 (s, 1H), a proton (OH) was not observed. ^{13}C NMR (100 MHz, CDCl$_3$): δ 29.7, 37.7, 40.5, 47.6, 59.9, 72.6, 85.0, 110.0, 111.5, 118.1, 118.9, 119.8, 119.9, 121.5, 123.5, 126.3, 128.1, 128.8, 137.1, 139.4, 142.9, a carbon in an aliphatic region was not observed, and the carbon binding to fluoride was not determined. HR-MS (ESI): Calcd for C$_{23}$H$_{20}$F$_3$N$_2$O$_5$S [M + H]$^+$: 493.1045. Found: 493.1058. Anal. Calcd for C$_{23}$H$_{19}$F$_3$N$_2$O$_5$S·MeOH: C, 54.85; H, 4.60; N, 5.33. Found C, 54.90; H, 4.73; N, 5.12.

6,7-Didehydro-4,5α-epoxy-17-(phenylsulfonyl)indolo[2′,3′:6,7]morphinan-3,14β-diol (**9c**)

Yield: 84%, white amorphous material, IR (film) cm^{-1}: 3395, 2961, 2874, 1719, 1638, 1457, 1323, 1273, 1159, 730. ^{1}H NMR (400 MHz, aceton-*d$_6$*): δ 1.69-1.76 (m, 1H), 2.59 (ddd, *J* = 5.4, 12.7, 12.7 Hz, 1H), 2.62 (dd, *J* = 1.0, 15.9 Hz, 1H), 2.67 (d, *J* = 18.6 Hz, 1H), 2.92 (ddd, *J* = 3.5, 12.8, 12.8 Hz, 1H), 2.94 (d, *J* = 15.9 Hz, 1H), 3.21 (dd, *J* = 6.4, 18.6 Hz, 1H), 3.73 (dd, *J* = 5.2, 12.8 Hz, 1H), 4.14 (s, 1H), 4.47 (d, *J* = 6.4 Hz, 1H), 5.59 (s, 1H), 6.39 (d, *J* = 8.1 Hz, 1H), 6.56 (d, *J* = 8.1 Hz, 1H), 6.96 (ddd, *J* = 0.9, 7.1, 8.0 Hz, 1H), 7.10 (ddd, *J* = 1.1, 7.1, 8.1 Hz, 1H), 7.35–7.39 (m, 2H), 7.59–7.67 (m, 3H), 7.84 (br s, 1H), 7.93-7.99 (m, 2H), 10.2 (br s, 1H). ^{13}C NMR (100 MHz, DMSO-*d$_6$*): δ 28.8, 29.0, 31.3, 38.5, 47.0, 58.2, 71.8, 71.9, 83.8, 109.5, 111.4, 117.3, 118.38, 118.44, 121.9, 123.1, 126.4, 126.9, 129.3, 129.5, 130.0, 132.6, 136.8, 140.3, 140.5, 143.2, two signals in the aromatic region would be overlapped. HR-MS (ESI): Calcd for C$_{28}$H$_{25}$N$_2$O$_5$S [M + H]$^+$: 501.1484. Found: 501.1474. Anal. Calcd for C$_{28}$H$_{24}$N$_2$O$_5$S·H$_2$O: C, 64.85; H, 5.05; N, 5.40. Found C, 64.92; H, 4.83; N, 5.31.

17-(Benzylsulfonyl)-6,7-didehydro-4,5α-epoxyindolo[2′,3′:6,7]morphinan-3,14β-diol (**9d**)

Yield: 84%, white amorphous material, IR (film) cm^{-1}: 3405, 1701, 1638, 1499, 1457, 1321, 1115, 1040, 862, 742, 700. ^{1}H NMR (400 MHz, acetone-*d$_6$*): δ 1.62 (dd, *J* = 2.3, 12.7 Hz, 1H), 2.58 (ddd, *J* = 5.5, 12.8, 12.8 Hz, 1H), 2.67 (dd, *J* = 0.9, 15.9 Hz, 1H), 2.95 (d, *J* = 15.9 Hz, 1H), 2.88-3.08 (m, 1H), 3.01 (d, *J* = 18.7 Hz, 1H), 3.38 (dd, *J* = 6.2, 18.7 Hz, 1H), 3.56 (dd, *J* = 5.3, 13.7 Hz, 1H), 4.28 (d, *J* = 6.2 Hz, 1H), 4.39 (s, 1H), 4.47 (d, *J* = 13.7 Hz, 1H), 4.56 (d, *J* = 13.7 Hz, 1H), 5.60 (s, 1H), 6.52 (d, *J* = 8.0 Hz, 1H), 6.62 (d, *J* = 8.0 Hz, 1H), 6.85–7.02 (m, 1H), 7.12 (ddd, *J* = 1.0, 7.0, 8.2 Hz, 1H), 7.24–7.42 (m, 5H), 7.53–7.59 (m, 2H), 7.87 (br s, 1H), 10.23 (s, 1H). ^{13}C NMR (100 MHz, CDCl$_3$): δ 29.4, 29.6, 32.9, 39.4, 47.8, 58.6, 59.0, 73.2, 85.0, 110.5, 111.5, 117.8 118.8, 119.5, 119.6, 123.1, 124.1, 126.4, 128.3, 128.9, 129.16, 129.21, 130.6, 137.1, 139.2, 142.8, 152.8. HR-MS (ESI): Calcd for C$_{29}$H$_{27}$O$_5$S [M + H]$^+$: 515.1641. Found: 515.1632. Anal. Calcd for C$_{29}$H$_{26}$N$_2$O$_5$S·2H$_2$O·EtOH: C, 62.40; H, 6.08; N, 6.69. Found C, 62.12; H, 5.75; N, 4.43.

6,7-Didehydro-4,5α-epoxy-17-((2-phenylethyl)sulfonyl)indolo[2′,3′:6,7]morphinan-3,14β-diol (**9e**)

Yield: 79%, white amorphous material, IR (film) cm^{-1}: 3407, 2923, 1504, 1455, 1319, 1146, 1041, 903, 736. ^{1}H NMR (400 MHz, CDCl$_3$): δ 1.78 (br d, *J* = 12.0 Hz, 1H), 2.47 (ddd, *J* = 5.2, 12.7, 12.7 Hz, 1H), 2.63 (d, *J* = 15.7 Hz, 1H), 2.64 (s, 1H), 2.87 (d, *J* = 15.7 Hz, 1H), 3.09–3.24 (m, 4H), 3.30–3.45 (m, 3H), 3.75 (dd, *J* = 4.9, 13.8 Hz, 1H), 4.34 (d, *J* = 6.4 Hz, 1H), 5.14 (br s, 1H), 5.59 (s, 1H), 6.57 (d, *J* = 8.2 Hz, 1H), 6.64 (d, *J* = 8.2 Hz, 1H), 7.06 (dd, *J* = 7.4, 7.4 Hz, 1 H), 7.17 (dd, *J* = 7.5, 7.5 Hz, 1H), 7.19–7.33 (m, 6H), 7.38 (d, *J* = 7.8 Hz, 1H), 8.31 (s, 1H) 1H). ^{13}C NMR (100 MHz, CDCl$_3$): δ 20.1, 29.6, 29.9, 33.4, 38.9, 48.1, 54.5, 58.4, 73.2, 84.9, 110.4, 111.5, 117.8, 118.9, 119.6, 119.8, 123.4, 124.2, 126.5, 126.9, 128.42, 128.45, 128.9, 129.2, 137.2, 138.2, 139.3, 145.0. HR-MS (ESI): Calcd for C$_{30}$H$_{28}$N$_2$NaO$_5$S [M + Na]$^+$: 551.1617. Found: 551.1623. Anal. Calcd for C$_{30}$H$_{28}$N$_2$O$_5$S·3.5H$_2$O·0.5CHCl$_3$: C, 56.24; H, 5.49; N, 4.30. Found C, 56.36; H, 5.71; N, 3.99.

17-(Cyclopropylsulfonyl)-6,7-didehydro-4,5α-epoxyindolo[2′,3′:6,7]morphinan-3,14β-diol (**9f**)

Yield: 96%, white amorphous material, IR (film) cm^{-1}: 3400, 2922, 1719, 1638, 1508, 1457, 1322, 1145, 1044, 899, 726, 499. ^{1}H NMR (400 MHz, aceton-*d$_6$*): δ 0.95–1.14 (m, 4H), 1.73 (dd, *J* = 2.0, 12.7 Hz, 1H), 2.659 (ddd, *J* = 5.4, 12.7, 12.7 Hz, 1H), 2.665 (d, *J* = 15.6 Hz, 1H), 2.74–2.83 (m, 1H), 2.94 (d, *J* = 15.6 Hz, 1H), 3.11 (ddd, *J* = 3.5, 13.1, 13.1 Hz, 1H), 3.25 (dd, *J* = 18.7 Hz, 1H), 3.43 (dd, *J* = 6.7, 18.7 Hz, 1H), 3.70 (dd, *J* = 5.4, 13.3 Hz, 1H), 4.23 (s, 1H), 4.35 (d, *J* = 6.7 Hz, 1H), 5.61 (s, 1H), 6.57 (d, *J* = 8.1 Hz, 1H), 6.63 (d, *J* = 8.1 Hz, 1H), 6.97 (ddd, *J* = 0.9, 7.1, 7.9 Hz, 1H), 7.11 (ddd, *J* = 1.0, 7.1, 8.2 Hz, 1H), 7.381

(br d, J = 8.2 Hz, 1H), 7.388 (br d, J = 8.3 Hz, 1H), 10.2 (s, 1H), a proton (OH) was not observed. ^{13}C NMR (100 MHz, CDCl$_3$): δ 5.3, 5.7, 29.2, 29.8, 30.0, 32.3, 38.9, 47.8, 58.8, 73.1, 85.2, 110.7, 111.4, 117.8, 118.9, 119.5, 119.6, 123.2, 123.9, 126.4, 128.2, 129.5, 137.1, 139.3, 142.9. HR-MS (ESI): Calcd for C$_{25}$H$_{24}$N$_2$NaO$_5$S [M + Na]$^+$: 487.1304. Found: 487.1283. Anal. Calcd for C$_{25}$H$_{24}$N$_2$O$_5$S·1.5H$_2$O·0.2CHCl$_3$: C, 58.72; H, 5.32; N, 5.43. Found C, 58.68; H, 5.16; N, 5.08.

6,7-Didehydro-4,5α-epoxy-17-(ethenylsulfonyl)indolo[2′,3′:6,7]morphinan-3,14β-diol (**9g**)

Yield: 71%, white amorphous material, IR (film) cm^{-1}: 3400, 1455, 1322, 1146, 903, 738. ^{1}H NMR (400 MHz, CDCl$_3$): δ 1.79 (dd, J = 2.1, 12.8 Hz, 1H), 2.46 (ddd, J = 5.3, 12.8, 12.8 Hz, 1H), 2.63 (d, J = 15.8 Hz, 1H), 2.78 (s, 1H), 2.90 (d, J = 15.8 Hz, 1H), 3.05 (ddd, J = 3.5, 13.1, 13.1 Hz, 1H), 3.14 (d, J = 18.7 Hz, 1H), 3.32 (dd, J = 6.5, 18.7 Hz, 1H), 3.63 (dd, J = 5.3, 13.3 Hz, 1H), 4.37 (d, J = 6.5 Hz, 1H), 5.12 (br s, 1H), 5.61 (s, 1H), 5.99 (d, J = 9.8 Hz, 1H), 6.32 (d, J = 16.4 Hz, 1H), 6.65 (d, J = 8.2 Hz, 1H), 6.639 (d, J = 8.2 Hz, 1H), 6.641 (dd, J = 9.8, 16.4 Hz, 1H), 7.06 (dd, J = 7.4, 7.4 Hz, 1H), 7.17 (dd, J = 7.5, 7.5 Hz, 1H), 7.25–7.29 (m, 1H), 7.39 (d, J = 7.9 Hz, 1H), 8.30 (s, 1H). ^{13}C NMR (100 MHz, CDCl$_3$): δ 29.4, 29.6, 32.5, 38.4, 47.9, 58.4, 73.1, 85.1, 110.7, 111.4, 117.8, 118.9, 119.5, 119.8, 123.4, 124.0, 126.5, 127.2, 128.3, 129.3, 135.6, 137.1, 139.3, 142.9. HR-MS (ESI): Calcd for C$_{24}$H$_{22}$N$_2$NaO$_5$S [M + Na]$_+$: 473.1147. Found: 473.1138. Anal. Calcd for C$_{24}$H$_{22}$N$_2$O$_5$S·EtOH·0.3CHCl$_3$: C, 59.33; H, 5.36; N, 5.26. Found C, 59.17; H, 5.22; N, 5.15.

3.3. Calculation of the Most Stable Conformations of Alkyl-, Amide-, and Sulfonamide-Type Piperidines

The initial geometries of the molecular models for density functional theory (DFT) calculations were prepared using Schrödinger suites (Schrödinger, LLC) [48–54]. Structural optimizations were performed for the prepared molecular models with ωB97XD/6-31G(d,p) level of theory, respectively. Their vibration frequencies were calculated at the same level to confirm their stationary structure. All of the DFT calculations were performed using the Gaussian09 program [55].

3.4. Bioassays

3.4.1. Membrane Preparation

The human MOR, DOR, or KOR recombinant CHO cell pellets were resuspended in 50 mM Tris–HCl buffer containing 5 mM MgCl$_2$, 1 mM ethylene glycol bis(2-aminoethyl ether)-*N,N,N,N*-tetraacetic acid (EGTA), pH 7.4. The cell suspensions were disrupted by use of a glassteflon homogeniser and centrifuged at 48,000× *g* for 15 min. The supernatant was discarded and the pellets were resuspended in buffer at a concentration of 5 mg protein/mL and stored at −80 °C until further use.

3.4.2. Competitive Binding Assays

Human MOR, DOR, or KOR recombinant CHO cell membranes were incubated for 2 h at 25 °C in 0.25 mL of the buffer containing with various concentrations of the tested compound, 2 nM [^{3}H] DAMGO, [^{3}H] DPDPE, or [^{3}H] U69,593 (PerkinElmer, Inc., MA, USA), respectively. The incubation was terminated by collecting membranes on Filtermat B filter (PerkinElmer, Inc.) using a FilterMate™ harvester (PerkinElmer, Inc.). The filters were then washed three times with 50 mM Tris–HCl buffer, pH 7.4. Then, MeltiLex scintillant (PerkinElmer, Inc.) was melted onto the dried filters. Radioactivity was determined by a MicroBeta scintillation counter (PerkinElmer, Inc.). Nonspecific binding was measured in the presence of 10 µM unlabeled DAMGO, DPDPE, or U-69,593 (PerkinElmer, Inc.). K_i and 95% CI values were calculated by Prism software (version 5.0).

3.4.3. [^{35}S]GTPγS Binding Assays

Human MOR, DOR, or KOR recombinant CHO cell membranes were incubated for 2 h at 25 °C in 0.25 mL of 50 mM Tris–HCl buffer containing 5 mM MgCl$_2$, 1 mM EGTA, 100 mM NaCl, pH 7.4 with various concentrations of the tested compound, 30 µM guanosine 5-diphosphate (GDP) and 0.1 nM

[^{35}S]GTPγS (PerkinElmer, Inc.). The incubation was terminated by collecting membranes on Filtermat B filter (PerkinElmer, Inc.) using a FilterMate™ harvester (Perkin Elmer, Inc.). The filters were then washed three times with 50 mM Tris–HCl buffer, pH 7.4. Then, MeltiLex scintillant (PerkinElmer, Inc.) was melted onto the dried filters. Radioactivity was determined by a MicroBeta scintillation counter (PerkinElmer, Inc.). EC_{50}, E_{max}, and 95% CI values were calculated by Prism software (version 5.0). Nonspecific binding was measured in the presence of 10 µM unlabeled GTPγS (PerkinElmer, Inc.). DPDPE and ICI-174,864 (PerkinElmer, Inc.) were used as the standard DOR full agonist and full inverse agonist, respectively.

4. Conclusions

We synthesized sulfonamide-type NTI derivatives to compare their functional activities for the DOR with those of the corresponding alkyl- and amide-type NTI derivatives. Among them, cyclopropylsulfonamide **9f** (SYK-839) was the most potent full inverse agonist. Its potency and efficacy were comparable to those of SYK-623, a previously reported amide-type full inverse agonist. On the other hand, phenethylsulfonamide **9e** (SYK-901) showed full agonist activity with moderate potency. Not only the sulfonamide-type NTI derivatives but also the alkyl- and amide-type derivatives, which induced activities for the DOR from full inverse agonist to full agonist, are expected to be useful compounds for investigation of the relationship among the interactions of ligands with the DOR, conformational changes of the DOR, and the induced functional activities.

Supplementary Materials: The following are available online. Synthesis of **5** hydrochloride, previously reported synthetic method of **7**, optimization of the reaction conditions for synthesis of **5**, synthesis of SYK-903, and ^{1}H and ^{13}C NMR spectra are available online.

Author Contributions: Conceptualization, S.H. and H.F.; methodology, H.F.; synthetic experiment, C.I., T.K., and S.I.; evaluation of compounds, S.H.; Analysis and data curation, C.I., A.H., S.H., and H.F.; conformational analysis, D.H. and H.G.; writing, H.G. and H.F. All authors have read and agreed to the published version of the manuscript.

Funding: This research received no external funding.

Acknowledgments: We also acknowledge the Institute of Instrumental Analysis of Kitasato University, School of Pharmacy for its facilities.

Conflicts of Interest: The authors declare no conflict of interest.

References

1. Chalmers, D.T.; Behan, D.P. The use of constitutively active gpcrs in drug discovery and functional genomics. *Nat. Rev. Drug Discov.* **2002**, *1*, 599–608. [CrossRef]
2. Costa, T.; Cotecchia, S. Historical review: Negative efficacy and the constitutive activity of G-protein coupled receptors. *Trends Pharmacol. Sci.* **2005**, *26*, 618–624. [CrossRef] [PubMed]
3. Bond, R.A.; IJzerman, A.P. Recent developments in constitutive receptor activity and inverse agonism, and their potential for GPCR drug discovery. *Trends Pharmacol. Sci.* **2006**, *27*, 92–96. [CrossRef] [PubMed]
4. Hirayama, S.; Fujii, H. δ Opioid Receptor Inverse Agonists and their In Vivo Pharmacological Effects. *Curr. Top. Med. Chem.* **2020**, in press. [CrossRef] [PubMed]
5. Recent examples (from ref. 5 to ref. 20), Cherney, R.J.; Cornelius, L.A.M.; Srivastava, A.; Weigelt, C.A.; Marcoux, D.; Duan, J.J.-W.; Shi, Q.; Batt, D.G.; Liu, Q.; Yip, S.; et al. Discovery of BMS-986251: A Clinically Viable, Potent, and Selective RORγt Inverse Agonist. *ACS Med. Chem. Lett.* **2020**, *11*, 1221–1227. [CrossRef]
6. Gege, C.; Albers, M.; Kinzel, O.; Kleymann, G.; Schlütera, T.; Steeneck, C.; Hoffmann, T.; Xue, X.; Cummingsc, M.D.; Spurlinoc, J.; et al. Optimization and biological evaluation of thiazole-bis-amide inverse agonists of RORγt. *Bioorg. Med. Chem. Lett.* **2020**, *30*, 127205. [CrossRef]
7. Nakajima, R.; Oono, H.; Sugiyama, S.; Matsueda, Y.; Ida, T.; Kakuda, S.; Hirata, J.; Baba, A.; Makino, A.; Matsuyama, R.; et al. Discovery of [1,2,4]Triazolo[1,5-*a*]pyridine Derivatives as Potent and Orally Bioavailable RORγt Inverse Agonists. *ACS Med. Chem. Lett.* **2020**, *11*, 528–534. [CrossRef]

8. Sun, N.; Ma, X.; Zhou, K.; Zhu, C.; Cao, Z.; Wang, Y.; Xu, J.; Fu, W. Discovery of novel N-sulfonamide-tetrahydroquinolines as potent retinoic acid receptor-related orphan receptor γt inverse agonists for the treatment of autoimmune diseases. *Eur. J. Med. Chem.* **2020**, *187*, 111984. [CrossRef]
9. Shrader, S.H.; Song, Z. Discovery of endogenous inverse agonists for G protein-coupled receptor 6. *Biochem. Biophys. Res. Commun.* **2020**, *522*, 1041–1045. [CrossRef]
10. Poli, G.; Dimmito, M.P.; Mollica, A.; Zengin, G.; Benyhe, S.; Zador, F.; Stefanucci, A. Discovery of Novel μ-Opioid Receptor Inverse Agonist from a Combinatorial Library of Tetrapeptides through Structure-Based Virtual Screening. *Molecules* **2019**, *24*, 3872. [CrossRef]
11. Sato, A.; Fukase, Y.; Kono, M.; Ochida, A.; Oda, T.; Sasaki, Y.; Ishii, N.; Tomata, Y.; Fukumoto, S.; Imai, Y.N. Design and Synthesis of Conformationally Constrained RORγt Inverse Agonists. *ChemMedChem* **2019**, *14*, 1917–1932. [CrossRef] [PubMed]
12. Shaikh, N.S.; Iyer, J.P.; Munot, Y.S.; Mukhopadhyay, P.P.; Raje, A.A.; Nagaraj, R.; Jamdar, V.; Gavhane, R.; Lohote, M.; Sherkar, P.; et al. Discovery and pharmacological evaluation of indole derivatives as potent and selective RORγt inverse agonist for multiple autoimmune conditions. *Bioorg. Med. Chem. Lett.* **2019**, *29*, 2208–2217. [CrossRef] [PubMed]
13. Lu, Z.; Duan, J.J.-W.; Xiao, H.; Neels, J.; Wu, D.; Weigelt, C.A.; Sack, J.S.; Khan, J.; Ruzanov, M.; An, Y.; et al. Identification of potent, selective and orally bioavailable phenyl ((R)-3-phenylpyrrolidin-3-yl)sulfone analogues as RORγt inverse agonists. *Bioorg. Med. Chem. Lett.* **2019**, *29*, 2265–2269. [CrossRef] [PubMed]
14. Amato, G.; Manke, A.; Wiethe, R.; Vasukuttan, V.; Snyder, R.; Yueh, Y.L.; Decker, A.; Runyon, S.; Maitra, R. Functionalized 6-(Piperidin-1-yl)-8,9-Diphenyl Purines as Peripherally Restricted Inverse Agonists of the CB1 Receptor. *J. Med. Chem.* **2019**, *62*, 6330–6345.
15. Amaudrut, J.; Argiriadi, M.A.; Barth, M.; Breinlinger, E.C.; Bressac, D.; Broqua, P.; Calderwood, D.J.; Chatar, M.; Cusac, K.P.; Gauld, S.B.; et al. Discovery of novel quinoline sulphonamide derivatives as potent, selective and orally active RORγ inverse agonists. *Bioorg. Med. Chem. Lett.* **2019**, *29*, 1799–1806. [CrossRef]
16. Tanis, V.M.; Venkatesan, H.; Cummings, M.D.; Albers, M.; Barbay, J.K.; Herman, K.; Kummer, D.A.; Milligan, C.; Nelen, M.I.; Nishimura, R.; et al. 3-Substituted Quinolines as RORγt Inverse Agonists. *Bioorg. Med. Chem. Lett.* **2019**, *29*, 1463–1470. [CrossRef]
17. Zhang, Y.; Wu, X.; Xue, X.; Li, C.; Wang, J.; Wang, R.; Zhang, C.; Wang, C.; Shi, Y.; Zou, L.; et al. Discovery and Characterization of XY101, a Potent, Selective, and Orally Bioavailable RORγ Inverse Agonist for Treatment of Castration-Resistant Prostate Cancer. *J. Med. Chem.* **2019**, *62*, 4716–4730.
18. Troxler, T.; Feuerbach, D.; Zhang, X.; Yang, C.R.; Lagu, B.; Perrone, M.; Wang, T.-L.; Briner, K.; Bock, M.G.; Auberson, Y.P. The Discovery of LML134, a Histamine H3 Receptor Inverse Agonist for the Clinical Treatment of Excessive Sleep Disorders. *ChemMedChem* **2019**, *14*, 1238–1247. [CrossRef]
19. Kim, J.; Song, J.; Ji, H.D.; Yoo, E.K.; Lee, J.-E.; Lee, S.B.; Oh, J.M.; Lee, S.; Hwang, J.S.; Yoon, H.; et al. Discovery of Potent, Selective, and Orally Bioavailable Estrogen-Related Receptor-γ Inverse Agonists To Restore the Sodium Iodide Symporter Function in Anaplastic Thyroid Cancer. *J. Med. Chem.* **2019**, *62*, 1837–1858.
20. Nirogi, R.; Shinde, A.; Mohammed, A.R.; Badange, R.K.; Reballi, V.; Bandyala, T.R.; Saraf, S.K.; Bojja, K.; Manchineella, S.; Achanta, P.K.; et al. Discovery and Development of N-[4-(1-Cyclobutylpiperidin-4-yloxy)phenyl]-2-(morpholin-4-yl)acetamide Dihydrochloride (SUVNG3031): A Novel, Potent, Selective, and Orally Active Histamine H_3 Receptor Inverse Agonist with Robust Wake-Promoting Activity. *J. Med. Chem.* **2019**, *62*, 1203–1217.
21. Costa, T.; Herz, A. Antagonists with negative intrinsic activity at δ opioid receptors coupled to GTP-binding proteins. *Proc. Natl. Acad. Sci. USA* **1989**, *86*, 7321–7325. [CrossRef] [PubMed]
22. Shaw, W.N. Long-term treatment of obese Zucker rats with LY255582 and other appetite suppressants. *Pharmacol. Biochem. Behav.* **1993**, *46*, 653–659. [CrossRef]
23. Emmerson, P.J.; McKinzie, J.H.; Surface, P.L.; Suter, T.M.; Mitch, C.H.; Statnick, M.A. Na^+ modulation, inverse agonism, and anorectic potency of 4-phenylpiperidine opioid antagonists. *Eur. J. Pharmacol.* **2004**, *494*, 121–130. [CrossRef] [PubMed]
24. Hirayama, S.; Iwai, T.; Higashi, E.; Nakamura, M.; Iwamatsu, C.; Itoh, K.; Nemoto, T.; Tanabe, M.; Fujii, H. Discovery of δ opioid receptor full inverse agonists and their effects on restraint stress induced cognitive impairment in mice. *ACS Chem. Neurosci.* **2019**, *10*, 2237–2242. [CrossRef] [PubMed]

25. Higashi, E.; Hirayama, S.; Nikaido, J.; Shibasaki, M.; Kono, T.; Honjo, A.; Ikeda, H.; Kamei, J.; Fujii, H. Development of novel δ opioid receptor inverse agonists without a basic nitrogen atom and their antitussive effects in mice. *ACS Chem. Neurosci.* **2019**, *10*, 3939–3945. [CrossRef] [PubMed]
26. Nemoto, T.; Iihara, Y.; Hirayama, S.; Iwai, T.; Higashi, E.; Fujii, H.; Nagase, H. Naltrindole derivatives with fluorinated ethyl substituents on the 17-nitrogen as δ opioid receptor inverse agonists. *Bioorg. Med. Chem. Lett.* **2015**, *25*, 2927–2930. [CrossRef]
27. Portoghese, P.S.; Sultana, M.; Nagase, H.; Takemori, A.E. Application of the message-address concept in the design of highly potent and selective non-peptide δ opioid receptor antagonists. *J. Med. Chem.* **1988**, *31*, 281–282. [CrossRef]
28. Portoghese, P.S.; Sultana, M.; Takemori, A.E. Design of peptidomimetic δ opioid receptor antagonists using the message-address concept. *J. Med. Chem.* **1990**, *33*, 1714–1720. [CrossRef]
29. Fujii, H.; Uchida, Y.; Shibasaki, M.; Nishida, M.; Yoshioka, T.; Kobayashi, R.; Honjo, A.; Itoh, K.; Yamada, D.; Hirayama, S.; et al. Discovery of δ opioid receptor full agonists lacking a basic nitrogen atom and their antidepressant-like effects. *Bioorg. Med. Chem. Lett.* **2020**, *30*, 127176. [CrossRef]
30. Casy, A.F.; Parfitt, R.T. *Opioid Analgesics: Chemistry and Receptors*; Plenum Press: New York, NY, USA, 1986; pp. 9–104.
31. Che, T.; Majumdar, S.; Zaidi, S.A.; Ondachi, P.; McCorvy, J.D.; Wang, S.; Mosier, P.D.; Uprety, R.; Vardy, E.; Krumm, B.E.; et al. Structure of the Nanobody-Stabilized Active State of the Kappa Opioid Receptor. *Cell* **2018**, *172*, 55–67. [CrossRef]
32. Huang, W.; Manglik, A.; Venkatakrishnan, A.J.; Laeremans, T.; Feinberg, E.N.; Sanborn, A.L.; Kato, H.E.; Livingston, K.E.; Thorsen, T.S.; Kling, R.C.; et al. Structural insights into μ-opioid receptor activation. *Nature* **2015**, *524*, 315–321. [CrossRef] [PubMed]
33. Fenalti, G.; Giguere, P.M.; Katritch, V.; Huang, X.-P.; Thompson, A.A.; Cherezov, V.; Roth, B.L.; Stevens, R.C. Molecular control of δ-opioid receptor signaling. *Nature* **2014**, *506*, 191–196. [CrossRef] [PubMed]
34. Granier, S.; Manglik, A.; Kruse, A.C.; Kobilka, T.S.; Thian, F.S.; Weis, W.I.; Kobilka, B.K. Structure of the δ-opioid receptor bound to naltrindole. *Nature* **2012**, *485*, 400–404. [CrossRef] [PubMed]
35. Manglik, A.; Kruse, A.C.; Kobilka, T.S.; Thian, F.S.; Mathiesen, J.M.; Sunahara, R.K.; Pardo, L.; Weis, W.I.; Kobilka, B.K.; Granier, S. Crystal structure of the μ-opioid receptor bound to a morphinan antagonist. *Nature* **2012**, *485*, 321–326. [CrossRef] [PubMed]
36. Mafi, A.; Kim, S.-K.; Goddard, W.A., III. The atomistic level structure for the activated human κ-opioid receptor bound to the full Gi protein and the MP1104 agonist. *Proc. Natl. Acad. Sci. USA* **2020**, *117*, 5836–5843. [CrossRef] [PubMed]
37. Koehl, A.; Hu, H.; Maeda, S.; Zhang, Y.; Qu, Q.; Paggi, J.M.; Latorraca, N.R.; Hilger, D.; Dawson, R.; Matile, H.; et al. Structure of the μ-opioid receptor–Gi protein complex. *Nature* **2018**, *558*, 547–552. [CrossRef]
38. Roth, B.L.; Baner, K.; Westkaemper, R.; Siebert, D.; Rice, K.C.; Steinberg, S.; Ernsberger, P.; Rothman, R.B. Salvinorin A: A potent naturally occurring non-nitrogenous κ opioid selective agonist. *Proc. Natl. Acad. Sci. USA* **2002**, *99*, 11934–11939. [CrossRef]
39. Yamaotsu, N.; Fujii, H.; Nagase, H.; Hirono, S. Identification of the three-dimensional pharmacophore of κ-opioid receptor agonists. *Bioorg. Med. Chem.* **2010**, *18*, 4446–4452. [CrossRef]
40. Olofson, R.A.; Martz, J.T.; Senet, J.P.; Piteau, M.; Malfroot, T. A New Reagent for the Selective, High-Yield N-Dealkylation of Tertiary Amines: Improved Syntheses of Naltrexone and Nalbuphine. *J. Org. Chem.* **1984**, *49*, 2081–2082. [CrossRef]
41. Olofson, R.A.; Schnur, R.C.; Bunes, L.; Pepe, J.P. Selective N-dealkylation of tertiary amines with vinyl chloroformate: An improved synthesis of naloxone. *Tetrahedron Lett.* **1977**, *18*, 1567–1570. [CrossRef]
42. Montzka, T.A.; Matiskella, J.D.; Partyka, R.A. 2,2,2-trichloroethyl chloroformate: A general reagent for demethylation of tertiary methylamines. *Tetrahedron Lett.* **1974**, *15*, 1325–1327. [CrossRef]
43. Fujii, H.; Imaide, S.; Watanabe, A.; Nemoto, T.; Nagase, H. Novel cleavage reaction of the C16–N17 bond in naltrexone derivatives. *Tetrahedron Lett.* **2008**, *49*, 6293–6296. [CrossRef]
44. Wuts, P.G.M. *Greene's Protective Groups in Organic Synthesis*, 5th ed.; John Wiley & Sons: Hoboken, NJ, USA, 2014; pp. 921–923.

45. McLamore, S.; Ullrich, T.; Rothman, R.B.; Xu, H.; Dersch, C.; Coop, A.; Davis, P.; Porreca, F.; Jacobson, A.E.; Rice, K.C. Effect of *N*-Alkyl and *N*-Alkenyl Substituents in Noroxymorphindole, 17-Substituted-6,7-dehydro-4,5α-epoxy-3,14-dihydroxy-6,7:2′,3′-indolomorphinans, on Opioid Receptor Affinity, Selectivity, and Efficacy. *J. Med. Chem.* **2001**, *44*, 1471–1474. [CrossRef] [PubMed]
46. Portoghese, P.S.; Larson, D.L.; Sultana, M.; Takemori, A.E. Opioid Agonist and Antagonist Activities of Morphindoles Related to Naltrindole. *J. Med. Chem.* **1992**, *35*, 4325–4329. [CrossRef] [PubMed]
47. Ishikawa, K.; Karaki, F.; Tayama, K.; Higashi, E.; Hirayama, S.; Itoh, K.; Fujii, H. *C*-Homomorphinan Derivatives as Lead Compounds to Obtain Safer and More Clinically Useful Analgesics. *Chem. Pharm. Bull.* **2017**, *65*, 920–929. [CrossRef] [PubMed]
48. Sastry, G.M.; Adzhigirey, M.; Day, T.; Annabhimoju, R.; Sherman, W. Protein and Ligand Preparation: Parameters, Protocols, and Influence on Virtual Screening Enrichments. *J. Comput.-Aided Mol. Des.* **2013**, *27*, 221–234. [CrossRef] [PubMed]
49. Bell, J.A.; Cao, Y.; Gunn, J.R.; Day, T.; Gallicchio, E.; Zhou, Z.; Levy, R.; Farid, R. PrimeX and the Schrödinger Computational Chemistry Suite of Programs. *Int. Tables Crystallogr.* **2012**, 534–538.
50. Jorgensen, W.L.; Tirado-Rives, J. The OPLS [Optimized Potentials for Liquid Simulations] Potential Functions for Proteins, Energy Minimizations for Crystals of Cyclic Peptides and Crambin. *J. Am. Chem. Soc.* **1988**, *110*, 1657–1666. [CrossRef]
51. Shivakumar, D.; Williams, J.; Wu, Y.; Damm, W.; Shelley, J.; Sherman, W. Prediction of Absolute Solvation Free Energies using Molecular Dynamics Free Energy Perturbation and the OPLS Force Field. *J. Chem. Theory Comput.* **2010**, *6*, 1509–1519. [CrossRef]
52. Harder, E.; Damm, W.; Maple, J.; Wu, C.; Reboul, M.; Xiang, J.Y.; Wang, L.; Lupyan, D.; Dahlgren, M.K.; Knight, J.L.; et al. OPLS3: A Force Field Providing Broad Coverage of Drug-like Small Molecules and Proteins. *J. Chem. Theory Comput.* **2016**, *12*, 281–296. [CrossRef]
53. Greenwood, J.R.; Calkins, D.; Sullivan, A.P.; Shelley, J.C. Towards the Comprehensive, Rapid, and Accurate Prediction of the Favorable Tautomeric States of Drug-Like Molecules in Aqueous Solution. *J. Comput.-Aided Mol. Des.* **2010**, *24*, 591–604. [CrossRef] [PubMed]
54. Shelley, J.C.; Cholleti, A.; Frye, L.; Greenwood, J.R.; Timlin, M.R.; Uchimaya, M. Epik: A Software Program for pKa Prediction and Protonation State Generation for Drug-Like Molecules. *J. Comput.-Aided Mol. Design* **2007**, *21*, 681–691. [CrossRef] [PubMed]
55. Frisch, M.J.; Trucks, G.W.; Schlegel, H.B.; Scuseria, G.E.; Robb, M.A.; Cheeseman, J.R.; Scalmani, G.; Barone, V.; Mennucci, B.; Petersson, G.A.; et al. *Gaussian 09, Revision D.01*; Gaussian, Inc.: Wallingford CT, UK, 2009.

Sample Availability: Samples of SYK-623, SYK-753, SYK-839, SYK-901, and SYK-903 are available from the authors.

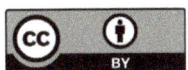

© 2020 by the authors. Licensee MDPI, Basel, Switzerland. This article is an open access article distributed under the terms and conditions of the Creative Commons Attribution (CC BY) license (http://creativecommons.org/licenses/by/4.0/).

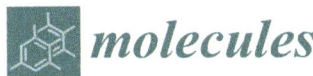

Article

β^2-*Homo*-Amino Acid Scan of μ-Selective Opioid Tetrapeptide TAPP

Dagmara Tymecka [1],*, Piotr F. J. Lipiński [2], Piotr Kosson [3] and Aleksandra Misicka [1],*

[1] Faculty of Chemistry, University of Warsaw, Pasteura 1, 02–093 Warsaw, Poland
[2] Department of Neuropeptides, Mossakowski Medical Research Centre Polish Academy of Sciences, Pawińskiego 5, 02–106 Warsaw, Poland; plipinski@imdik.pan.pl
[3] Toxicology Research Laboratory, Mossakowski Medical Research Centre Polish Academy of Sciences, Pawińskiego 5, 02–106 Warsaw, Poland; pkosson@imdik.pan.pl
* Correspondence: dulok@chem.uw.edu.pl (D.T.); misicka@chem.uw.edu.pl (A.M.)

Academic Editors: Mariana Spetea, Raffaele Capasso and Andrea Trabocchi
Received: 28 April 2020; Accepted: 22 May 2020; Published: 25 May 2020

Abstract: TAPP (H-Tyr-D-Ala-Phe-Phe-NH$_2$) is a potent, μ-selective opioid ligand. In order to gain further insights into pharmacophoric features of this tetrapeptide, we have performed a β^2-*Homo*-amino acid (β^2hAA) scan of the TAPP sequence. To this aim, 10 novel analogues have been synthesized and evaluated for μ-opioid and δ-opioid receptor affinity as well as for stability in human plasma. The derivatives included compounds in which a (R)- or (S)-β^2-*Homo*-Homologue replaced the amino acids in the TAPP sequence. The derivatives with (R)- or (S)-β^2hPhe^4 turned out to bind μOR with affinities equal to that of the parent. β^2hAAs in position 1 and 3 resulted in rather large affinity decreases, but the change differed depending on the stereochemistry. β^2-*Homo*logation in the second position gave derivatives with very poor μOR binding. According to molecular modelling, the presented α/β-peptides adopt a variety of binding poses with their common element being an ionic interaction between a protonable amine of the first residue and Asp147. A feature required for high μOR affinity seems the ability to accommodate the ring in the fourth residue in a manner similar to that found for TAPP. Contrary to what might be expected, several compounds were significantly less stable in human plasma than the parent compound.

Keywords: β^2-amino acids; β^2-*Homo*-amino acids; μ-opioid receptor; opioid peptides; TAPP; racemic synthesis of β^2-amino acids

1. Introduction

There is a rich repertoire of structural modifications that a medicinal chemist can use when exploring structure-activity relationships of peptide active compounds or working on the improvement of their physicochemical properties. This repertoire includes, e.g., backbone cyclization, introduction of peptide bond isosteres, incorporation of D-amino acids, α,α-disubstituted amino acids, residues with substituted or constrained side-chains, and other unnatural amino acids [1]. In the latter group, a prominent place is occupied by β-amino acids (β-AAs) [2,3]. The amino acids of this class have two carbon atoms between the carboxylic and amino groups. With both mono-substitutions and poly-substitutions being possible in different combinations and stereochemistries (Figure 1), β-AAs constitute a family of building blocks of enormous structural diversity.

β-Amino acids can be used to construct full β-peptides (solely made of β-AAs), but it is also possible to create mixed α/β-peptides in which one or more β-residues are incorporated instead of some α-amino acids. There are three main structural consequences of introducing a β-residue into a peptide backbone. First, each β-AA elongates the backbone by one methylene unit. Furthermore, it adds one freely rotating sp^3-sp^3 C-C bond, which increases the backbone flexibility. Lastly, in topographical terms, the position of side-chains of the residues that follow a β-residue is shifted toward the C-terminus. All these changes can have critical impact on activity and other properties (e.g., stability) of a peptide sequence and this is why β-AAs are useful means in medicinal chemistry research.

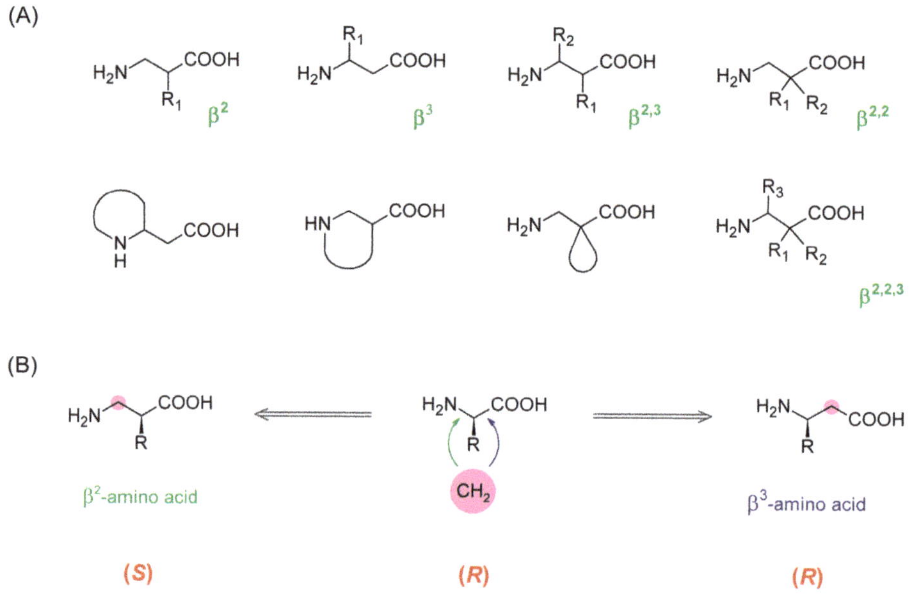

Figure 1. (**A**) Examples of diverse possible types of β-amino acids. (**B**) Comparison of absolute configuration of α-, $β^2$-, and $β^3$-amino acids.

Peptides are endogenous ligands for all types of opioid receptors (μ, δ, κ, and nociceptin) [4]. Among these receptors, the μ type (μ-opioid receptor, μOR) constitutes a major molecular target for the treatment of pain, but the medicinal potential of the remaining ORs has been increasingly acknowledged [5]. Over the years, both natural and synthetic peptides as well as peptide-inspired organic analogues have continued to be key compounds in the research on the opioid receptors.

In attempts to decipher structure-activity relationships of opioid peptides, or in search for more stable analogues, the researchers also used β-AAs. All-β analogues (that is with $β^3$-*Homo*-AA in every position) of deltorphin I, Leu-enkephalin, and dermorphin were reported by Wilczyńska et al. [6]. The same paper presented several α/β-hybrides of deltorphin I. Alicyclic β-amino acids as proline mimics were used for studying conformational requirements in endomorphin-1/-2 analogues [7,8]. Other authors replaced proline for β-alanine [9]. Earlier, cyclic β-AAs were applied in studies on morphiceptin [10,11] and dermorphin [12]. Cardillo et al. conducted a systematic β-AA [13] and $β^3$-*Homo*-AA scan of endomorphin-1 [14], exchanging each single AA in the sequence for its β-isomer or $β^3$-Homologue. In another work, $β^3$-*Homo* and $β^2$-*Homo* aromatic amino acids were introduced alone or in combination in positions 3 or/and 4 of endomorphin sequence [15,16]. Mollica et al. performed a $β^3$-*Homo*-AA scan of a dimeric peptide, biphalin [17]. Several derivatives of this peptide with $β^3$hPhe or $β^3$-*Homo*-p-NO_2-Phe were reported by Frączak et al. [18]. Dimeric derivatives of dermorphin were probed with $β^3$-hAAs as well [19]. Recently, Adamska-Bartłomiejczyk et al. incorporated β-AAs into the structure of a cyclic endomorphin derivative, Tyr-c[D-Lys-Phe-Phe-Asp]NH_2 [20]. It is also polysubstituted β-AAs that were used in the opioid field. For example, several recent papers dealt with endomorphin-1/-2 analogues containing one or more $β^{2,3}$-AAs [21–25].

An interesting µOR selective opioid peptide is TAPP (H-Tyr-D-Ala-Phe-Phe-NH$_2$, **1**) [26]. Structurally, it resembles endomorphin-2 (H-Tyr-Pro-Phe-Phe-NH$_2$) in having Phe-Phe in positions 3 and 4, but it is also similar to some enkephalin-based derivatives, such as DAMGO (H-Tyr-D-Ala-Gly-*N*-MePhe-Gly-ol), in having D-Ala in the second position. The TAPP sequence was probed by a β^3-*Homo*-AA scan by Podwysocka et al. [27]. In the presented research, we wanted to complement their work by conducting a β^2-*Homo*-AA scan. To this aim, we have synthesized, tested for receptor affinity, and plasma stability as well as subjected to molecular modelling 10 novel TAPP analogues. In these, α-AAs in each position were replaced by their β^2-Homologues. Additionally, β^{2}h-*m*-Tyr was used in the first position. As we employed both (*R*)-isomers and (*S*)-isomers of β^{2}h-AAs, we were able to probe the effect of backbone expansion with the concomitant retention or reversion of side-chain spatial positioning. In this case, it is worth noting that, in β^2-AAs, the very same spatial arrangement of substituents at the asymmetric carbon as in α-AAs or β^3-AAs gives usually different absolute configurations (Figure 1B). In addition, a direct β^2-*Homo*-counterpart (in terms of side-chain location) of (*S*)-Phe is (*R*)-β^{2}hPhe (exceptions are β^{2}hCys, β^{2}hThr, and β^{2}hSer).

2. Results and Discussion

2.1. Chemistry

The planned modifications of the TAPP structure required preparation of β^2-*Homo*-amino acids. Since chiral synthesis of β^2-amino acids is labour-intensive (several stages of synthesis), we decided to start with β^2-amino acids in the racemic form. These were prepared in two-step syntheses (Scheme 1), starting from methyl cyanoacetate (**2**). This substrate was either alkylated with methyl iodide to form methyl α-methyl cyanoacetate (**3a**, alanine analogue path) or transformed into Z/E isomers of methyl α-cyano-cinnamates (**3b–d**) via Knoevenagel condensation with aromatic aldehydes (aromatic analogues path). In the second step, the intermediates **3a–d** were subject to simultaneous one-pot reduction of nitrile groups and double bonds along with Boc-protection. This was possible due to using CoCl$_2$-NaBH$_4$ combination in anhydrous methanol with di-tert-butyl dicarbonate as a trapping (to prevent dimerization into secondary amines) and a protective agent [28,29]. Thus, fully *N*-protected and *C*-protected racemic β^2-*Homo*-amino acids (**4a–d**) were obtained in moderately good yields.

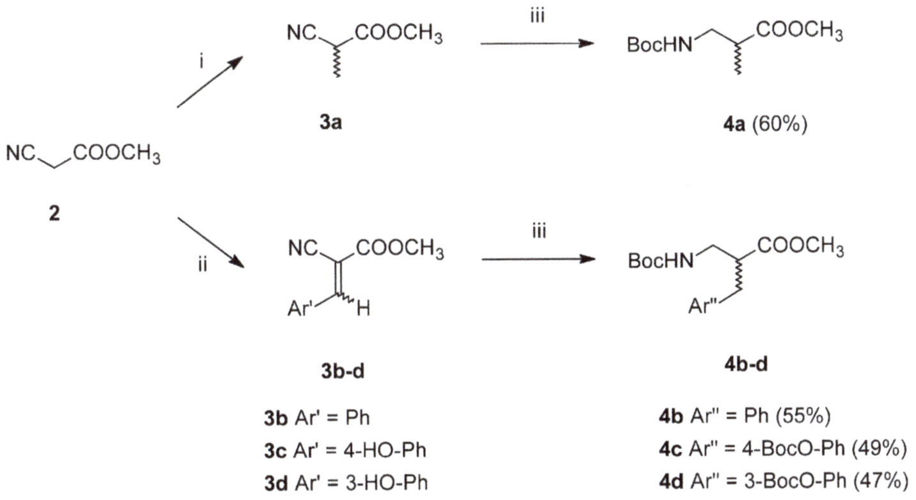

Scheme 1. Synthesis of racemic β^2-*Homo*-amino acids. Reagents and conditions (i) MeI, K$_2$CO$_{3(dry)}$, -*N,N* dimethylformamide (DMF), (ii) Ar'CHO, piperidine, MeOH, (iii) CoCl$_2$·6H$_2$O, NaBH$_4$, Boc$_2$O, MeOH$_{(dry)}$.

Furthermore, an attempt was made to separate pure enantiomers (Scheme 2). After C-deprotection, the acids (**5a–d**) were derivatized by coupling with (S)-(−)-α-methylbenzylamine. In the case of alanine and phenylalanine analogues, the resulting diastereoisomeric amide pairs (**6a–b**) were separated with column chromatography and further hydrolysed with 6M HCl. After purification (ion-exchange chromatography), the absolute configuration of the products (**7a–b**) was determined by measuring specific rotation and comparing it to the literature values. Regarding diastereoisomeric pairs of amides of β²h-Tyr and β²h-m-Tyr (**6c–d**), it was possible to separate them using preparative high performance liquid chromatography (HPLC). However, hydrolysis and isolation of the expected products failed.

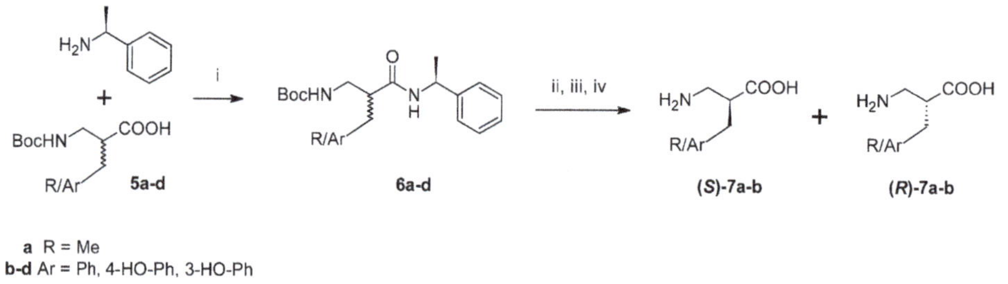

Scheme 2. Separation of racemic β²-*Homo*-amino acids. Reagents and conditions (i) coupling reagent TBTU, diisopropylethylamine (DIPEA), DMF, (ii) column chromatography: hexane (or CHCl₃)/AcOEt, (iii) 6M HCl reflux, (iv) ion exchange chromatography (Dowex 50W-X12), NH₃ aq.

The planned α/β-tetrapeptides (**8–17**) were then synthesized in solution. First, dipeptides were formed from respective α- or β²-*Homo* amino acid derivatives. Then, the dipeptides were coupled to yield the tetrapeptides, which was followed by ammonolysis to obtain the desired tetrapeptide amides. In the case of analogues containing β²hTyr and β²h-m-Tyr, diastereoisomeric mixtures were used for dipeptide syntheses and, therefore, diastereoisomeric mixtures of tetrapeptides were obtained. It was possible to separate single isomers by preparative HPLC. The absolute configurations of these derivatives were assigned based on HPLC retention times, per analogiam to isomers of β²hPhe-D-Ala-Phe-Phe-NH₂ (**18–19**), on the assumption that the presence of meta-phenol or para-phenol groups does not influence the elution order of diastereoisomers. The names of the analogues for which such an assignment procedure was performed will be further on marked with an asterisk: [(R)-β²hTyr]-TAPP*, [(S)-β²hTyr]-TAPP* etc.

2.2. Opioid Receptor Affinity

The parent compound (TAPP, **1**) and the synthesized α/β-peptides (**8–17**) were tested for binding affinity to μ-opioid and δ-opioid receptors. The determinations were performed by a competitive radioligand displacement assay with selective radioligands. The results are presented in Table 1 (μOR) and Table SM-BIN-1 in the Supplementary Materials (δOR) as half-maximal inhibitory concentration (IC_{50}) with standard errors of the mean (S.E.M).

The parent peptide (TAPP) was found to have high affinity for μOR (IC_{50} = 5.1 ± 3.5 nM) and only low binding to δOR, which is consistent with the data in the original TAPP report by Schiller et al. [30]. Introduction of an additional -CH₂- unit into the TAPP backbone resulted in diverse changes in μOR affinity, depending on the position where the backbone was expanded. Position 4 does not seem sensitive for this modification at all. Derivative [(R)-β²hPhe⁴]-TAPP (**12**) exhibited IC_{50} of 1.9 ± 2.4 nM, which is equal to (not significantly different than) the value found for TAPP. In position 3, the additional methylene ([(R)-β²hPhe³]-TAPP, **11**) brought about a more than 10-fold decrease in μOR binding. An even greater drop in affinity was observed for a derivative with the expansion in position 2. For this compound ([(S)-β²hAla²]-TAPP, **10**) the IC_{50} value was greater than 1000 nM, which means that it is at least a 200-times weaker ligand than the parent. The backbone expansion in the first position decreased the affinity about 15-times ([(R)-β²hTyr¹]-TAPP*, **8**). However, in this case, the binding strength may be partially restored if the expansion is accompanied by meta-positioning of the phenol group ([(R)-β²h-*m*-Tyr¹]-TAPP*, **9**).

Table 1. Binding affinity of the studied compounds.

No.	Compound	$IC_{50} \pm$ S.E.M. [nM] [1] μOR [2]
1	TAPP	5.1 ± 3.5
Backbone Expansion without Changing the Spatial Positioning of the Side-Chain		
8	[(R)-β²hTyr¹]-TAPP*	77.6 ± 2.4
9	[(R)-β²h-*m*-Tyr¹]-TAPP*	48.9 ± 2.3
10	[(S)-β²hAla²]-TAPP	> 1000
11	[(R)-β²hPhe³]-TAPP	95.4 ± 2.5
12	[(R)-β²hPhe⁴]-TAPP	1.9 ± 2.4
Backbone Expansion with Changing the Spatial Positioning of the Side-Chain		
13	[(S)-β²hTyr¹]-TAPP *	338.8 ± 5.1
14	[(S)-β²h-*m*-Tyr¹]-TAPP*	11.2 ± 6.3
15	[(R)-β²hAla²]-TAPP	954.9 ± 2.9
16	[(S)-β²hPhe³]-TAPP	15.5 ± 2.5
17	[(S)-β²hPhe⁴]-TAPP	7.8 ± 4.0

[1] $IC_{50} \pm$ S.E.M. Half-maximal inhibitory concentration ± standard error of the mean. Mean of three determinations in duplicate. [2] Radioligand: 0.5 nM [³H]DAMGO.

If simultaneously with the introduction of a methylene unit into the backbone, side chain positioning was inverted, the observed trends in affinity were not parallel to those in the former series. Position four is the least sensitive one, and the derivative [(S)-β²hPhe⁴]-TAPP (**17**) exhibited similar μOR binding strength as TAPP. Not much worse was the analogue with (S)-β²hPhe in position 3 (**16**), which is in contrast to the former series where (R)-β²hPhe in this position (**16**) brought a more pronounced decrease in affinity. Introduction of (R)-β²hAla in position 2 produced a derivative with very low affinity (**15**, $IC_{50} = 954.9 \pm 2.9$ nM). With respect to position 1, backbone expansion accompanied with an inversion of the side-chain positioning was associated with a large decline in μOR affinity ([(S)-β²hTyr¹]-TAPP*, **13**, $IC_{50} = 338.8 \pm 5.1$ nM). Notably, if additionally the phenol group was switched to the *meta*-position, the binding strength was restored and equal to that of the parent peptide ([(S)-β²h-*m*-Tyr¹]-TAPP*, **14**, $IC_{50} = 11.2 \pm 6.3$ nM).

As to the δOR affinity (Table SM-BIN-1), derivatives with modifications in positions 1 and 2 (**8**, **9**, **10**, **13**, **14**, **15**) did not exhibit any measurable binding for the δ opioid receptor. Expansion of the backbone in the fourth position accompanied by inversion of the side chain location ([(S)-β²hPhe⁴]-TAPP, **17**) brought about a slight improvement in δOR affinity when compared to the parent peptide, but the IC_{50} value reads in the high-middle nanomolar range. The remaining three derivatives (**11**, **12**, **16**) exhibited δOR binding at a level similar to the parent TAPP.

Comparing these results to the work by Podwysocka et al. [27], a disparity of trends is noticed. β³-*Homo*-AAs in position 1 and 3 gave completely inactive derivatives, irrespectively of the stereochemistry, while, in our work, β²-*Homo*-AAs in these positions produced smaller μOR affinity decreases that varied with stereochemistry and [(S)-β²hPhe³]-TAPP can be considered as only a slightly worse binder than the parent compound. On the contrary, β³-*Homo*logation in position 2 gave a derivative with nanomolar affinity, and, in our work, analogues with β²hAla² did not have appreciable μOR binding. Furthermore, in our report, derivatives with β³h-AA in the fourth position are essentially equipotent to the parent, but, for β²-hAA⁴ analogues, an affinity decrease by about six times was reported.

2.3. Molecular Modelling

In order to understand the observed structure-activity trends in terms of ligand-receptor interactions, the compounds **1** and **8–17** were docked into the μ-opioid receptor structure (PDB accession code: 6DDF [31]) using AutoDock 4.2.6 [32].

The best scored pose for the parent TAPP (**1**) is presented in Figure 2A. Docking predicts that TAPP binds μOR with the N-terminal Tyr^1 directed toward the intracellular part of the receptor. The complex is stabilized by a canonical ionic interaction of protonated Tyr^1 amine with Asp147. The phenol group of this residue is involved in hydrogen bonding with His297. Furthermore, the aromatic ring forms several dispersive (π-alkyl) contacts with side chains of Met151, Ile296, and Val300. At the C-terminus, the terminal amide interacts with Thr218 via the hydrogen bond. The Phe^4 is located in a hydrophobic subsite formed by several residues of transmembrane helix 3 (TM3) and extracellular loops 1 and 2 (ECL1 and ECL2). There the aromatic ring participates in dispersive (π-alkyl) interactions with Trp133, Ile144, and Cys217. The Phe^3 is positioned close to Asn127 and His319. Some other receptor residues present in the vicinity of TAPP are shown in Figure 2B. Furthermore, an intramolecular hydrogen bond between C=O of D-Ala^2 and N-H of Phe^4 was predicted by docking.

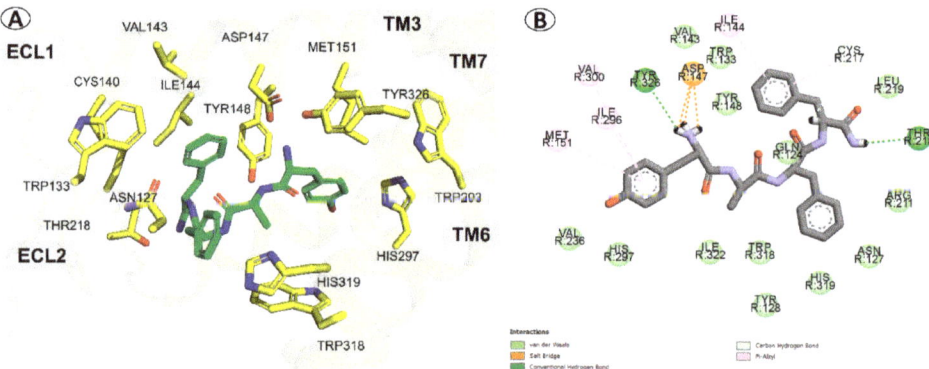

Figure 2. μOR binding mode of the parent compound (TAPP, **1**) as predicted by docking. (**A**) The peptide (green sticks) in the binding site of the receptor (yellow). Side chains of only several residues are shown. (**B**) The interactions scheme.

This binding mode is highly similar (Figure 3) to the one experimentally found for DAMGO in 6DDE and 6DDF structures [31]. In particular, both modes share (i) the canonical ionic interaction with Asp147, (ii) similar positioning of Tyr^1 ring, and (iii) location of Phe^4 ring in the same hydrophobic subsite. On the other hand, the D-Ala^2 in TAPP is shifted more towards TM7 and to the binding site outlet when compared to DAMGO. The placement of TAPP's Phe^4 aromatic ring is also similar to the location of aromatic rings in small molecular ligands like BU72 (as found in crystallography [33]) or fentanyl (as found by molecular modelling [34,35]).

For the herein reported α/β-peptides (**8–17**), the docking predicts that they do not necessarily adopt the binding mode found for TAPP. The obtained binding poses are presented in Figure 4 and they are summarized in detail in Table SM-MOD-1 in Supplementary Materials. A feature common for all studied derivatives is the presence of the canonical ionic interaction with Asp147. On the other hand, the side chain of Tyr^1 may be displaced in comparison to TAPP or DAMGO, participating in different sets of interactions. Furthermore, in some cases, docking predicts that the peptide bond elements may form hydrogen bonding to Tyr148. The aromatic ring in position three can be located either closer to TM7 (as in TAPP) or closer to ECL2 and TM2. With regard to position four, for majority of the derivatives, the aromatic ring is situated in the hydrophobic pocket formed by TM3, ECL1, and ECL2, as in the case of TAPP and DAMGO. However, the position of the ring can be more or less displaced in comparison to these ligands and utterly different positions are found as well. Furthermore, the interactions of the C-terminal amide are also predicted to vary depending on the derivative.

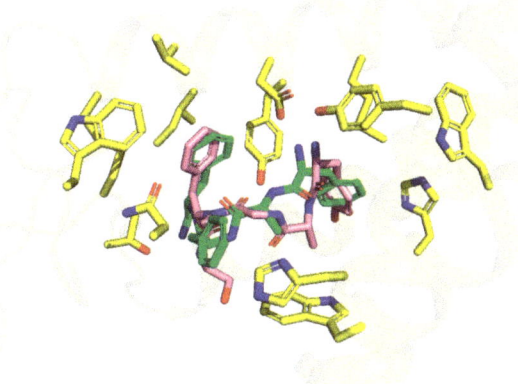

Figure 3. Comparison of the binding modes of DAMGO (from 6DDF PDB structure [31], pink sticks) and TAPP (from docking, green sticks). The picture is oriented in the same projection as Figure 2. Only several side-chains of the receptor binding site (yellow sticks) are shown.

Among this diversity of binding poses, it is hard to establish a coherent relationship between the modification in the peptide structure and the change in the peptide-receptor interactions. The considered expansions of the backbone affect, in most cases, more than one interaction site. Unfortunately, in quantitative terms, the scoring function used for docking is not able to provide a predictive tool for foreseeing the effects of such modest structural changes since no correlation was found between the scoring value and the experimental affinity (Figure SM-MOD-1 and SM-MOD-2 in Supplementary Materials). The analysis of the binding poses in qualitative terms allowed however for detection of an interesting relationship between the position of the Xxx^4 side chain (according to docking) and the affinity. The derivatives with the worst binding results are predicted to have the aromatic ring of the fourth residue significantly displaced when compared to DAMGO or TAPP. This can be quantitatively expressed in the form of a correlation equation (Figure 5A) where the independent variable standing for the ring displacement is the root mean square deviation (RMSD) of Xxx^4 atoms' positions of a considered derivative when compared to DAMGO in the 6DDF structure [31]. It turns out that this computational value correlates with the experimental affinity with a coefficient of determination (R^2) of 0.67, which can be considered a fairly good explanatory power for such a model.

We were then curious to see whether this relationship (of Xxx^4 position and affinity) might have some general validity. In order to check it, we have docked another 12 H-Tyr-Xxx-Yyy-Phe-NH$_2$ derivatives (Xxx = Ala, D-Ala, β-Ala, N-MeAla, N-MeGly, Yyy = Phe or Trp) that were experimentally tested for µOR affinity by Perlikowska et al. [9]. For these compounds, the Xxx^4 ring RMSD correlated against affinity with R^2 = 0.60 (Figure 5B). In light of these results, it seems reasonable to conclude that, for closer or more remote TAPP derivatives, a critical requirement for high µOR affinity is the ability to place the Xxx^4 ring in the manner similar to that of DAMGO (that is, in the hydrophobic subpocket formed by residues of TM3, ECL1, and ECL2).

A pair of derivatives that deserves a closer structural look are [(S)-β^{2}hTyr^1]-TAPP* (**13**, IC$_{50}$ = 338.8 ± 5.1 nM) and [(S)-β^{2}h-m-Tyr^1]-TAPP* (**14**, IC$_{50}$ = 11.2 ± 6.3 nM). In this case, the minute difference in positioning of the phenol group (*para*- vs. *meta*-) is associated with over a thirty-fold difference in affinity. Our modelling seems to provide explanation for this effect. Figure 6 gives a comparison of the binding poses of **13** and **14**. β^2-*Hom*ologation in the first position backbone accompanied with the inversion of the side chain spatial positioning causes the peptide **13** to adopt the binding pose of an apparently higher energetics than the parent. This can be associated with an additional rotor being penalized for entropy and no novel interactions being created. On the other hand, if the phenol group is shifted to the meta-position of the aromatic ring ([(S)-β²h-m-Tyr¹]-TAPP*, **14**), it allows for forming an H-bond to backbone carbonyl of Ile296 and this restores the affinity.

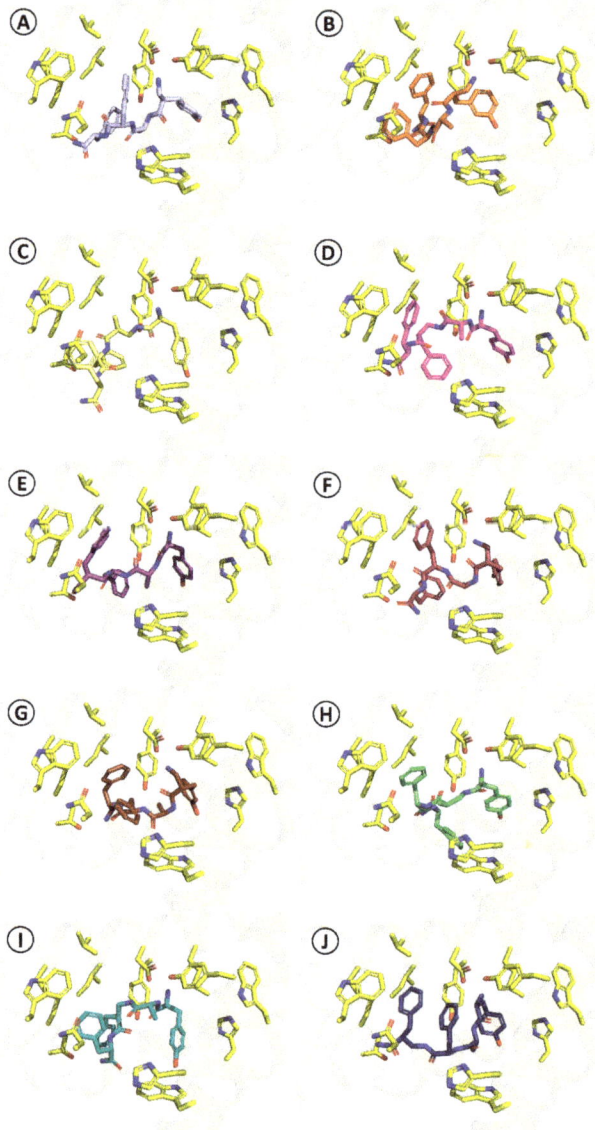

Figure 4. Binding modes of compounds **8–17** as predicted by docking. The pictures are oriented in the same projection as Figure 2. Only several side-chains of the receptor binding site (yellow sticks) are shown. (**A**) [(R)-β²hTyr¹]-TAPP*, **8**, (**B**) [(R)-β²h-m-Tyr¹]-TAPP*, **9**, (**C**) [(S)-β²hAla²]-TAPP, **10**, (**D**) [(R)-β²hPhe³]-TAPP, **11**, (**E**) [(R)-β²hPhe⁴]-TAPP, **12**, (**F**) [(S)-β²hTyr¹]-TAPP*, **13**, (**G**) [(S)-β²h-m-Tyr¹]-TAPP*, **14**, (**H**) [(R)-β²hAla²]-TAPP, **15**, (**I**) [(S)-β²hPhe³]-TAPP, **16**, (**J**) [(S)-β²hPhe⁴]-TAPP, **17**.

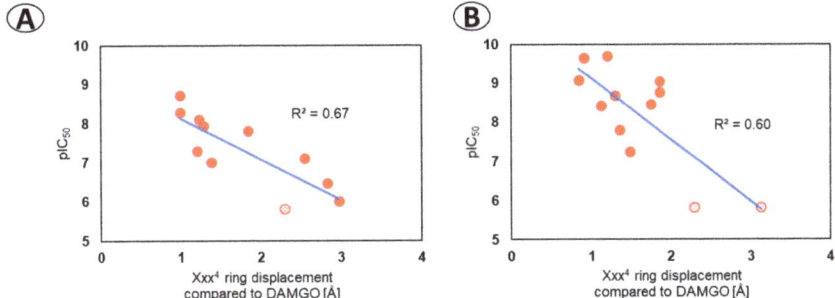

Figure 5. Correlation between the displacement of the ring of the fourth residue predicted by docking and the experimental μOR affinity. The relationship for (**A**) the α/β-peptides reported in this work, (**B**) derivatives reported in Reference [9]. The ring displacement is expressed as the RMSD of Xxx^4 ring in the considered derivative (as predicted by docking) compared to N-Me-Phe^4 ring in DAMGO (6DDF structure [31]). The points marked with dotted texture are arbitrarily chosen 5.82 for pIC$_{50}$ being less than 6.

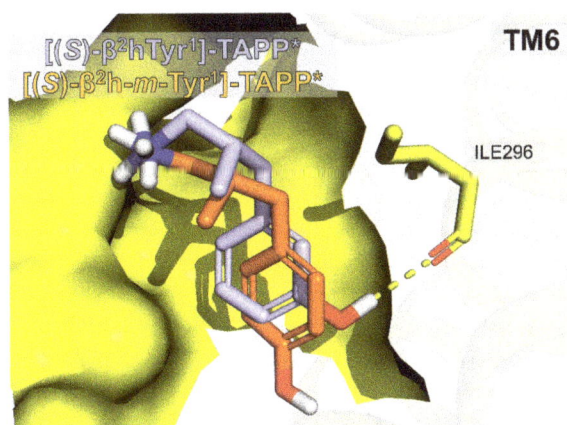

Figure 6. Comparison of binding poses of compounds [(S)-β^{2}hTyr^1]-TAPP*, **13** (orange) and [(S)-β^{2}h-*m*-Tyr^1]-TAPP*, **14** (light blue). Only the first residues of the peptides are shown. The receptor is partially represented as a surface representing the binding site. Only Ile296 side-chain (yellow sticks) is explicitly shown.

2.4. Stability Against Proteolysis in Plasma

The parent peptide (**1**) and the analogues (**8**–**17**) were tested as to stability against proteolysis in human plasma by a HPLC/MS method [19]. The results are graphically presented in Figure 7 and the representative HPLC chromatograms are given in Figures SM-STAB-1 to SM-STAB-22 in Supplementary Materials. TAPP turned out to be resistant to proteolysis. After 96 h, more than 90% of the initial peptide concentration (C$_{96h}$ > 90%) remained in the test sample. This is in marked contrast to endomorphin-2 (Tyr-Pro-Phe-Phe-NH$_2$) that, in the very same conditions, is rapidly degraded with half-life time (T$_{1/2}$) of only 30 min. For TAPP, the first proteolytic cleavage occurs at the C-terminal amide (deamidation).

Several of the studied analogues were much less stable when compared to the parent compound. In particular, replacement of D-Ala (**1**) for both (S)-β^{2}hAla (**10**) or (R)-β^{2}hAla (**15**) in position 2 gave compounds prone to proteolysis with T$_{1/2}$ of about 4.5 h. Derivatives with β^{2}hPhe in the third position were also less stable than the parent, but different rates of cleavage were observed for the stereoisomers. [(R)-β²hPhe³]-TAPP (**11**) was found to have half-life time of about 40 h, while, in the case of [(S)-β²hPhe³]-TAPP (**16**), more than 65% of the initial peptide concentration remained in the test solution after 96 h. When modifications in the fourth position are considered, again the isomer with (R)-β²hPhe (**12**) was less stable (C_{96h} = 55%) than the peptide with reverse configuration in this position (**17**, C_{96h} ~ 90%). The latter was equally resistant to proteolysis as the parent. All derivatives with β²-*Homo*-amino acids in positions 2, 3, and 4 were cleaved at the peptide bond between the Tyr¹ and the second residue (the site of the first proteolytic cleavage).

On the contrary, for the analogues modified in the first position, the first cleavage occurred at the C-terminal amide (deamidation) in the case of the parent compound. All they (**8, 9, 13, 14**) exhibited stability similar to TAPPs.

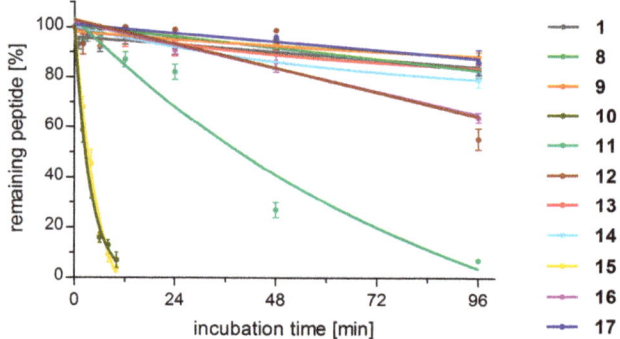

Figure 7. Results of stability determinations for compounds **1** and **8–17** expressed as percent of the initial peptide concentration remaining in the test solution at a certain time-point. Each point is an average result ± standard deviation calculated from three independent experiments.

3. Materials and Methods

3.1. Chemistry

All materials (solvents and reagents) were purchased from commercial suppliers and used without further purification. The NMR spectra were recorded on a Varian Unity Plus 200 spectrometer operating at 200 MHz for ¹H-NMR and 50 MHz for ¹³C-NMR. The spectra were measured in CDCl₃ or CD₃OD or acetone d₆ and are given as δ values (in ppm) relative to TMS. Melting points were determined on a Melting Point Meter KSP1D (A. Krüss Optronic, Hamburg, Germany). TLC analyses were performed on silica gel plates (Merck Kiesegel GF254, Merck, Darmstadt, Germany) and visualized using UV light or iodine vapour or ninhydrin test. Column chromatography was carried out (at atmospheric pressure) using Silica Gel 60 (230–400 mesh, Merck, Darmstadt, Germany) using appropriate eluents. The crude final peptides were purified using reversed-phase high performance liquid chromatography (RP-HPLC) on a preparative C-12 column (Phenomenex, Jupiter 4u Proteo 90A, AXIA 250 × 21.20 mm) using 0.1% trifluoroacetic acid (TFA) in water/acetonitrile as a solvent system with UV detection (214 nm). The peptide purity was estimated by analytical HPLC using a C-12 column (Jupiter 4u Proteo 90A, 250 × 4.6 mm) and the same solvent system and UV detection as above, and then confirmed in a second solvent system 0.1% TFA in water/methanol. High resolution mass spectra (also low resolution) were acquired on the Shimadzu LCMS-IT TOF mass spectrometer with electrospray ionization (ESI).

3.2. Synthesis of β²-Homo-Amino Acids

3.2.1. Methyl α-methyl-cyanoacetate (**3a**)

To a stirred solution of methyl cyanoacetate **2** (30 mmol, 1 equiv) and anhydrous potassium carbonate (30 mmol, 1 equiv) in dimethylformamide, methyl iodide (30 mmol, 1 equiv) was added.

Then the reaction mixture was stirred overnight. Next, the reaction mixture was diluted with water and extracted with diethyl ether (4×). The combined organic layers successively washed with water (2×), brine solution (3×), dried over anhydrous Na_2SO_4, and evaporated under vacuum. The crude compound was purified by column chromatography on silica gel (hexane/ethyl acetate). Pure product **3a** was obtained as colourless, low-density oil (1.42 g, 42%).

^{1}H NMR (200 MHz, CDCl$_3$) δ: 3.82 (s, 3H), 3.42 (q, *J* = 7.6 Hz, 1H), 1.37 (d, *J* = 7.6 Hz, 3H). ^{13}C NMR (50 MHz, CDCl$_3$) δ: 165.9, 117.35, 53.24, 30.57, 15.30.

3.2.2. General Procedure (GP1) of Methyl α-cyano-cinnamates Synthesis via Knoevenagel Condensation (**3b–d**)

The benzaldehyde (30 mmol, 1 equiv) or 3- or 4-hydroxybenzaldehyde, methyl cyanoacetate **2** (30 mmol, 1 equiv) and piperidine (0.2 mmol, 0.007 equiv) were heated under reflux for 8–12 h in methanol. The reaction mixture was allowed to reach room temperature. Then volatiles were evaporated. The crude compounds **3b–d** were purified by column chromatography (hexane/ethyl acetate) or crystallization from methanol.

Methyl α-cyanocinnamate (**3b**)

The desired product was isolated by column chromatography (hexane/ethyl acetate) or crystallization (methanol) as white solid (4.98 g, 89%), mp = 90–91 °C [lit. 89–90 °C] [36].

^{1}H NMR (200 MHz, CDCl$_3$) δ: 8.27 (s, 1H), 8.06–7.88 (m, 2H), 7.60–7.42 (m, 3H), 3.94 (s, 3H). ^{13}C NMR (50 MHz, CDCl$_3$) δ: 162.94, 155.28, 133.38, 131.33, 131.06, 129.25, 115.41, 102.47, 53.36.

Methyl α-cyano-4-hydroxycinnamate (**3c**)

The desired product was isolated by crystallization (twice from methanol) as a pale yellow solid (4.63 g, 76%), mp = 210–212 °C [lit. 208–210 °C] [37].

^{1}H NMR (200 MHz, CD$_3$OD) δ: 8.21 (s, 1H), 7.98–7.88 (m, 2H), 6.95–6.87 (m, 2H), 3.88 (s, 3H). ^{13}C NMR (50 MHz, CD$_3$OD) δ: 165.09, 164.46, 156.13, 135.17, 124.49, 117.30, 115.45, 98.58, 53.50.

Methyl α-cyano-3-hydroxycinnamate (**3d**)

The desired product was isolated by crystallization (twice from methanol) as a yellow solid (4.81 g, 79%), mp = 139–140 °C [lit. 142–143 °C] [38].

^{1}H NMR (200 MHz, CD$_3$OD) δ: 8.21 (s, 1H), 7.47–7.34 (m, 3H), 7.05–6.99 (m, 1H), 3.90 (s, 3H). ^{13}C NMR (50 MHz, CD$_3$OD) δ: 164.41, 159.42, 156.61, 134.21, 131.48, 124.04, 121.93, 117.90, 116.48, 103.57, 53.91.

3.2.3. (*R,S*)-*N*-Boc-β^2-*Homo*-Alanine Methyl Ester (**4a**)

To a stirred solution of the methyl α-methyl-cyanoacetate **3a** (10 mmol, 1 equiv), Boc anhydride (20 mmol, 2 equiv), CoCl$_2$·6H$_2$O (2 mmol, 0.2 equiv) in dry methanol at 0 °C, sodium borohydride (70 mmol, 7 equiv) were added gradually over 30 min. The reaction mixture was then stirred overnight at room temperature. Then, triethylamine (10 mmol, 1 equiv) was added and stirring was continued for 30 min. Next, the solvent was evaporated and the residue was diluted with ethyl acetate and extracted with saturated aqueous NaHCO$_3$ (3 ×). The organic layer was washed with brine solution and dried over anhydrous Na$_2$SO$_4$, and then evaporated under vacuum. The product (Boc-β^{2}hAla-OMe, **4a**) was isolated by column chromatography on silica gel (hexane/ethyl acetate) as solidifying, colorless oil (1.30 g, 60%).

^{1}H NMR (200 MHz, CDCl$_3$) δ: 4.86 (br s, 1H), 3.71 (s, 3H), 3.54–3.12 (dm, 2H), 2.54–2.36 (m, 1H), 1.43 (s, 9H), 1.12 (d, *J* = 7 Hz, 3H). ^{13}C NMR (50 MHz, CDCl$_3$) δ: 175.07, 155.77, 79.24, 52.15, 43.18, 39.58, 28.31, 15.91. LR–MS *m/z*: 140 [M–Boc + Na]$^+$, 240 [M + Na]$^+$.

3.2.4. General Procedure (GP2) of Aromatic β²-*Homo*-Amino Acid Synthesis, Boc-β²hXaa-OMe (**4b–d**)

To a stirred solution of the suitable methyl α-cyano-cinnamate derivative **3b–d** (10 mmol, 1 equiv), Boc anhydride (40 mmol, 4 equiv), $CoCl_2 \cdot 6H_2O$ (4 mmol, 0.4 equiv) in dry methanol at 0 °C, and sodium borohydride (140 mmol, 14 equiv) were added gradually over 30 min. The reaction mixture was then stirred overnight. Then, triethylamine (20 mmol, 2 equiv) was added and stirring was continued for 30 min. Next, the solvent was evaporated and the residue was diluted with ethyl acetate and extracted with saturated aqueous $NaHCO_3$ (3 ×). The organic layer was washed with brine solution, dried over anhydrous Na_2SO_4, and then evaporated under vacuum. The crude products **4b–d** were isolated by column chromatography on silica gel (hexane or chloroform/ethyl acetate).

(*R,S*)-*N*-Boc-β²-*Homo*-phenylalanine methyl ester (**4b**)

The desired product (Boc-β²hPhe-OMe, **4b**) was purified by column chromatography (hexane/ethyl acetate) as a solidifying oil (1.61 g, 55%).

^{1}H NMR (200 MHz, $CDCl_3$) δ: 7.33–7.13 (m, 5H), 4.86 (br s, 1H,), 3.64 (s, 3H), 3.48–3.16 (m, 2H), 3.10–2.74 (m, 3H), 1.42 (s, 9H). ^{13}C NMR (50 MHz, $CDCl_3$) δ: 174.61, 155.73, 138.22, 128.80, 128.49, 126.56, 79.38, 51.77, 47.35, 41.48, 35.85, 28.30. LR-MS *m/z*: 316.2 $[M + Na]^+$.

(*R,S*)-*N*-Boc-β²-*Homo*-*O*-tert-butyloxycarbonyl-tyrosine methyl ester (**4c**)

The desired product (Boc-β²hTyr(Boc)-OMe, **4c**) was purified by column chromatography (chloroform/ethyl acetate) as a solidifying oil (2.01 g, 49%).

^{1}H NMR (200 MHz, acetone d$_6$) δ: 7.32–7.16 (m, 2H), 7.16–6.96 (m, 2H), 6.14 (br s, 1H), 3.57 (s, 3H), 3.38–3.20 (m, 2H), 3.0–2.76 (m, 3H), 1.52 (s, 9H), 1.40 (s, 9H). ^{13}C NMR (50 MHz, acetone d$_6$) δ: 174.59, 152.66, 150.81, 137.62, 130.71, 122.07, 83.50, 79.38, 51.89, 48.81, 42.84, 35.61, 28.64, 27.83. LR-MS *m/z*: 432.2 $[M + Na]^+$.

(*R,S*)-*N*-Boc-β²-*Homo*-*O*-tert-butyloxycarbonyl-*meta*-tyrosine methyl ester (**4d**)

The desired product (Boc-β²h-*m*-Tyr(Boc)-OMe, **4d**) was purified by column chromatography (chloroform/ethyl acetate) as a solidifying oil (1.92 g, 47%).

^{1}H NMR (200 MHz, acetone d$_6$) δ: 7.38–7.20 (m, 1H), 7.16–6.90 (m, 3H), 6.14 (br s, 1H), 3.57 (s, 3H), 3.38–3.24 (m, 2H), 3.0–2.78 (m, 3H), 1.52 (s, 9H), 1.40 (s, 9H). ^{13}C NMR (50 MHz, acetone d$_6$) δ: 176.59, 156.37, 150.81, 143.25, 142.08, 130.61), 127.65, 121.93, 118.07, 83.63, 79.10, 51.70, 48.81, 42.84, 35.35, 28.31, 27.80. LR-MS *m/z*: 432.2 $[M + Na]^+$, 841.4 $[2M + Na]^+$.

3.3. *Separation of Racemic β²-Homo-Amino Acids (7a–b)*

Boc-protected β²-*Homo*-amino acids **5a–b** (also **5c–d**) were obtained according to the GP4. To a stirred solution of **5a–b** (5 mmol, 1 equiv) in DMF (10 mL), TBTU (5 mmol, 1 equiv), HOBt (5 mmol, 1 equiv), and DIPEA (10 mmol, 2 equiv) were added. After stirring the mixture at 0 °C for 10 min, the (*S*)-(−)-α-methylbenzylamine (5 mmol, 1 equiv) was added. The reaction mixture was then stirred overnight (allowing to reach to room temperature). Next, the mixture was diluted with 5% $NaHCO_3$ and washed several times with ethyl acetate. The combined organic layers successively washed with 5% $NaHCO_3$ (2 ×), 1M $KHSO_4$ (3 ×), brine solution (3 ×), and dried over anhydrous Na_2SO_4 and evaporated under vacuum. The resulting diastereoisomeric amide pairs (**6a–b**) were separated by column chromatography (supplemented by an additional re-chromatography of partially separated fractions) using as eluent $CHCl_3$/AcOEt for **6a** or hexane/AcOEt for **6b**. The individual amide diastereoisomers were heated under reflux in 6M HCl for 12 to 18 h. The reaction progress was monitored by TLC. After the reaction, the mixture was concentrated, and respective (*R*)- or (*S*)-**7a–b** enantiomers were isolated using cation exchange ion chromatography (Dowex 50W X12). A 0.2 M ammonia solution was used as an eluent. After evaporation, white solids of individual isomers were obtained and dried over NaOH.

3.3.1. (R)-(−)-β²-Homo-alanine, (R)-(−)-7a

The desired product (R)-(−)-β²hAla was obtained as white solid, mp 186–187 °C [lit. 185–187 °C] [39]; $[α]^{20}_D$ − 10.7 (c 1.0, 1M HCl) [lit. $[α]^{29}_D$ − 11.8 (c 1.0, 1M HCl)] [39].
¹H NMR (200 MHz, CD₃OD) δ: 3.26–3.10 (dd, J = 8.6 Hz, J =12.8 Hz, 1H), 3.10–2.96 (dd, J = 4.8 Hz, J = 12.8 Hz, 1H), 2.96–2.76 (m, 1H), 1.31 (d, J = 7.0 Hz, 3H). ¹³C NMR (50 MHz, CD₃OD) δ: 176.71, 42.68, 38.18, 15.33. LR–MS m/z: 104.1 [M + H]⁺, 207.2 [2M + H]⁺.

3.3.2. (S)-(+)-β²-Homo-alanine, (S)-(+)-7a

The desired product (S)-(+)-β²hAla was obtained as a white solid, mp 187–188 °C [lit. 184–188 °C] [39]; $[α]^{20}_D$ + 10.2 (c 0.96, 1M HCl) [lit. $[α]^{29}_D$ + 11.6 (c 1.0, 1M HCl)] [39].
¹H NMR (200 MHz, CD₃OD) δ: 3.30–3.12 (dd, J = 8.4 Hz, J = 13 Hz, 1H), 3.10–2.92 (dd, J = 5 Hz, J = 13 Hz, 1H), 2.92–2.80 (m, 1H), 1.27 (d, J = 7.0 Hz, 3H). ¹³C NMR (50 MHz, CD₃OD) δ: 176.76, 42.88, 38.98, 15.43. LR-MS m/z: 104.1 [M + H]⁺, 207.2 [2M + H]⁺.

3.3.3. (R)-(+)-β²-Homo-phenylalanine, (R)-(+)-7b

The desired product (R)-(+)-β²hPhe was obtained as a white solid, mp 210–212 °C [lit. 225–226 °C] [39]; $[α]^{20}_D$ + 13.8 (c 1.083, 1M HCl) [lit. $[α]^{29}_D$ + 11.3 (c 1.0, 1M HCl)] [39].
¹H NMR (200 MHz, CD₃OD) δ: 7.35–7.28 (m, 2H), 7.20–6.87 (m, 3H), 3.12–2.90 (m, 3H), 2.80–2.54 (m, 2H). ¹³C NMR (50 MHz, CD₃OD) δ: 176.61, 138.22, 129.80, 128.49, 126.56, 46.35, 40.48, 36.85. LR-MS m/z: 180.1 [M + H]⁺, 359.2 [2M + H]⁺.

3.3.4. (S)-(−)-β²-Homo-phenylalanine, (S)-(−)-7b

The desired product (S)-(−)-β²hPhe was obtained as a white solid, mp 212–214 °C [lit. 224–225 °C] [39]; $[α]^{20}_D$ − 9.8 (c 0.835, 1M HCl) [lit. $[α]^{29}_D$ − 11.0 (c 1.0, 1M HCl)] [39].
¹H NMR (200 MHz, CD₃OD) δ: 7.37–7.28 (m, 2H), 7.30–6.95 (m, 3H), 3.14–2.90 (m, 3H), 2.80–2.56 (m, 2H). ¹³C NMR (50 MHz, CD₃OD) δ: 177.61, 139.20, 128.80, 128.59, 127.56, 45.35, 41.44, 36.67. LR-MS m/z: 180.1 [M + H]⁺, 359.2 [2M + H]⁺.

3.4. Synthesis of the Peptides

All planned tetrapeptides (1, 8–17) were obtained according to the following steps of the synthesis: (I) preparation of Boc-protected N-terminal dipeptide methyl ester by the GP3, (II) preparation of Boc-protected C-terminal dipeptide methyl ester using the GP3, (III) hydrolysis of the methyl ester of the product of step (I) according to GP4, (IV) Boc-deprotection of Boc-protected C-terminal dipeptide methyl ester (step II) using GP5, (V) coupling of Boc-protected N-terminal dipeptide to C-terminal dipeptide methyl ester according to GP3, (VI) aminolysis of Boc-protected tetrapeptide methyl ester by the GP6. (VII) purification by RP-HPLC, confirmation of purity (≥ 96%) by analytical RP-HPLC and confirmation of molecular weight by mass spectrometry (3.1. Chemistry). HR-MS: for TAPP (1) 546.2715 (calcd for $C_{30}H_{35}N_5O_5$, 546.2711), for [(R)-β²hTyr¹]-TAPP* (8) 560.2885, for [(R)-β²h-m-Tyr¹]-TAPP* (9) 560.2885, for [(S)-β²hAla²]-TAPP (10) 560.2893, for [(R)-β²hPhe³]-TAPP (11) 560.2879, for [(R)-β²hPhe⁴]-TAPP (12) 560.2889, for [(S)-β²hTyr¹]-TAPP* (13) 560.2874, for [(S)-β²h-m-Tyr¹]-TAPP* (14) 560.2879, for [(R)-β²hAla²]-TAPP (15) 560.2880, for [(S)-β²hPhe³]-TAPP (16) 560.2879, for [(S)-β²hPhe⁴]-TAPP (17) 560.2882 (for 8–17 calcd for $C_{31}H_{37}N_5O_5$, 560.2867). The analytical data for compounds 1 and 8–17 are summarized in Supplementary Materials (Table SM-SYN-1).

3.4.1. General Procedure (GP3) for Synthesis of Protected Dipeptides and Tetrapeptides

To stirred solution of Boc-amino acid or Boc-dipeptide acid (10 mmol) in DMF (10mL), TBTU (10 mmol, 1 equiv), HOBt (10 mmol, 1 equiv), and DIPEA (30 mmol, 3 equiv) were added. After stirring the mixture at 0 °C for 10 min, the amine component or dipeptide methyl ester (10 mmol, 1 equiv) was added. The reaction mixture was then stirred overnight (allowing to reach the room temperature). Next, the mixture was diluted with 5% NaHCO$_3$ and washed several times with ethyl acetate. The combined organic layers successively washed with 5% NaHCO$_3$ (2 ×), 1M KHSO$_4$ (3 ×), brine solution (3 ×), and dried over anhydrous Na$_2$SO$_4$ and evaporated under vacuum. The crude peptides were used for the next step without further purification.

3.4.2. General Procedure (GP4) for Methyl ester Removal

To a stirred solution of Boc-protected dipeptide methyl ester (10 mmol, 1 equiv) in MeOH, LiOH·H$_2$O (50 mmol, 5 equiv) was added. The reaction mixture was stirred at 0 °C for 4–8 h with TLC-monitoring of the reaction progress. Next, the solvent was evaporated under reduced pressure. The residue was diluted with water and washed with diethyl ether (2 ×), acidified up to pH = 3 with 10% citric acid (aq.), and extracted with ethyl acetate (3 ×). The organic layer was dried over anhydrous MgSO$_4$, and concentrated under vacuum and used for the next step without further purification.

3.4.3. General Procedure (GP5) for Boc-Deprotection

Boc-protected dipeptide methyl ester (10 mmol, 1 equiv) was deprotected by 1N HCl(g) in ethyl acetate (8–10 mL). The Boc-tetrapeptide amide was deprotected by 1N HCl(g) in acetic acid (8–10 mL) at room temperature for 2–3 h (TLC-monitoring). Then, the excess of cold ethyl ether was added to the reaction mixture. Precipitated product was filtered off, washed with diethyl ether, and used for the next step without further purification.

3.4.4. General Procedure (GP6) for Aminolysis of Methyl ester

The Boc–protected tetrapeptide methyl ester (20 mmol, 1 equiv) was dissolved in ammonia solution in methanol (7N, 10 mL) and stirred for 3 to 10 days. The progress of the reaction was monitored by HPLC. The solution was evaporated under reduced pressure and the crude product was used for the next step without further purification.

3.5. Binding Affinity Determinations

The binding affinity of compounds **1** and **8–17** for µOR and δOR was determined in competitive radioligand binding assays following the previously described method [19,40]. Membrane fractions of rat brain *Homo*genate were incubated at 25 °C for 60 mins in the presence of radioligands (0.5 nM) specific for each receptor (µOR: [^{3}H]DAMGO and δOR: [^{3}H]DELT II, obtained as a generous gift from Prof. Géza Tóth [41]) and the increasing concentrations of the tested compounds (10^{-11} up to 10^{-5} M, each concentration in duplicate). For measuring non-specific binding, 10 µM naloxone was used as the competitor. The assay buffer contained 50mM Tris-HCl (pH 7.4), bovine serum albumin (0.1 mg/mL), bacitracin (30 µg/mL), bestatin (30 µM), captopril (10 µM), and phenylmethylsulfonyl fluoride (0.1 mM) in the total reaction volume of 1 mL. After the incubation, the binding reactions were terminated by rapid filtration with M-24 Cell Harvester (Brandel/USA) through GF/B Whatman glass fibre strips. The filters were pre-soaked with 0.5% PEI before harvesting in order to minimize non-specific binding. Filter discs were placed separately in 24-well plates and immersed with the Optiphase Supermix scintillation cocktail (Perkin Elmer, Waltham, MA, USA). Radioactivity was measured using a MicroBeta LS Trilux scintillation counter (PerkinElmer, Waltham, MA, USA). The experiments were repeated three times in duplicate and the results are presented as mean half-maximal inhibitory concentrations (IC$_{50}$) with standard errors of the mean.

3.6. Molecular Modelling

The compounds **1** and **8–17** were docked into activated µOR structure (PDB accession code: 6DDF [31]) using AutoDock 4.2.6 [32]. The studied derivatives were sketched in Biovia Discovery Studio Visualizer [42] and minimized with a Dreiding-like force field. Furthermore, they and the protein structure were processed in AutoDock Tools 4 [32]. Protonation states were set as expected at physiological pH. The G-protein was removed from the receptor structure. The ligands were considered flexible (except for amide bonds of the backbone) and the receptor was set as rigid. The docking box was centered around the position of DAMGO in the 6DDF structure [31] and its size was extended to cover the binding pocket and the extracellular part of the binding pocket entry. Grids were calculated with AutoGrid and the docking was performed using Lamarckian Genetic Algorithm with pseudo-Solis and Wets local searches (300 runs). A genetic algorithm was set to work with a population of 3000 individuals with a maximum number of generations being 37,000, mutation rate of 0.02, crossover rate of 0.8, and one individual surviving to the next generation. The probability of local search on the individual was set to 0.1. The results of each run were clustered and representative poses from several top-scored clusters of each ligand were visually inspected. A criterion for selecting the binding poses was their conformity to known literature data on ligand-µOR interactions, i.e., presence of the interaction of protonated amine in position 1 with Asp147. Molecular graphics were prepared in PyMOL [43].

In order to validate the relationship presented in Figure 5, a further 12 derivatives [9] were docked to the µOR structure using the very same procedure as described above.

3.7. Stability Determinations

The determination of plasma stability was performed according to a previously described protocol with minor modifications [19]. Human plasma for testing was obtained from a healthy donor. Compounds **1** and **8–17** (0.7 µmol) were dissolved in water to obtain 1 mL of stock solution. Portions of the plasma (100 µL) were dispensed into Eppendorf tubes and equilibrated at 37 ± 1 °C for 5 min, before adding 100 µL of the stock solution of each tested peptide. Samples of the test solution were taken and analyzed at several time points (0, 1, 2, 3, 4, 5, 6, 12, 24, 48, and 96 h of the experiment).

In order to precipitate the plasma proteins, 400 µL ethanol (98%) was added to the samples, whereafter shaking (1 min) and cooling in 4 °C (5 min) followed. Subsequently, the samples were centrifuged for 10 min at 2000 g. The supernatant (20 µL) was immediately analyzed by HPLC/MS using the LCMS-2010EV Shimadzu apparatus with a Phenomenex Jupiter 4u Proteo 90A, C12 (25 cm × 2 mm × 4 µm) column. The chromatography was performed in reversed-phase system (solvents A: 0.05% FA in water, B: 0.05% FA in acetonitrile) with a non-linear gradient was used (1–31% B in 20 min followed by an increase to 97% B from 20 to 30 min) at a solvent flow of 0.5 mL/min. The activity of the plasma was confirmed by using endomorphin-2 (0.7 µM/mL) as a control sample. The results of the HPLC/MS analyses allowed for quantitative determination of the concentration changes of the tested peptides. Furthermore, it was possible to indicate the location of the first proteolytic cleavage.

4. Conclusions

In conclusion, we have presented in this paper the results of β^2hAA scan of the TAPP sequence. Ten novel analogues were synthesized as well as tested for opioid binding and stability. None of the new compounds bound the µOR better than the parent, but the compounds modified at position four had equally good affinity as TAPP. On the contrary, β^2-*Homo*logation in the second position gave derivatives with very low binding strength. If the third position was modified, the (*R*)-isomer was weaker than TAPP, but, in the case of the (*S*)-isomer, the decrease was only minor. β^2hTyr in the first position caused affinity decreases (more pronounced with the (*S*)-isomer), but interestingly shifting the phenol group to the *meta*-position (β^2h-*m*-Tyr) gave restoration of binding strength. It was particularly noticeable with [(*S*)-β^2h-*m*-Tyr^1]-TAPP whose IC$_{50}$ value was statistically equal to that of TAPP and 30 times lower than that of [(*S*)-β^2hTyr^1]-TAPP.

The presented α/β-peptides and their parent, TAPP, were docked into the µOR structure. According to modelling, TAPP binds the receptor by a canonical ionic interaction with Asp147 and by anchoring the Phe^4 ring in a hydrophobic subsite formed by residues of TM3, ECL1, and ECL2, while placing the Phe^3 ring closer to TM7. For the novel analogues, docking does not predict a uniform binding mode, but a rather multitude of poses that vary at several subsites. No straightforward correlation can be found between the site of backbone expansion and the change in receptor-ligand interactions. There is also no correlation between the experimental binding affinity and the scoring value. Yet, it is possible to find a relationship between the experimental binding and the positioning of the Xxx^4 aromatic ring and this relationship can be even expressed quantitatively. Furthermore, this correlation was validated to hold for some opioid tetrapeptides reported earlier by other authors.

With regard to stability in human plasma, TAPP turned out to be fairly stable (C_{96h} > 90% of the initial concentration). Surprisingly, the α/β-analogues were not necessarily so. For example, those with (R/S)-β^{2}hAla in position 2 turned out to have half-life times of less than 5 h. Modifications in position 3 produced derivatives that were less stable than the parent. On the contrary, β^{2}hAAs in the first position gave analogues equally stable to the parent.

The presented results enhance our understanding of structure-activity (stability) relationships of opioid peptides, and, in particular, of the TAPP sequence. Thus, they will be useful for further design of peptide analgesics.

Supplementary Materials: The following are available online. SM file is divided into sections that contain data pertaining to particular analysis subjects. Items in each section are independently numbered. The sections are: **SM-SYN** (analytical data for the synthesized peptides, 1 Table), **SM-MOD** (minor data coming from modelling, 1 Table, 2 Figures), **SM-STAB** (data from stability determinations, 22 Figures).

Author Contributions: Conceptualization, A.M. and D.T. Data curation, D.T., P.F.J.L., and P.K. Funding acquisition, A.M. Investigation, D.T., P.F.J.L., and P.K. Methodology, D.T., P.F.J.L., and P.K. Project administration, A.M. Supervision, A.M. Writing-original draft, D.T. and P.F.J.L. Writing-review & editing, A.M., D.T., P.F.J.L., and P.K. All authors have read and agreed to the published version of the manuscript.

Funding: The European Union Grant NORMOLIFE (LSHC-CT-2006–037733) supported this work.

Acknowledgments: The calculations were performed at Świerk Computing Centre, National Centre for Nuclear Research, Świerk, Poland. Prof. Géza Tóth (Biological Research Centre, Hungarian Academy of Sciences, Szeged, Hungary) is gratefully acknowledged for providing tritiated radioligands. This work was co-financed by the EU from the European Regional Development Fund under the Operational Programme Innovative Economy, 2007–2013, and with the use of CePT infrastructure financed by the same EU program.

Conflicts of Interest: The authors declare no conflict of interest.

References

1. Henninot, A.; Collins, J.C.; Nuss, J.M. The Current State of Peptide Drug Discovery: Back to the Future? *J. Med. Chem.* **2018**, *61*, 1382–1414. [CrossRef]
2. Steer, D.; Lew, R.; Perlmutter, P.; Smith, A.; Aguilar, M.-I. β-Amino Acids: Versatile Peptidomimetics. *Curr. Med. Chem.* **2002**, *9*, 811–822. [CrossRef] [PubMed]
3. Cabrele, C.; Martinek, T.A.; Reiser, O.; Berlicki, Ł. Peptides Containing β-Amino Acid Patterns: Challenges and Successes in Medicinal Chemistry. *J. Med. Chem.* **2014**, *57*, 9718–9739. [CrossRef] [PubMed]
4. Janecka, A.; Fichna, J.; Janecki, T. Opioid Receptors and their Ligands. *Curr. Top. Med. Chem.* **2004**, *4*, 1–17. [CrossRef] [PubMed]
5. Pradhan, A.A.; Befort, K.; Nozaki, C.; Gavériaux-Ruff, C.; Kieffer, B.L. The delta opioid receptor: An evolving target for the treatment of brain disorders. *Trends Pharmacol. Sci.* **2011**, *32*, 581–590. [CrossRef] [PubMed]
6. Wilczyńska, D.; Kosson, P.; Kwasiborska, M.; Ejchart, A.; Olma, A. Synthesis and receptor binding of opioid peptide analogues containing β 3 – Homo –amino acids. *J. Pept. Sci.* **2009**, *15*, 777–782. [CrossRef]
7. Mallareddy, J.R.; Borics, A.; Keresztes, A.; Kövér, K.E.; Tourwé, D.; Tóth, G. Design, Synthesis, Pharmacological Evaluation, and Structure–Activity Study of Novel Endomorphin Analogues with Multiple Structural Modifications. *J. Med. Chem.* **2011**, *54*, 1462–1472. [CrossRef]
8. Keresztes, A.; Szűcs, M.; Borics, A.; Kövér, K.E.; Forró, E.; Fülöp, F.; Tömböly, C.; Péter, A.; Páhi, A.; Fábián, G.; et al. New Endomorphin Analogues Containing Alicyclic β-Amino Acids: Influence on Bioactive Conformation and Pharmacological Profile. *J. Med. Chem.* **2008**, *51*, 4270–4279. [CrossRef]
9. Perlikowska, R.; Fichna, J.; Wyrębska, A.; Poels, J.; Vanden Broeck, J.; Toth, G.; Storr, M.; do Rego, J.-C.; Janecka, A. Design, Synthesis and Pharmacological Characterization of Endomorphin Analogues with Non-Cyclic Amino Acid Residues in Position 2. *Basic Clin. Pharmacol. Toxicol.* **2010**, *106*, 106–113. [CrossRef]

10. Yamazaki, T.; Pröbstl, A.; Schiller, P.W.; Goodman, M. Biological and conformational studies of [Val4]morphiceptin and [D-Val4]morphiceptin analogs incorporating cis-2-aminocyclopentane carboxylic acid as a peptidomimetic for proline. *Int. J. Pept. Protein Res.* **1991**, *37*, 364–381. [CrossRef]
11. Mierke, D.F.; Nößner, G.; Schiller, P.W.; Goodman, M. Morphiceptin analogs containing 2-aminocyclopentane carboxylic acid as a peptidomimetic for proline. *Int. J. Pept. Protein Res.* **1990**, *35*, 35–45. [CrossRef] [PubMed]
12. Bozü, B.; Fülöp, F.; Tóth, G.; Tóth, G.; Szücs, M. Synthesis and opioid binding activity of dermorphin analogues containing cyclic β-amino acids. *Neuropeptides* **1997**, *31*, 367–372.
13. Cardillo, G.; Gentilucci, L.; Melchiorre, P.; Spampinato, S. Synthesis and binding activity of endomorphin-1 analogues containing β-amino acids. *Bioorg. Med. Chem. Lett.* **2000**, *10*, 2755–2758. [CrossRef]
14. Cardillo, G.; Gentilucci, L.; Qasem, A.R.; Sgarzi, F.; Spampinato, S. Endomorphin-1 Analogues Containing β-Proline Are μ-Opioid Receptor Agonists and Display Enhanced Enzymatic Hydrolysis Resistance. *J. Med. Chem.* **2002**, *45*, 2571–2578. [CrossRef]
15. Lesma, G.; Salvadori, S.; Airaghi, F.; Bojnik, E.; Borsodi, A.; Recca, T.; Sacchetti, A.; Balboni, G.; Silvani, A. Synthesis, pharmacological evaluation and conformational investigation of endomorphin-2 hybrid analogues. *Mol. Divers.* **2013**, *17*, 19–31. [CrossRef]
16. Lesma, G.; Salvadori, S.; Airaghi, F.; Murray, T.F.; Recca, T.; Sacchetti, A.; Balboni, G.; Silvani, A. Structural and Biological Exploration of Phe 3 – Phe 4 – Modified Endomorphin-2 Peptidomimetics. *ACS Med. Chem. Lett.* **2013**, *4*, 795–799. [CrossRef]
17. Mollica, A.; Pinnen, F.; Costante, R.; Locatelli, M.; Stefanucci, A.; Pieretti, S.; Davis, P.; Lai, J.; Rankin, D.; Porreca, F.; et al. Biological Active Analogues of the Opioid Peptide Biphalin: Mixed α/β 3 – Peptides. *J. Med. Chem.* **2013**, *56*, 3419–3423. [CrossRef]
18. Frączak, O.; Lasota, A.; Kosson, P.; Lesniak, A.; Muchowska, A.; Lipkowski, A.W.; Olma, A. Biphalin analogs containing β3-*Homo*-amino acids at the 4,4' positions: Synthesis and opioid activity profiles. *Peptides* **2015**, *66*, 13–18. [CrossRef]
19. Frączak, O.; Lasota, A.; Tymecka, D.; Kosson, P.; Muchowska, A.; Misicka, A.; Olma, A. Synthesis, binding affinities and metabolic stability of dimeric dermorphin analogs modified with β 3 – *Homo* –amino acids. *J. Pept. Sci.* **2016**, *22*, 222–227. [CrossRef]
20. Adamska-Bartłomiejczyk, A.; Lipiński, P.F.J.; Piekielna-Ciesielska, J.; Kluczyk, A.; Janecka, A. Pharmacological profile and molecular modeling of cyclic opioid analogs incorporating various phenylalanine derivatives. *sent* **2020**.
21. Wang, Y.; Yang, J.; Liu, X.; Zhao, L.; Yang, D.; Zhou, J.; Wang, D.; Mou, L.; Wang, R. Endomorphin-1 analogs containing α-methyl-β-amino acids exhibit potent analgesic activity after peripheral administration. *Org. Biomol. Chem.* **2017**, *15*, 4951–4955. [CrossRef] [PubMed]
22. Wang, Y.; Xing, Y.; Liu, X.; Ji, H.; Kai, M.; Chen, Z.; Yu, J.; Zhao, D.; Ren, H.; Wang, R. A New Class of Highly Potent and Selective Endomorphin-1 Analogues Containing α-Methylene-β-aminopropanoic Acids (Map). *J. Med. Chem.* **2012**, *55*, 6224–6236. [CrossRef] [PubMed]
23. Zhao, L.; Luo, K.; Wang, Z.; Wang, Y.; Zhang, X.; Yang, D.; Ma, M.; Zhou, J.; Cui, J.; Wang, J.; et al. Design, synthesis, and biological activity of new endomorphin analogs with multi-site modifications. *Bioorg. Med. Chem.* **2020**, *28*, 115438. [CrossRef] [PubMed]
24. Liu, X.; Wang, Y.; Xing, Y.; Yu, J.; Ji, H.; Kai, M.; Wang, Z.; Wang, D.; Zhang, Y.; Zhao, D.; et al. Design, Synthesis, and Pharmacological Characterization of Novel Endomorphin-1 Analogues as Extremely Potent μ-Opioid Agonists. *J. Med. Chem.* **2013**, *56*, 3102–3114. [CrossRef] [PubMed]
25. Hu, M.; Giulianotti, M.A.; McLaughlin, J.P.; Shao, J.; Debevec, G.; Maida, L.E.; Geer, P.; Cazares, M.; Misler, J.; Li, L.; et al. Synthesis and biological evaluations of novel endomorphin analogues containing α-hydroxy-β-phenylalanine (AHPBA) displaying mixed μ/δ opioid receptor agonist and δ opioid receptor antagonist activities. *Eur. J. Med. Chem.* **2015**, *92*, 270–281. [CrossRef] [PubMed]
26. Schiller, P.W.; Dung, N.T.M.; Chung, N.N.; Lemieux, C. Dermorphin analogs carrying an increased positive net charge in their "message" domain display extremely high. mu.-opioid receptor selectivity. *J. Med. Chem.* **1989**, *32*, 698–703. [CrossRef] [PubMed]
27. Podwysocka, D.; Kosson, P.; Lipkowski, A.W.; Olma, A. TAPP analogs containing β3-*Homo*-amino acids: Synthesis and receptor binding. *J. Pept. Sci.* **2012**, *18*, 556–559. [CrossRef]
28. Caddick, S.; de, K.; Haynes, A.K.; Judd, D.B.; Williams, M.R. Convenient synthesis of protected primary amines from nitriles. *Tetrahedron Lett.* **2000**, *41*, 3513–3516. [CrossRef]

29. Caddick, S.; Judd, D.B.; Lewis, A.K.d.K.; Reich, M.T.; Williams, M.R. A generic approach for the catalytic reduction of nitriles. *Tetrahedron* **2003**, *59*, 5417–5423. [CrossRef]
30. Kim, F.J.; Kovalyshyn, I.; Burgman, M.; Neilan, C.; Chien, C.-C.; Pasternak, G.W. σ 1 Receptor Modulation of G-Protein-Coupled Receptor Signaling: Potentiation of Opioid Transduction Independent from Receptor Binding. *Mol. Pharmacol.* **2010**, *77*, 695–703. [CrossRef]
31. Koehl, A.; Hu, H.; Maeda, S.; Zhang, Y.; Qu, Q.; Paggi, J.M.; Latorraca, N.R.; Hilger, D.; Dawson, R.; Matile, H.; et al. Structure of the μ-opioid receptor–Gi protein complex. *Nature* **2018**, *558*, 547–552. [CrossRef] [PubMed]
32. Morris, G.M.; Huey, R.; Lindstrom, W.; Sanner, M.F.; Belew, R.K.; Goodsell, D.S.; Olson, A.J. AutoDock4 and AutoDockTools4: Automated docking with selective receptor flexibility. *J. Comput. Chem.* **2009**, *30*, 2785–2791. [CrossRef] [PubMed]
33. Huang, W.; Manglik, A.; Venkatakrishnan, A.J.; Laeremans, T.; Feinberg, E.N.; Sanborn, A.L.; Kato, H.E.; Livingston, K.E.; Thorsen, T.S.; Kling, R.C.; et al. Structural insights into μ-opioid receptor activation. *Nature* **2015**, *524*, 315–321. [CrossRef] [PubMed]
34. Lipiński, P.F.J.; Jarończyk, M.; Dobrowolski, J.C.; Sadlej, J. Molecular dynamics of fentanyl bound to μ-opioid receptor. *J. Mol. Model.* **2019**, *25*, 144. [CrossRef] [PubMed]
35. Lipiński, P.; Kosson, P.; Matalińska, J.; Roszkowski, P.; Czarnocki, Z.; Jarończyk, M.; Misicka, A.; Dobrowolski, J.; Sadlej, J. Fentanyl Family at the Mu-Opioid Receptor: Uniform Assessment of Binding and Computational Analysis. *Molecules* **2019**, *24*, 740. [CrossRef] [PubMed]
36. Texier-Boullet, F.; Foucaud, A. Knoevenagel condensation catalysed by aluminium oxide. *Tetrahedron Lett.* **1982**, *23*, 4927–4928. [CrossRef]
37. Sipilä, J.; Nurmi, H.; Kaukonen, A.M.; Hirvonen, J.; Taskinen, J.; Yli-Kauhaluoma, J. A modification of the Hammett equation for predicting ionisation constants of p-vinyl phenols. *Eur. J. Pharm. Sci.* **2005**, *25*, 417–425. [CrossRef]
38. Yang, P.; Liu, Y.; Chai, L.; Lai, Z.; Fang, X.; Liu, B.; Zhang, W.; Lu, M.; Xu, Y.; Xu, H. Nmp-based ionic liquids: Recyclable catalysts for both hetero-Michael addition and Knoevenagel condensation in water. *Synth. Commun.* **2018**, *48*, 1060–1067. [CrossRef]
39. Juaristi, E.; Quintana, D.; Balderas, M.; García-Pérez, E. Enantioselective synthesis of β-amino acids. 7. Preparation of enantiopure α-substituted β-amino acids from 1-benzoyl-2(S)-tert-butyl-3-methylperhydropyrimidin-4-one.1,2. *Tetrahedron Asymmetry* **1996**, *7*, 2233–2246. [CrossRef]
40. Matalińska, J.; Lipiński, P.F.J.; Kotlarz, A.; Kosson, P.; Muchowska, A.; Dyniewicz, J. Evaluation of Receptor Affinity, Analgesic Activity and Cytotoxicity of a Hybrid Peptide, AWL3020. *Int. J. Pept. Res. Ther.* **2020**. [CrossRef]
41. Tóth, G.; Lovas, S.; Ötvös, F. Tritium Labeling of Neuropeptides. In *Neuropeptide Protocols*; Humana Press: New Jersey, NJ, USA, 1997; pp. 219–230.
42. Biovia Discovery Studio Visualizer Biovia Discovery Studio Visualizer 2018. Available online: www.3dsbiovia.com (accessed on 20 April 2020).
43. Schrödinger LLC The PyMOL Molecular Graphics System 2018. The PyMOL Molecular Graphics System. Available online: www.pymol.org (accessed on 20 April 2020).

Sample Availability: Samples of the compounds **1** and **8–17** are available from the authors.

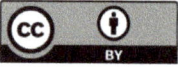

© 2020 by the authors. Licensee MDPI, Basel, Switzerland. This article is an open access article distributed under the terms and conditions of the Creative Commons Attribution (CC BY) license (http://creativecommons.org/licenses/by/4.0/).

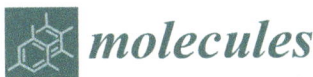

Article

Mechanistic Understanding of Peptide Analogues, DALDA, [Dmt¹]DALDA, and KGOP01, Binding to the Mu Opioid Receptor

Maria Dumitrascuta [1,†], Marcel Bermudez [2,†], Steven Ballet [3], Gerhard Wolber [2,*] and Mariana Spetea [1,*]

1. Department of Pharmaceutical Chemistry, Institute of Pharmacy and Center for Molecular Biosciences Innsbruck (CMBI), University of Innsbruck, Innrain 80-82, 6020 Innsbruck, Austria; maria.dumitrascuta@uibk.ac.at
2. Institute of Pharmacy, Freie Universität Berlin, Königin-Luise-Str. 2+4, D-14195 Berlin, Germany; m.bermudez@fu-berlin.de
3. Research Group of Organic Chemistry, Departments of Chemistry and Bioengineering Sciences, Vrije Universiteit Brussel, Pleinlaan 2, B-1050 Brussels, Belgium; Steven.Ballet@vub.be
* Correspondence: gerhard.wolber@fu-berlin.de (G.W.); mariana.spetea@uibk.ac.at (M.S.)
† Contributed equally to this work.

Academic Editor: Derek J. McPhee
Received: 8 April 2020; Accepted: 27 April 2020; Published: 29 April 2020

Abstract: The mu opioid receptor (MOR) is the primary target for analgesia of endogenous opioid peptides, alkaloids, synthetic small molecules with diverse scaffolds, and peptidomimetics. Peptide-based opioids are viewed as potential analgesics with reduced side effects and have received constant scientific interest over the years. This study focuses on three potent peptide and peptidomimetic MOR agonists, DALDA, [Dmt¹]DALDA, and KGOP01, and the prototypical peptide MOR agonist DAMGO. We present the first molecular modeling study and structure–activity relationships aided by in vitro assays and molecular docking of the opioid peptide analogues, in order to gain insight into their mode of binding to the MOR. In vitro binding and functional assays revealed the same rank order with KGOP01 > [Dmt¹]DALDA > DAMGO > DALDA for both binding and MOR activation. Using molecular docking at the MOR and three-dimensional interaction pattern analysis, we have rationalized the experimental outcomes and highlighted key amino acid residues responsible for agonist binding to the MOR. The Dmt (2′,6′-dimethyl-L-Tyr) moiety of [Dmt¹]DALDA and KGOP01 was found to represent the driving force for their high potency and agonist activity at the MOR. These findings contribute to a deeper understanding of MOR function and flexible peptide ligand–MOR interactions, that are of significant relevance for the future design of opioid peptide-based analgesics.

Keywords: mu opioid receptor; opioid peptides and peptidomimetics; DAMGO; DALDA; [Dmt¹]DALDA; KGOP01; binding; molecular docking; structure-activity relationships

1. Introduction

Opioids are the mainstay in the management of moderate to severe pain, and remain the most efficacious analgesics currently available [1]. The opioid receptors, mu (MOR), delta (DOR), and kappa (KOR), are G protein-coupled receptors (GPCRs) and molecular targets for opioid analgesics [2], that modulate nociception pathways in the central and peripheral nervous systems (CNS and PNS) [2–4]. Over the years, the MOR received a constant attention as the most important opioid receptor subtype responsible for opioid-induced analgesia, but concomitantly is also most responsible for the unwanted side effects (e.g., respiratory depression, constipation, sedation, dependence, and tolerance) of opioid analgesics [1,2]. All major clinically used opioid drugs, including morphine, oxycodone, and fentanyl, are agonists at the MOR [1,5]. In the past decade, abuse and misuse of opioids became a significant public health concern due to the huge rise in overdose morbidity and mortality [6,7]. In this view, the development of effective and safer analgesics represents a key research goal for 21st century analgesic drug discovery and pain medicine.

MOR mediates not only the analgesic effect of morphine, structurally related compounds, and other opioid drugs, but it is also the endogenous target of naturally occurring peptides [3,4]. Under physiological conditions, the MOR is activated by β-endorphins, enkephalins, endomorphins, and dermorphins, as endogenous neurotransmitters that have been extensively studied since their discovery [8–10]. Although there is a strong evidence for their role in pain regulation and potential use as analgesics, their poor enzymatic stability and difficulties in penetrating the blood–brain barrier (BBB) after systemic administration have limited their clinical applicability [8–14]. Generation of potent, stable peptidomimetics with improved pharmacodynamics and pharmacokinetics entails a systematic understanding of the structure-activity relationships (SAR), where the function of key residues can be determined using different strategies, such as amino acid substitution, deletion or addition of natural or unnatural amino acids, conformational restriction through peptide main chain or side chain cyclization, peptide bond replacement, or design of bi- or multifunctional peptide ligands [11–17]. A diversity of opioid peptide-based analgesics with reduced adverse effects was made available through chemical synthesis and appraised as prospective therapeutic agents or research tools [5,11,13–15,17].

Since the breakthrough of GPCR crystallization one decade ago, the understanding of the complex biology of GPCR activation and signaling has dramatically increased [16–19]. Substantial advances in structural biology of GPCRs were possible by means of innovative methodological and powerful computational systems [20–22]. Due to its therapeutic relevance, the MOR is among the few GPCRs determined in different activation states, with the first X-ray crystal structure of the murine MOR published in 2012 in complex with the irreversible morphinan antagonist β-funaltrexamine (PDB ID: 4DKL) [23], and the 3D-structure in the active conformation reported in 2015, where the receptor was co-crystallized with the morphinan agonist BU72 (PDB ID: 5C1M) [24]. Recently, the high resolution cryo-electron microscopy (cryo-EM) structure of the MOR (PDB ID: 6DDF) bound to the agonist peptide DAMGO (Figure 1) was reported [25], offering an important view on the structural features that contribute to the G_i protein-coupling specificity of the MOR. The available crystal structures of the MOR together with efficient computational methods (i.e., molecular docking and molecular dynamics simulations) provide essential insights into binding modes of ligands to the receptor, with the gained knowledge being successfully translated into the discovery of novel bioactive molecules [22,26,27]. Most of molecular modeling reports on the active and inactive structures of the MOR targeted small molecules as ligands, with only few studies employing peptides, mostly DAMGO, as the prototypical MOR selective synthetic analogue of the natural peptides enkephalin [25,28,29], endomorphin-2, and dermorphin, as endogenous opioid ligands for the MOR [30,31].

DAMGO	H-Tyr-*D*Ala-Gly-*N*MePhe-Gly-OH
DALDA	H-Tyr-*D*Arg-Phe-Lys-NH$_2$
[Dmt^1]DALDA	H-Dmt-*D*Arg-Phe-Lys-NH$_2$
KGOP01	H-Dmt-*D*Arg-Aba-βAla-NH$_2$

Figure 1. Sequence of investigated opioid peptide analogues. Dmt: 2′,6′-dimethyl-L-tyrosine; Aba: 4-amino-tetrahydro-2-benzazepinone.

In this report, we have addressed for the first time a structure-based docking study at the active conformation of the MOR of three peptide and peptidomimetic, potent MOR agonists, DALDA, [Dmt^1]DALDA, and KGOP01 (Figure 1). Merging experimental (in vitro assays) with computational (in silico methods) approaches, we aimed to explain the molecular basis for their binding to the

MOR, in terms of understanding the structural correlations as well as interpreting the related SARs. The two peptides DALDA [32] and [Dmt^1]DALDA [33] are synthetic analogues of the naturally-occurring dermorphin, having high enzymatic stability due to the presence of D-Arg in the second position of the peptide sequence (instead of D-Ala in dermorphin), and a modified Tyr^1, Dmt (2′,6′-dimethyl-L-Tyr), in [Dmt^1]DALDA (Figure 1). While DALDA does not cross the BBB to a significant extent, [Dmt^1]DALDA was demonstrated to be able to pass the BBB to produce analgesia in animals after systemic administration [13]. KGOP01 is a new tetrapeptide, CNS penetrant, and stable analogue of [Dmt^1]DALDA with two unnatural amino acids, 4-amino-tetrahydro-2-benzazepinone (Aba) at position 3 and βAla at position 4 [34]. The rationale for the selection of these peptide analogues is based on the numerous in vitro and in vivo studies that have established them as stable, potent MOR agonists and effective analgesics in animal pain models with an interesting pharmacology, as well as based on their value as leads in the development of new peptide ligands [13,34–43]. However, binding behavior of DALDA, [Dmt^1]DALDA, and KGOP01 to their primary target, the MOR, using computational approaches has not been investigated up to now. The findings of this study provide structural insights into flexible peptide ligand–MOR interactions that are of significant relevance for further understanding MOR function and pharmacology, and the future design of new generation analgesics.

2. Results and Discussions

2.1. Comparison of In Vitro Binding and Activation Profiles of DALDA, [Dmt^1]DALDA, and KGOP01 to the MOR

We have initially performed a direct comparison of in vitro activity profiles of targeted opioid peptide analogues, DALDA, [Dmt^1]DALDA, and KGOP01 (Figure 1) at the human MOR, in terms of receptor binding and activation. For comparison purposes, the opioid binding profile of DAMGO [44], as the standard MOR agonist, is also presented. Whereas specific binding of DALDA and [Dmt^1]DALDA to the MOR in the rat brain has been reported previously [32], with both ligands showing high affinity and selectivity for the MOR, in the present study the first data on binding affinity to the human MOR is reported. Binding to the human MOR was evaluated using in vitro competitive radioligand binding assays with membrane preparations from Chinese hamster ovary cells stably expressing the human MOR (CHO-hMOR cells) and the specific MOR radioligand [^{3}H]DAMGO, according to the published procedures [43]. All three peptides displayed high capability to inhibit [^{3}H]DAMGO binding to the human MOR in a concentration-dependent manner (Figure 2A), with binding affinities (as K_i values) in the low nanomolar to subnanomolar range (Table 1).

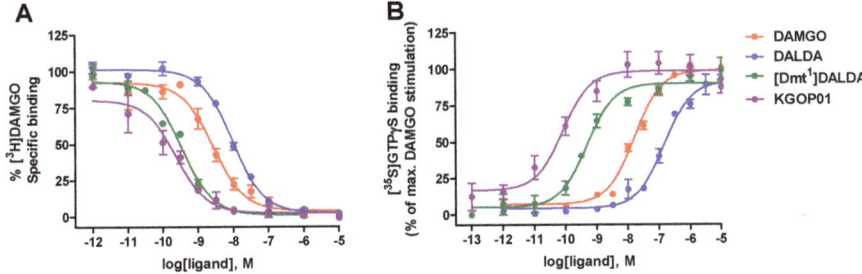

Figure 2. In vitro activity profiles of DAMGO, DALDA, [Dmt^1]DALDA, and KGOP01 to the human MOR (hMOR). (**A**) Binding of tested peptides to the MOR was determined in competitive radioligand binding assays using CHO-hMOR cell membranes. (**B**) Stimulation of [^{35}S]GTPγS binding by tested peptides was determined in the [^{35}S]GTPγS binding assay using CHO-hMOR cell membranes. Values are expressed as the mean ± SEM (n = 3–4 independent experiments).

The high binding affinities to the human recombinant MOR expressed in CHO cells showed by DALDA and [Dmt¹]DALDA confirms earlier data at the rat MOR in the brain tissue (K_i values of 1.69 nM for DALDA, and 0.143 nM for [Dmt¹]DALDA) [32]. As shown in Table 1, replacement of the Tyr¹ residue in DALDA with Dmt¹ in [Dmt¹]DALDA led to a significant increase (27-fold) in binding affinity to the human MOR, an observation that is in good agreement with findings at the rat MOR [32]. Additionally, exchanging Phe³-Lys⁴ residues in [Dmt¹]DALDA with an unnatural, uncommon amino acid, respectively, in the Aba³-βAla⁴ sequence lead to in a new analogue, KGOP01 [34], which exhibited a further increase (ca. 2-fold) in the MOR affinity than [Dmt¹]DALDA, and a 13-fold better MOR affinity than DAMGO (Table 1, Figure 2A).

Table 1. In vitro binding and agonist activity of opioid peptide analogues at the human MOR.

Opioid Peptide	Binding Affinity [a]	Agonist Activity [b]	
	K_i (nM)	EC_{50} (nM)	% stim.
DAMGO	1.46 ± 0.37	18.1 ± 2.0	100
DALDA	6.36 ± 0.24	149 ± 28	92 ± 2
[Dmt¹]DALDA	0.23 ± 0.02	0.51 ± 0.06	90 ± 4
KGOP01	0.11 ± 0.05	0.10 ± 0.02	99 ± 6

[a] Determined in competitive radioligand binding assays using membrane from CHO expressing the human MOR (CHO-hMOR). [b] Determined in the [³⁵S]GTPγS binding assay using CHO-hMOR cell membranes. Percentage stimulation (% stim.) relative to DAMGO (reference MOR full agonist). Values are means ± SEM (n = 3-4 independent experiments).

Next, we have compared in vitro functional activities of DALDA, [Dmt¹]DALDA and KGOP01 at the human MOR in the guanosine-5'-O-(3-[³⁵S]thio)-triphosphate ([³⁵S]GTPγS) binding assay using membranes from CHO cells stably expressing the human MOR, performed as described [43]. All tested peptides produced a concentration-dependent increase in the [³⁵S]GTPγS binding with different levels of potencies (Figure 2B). Whereas DALDA and [Dmt¹]DALDA showed full efficacy at the MOR, [Dmt¹]DALDA had a considerable increased (292-fold) in agonist potency than DALDA in inducing MOR-mediated G protein activation (Table 1). Additionally, [Dmt¹]DALDA had higher agonist potency (35-fold) than that of DAMGO. Previous in vitro bioassays using guinea-pig ileum (GPI) preparations established [Dmt¹]DALDA as a more potent MOR agonist (180-fold) than DALDA [32]. Further, an enhanced MOR agonist potency by 5-fold was measured in the present study for KGOP01 as compared to [Dmt¹]DALDA in the [³⁵S]GTPγS binding assay (Table 1). The potent MOR agonist profile of KGOP01 was established previously in the GPI bioassay (IC_{50} = 0.8 nM) [34] and cAMP accumulation assay with HEK293 cells expressing the human MOR (EC_{50} = 0.204 nM) [42]. The outcomes derived from functional assays correlate well with the results obtained in binding studies at the MOR and structural features of investigated peptide analogues, where [Dmt¹]DALDA and KGOP01 show a better in vitro profile than DALDA, with KGOP01 being the most potent MOR agonist of the series.

2.2. In Silico Investigation of DALDA, [Dmt¹]DALDA, and KGOP01 Binding to the MOR

The observed differences in the in vitro activity profiles of DALDA, [Dmt¹]DALDA, and KGOP01 (Table 1) encouraged in silico investigations of their binding modes at the MOR. The recently published crystal structure of the active conformation of the MOR (PDB ID: 5C1M; resolution: 2.1 Å) [24] provides the structural basis for understanding important aspects of MOR pharmacology and its function [22,24,45]. In order to examine possible binding conformations of the targeted peptide analogues to the MOR, docking experiments were performed using GOLD [46], and LigandScout [47] was used to analyze differences in receptor–ligand interactions. We used the numbering scheme from the PDB together with Ballosteros–Weinstein nomenclature.

Since the available crystal structure of the active MOR (PDB ID: 5C1M) [24] represents the murine receptor, a structural model of the human MOR was built by in silico mutations of differing residues. Interestingly, six out of seven differing amino acid residues are located in the extracellular region.

The high similarity in the receptor core region and the intracellular side suggests a conserved receptor activation mechanism, but potential differences for ligand recognition (Figure 3). However, only one of these residues turned out to directly point to the ligand binding site. Instead of a histidine at position 54 in the murine MOR, the human receptor has an aspartic acid at this position. Notable, the recently reported cryo-EM structure of the MOR (PDB ID: 6DDF; resolution: 3.5 Å) [25] bound to the agonist peptide DAMGO misses the N-terminal region and unveils a binding mode for DAMGO, which is not compatible with the previous crystal structure [24] (Figure 4), indicating that DAMGO might bind differently in the truncated vs. untruncated receptor. Due to the fact that the cryo-EM structure presents the MOR bound to DAMGO, this structure was subsequently used for binding mode investigations of DALDA, [Dmt¹]DALDA, and KGOP01, with the same in silico mutations as in the abovementioned structural model of the human MOR. The discrepancies between the crystal structure and the cryo-EM structure with regard to the N-terminus suggests an important, but different role in binding of non-peptide ligands, such as morphinan-based agonists and peptide ligands. We would like to note that binding mode predictions are always of hypothetic nature and in this specific case the reliability of our proposed interaction pattern strongly depends on the receptor region. Whereas the C-terminal parts of the studied peptides, located in the receptor core region are more reliable, the missing structural information for the N-terminus of the receptor makes the binding orientations of the N-terminal parts of the studied peptides and resulting interactions more speculative.

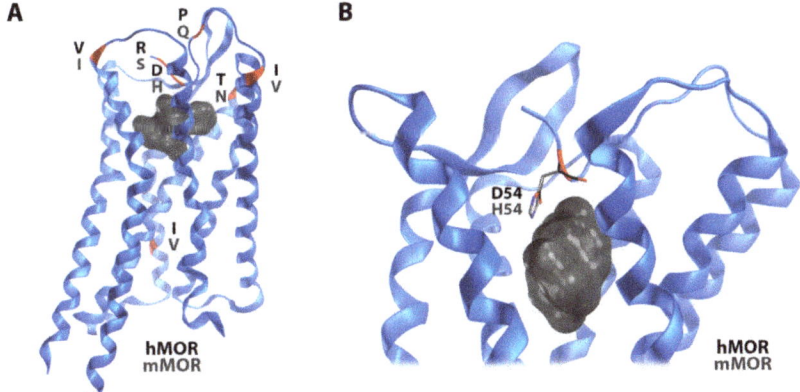

Figure 3. The murine (PDB ID: 5C1M) and the human MOR model differ only in seven amino acid residues as illustrated in red (**A**). Only one of these differing residues is directly pointing to the ligand binding site (**B**, grey surface). Whereas a histidine residue is at position 54 in the murine MOR, the human receptor has an aspartic acid at this position.

Docking of DAMGO, DALDA, [Dmt¹]DALDA, and KGOP01 to the structural model of the human MOR (PDB ID: 6DDF) resulted in comparable binding orientations for the four peptides (Figure 5). Several receptor–ligand interactions were observed in all complexes (Figure 6), and an overview of detected receptor–ligand interactions is presented in Figure 7. Due to missing information on the role of the receptor's N-terminus for ligand binding and the high flexibility of the peptide ligands, the interactions with the extracellular loop regions are more speculative than the interactions within the inner core region. As expected, D147$^{3.32}$ forms a charge interaction with the primary amine of the tyrosine (in DAMGO and DALDA) or the Dmt (in [Dmt¹]DALDA and KGOP01). Additionally, this primary amine of the tyrosine of DALDA and [Dmt¹]DALDA forms a π–cation interaction with Y148$^{3.33}$. The central role of D147$^{3.32}$ and Y148$^{3.33}$ for binding of DAMGO, morphine and morphinan ligands, and other small molecules to the MOR is well-recognized [23–28,48]. The phenol moieties of all ligands are pointing towards I296$^{6.51}$ and form a hydrogen bond except for DAMGO. In theory, the phenol moieties could also form hydrogen bonds to water molecules as observed in the MOR crystal structure (PDB ID: 5C1M), but the role of water-mediated interaction networks for peptide ligands is still not clear. The phenyl rings of the phenylalanine (in DAMGO, DALDA, and [Dmt^1]DALDA) fill a hydrophobic pocket that comprises the aliphatic chain of I144$^{3.29}$ residues. While the Aba moiety of KGOP01 only reaches I144$^{3.29}$, it also makes KGOP01 more rigid and thereby allows for a potentially highly favorable hydrogen bond with K303$^{6.58}$. Interestingly, the methyl group of the alanine of DAMGO shows unique lipophilic contacts with W318$^{7.34}$ and I322$^{7.38}$ residues, which could not be observed for the other peptides. In comparison, DAMGO and KGOP01 are more similar in terms of their hydrogen bonding pattern including T218^{ECL2} and K303$^{6.58}$. Further, DALDA and [Dmt^1]DALDA only differ in the additional lipophilic contact of [Dmt^1]DALDA with Y326$^{7.42}$. Overall, the four targeted opioid peptides show comparable binding modes to the MOR. The tyrosine/Dmt ring of all four peptides shows lipophilic contacts with M151$^{3.36}$, I296$^{6.51}$, and V300$^{6.55}$ residues. The two methyl groups of the Dmt moiety in [Dmt^1]DALDA and KGOP01 show additional lipophilic contacts with Y148$^{3.33}$ and Y326$^{7.42}$ residues, which might lower the entropic penalty upon binding (Figure 8). The latter rigidification effect might also strengthen the hydrogen bond with I296$^{6.51}$ residue (Figure 6).

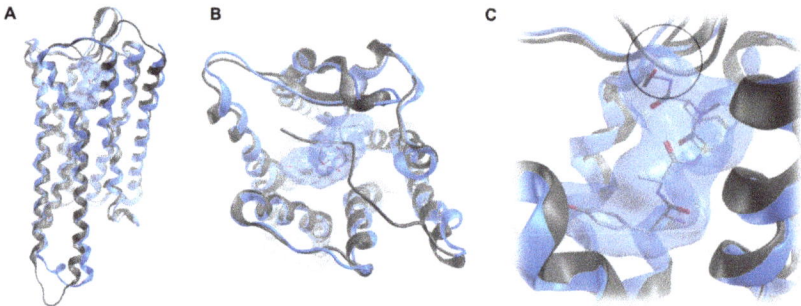

Figure 4. Superimposition of the crystal structure of the MOR (PDB ID: 5C1M) with co-crystallized BU72 (grey), and the recently available cryo-EM structure (PDB ID: 6DDF) with bound DAMGO (blue) in a transmembrane (**A**) and extracellular view (**B**). The close-up view on DAMGO (blue surface) in the binding site (**C**) unveils a sterical clash (circle) of the peptide with the N-terminus resolved in the active crystal structure.

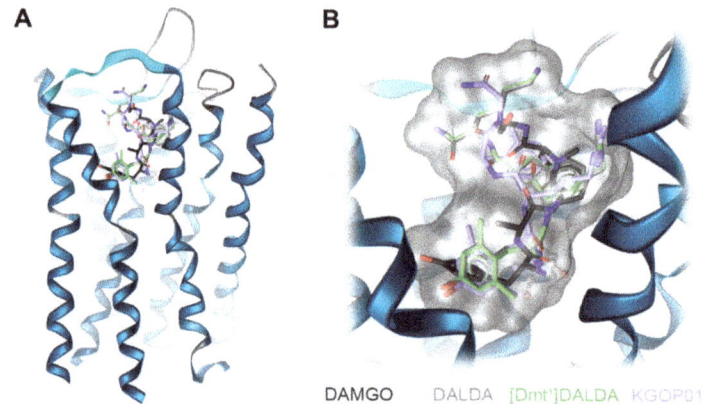

Figure 5. Investigated opioid peptides DAMGO, DALDA, [Dmt^1]DALDA, and KGOP01 show a comparable binding orientation in the inner core region of the human MOR model (based on PDB ID: 6DDF) (**A**). Aspartic acid D147$^{3.32}$ plays a major role in ligand binding through a charge interaction with the opioid peptides (**B**).

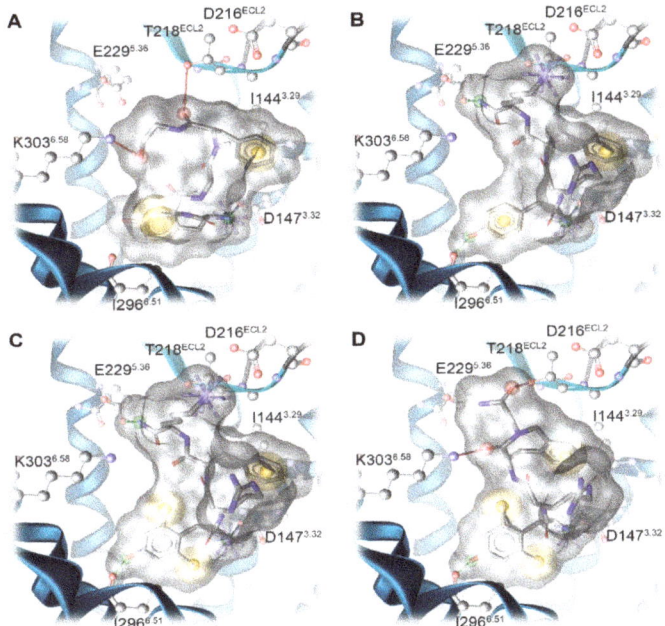

Figure 6. Predicted binding modes at the human MOR model (based on PDB ID: 6DDF) and receptor–ligand interaction patterns of opioid peptides (**A**) DAMGO, (**B**) DALDA, (**C**) [Dmt^1]DALDA, and (**D**) KGOP01. Yellow spheres indicate lipophilic contacts, red arrows hydrogen bond acceptors, green arrows hydrogen bond donors, and positively charged centers are shown as blue spheres.

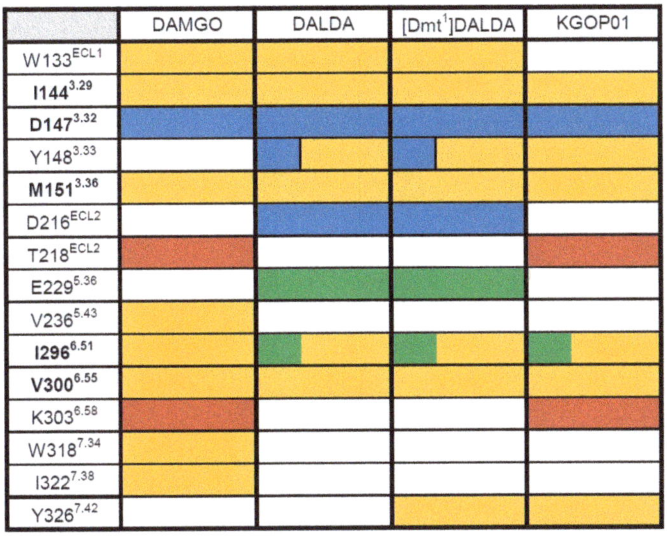

	DAMGO	DALDA	[Dmt^1]DALDA	KGOP01
W133^{ECL1}	yellow	yellow	yellow	yellow
I144$^{3.29}$	yellow	yellow	yellow	yellow
D147$^{3.32}$	blue	blue	blue	blue
Y148$^{3.33}$		blue/yellow	blue/yellow	yellow
M151$^{3.36}$	yellow	yellow	yellow	yellow
D216^{ECL2}		blue	blue	
T218^{ECL2}	red			red
E229$^{5.36}$	yellow	green	green	yellow
V236$^{5.43}$	yellow	yellow	yellow	yellow
I296$^{6.51}$	yellow	green/yellow	green/yellow	green/yellow
V300$^{6.55}$	yellow	yellow	yellow	yellow
K303$^{6.58}$	red			red
W318$^{7.34}$	yellow			yellow
I322$^{7.38}$	yellow			yellow
Y326$^{7.42}$	yellow		yellow	yellow

Figure 7. Ligand–MOR interaction pattern derived from molecular docking solutions of opioid peptides DAMGO, DALDA, [Dmt^1]DALDA, and KGOP01. Yellow fields indicate lipophilic contacts, red fields hydrogen bond acceptors, green fields hydrogen bond donors, and positively charged centers are shown as blue fields. White fields indicate the absence of an interaction with that residue. Residues which show the same type of interaction for all morphinan ligands are marked in bold.

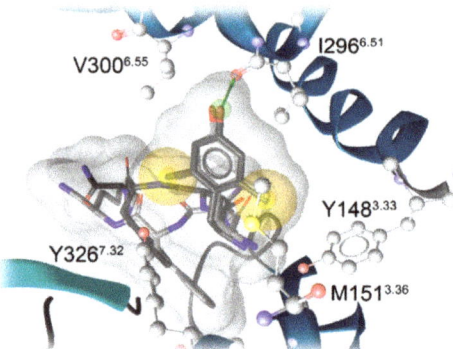

Figure 8. Hydrophobic environment of Dmt moieties of [Dmt^1]DALDA (light grey) and KGOP01 (dark grey). The two methyl groups show additional hydrophobic contacts with Y148$^{3.33}$ and Y326$^{7.32}$, respectively, which are not observable for DAMGO or DALDA. Yellow spheres indicate lipophilic contacts and green arrows hydrogen bond donors. For clarity, only interactions of the Dmt moiety are shown.

3. Materials and Methods

3.1. Chemicals and Materials

Cell culture media and supplements were obtained from Sigma-Aldrich Chemicals (St. Louis, MO, USA). Radioligands [^{3}H]DAMGO (50 Ci/mmol) and [^{35}S]GTPγS (1250 Ci/mmol) were purchased from PerkinElmer (Boston, MA, USA). DAMGO, unlabeled GTPγS, and guanosine diphosphate (GDP) were obtained from Sigma-Aldrich Chemicals (St. Louis, MO, USA). All other chemicals were of analytical grade and obtained from standard commercial sources.

3.2. Peptide and Peptidomimetic Ligands

DALDA [32], [Dmt^1]DALDA [33], and KGOP01 [34] were synthesized as described previously [34], with purities >98%. DAMGO was obtained from Sigma-Aldrich Chemicals (St. Louis, MO, USA). Test peptides were prepared as 1 mM stocks in water, and further diluted to working concentrations in the appropriate medium.

3.3. Cell Culture

CHO cells stably expressing the human MOR were kindly provided by Dr. Lawrence Toll (SRI International, Menlo Park, CA, USA). The CHO-hMOR cell line was grown in Dulbecco's Minimal Essential Medium (DMEM)/Ham's F-12 medium supplemented with fetal bovine serum (FBS, 10%), penicillin/streptomycin (0.1%), L-glutamine (2 mM), and geneticin (400 μg/mL). Cells were maintained at 37 °C in 5% CO_2 humidified air.

3.4. Competitive Radioligand Binding Assays

Binding assays were conducted on human MOR stably transfected into CHO cells (CHO-hMOR) according to the published procedure [43]. Cell membranes were prepared as described previously, and stored at −80 °C until use [43]. Protein concentration of cell membrane preparations was determined by the method of Bradford using bovine serum albumin as the standard [49]. Cell membranes (15–20 μg) were incubated in 50 mM Tris-HCl buffer (pH 7.4) with [^{3}H]DAMGO (1 nM) and various concentrations of test peptides in a final volume of 1 mL, for 60 min at 25 °C. Non-specific binding was determined using 10 μM of unlabeled DAMGO. After incubation, reactions were terminated by rapid filtration through Whatman glass GF/C fiber filters. Filters were washed three times with 5 mL of ice-cold 50 mM Tris-HCl buffer (pH 7.4) using a Brandel M24R cell harvester (Gaithersburg, MD, USA). Radioactivity retained on the filters was counted by liquid scintillation counting using a Beckman Coulter LS6500 (Beckman Coulter Inc., Fullerton, CA, USA). The inhibitory constant (K_i, in nM) values were calculated from the competition binding curves by nonlinear regression analysis and the Cheng–Prusoff equation [50]. All experiments were performed in duplicate and repeated at least three times.

3.5. $[^{35}S]GTP\gamma S$ Binding Assays

Binding of $[^{35}S]GTP\gamma S$ to membranes from CHO cells stably expressing the human MOR(CHO-hMOR) was conducted according to the published procedure [43]. Cell membranes (5-10 μg) in 20 mM HEPES, 10 mM $MgCl_2$, and 100 mM NaCl, pH 7.4 were incubated with 0.05 nM $[^{35}S]GTP\gamma S$, 10 μM GDP and various concentrations of test peptides in a final volume of 1 mL, for 60 min at 25°C. Non-specific binding was determined using 10 μM $GTP\gamma S$, and the basal binding was determined in the absence of test ligand. Samples are filtered over glass Whatman glass GF/B fiber filters and counted as described for binding assays. In each individual experiment, the increase in $[^{35}S]GTP\gamma S$ binding produced by the test peptides were normalized to the maximal stimulation of the reference full MOR agonist, DAMGO and nonlinear regression performed on each individual curve were averaged to yield potency (EC_{50}, in nM) and efficacy (as % stim.) values. All experiments were performed in duplicate and repeated at least three times.

3.6. Data Analysis

Experimental data were analyzed and graphically processed using the GraphPad Prism 5.0 Software (GraphPad Prism Software Inc., San Diego, CA, USA), and are presented as means ± SEM

3.7. Molecular Modeling

The structure of the human MOR was remodeled based on the crystal structure of the murine MOR (PDB ID: 5C1M) [24] by using the mutation tool of Molecular Operating Environment (MOE, 2019.0101; Chemical Computing Group Inc., Montreal, QC, Canada) with subsequent sidechain optimization. Complementary, the cryo-EM structure of the MOR with bound DAMGO (PDB ID: 6DDF) [25] was used. All receptor-ligand docking experiments were performed with the CCDCs software GOLD version 5.7.0 [46]. Water molecules and ligands were removed. Assignment of protonation states and protein preparation were performed using Protonate3D [51] (implemented in MOE 2019.1, Chemical Computing Group, Montreal, QC, Canada). All residues of the inner receptor core region and the C-terminal domain were defined as potential binding site (12 Å around the γ-carbon atom of D147; PDB ID: 6DDF) [25]. For receptor-ligand docking, default settings were applied and GoldScore served as primary scoring function with DAMGO as reference ligand. All obtained docking poses and receptor–ligand interactions were analyzed using LigandScout 4.4 [47] using a 3D-pharmacophore approach [52].

4. Conclusions

Given the essential clinical role of the MOR in mediating pain inhibition and other physiological activities, with endogenous peptides as natural agonists of the MOR, a basic understanding of the binding mechanism of opioid peptides to the MOR is required for their further development as potential analgesics and drugs for pain treatment and other human disorders. The peptidic nature of endogenous MOR agonists provides a variety of modification possibilities to design specific and stable MOR agonists. In this study, we have reported on a set of peptide analogues, DAMGO, DALDA, [Dmt[1]]DALDA, and KGOP01, for which in silico binding modes and in vitro activities at the MOR were correlated. The present results evidence the consequence of the modified Tyr[1], Dmt, in [Dmt[1]]DALDA and KGOP01 on the pharmacological profile with molecular docking studies offering a structural basis for the observed MOR activities. In vitro receptor binding and functional assays revealed the same rank order with KGOP01 > [Dmt^1]DALDA > DAMGO > DALDA for both binding and MOR activation. In silico binding mode investigations indicated the important contribution of the Dmt moiety for binding and MOR activation, specifically, with the two methyl groups of the Dmt moiety in [Dmt^1]DALDA and KGOP01 showing additional lipophilic contacts with Y148$^{3.33}$ and Y326$^{7.42}$ residues. Generally, the limited CNS penetration of peptides often impairs their development as therapeutics. Furthermore, the feasibility of peptides for clinical application is much precluded by their enzymatic degradation. DALDA, [Dmt^1]DALDA, and KGOP01 have high stability against enzymatic degradation, due to the presence of certain structural modifications, i.e., unnatural and synthetic amino acids. While DALDA does not cross the BBB, the [Dmt^1]DALDA and KGOP01 can enter the CNS [13,42]. The gained knowledge from this study on which molecular interactions with the MOR these opioid peptides share and distinguish them, with Y148$^{3.33}$ and Y326$^{7.42}$ sites being of significance, may also help to understand the differences in the pharmacokinetics between these peptides. Our findings offer structural insights into flexible peptide ligand–MOR interactions that are important for further understanding of MOR function and pharmacology, and the future design of peptide-based analgesics.

Author Contributions: M.D. and M.B. contributed equally to the work; M.S. and G.W. conceived and designed the study; M.D. and M.B. performed the research; S.B. provided compounds; M.D., M.B., G.W., and M.S. analyzed the data; M.D., M.B., G.W., and M.S. wrote the manuscript with inputs from S.B. All authors have read and agreed to the published version of the manuscript.

Funding: This research was funded by the Austrian Science Fund (FWF: I2463-B21), the German Research Foundation (DFG: 407626949), and the Research Foundation Flanders (FWO Vlaanderen).

Conflicts of Interest: The authors declare no conflict of interest.

References

1. Pasternak, G.W. Mu opioid pharmacology: 40 years to the promised land. *Adv. Pharmacol.* **2018**, *82*, 261–291. [PubMed]
2. Stein, C. Opioid receptors. *Annu. Rev. Med.* **2016**, *67*, 433–451. [CrossRef] [PubMed]
3. Corder, G.; Castro, D.C.; Bruchas, M.R.; Scherrer, G. Endogenous and exogenous opioids in pain. *Annu. Rev. Neurosci.* **2018**, *41*, 453–473. [CrossRef]
4. Darcq, E.; Kieffer, B.L. Opioid receptors: Drivers to addiction. *Nature* **2018**, *19*, 499–514. [CrossRef] [PubMed]
5. Spetea, M.; Asim, M.F.; Wolber, G.; Schmidhammer, H. The μ opioid receptor and ligands acting at the μ opioid receptor, as therapeutics and potential therapeutics. *Curr. Pharm. Des.* **2013**, *19*, 7415–7434. [CrossRef] [PubMed]
6. Volkow, N.D.; Jones, E.B.; Einstein, E.B.; Wargo, E.M. Prevention and treatment of opioid misuse and addiction: A review. *JAMA Psychiatry* **2019**, *76*, 208–216. [CrossRef] [PubMed]
7. Epstein, D.H.; Heilig, M.; Shaham, Y. Science-based actions can help address the opioid crisis. *Trends Pharmacol. Sci.* **2018**, *39*, 911–916. [CrossRef]
8. Berezniuk, I.; Fricker, L.D. Endogenous opioids. In *The Opiate Receptors*, 2nd ed.; Pasternak, G.W., Ed.; Humana Press: Totowa, NJ, USA, 2011; pp. 93–120.
9. Fichna, J.; Janecka, A.; Constentin, J.; Do Rego, J.C. The endomorphin system and its evolving neurophysiological role. *Pharmacol. Rev.* **2007**, *59*, 88–123. [CrossRef]
10. Negri, L.; Melchiorri, P.; Lattanzi, R. Pharmacology of amphibian opiate peptides. *Peptides* **2000**, *21*, 1639–1647. [CrossRef]
11. Aldrich, J.V.; McLaughlin, J.P. Opioid peptides: Potential for drug development. *Drug Discov. Today Technol.* **2012**, *9*, e23–e31. [CrossRef]
12. Bryant, S.D.; Jinsmaa, Y.; Salvadori, S.; Okada, Y.; Lazarus, L.H. Dmt and opioid peptides: A potent alliance. *Pept. Sci.* **2003**, *71*, 86–102. [CrossRef] [PubMed]
13. Schiller, P.W. Opioid peptide-derived analgesics. In *Drug Addiction: From Basic Research to Therapy*; Rapaka, R.S., Sadee, W., Eds.; Springer: New York, NY, USA, 2008; pp. 357–366.

14. Janecka, A.; Perlikowska, R.; Gach, K.; Wyrebska, A.; Fichna, J. Development of opioid peptide analogs for pain relief. *Curr. Pharm. Des.* **2010**, *16*, 1126–1135. [CrossRef] [PubMed]
15. Janecka, A.; Gentilucci, L. Cyclic endomorphin analogs in targeting opioid receptors to achieve pain relief. *Future Med. Chem.* **2014**, *6*, 2093–2101. [CrossRef] [PubMed]
16. De Marco, R.; Janecka, A. Strategies to improve bioavailability and in vivo efficacy of the endogenous opioid peptides endomorphin-1 and endomorphin-2. *Curr. Top. Med. Chem.* **2015**, *16*, 141–155. [CrossRef] [PubMed]
17. Giri, A.K.; Hruby, V.J. Investigational peptide and peptidomimetic μ and δ opioid receptor agonists in the relief of pain. *Expert Opin. Investig. Drugs* **2014**, *23*, 227–241. [CrossRef]
18. Shonberg, J.; Kling, R.C.; Gmeiner, P.; Löber, S. GPCR crystal structures: Medicinal chemistry in the pocket. *Bioorganic Med. Chem.* **2015**, *23*, 3880–3906. [CrossRef]
19. Weis, W.I.; Kobilka, B.K. The molecular basis of G protein-coupled receptor activation. *Annu. Rev. Biochem.* **2018**, *87*, 897–919. [CrossRef]
20. Hilger, D.; Masureel, M.; Kobilka, B.K. Structure and dynamics of GPCR signaling complexes. *Nat. Struct. Mol. Biol.* **2018**, *25*, 4–12. [CrossRef]
21. Bermudez, M.; Nguyen, T.N.; Omieczynski, C.; Wolber, G. Strategies for the discovery of biased GPCR ligands. *Drug Discov. Today* **2019**, *24*, 1031–1037. [CrossRef]
22. Ribeiro, J.M.L.; Filizola, M. Insights from molecular dynamics simulations of a number of G-protein coupled receptor targets for the treatment of pain and opioid use disorders. *Front. Mol. Neurosci.* **2019**, *12*, 207. [CrossRef]
23. Manglik, A.; Kruse, A.C.; Kobilka, T.S.; Thian, F.S.; Mathiesen, J.M.; Sunahara, R.K.; Pardo, L.; Weis, W.I.; Kobilka, B.K.; Granier, S. Crystal structure of the mu-opioid receptor bound to a morphinan antagonist. *Nature* **2012**, *485*, 321–326. [CrossRef] [PubMed]
24. Huang, W.; Manglik, A.; Venkatakrishnan, A.J.; Laeremans, T.; Feinberg, E.N.; Sanborn, A.L.; Kato, H.E.; Livingston, K.E.; Thorsen, T.S.; Kling, R.C.; et al. Structural insights into μ-opioid receptor activation. *Nature* **2015**, *524*, 315–321. [CrossRef] [PubMed]
25. Koehl, A.; Hu, H.; Maeda, S.; Zhang, Y.; Qu, Q.; Paggi, J.M.; Latorraca, N.R.; Hilger, D.; Dawson, R.; Matile, H.; et al. Structure of the μ-opioid receptor–Gi protein complex. *Nature* **2018**, *558*, 547–552. [CrossRef] [PubMed]
26. Manglik, A.; Lin, H.; Aryal, D.K.; McCorvy, J.D.; Dengler, D.; Corder, G.; Levit, A.; Kling, R.C.; Bernat, V.; Hübner, H.; et al. Structure-based discovery of opioid analgesics with reduced side effects. *Nature* **2016**, *537*, 185–190. [CrossRef] [PubMed]
27. Kaserer, T.; Lantero, A.; Schmidhammer, H.; Spetea, M.; Schuster, D. μ Opioid receptor: Novel antagonists and structural modeling. *Sci. Rep.* **2016**, *6*, 21548. [CrossRef]
28. Cui, X.; Yeliseev, A.; Liu, R. Ligand interaction, binding site and G protein activation of the mu opioid receptor. *Eur. J. Pharmacol.* **2013**, *702*, 309–315. [CrossRef]
29. Bartuzi, D.; Kaczor, A.A.; Matosiuk, D. Activation and allosteric modulation of human μ opioid receptor in molecular dynamics. *J. Chem. Inf. Model.* **2015**, *55*, 2421–2434. [CrossRef]
30. Wtorek, K.; Artali, R.; Piekielna-Ciesielska, J.; Koszuk, J.; Kluczyk, A.; Gentilucci, L.; Janecka, A. Endomorphin-2 analogs containing modified tyrosines: Biological and theoretical investigation of the influence on conformation and pharmacological profile. *Eur. J. Med. Chem.* **2019**, *179*, 527–536. [CrossRef]
31. Strack, M.; Bedini, A.; Yip, K.T.; Lombardi, S.; Siegmund, D.; Stoll, R.; Spampinato, S.M.; Metzler-Nolte, N. A blocking group scan using a spherical organometallic complex identifies an unprecedented binding mode with potent activity in vitro and in vivo for the opioid peptide dermorphin. *Chemistry* **2016**, *22*, 14605–14610. [CrossRef]
32. Schiller, P.W.; Nguyen, T.M.; Chung, N.N.; Lemieux, C. Dermorphin analogues carrying an increased positive net charge in their "message" domain display extremely high mu opioid receptor selectivity. *J. Med. Chem.* **1989**, *32*, 698–703. [CrossRef]
33. Schiller, P.W.; Nguyen, T.M.; Berezowska, I.; Dupuis, S.; Weltrowska, G.; Chung, N.N.; Lemieux, C. Synthesis and in vitro opioid activity profiles of DALDA analogues. *Eur. J. Med. Chem.* **2000**, *35*, 895–901. [CrossRef]
34. Guillemyn, K.; Kleczkowska, P.; Lesniak, A.; Dyniewicz, J.; Van der Poorten, O.; Van den Eynde, I.; Keresztes, A.; Varga, E.; Lai, J.; Porreca, F.; et al. Synthesis and biological evaluation of compact, conformationally constrained bifunctional opioid agonist—Neurokinin-1 antagonist peptidomimetics. *Eur. J. Med. Chem.* **2015**, *92*, 64–77. [CrossRef]

35. Shimoyama, M.; Shimoyama, N.; Zhao, G.M.; Schiller, P.W.; Szeto, H.H. Antinociceptive and respiratory effects of intrathecal H-Tyr-D-Arg-Phe-Lys-NH2 (DALDA) and [Dmt¹] DALDA. *J. Pharmacol. Exp. Ther.* **2001**, *297*, 364–371.
36. Neilan, C.L.; Nguyen, T.M.; Schiller, P.W.; Pasternak, G.W. Pharmacological characterization of the dermorphin analog [Dmt¹]DALDA, a highly potent and selective mu-opioid peptide. *Eur. J. Pharmacol.* **2001**, *419*, 15–23. [CrossRef]
37. Riba, P.; Ben, Y.; Nguyen, T.M.; Furst, S.; Schiller, P.W.; Lee, N.M. [Dmt¹)]DALDA is highly selective and potent at mu opioid receptors, but is not cross-tolerant with systemic morphine. *Curr. Med. Chem.* **2002**, *9*, 31–39. [CrossRef]
38. Schiller, P.W. Bi- or multifunctional opioid peptide drugs. *Life Sci.* **2010**, *86*, 598–603. [CrossRef]
39. Shimoyama, M.; Schiller, P.W.; Shimoyama, N.; Toyama, S.; Szeto, H.H. Superior analgesic effect of H-Dmt-D-Arg-Phe-Lys-NH2 ([Dmt¹]DALDA), a multifunctional opioid peptide, compared to morphine in a rat model of neuropathic pain. *Chem. Biol. Drug Des.* **2012**, *80*, 771–774. [CrossRef]
40. Cai, Y.; Lu, D.; Chen, Z.; Ding, Y.; Chung, N.N.; Li, T.; Schiller, P.W. [Dmt¹]DALDA analogues modified with tyrosine analogues at position 1. *Bioorganic Med. Chem. Lett.* **2016**, *26*, 3629–3631. [CrossRef]
41. Kokubu, S.; Eddinger, K.A.; Yamaguchi, S.; Huerta-Esquivel, L.L.; Schiller, P.W.; Yaksh, T.L. Characterization of analgesic actions of the chronic intrathecal infusion of H-Dmt-D-Arg-Phe-Lys-NH2 in rat. *Neuromodulation* **2019**, *22*, 781–789. [CrossRef]
42. Drieu la Rochelle, A.; Guillemyn, K.; Dumitrascuta, M.; Martin, C.; Utard, V.; Quillet, R.; Schneider, S.; Daubeuf, F.; Willemse, T.; Mampuys, P.; et al. A bifunctional-biased mu-opioid agonist-neuropeptide FF receptor antagonist as analgesic with improved acute and chronic side effects. *Pain* **2018**, *159*, 1705–1718.
43. Martin, C.; Dumitrascuta, M.; Mannes, M.; Lantero, A.; Bucher, D.; Walker, K.; Van Wanseele, Y.; Oyen, E.; Hernot, S.; Van Eeckhaut, A.; et al. Biodegradable amphipathic peptide hydrogels as extended-release system for opioid peptides. *J. Med. Chem.* **2018**, *61*, 9784–9789. [CrossRef] [PubMed]
44. Handa, B.K.; Lane, A.C.; Lord, J.A.H.; Morgan, B.A.; Rance, M.J.; Smith, C.F.C. Analogues of β-LPH61–64 possessing selective agonist activity at μ-opiate receptors. *Eur. J. Pharmacol.* **1981**, *70*, 531–540. [CrossRef]
45. Marino, K.A.; Shang, Y.; Filizola, M. Insights into the function of opioid receptors from molecular dynamics simulations of available crystal structures. *Br. J. Pharmacol.* **2018**, *175*, 2834–2845. [CrossRef]
46. Jones, G.; Willet, P.; Glen, R.C.; Leach, A.R.; Taylor, R. Development and validation of a genetic algorithm for flexible docking. *J. Mol. Biol.* **1997**, *267*, 727–748. [CrossRef]
47. Wolber, G.; Langer, T. LigandScout: 3-D Pharmacophores derived from protein-bound ligands and their use as virtual screening filters. *J. Chem. Inf. Modeling* **2005**, *45*, 160–169. [CrossRef]
48. Dumitrascuta, M.; Ben Haddou, T.; Guerrieri, E.; Noha, S.M.; Schläfer, L.; Schmidhammer, H.; Spetea, M. Synthesis, pharmacology, and molecular docking studies on 6-desoxo-*N*-methylmorphinans as potent μ-opioid receptor agonists. *J. Med. Chem.* **2017**, *60*, 9407–9412. [CrossRef]
49. Bradford, M.M. A rapid and sensitive method for the quantification of microgram quantities of protein utilizing the principle of protein-dye binding. *Anal. Biochem.* **1976**, *72*, 248–254. [CrossRef]
50. Cheng, Y.; Prusoff, W.H. Relationship between the inhibition constant (k1) and the concentration of inhibitor which causes 50 per cent inhibition (i50) of an enzymatic reaction. *Biochem. Pharmacol.* **1973**, *22*, 3099–3108.
51. Labute, P. Protonate3D: Assignment of ionization states and hydrogen coordinates to macromolecular structures. *Proteins* **2009**, *75*, 87–205. [CrossRef]
52. Schaller, D.; Šribarn, D.; Noonan, T.; Deng, L.; Nguyen, T.N.; Pach, S.; Machalz, D.; Bermudez, M.; Wolber, G. Next generation 3D pharmacophore modeling. *WIREs Comput. Mol. Sci.* **2020**, e1468. [CrossRef]

© 2020 by the authors. Licensee MDPI, Basel, Switzerland. This article is an open access article distributed under the terms and conditions of the Creative Commons Attribution (CC BY) license (http://creativecommons.org/licenses/by/4.0/).

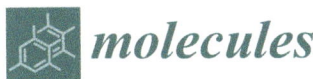

Article

The Meta-Position of Phe[4] in Leu-Enkephalin Regulates Potency, Selectivity, Functional Activity, and Signaling Bias at the Delta and Mu Opioid Receptors

Robert J. Cassell [1,†], Krishna K. Sharma [2,†], Hongyu Su [1], Benjamin R. Cummins [3], Haoyue Cui [4], Kendall L. Mores [1], Arryn T. Blaine [1], Ryan A. Altman [2,*] and Richard M. van Rijn [1,5,6,*]

1. Department of Medicinal Chemistry and Molecular Pharmacology, College of Pharmacy, Purdue University, West Lafayette, IN 47907, USA; rcassell@purdue.edu (R.J.C.); Su147@purdue.edu (H.S.); kmores@purdue.edu (K.L.M.); harri374@purdue.edu (A.T.B.)
2. Department of Medicinal Chemistry, The University of Kansas, Lawrence, KS 66045, USA; sharma.979@osu.edu
3. Department of Chemistry, Purdue University, West Lafayette, IN 47907, USA; bcummins96@gmail.com
4. College of Wuya, Shenyang Pharmaceutical University, Shenyang 110016, China; Cuihy1@shanghaitech.edu.cn
5. Purdue Institute for Drug Discovery, Purdue University, West Lafayette, IN 47907, USA
6. Purdue Institute for Integrative Neuroscience, Purdue University, West Lafayette, IN 47907, USA
* Correspondence: raaltman@ku.edu (R.A.A.); rvanrijn@purdue.edu (R.M.v.R.)
† These authors contributed equally to this work.

Academic Editors: Mariana Spetea and Helmut Schmidhammer
Received: 20 November 2019; Accepted: 10 December 2019; Published: 12 December 2019

Abstract: As tool compounds to study cardiac ischemia, the endogenous δ-opioid receptors (δOR) agonist Leu[5]-enkephalin and the more metabolically stable synthetic peptide (D-Ala[2], D-Leu[5])-enkephalin are frequently employed. However, both peptides have similar pharmacological profiles that restrict detailed investigation of the cellular mechanism of the δOR's protective role during ischemic events. Thus, a need remains for δOR peptides with improved selectivity and unique signaling properties for investigating the specific roles for δOR signaling in cardiac ischemia. To this end, we explored substitution at the Phe[4] position of Leu[5]-enkephalin for its ability to modulate receptor function and selectivity. Peptides were assessed for their affinity to bind to δORs and μ-opioid receptors (μORs) and potency to inhibit cAMP signaling and to recruit β-arrestin 2. Additionally, peptide stability was measured in rat plasma. Substitution of the meta-position of Phe[4] of Leu[5]-enkephalin provided high-affinity ligands with varying levels of selectivity and bias at both the δOR and μOR and improved peptide stability, while substitution with picoline derivatives produced lower-affinity ligands with G protein biases at both receptors. Overall, these favorable substitutions at the meta-position of Phe[4] may be combined with other modifications to Leu[5]-enkephalin to deliver improved agonists with finely tuned potency, selectivity, bias and drug-like properties.

Keywords: Leu-enkephalin; beta-arrestin; mu opioid receptor; delta opioid receptor; biased signaling; DADLE; ischemia; plasma stability

1. Introduction

Leu[5]-enkephalin (Tyr[1]-Gly[2]-Gly[3]-Phe[4]-Leu[5], Figure 1) is an endogenous opioid peptide produced in vertebrate species including rodents, primates and humans [1–4] that results from the metabolism of proenkephalin or dynorphin [5]. Pharmacologically, Leu^5-enkephalin agonizes the δ opioid receptor (δOR) with moderate selectivity over the μ opioid receptor (μOR), but does not significantly interact with the κ opioid receptor [6]. As a neurotransmitter in pain circuits, Leu^5-enkephalin possesses antinociceptive properties [7], whereas peripherally, the peptide demonstrates cardiovascular effects [8]. Over the last two decades, improved pharmacological characterization of opioid pathways has revealed that activation of an opioid receptor can trigger two distinct pathways, β-arrestin-dependent or β-arrestin-independent (i.e., G protein-mediated) and that these pathways differentially modulate antinociception and side effect profiles [9]. Despite the increasing number of studies that implicate δOR mediated β-arrestin recruitment with various (patho)physiological effects, such as tolerance [10], alcohol intake [11,12] and δOR agonist-induced seizures [10], the role of β-arrestin recruitment towards δOR-induced cardioprotection remains unclear.

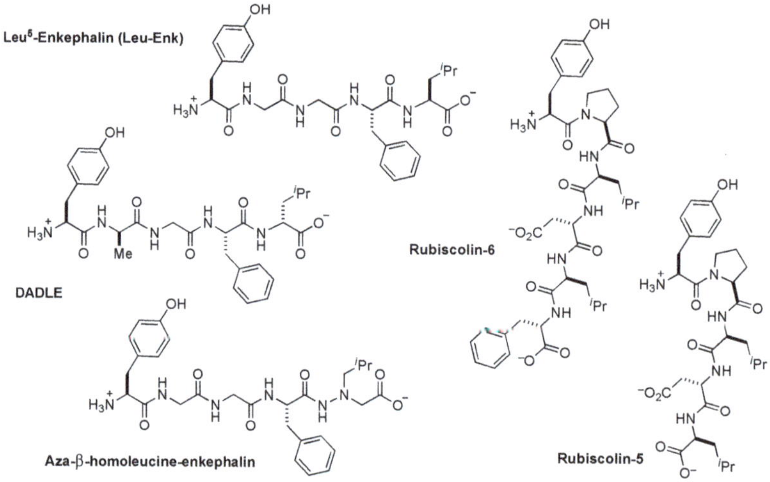

Figure 1. Overview of unbiased (Leu^5-enkephalin and **DADLE**) and biased (Aza-β-Homoleucine-Enkephalin, Rubiscolin-5 and -6) δOR peptides.

From a translational perspective, peptide-based probes provide an ideal tool for studying the cardioprotective effects of the δOR, given their low brain penetration. While numerous enkephalin-like peptides have been synthesized that interact with excellent potency and selectivity for δORs and μORs [13], a majority of studies [14] investigating δOR involvement in ischemia have utilized the synthetic peptide D-Ala^2, D-Leu^5-enkephalin (**DADLE**, Figure 1) [15,16], because **DADLE** possesses improved proteolytic stability and improved selectivity for δORs over μORs relative to Leu^5-enkephalin [6,17]. However, **DADLE**'s discovery in 1977 [18], predated identification of β-arrestin as a modulator of opioid signaling [14,19–21], With the use of contemporary cellular assays it is now apparent that **DADLE** pharmacologically signals similarly to Leu^5-enkephalin, though it recruits β-arrestin 2 (arrestin 3) slightly more efficaciously. Given the similarities between **DADLE** and Leu^5-enkephalin, it is unclear to what degree β-arrestin recruitment contributes to or detracts from these peptides' in vivo cardioprotective efficacy, and new analogs with distinct pharmacoloogical profiles are necessary to probe these contributions.

To better investigate the role of δOR-mediated β-arrestin signaling in ischemic protection, the development of δOR selective agonists that have either low, intermediate or high β-arrestin is desired; however, reports of δOR selective peptide-based biased ligands remain limited. Recently, the naturally occurring peptides rubiscolin-5 and -6 (Figure 1) were classified as G protein-biased (β-arrestin 2 efficacy = 15% and 20%, respectively; δOR bias factor = 2.0) δOR selective peptides, albeit with only micromolar potencies [22]. While a number of synthetic peptides display nanomolar potencies at δORs, such as aza-β-homoleucine-enkephalin (β-arrestin 2 efficacy = 64%; δOR bias factor = 5.2) [23] and Dmt-Tic analogs [24], these peptides all recruit β-arrestin 2 far more efficaciously than the rubiscolins (UFP-512: cAMP potency 0.4 nM, β-arrestin 2 potency = 20 nM, efficacy = 60%) [23–25]. Additionally, these latter biased compounds, including aza-β-homoleucine-enkephalin and Dmt-Tic-Gly-NH-Ph, have at best 10-fold selectivity for δORs over μORs and actually super-recruit β-arrestin 2 at μOR [23,24], which is likely to cause adverse, undesired in vivo effects [26,27]. As such, our goal was to identify novel and potent δOR peptide agonists with varying degrees of β-arrestin recruitment efficacy, and that importantly have improved δOR selectivity over μOR while limiting β-arrestin recruitment at μOR.

A collection of previously published structure activity relationship studies on Leu^5-enkephalin directed us to Phe^4 as a position that can modulate δOR and μOR potency and selectivity (Figure 2A) [28]. Specifically, ortho and para substitutions on Phe^4 can modulate binding affinity and selectivity between opioid receptors [28], and halogenation of the para-position of Leu^5-enkephalin and endomorphin 1 in particular appears to enhance δOR affinity while reducing μOR affinity [28]. Corroborating research has further shown that halogenation of the para position of Phe^4 of [D-Pen^2,D-Pen^5]enkephalin (DPDPE) enhanced δOR selectivity, potency, peptide stability, central nervous system (CNS) distribution, and antinociceptive potency compared to unsubstituted DPDPE [29–31]. Thus, halogenation at Phe^4 may provide Leu^5-enkephalin derivatives that can be used to study not only cardiac but also cerebral ischemia [32,33]. We herein report structure-activity-relationship trends at the meta-position of Phe^4 of Leu^5-enkephalin (Figure 2B), demonstrating that substitution at this position variously regulates δOR and μOR affinity and G-protein activity, enables the fine-tuning of β-arrestin 2 recruitment to both δOR and μOR, and further increases the plasma stability of the derived peptides. Combined, these features provide a clear direction for designing the next-generation of Leu^5-enkephalin analogs with well-defined biases and improved stabilities.

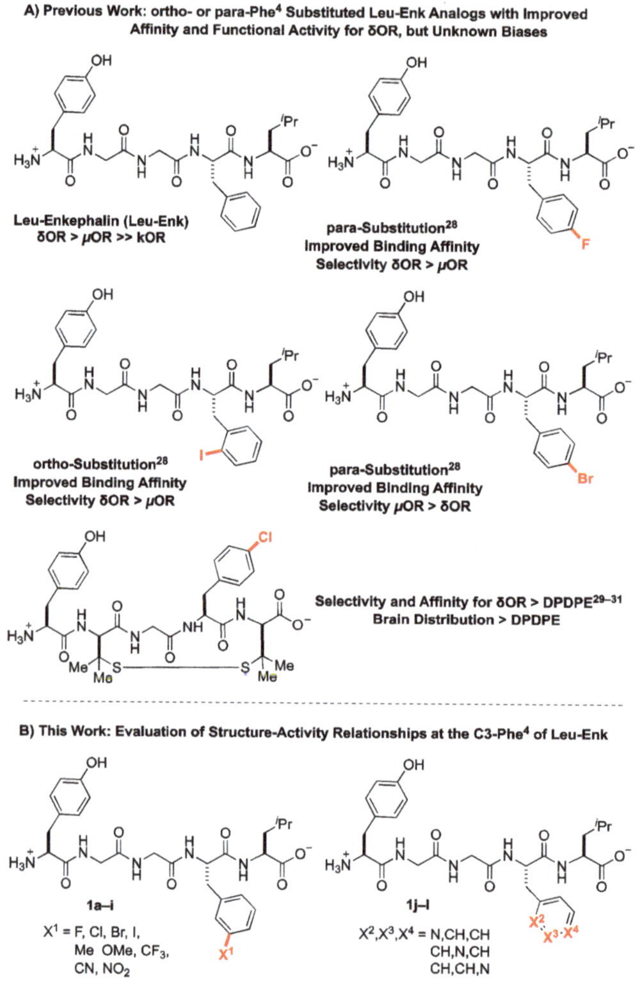

Figure 2. Substituents of Phe[4] of Leu[5]-enkephalin Affect Pharmacodynamic, Stability, and Distribution Properties.

2. Results and Discussion

2.1. Design Considerations

To probe the meta position of Phe[4], we initially considered known structure-activity-relationship trends at the ortho and para positions of this residue. Considering that halogenated substituents at these positions perturbed binding affinity, δOR selectivity, and stability properties of the Leu[5]-enkephalin [28], we initially hypothesized that meta-halogenated analogs might similarly perturb the parent scaffold (Figure 3A, **1a–1d**). An additional set of analogs bearing electron-donating (**1e–1f**) and -withdrawing groups (**1g–1i**) would further probe interactions at this site, including the electronic character of the Phe[4] ring. Finally, pyridine analogs (**1j–1l**) would present H-bond accepting contacts about the ring, as well as provide analogs that present dipoles at similar vectors as to previously successful halogenated substituents.

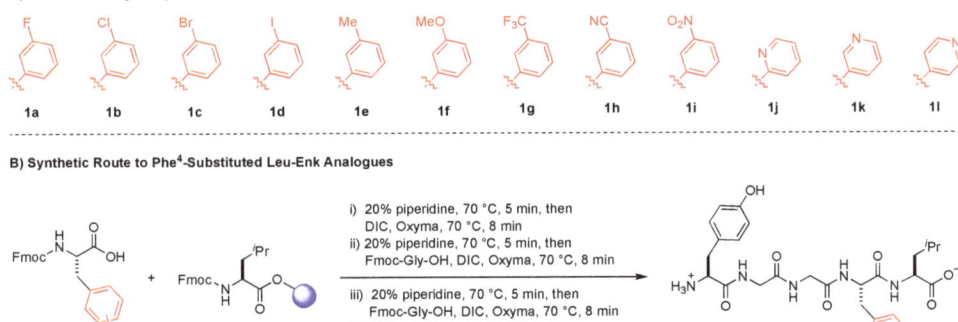

Figure 3. Peptide Synthesis of Phe[4]-Substituted Analogs of Leu[5]-enkephalin.

2.2. Solid Phase Synthesis of Peptides

All peptides were synthesized using a rapid solid phase peptide synthesis protocol on an automated peptide synthesizer using an Fmoc protection strategy [34,35] and N,N'-diisopropylcarbodiimide and oxyma as the coupling reagents (Figure 3B). Fmoc-Leu-Wang resin was utilized as a starting template for this synthetic protocol. All coupling steps and Fmoc-deprotection steps were carried out at 70 °C under an atmosphere of N_2. Cleavage from the resin was performed using TFA/triisopropylsilane/H_2O. Purification of the synthesized peptides was performed by reverse-phase high performance liquid chromatography (RP-HPLC), and analysis of purity was performed using ultra-performance liquid chromatography (UPLC). All desired peptides were obtained in ≥95% purity before submitting for pharmacological evaluation.

2.3. Pharmacological Characterization

To characterize our substituted analogs, we assessed binding affinity by competition radioligand binding, G protein potency and efficacy using a cAMP GloSensor assay and β-arrestin 2 recruitment via PathHunter assays at both the δOR and μOR. Using Leu[5]-enkephalin as well as DAMGO (for μOR), as reference compounds, substitution of the meta position of Phe[4] (**1a–1i**) generally increased binding affinity for the δOR (Table 1, K_i = 0.023–0.93 nM; Leu[5]-enkephalin = 1.26 nM) and μOR (K_i = 0.059–0.98 nM; Leu[5]-enkephalin = 1.7 nM). The improved binding affinity correlated with improved functional activation of the G protein pathway at both the δOR and μOR, while providing near-full agonist activity at the δOR (Table S1, 92–100% efficacy) relative to Leu[5]-enkephalin, and mostly near-full agonist activities at the μOR (Table S1, 85–105% efficacy; Leu[5]-enkephalin = 100% efficacy vs. DAMGO).

At the δOR, meta-substituted analogs recruited β-arrestin 2 with a range of potencies (Table 2, EC_{50}: 0.56–49 nM; Leu[5]-enkephalin = 8.9 nM) with near-full efficacies (Table 2, 91–130%; Leu-enkephalin = 100%), and likewise at the μOR, analogs recruited β-arrestin 2 with a broad range of potencies (Table 2, EC_{50}: 36–589 nM; Leu[5]-enkephalin = 977 nM) and efficacies (Table 2, 60–96% relative to DAMGO; Leu[5]-enkephalin = 60%; Figure 4). Interestingly, **DADLE** recruited β-arrestin 2 more efficaciously than Leu[5]-enkephalin at both δOR (126%) and μOR (99%). Picoline analogs **1j–1l**, generally showed reduced affinity at both receptors (Table 1, δOR K_i = 6.2–33 nM; μOR K_i = 9–158 nM), which further correlated with decreased G protein activation of the receptors (Table 2, δOR IC_{50} = 4.6–48 nM; μOR IC_{50} = 41–302 nM). At the δOR, the low affinity of pyridyl-substituted analogs correlated with low β-arrestin 2 recruitment (Table 2, EC_{50} = 100–1122 nM; 84–98% efficacy), though these substitutions drastically affected β-arrestin 2 recruitment though the μOR (Table 2, EC_{50} = 1.3–41.6 μM; 36–70% efficacy).

Table 1. Meta Substituted Phe[4] Analogs of Leu[5]-enkephalin Increase Affinity at δOR and μOR.

	$pK_i \pm$ SEM (δOR)	K_i (nM)	$pK_i \pm$ SEM (μOR)	K_i (nM)	Binding Selectivity (δOR vs μOR)
1a (F)	9.48 ± 0.1	0.33	9.12 ± 0.4	0.76	2.3
1b (Cl)	9.87 ± 0.1	0.13	10.14 ± 0.2	0.072	0.55
1c (Br)	10.35 ± 0.2	0.045	9.90 ± 0.3	0.13	2.9
1d (I)	10.64 ± 0.2	0.023	9.86 ± 0.5	0.14	6.1
1e (Me)	9.86 ± 0.1	0.14	9.86 ± 0.1	0.14	1.0
1f (OMe)	9.31 ± 0.1	0.49	9.07 ± 0.1	0.85	1.7
1g (CF$_3$)	9.93 ± 0.1	0.12	10.23 ± 0.3	0.059	0.49
1h (CN)	9.17 ± 0.3	0.68	9.52 ± 0.1	0.30	0.44
1i (NO$_2$)	9.03 ± 0.2	0.93	9.01 ± 0.1	0.98	1.05
1j (2-pyr)	8.21 ± 0.1	6.17	8.04 ± 0.2	9.12	1.5
1k (3-pyr)	7.48 ± 0.1	33.1	6.80 ± 0.1	158	4.8
1l (4-pyr)	7.69 ± 0.1	20.4	7.41 ± 0.1	38.9	1.9
DADLE	9.01 ± 0.1	0.98	8.80 ± 0.1	1.58	1.6
Leu[5]-enkephalin	8.90 ± 0.1	1.26	8.77 ± 0.1	1.70	1.3
DAMGO	-	-	9.01 ± 0.1	0.98	-

All compounds were tested in three independent trials.

Table 2. Meta-substituted Phe[4] Analogs of Leu[5]-enkephalin Display Enhanced δOR and μOR Potency for cAMP Inhibition and β-arrestin 2 Recruitment, But Vary in β-arrestin Recruitment Efficacy.

	cAMP				β-Arrestin 2				
Compound	$pIC_{50} \pm$ SEM (δOR)	IC_{50} (nM)	$pIC_{50} \pm$ SEM (μOR)	IC_{50} (nM)	$pEC_{50} \pm$ SEM (δOR)	EC_{50} (nM)	δOR Efficacy (% ± SEM)	$pEC_{50} \pm$ SEM (μOR)	EC_{50} (nM)	μOR Efficacy (% + SEM)
1a (F)	9.47 ± 0.2	0.39	8.10 ± 0.2	7.94	8.01 ± 0.2	9.77	107 ± 9	6.24 ± 0.1	575	75 ± 13
1b (Cl)	10.66 ± 0.3	0.022	7.52 ± 0.1	30.2	8.77 ± 0.2	1.70	130 ± 10	7.17 ± 0.2	67.6	96 ± 8
1c (Br)	10.52 ± 0.3	0.030	8.00 ± 0.4	10	9.25 ± 0.2	0.56	116 ± 7	7.45 ± 0.2	35.5	79 ± 6
1d (I)	10.61 ± 0.2	0.025	8.37 ± 0.3	4.27	8.95 ± 0.2	1.12	111 ± 7	7.33 ± 0.2	46.8	70 ± 3
1e (Me)	10.41 ± 0.3	0.039	8.43 ± 0.3	3.72	8.46 ± 0.2	3.46	105 ± 5	6.73 ± 0.2	186	71 ± 3
1f (OMe)	9.84 ± 0.3	0.14	8.09 ± 0.3	8.12	7.93 ± 0.2	11.7	106 ± 5	6.23 ± 0.1	589	67 ± 3
1g (CF$_3$)	9.97 ± 0.4	0.11	8.61 ± 0.4	2.45	8.39 ± 0.2	4.07	108 ± 9	7.25 ± 0.2	56.2	71 ± 3
1h (CN)	9.46 ± 0.3	0.35	7.92 ± 0.3	12.0	7.77 ± 0.2	17.0	91 ± 5	6.8 ± 0.2	158	68 ± 4
1i (NO$_2$)	9.33 ± 0.3	0.47	7.31 ± 0.4	49.0	7.31 ± 0.2	49.0	96 ± 6	6.27 ± 0.1	537	60 ± 6
1j (2-pyr)	8.34 ± 0.2	4.57	7.39 ± 0.4	40.7	7.00 ± 0.2	100	92 ± 13	5.87 ± 0.1	1349	70 ± 4
1k (3-pyr)	7.32 ± 0.2	47.9	6.63 ± 0.4	234	5.95 ± 0.1	1122	85 ± 6	4.38 ± 0.1	41687	36 ± 7
1l (4-pyr)	7.52 ± 0.2	30.2	6.52 ± 0.3	302	6.40 ± 0.2	398	98 ± 6	4.43 ± 0.1	37153	64 ± 11
DADLE	9.09 ± 0.2	0.81	7.45 ± 0.1	35.5	7.92 ± 0.4	12.0	126 ± 10	6.33 ± 0.1	468	99 ± 3
Leu[5]-enkephalin	8.99 ± 0.1	1.02	7.34 ± 0.2	45.7	8.05 ± 0.1	8.91	100	6.01 ± 0.1	977	61 ± 3
DAMGO	5.91 ± 0.2	1230	7.82 ± 0.1	15.1	<5		-	6.80 ± 0.1	158	100

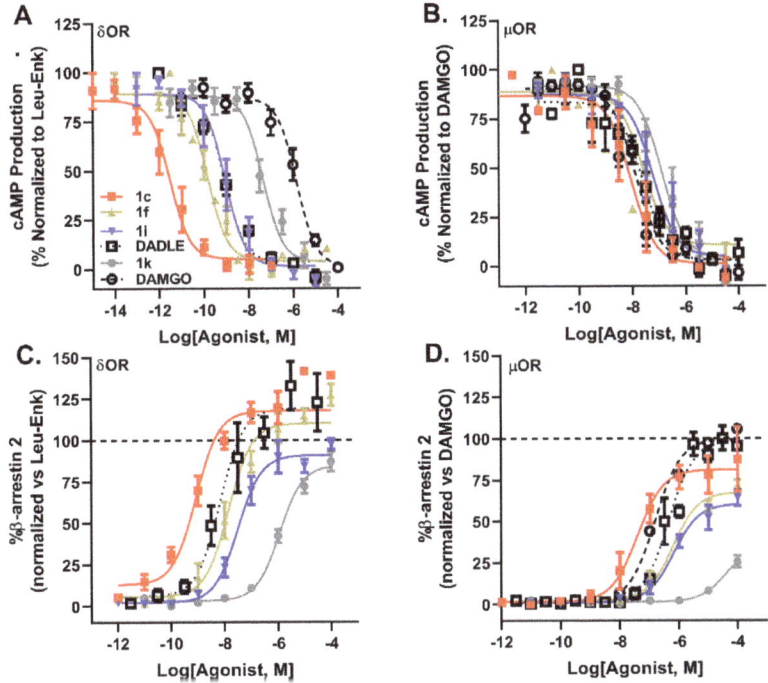

Figure 4. Modifications of Phe[4] of Leu[5]-enkephalin Produces Analogs with Divergent and Distinct Signaling Profiles. Inhibition of cAMP production by **1c** (■), **1f** (▲), **1i** (▼), **1k** (●), Leu[5]-enkephalin (□) and DAMGO (○) in HEK cells expressing δOR (**A**) and µOR (**B**). Recruitment of β-arrestin 2 by **1c**, **1f**, **1i**, **1k**, Leu-Enk and DAMGO in CHO cells expressing δOR (**C**) and µOR (**D**).

Within these overall trends, specific analogs show unique profiles. Meta– chlorination, –bromination, or –iodination (**1b–1d**) produced high-affinity analogs of Leu[5]-enkephalin that super-recruited β-arrestin 2 and that drastically increased functional selectivity (Table 3). These increases in affinity at δOR linearly correlate (R^2 = 0.998) with the atomic van der Waals radii (H, 1.20 Å; Cl, 1.77 Å; Br, 1.92 Å; I, 2.06 Å) [36], and might suggest a halogen bonding interaction similar to those previously explored at the ortho position of Phe[4] [28]. However, the distinct vectors at which a sigma-hole would present from the ortho vs. meta positions suggest that the specific residues engaged through meta-substitution are likely distinct from those previously identified through ortho-substitution [28], and future computational collaborative work might enable a better understanding of the unique binding interactions between the δOR and meta-halogenated analogs of Leu[5]-enkephalin. Notably, the meta-chlorinated and –brominated analogs (**1b**, and **1c**) are 500–900-fold more potent in cAMP assays at δOR than at µOR, despite exhibiting little differences in binding affinity at δOR relative to µOR (Table 1). Interestingly, the meta-Cl analog (**1b**) had stronger bias towards G protein-signaling at δOR (Table 3, bias factor 1.6), but towards β-arrestin 2 recruitment at µOR relative to Leu[5]-enkephalin (Table 3, bias factor 0.004) as well as DAMGO (Table 3, bias factor 0.3), which provides a unique pharmacological profile for future uses. In contrast, meta-F and –CN and –NO$_2$-substitutions (**1a,h,i**) improved δOR functional selectivity (Table 3), but lost β-arrestin 2 potency at δOR relative to Leu[5]-enkephalin. Additionally, meta-OMe and –NO$_2$ substitution (**1f**, **1i**) provided both potent and biased analogs, with G protein coupling activities comparable to Leu[5]-enkephalin (Table 2, IC$_{50}$ = 0.14–0.47 nM vs. 1.02 nM), but with improved bias factors relative to Leu[5]-enkephalin at both δOR (Table 3, bias factor 6.9–7.5) and µOR (Table 3, bias factor 8.4–11.1). Of these two analogs, the -NO$_2$-substituted analog **1i** exhibited higher δOR functional G protein selectivity (Table 3, 104-fold δOR selectivity) relative to the –OMe analog **1f** (Table 3, 58-fold δOR selectivity). Though pyridyl-substituted analogs (**1j–1l**) showed poor potency and efficacy for the δOR and μOR relative to Leu^5-enkephalin (Table 2), the 3- and 4-pyridyl analogs (**1k–1l**) showed strong bias at μOR (Table 3, bias factor 17–331), when compared to the full agonist DAMGO. However, if instead of DAMGO, Leu^5-enkephalin was used as the reference compound, most analogs, with the exception of **1k** and **1l** lost G protein bias (Table 3, bias factor < 1), because the analogs generally were more potent and efficacious than Leu^5-enkephalin in recruiting β-arrestin 2 at μOR (Table 2), with the exception of **1k** (Table 2, 36% recruitment efficacy). Given that exogenous Leu^5-enkephalin analogs in vivo would compete with endogenous Leu^5-enkephalin and not DAMGO, our results highlight the limitations of interpreting bias factors (particularly using an unnatural compound, such as DAMGO, as a reference) and the associated risk of using bias factor as a major driver of lead optimization.

Table 3. Meta-substituted Phe^4 Analogs of Leu^5-enkephalin Display a Range of Selectivity and Bias Profiles.

Compound	G Protein Selectivity (δOR vs μOR)	Bias Factor		
		δOR	μOR (DG = Ref)	μOR (LE = Ref)
1a (F)	20	1.8	22.2	0.36
1b (Cl)	1372	3.2	0.3	0.004
1c (Br)	333	1.3	1.2	0.02
1d (I)	171	3.5	3.2	0.05
1e (Me)	95	4.3	11.5	0.19
1f (OMe)	58	7.5	8.4	0.14
1g (CF$_3$)	22	2.0	4.3	0.07
1h (CN)	34	6.8	5.4	0.09
1i (NO$_2$)	104	6.9	11.1	0.18
1j (2-pyr)	8.9	4.0	17.2	0.27
1k (3-pyr)	4.9	6.7	331.1	5.89
1l (4-pyr)	10	2.2	63.7	1.08
DADLE	44	0.5	2.3	0.035
Leu^5-enkephalin	45	1	4.9	1
DAMGO	0.012	-	1	0.003
Aza-β-homoleucine ¶	9.9 [23]	5.2 ¶	-	1.2
Rubiscolin-5	-	2.0 [22]	-	-

¶ from reference 26 using BRET (β-arrestin 2) and EPAC (cAMP) assays. DG = DAMGO, LE = Leu^5-enkephalin.

Compared to **DADLE**, the Leu^5-enkephalin analogs **1b** and **1c** displayed a similar signaling bias profile, but were more potent and selective for δOR, and thus may provide a better tool compound to target δORs for the treatment of cardiac ischemia. However, compounds **1b** and **1c** are also more potent than **DADLE** at recruiting β-arrestin 2 to μOR, resulting in a lower bias factor (Figure 4). In contrast, analog **1i** has a favorable pharmacology relative to **DADLE**, with similar selectivity as **1c**, but improved G-protein bias at δOR and μOR relative to **DADLE**. Given the potential adverse effects associated with strong μOR-mediated β-arrestin 2 recruitment, analog **1k** is potentially useful, as it exhibited weak β-arrestin 2 recruitment (36% efficacy) and concomitant strong bias factor for G-protein signaling. However, cAMP potency for **1k** at δOR was more than one log unit weaker than **DADLE**, and thus it may be necessary further optimize the ligand by increasing δOR potency in the cAMP assay, while retaining the low μOR β-arrestin 2 recruitment efficacy (Figure 4).

2.4. Stability

The stability of all compounds to Sprague Dawley rat plasma was assessed to study the influence of the meta– and picoline/pyridine-substitutions at Phe^4 relative to Leu^5-enkephalin (Table 4). For this parent compound, the predominant known routes of metabolism and clearance occur through cleavage of Tyr^1-Gly^2 by aminopeptidase N [37,38], and of Gly^3-Phe^4 by angiotensin converting enzyme [39], and combined, the plasma metabolism occurs with a half-life ($t_{1/2}$) of < 10 min. In general, meta substituted Phe^4 analogs exhibited improved plasma stability compared with Leu^5-enkephalin with half-lives typically >20 min. The 3-fluoro derivative (**1a**) was the most stable analog with a half-life of 82.3 min. From UPLC-mass spectrometry analysis of degradation fragments, meta-substitution did not greatly impede the proteolysis at the Tyr^1-Gly^2 site, but instead slowed digestion at the Gly^3-Phe^4 site (Table 4). Thus, the improved stability of our Phe^4-substituted analogs presumably derived from perturbation/deceleration of angiotensin-converting enzyme activity. Picoline peptides also displayed improved stability though interestingly, UPLC-mass spectrometry analysis indicated that degradation of all pyridyl-substituted analogs (**1j–1l**) predominantly occurred through Tyr^1-Gly^2 as opposed to meta-substituted analogs **1a–1i** that degraded through cleavage of Gly^3-Phe^4.

Table 4. Rat Plasma Stability of Leu^5-enkephalin and Its Analogs.

Compound	Half-Life (min)	95% CI	Degradation Products (First Appearance)
Leu^5-enkephalin	9.4	6.3–4.5	Gly-Gly-Phe-Leu (5 min) Phe-Leu (10 min)
1a (F)	82.3	68.0–102.6	Gly-Gly-(meta-F)Phe-Leu (5 min) (meta-F)Phe-Leu (60 min)
1b (Cl)	37.8	26.5–56.6	Gly-Gly-(meta-Cl)Phe-Leu (5 min) (meta-Cl)Phe-Leu (30 min)
1c (Br)	21.5	12.7–38.7	Gly-Gly-(meta-Br)Phe-Leu (5 min) (meta-Br)Phe-Leu (15 min)
1d (I)	13.2	11.4–15.2	Gly-Gly-(meta-I)Phe-Leu (5 min) (meta-I)Phe-Leu (15 min)
1e (Me)	39.5	30.0–53.5	Gly-Gly-(meta-Me)Phe-Leu (5 min) (meta-Me)Phe-Leu (20 min)
1f (OMe)	46.1	30.4–75.6	Gly-Gly-(meta-OMe)Phe-Leu (5 min) (meta-OMe)Phe-Leu (20 min)
1g (CF$_3$)	44.5	35.0–59.1	Gly-Gly-(meta-CF$_3$)Phe-Leu (5 min) (meta- CF$_3$)Phe-Leu (30 min)
1h (CN)	33.0	24.0–47.0	Gly-Gly-(meta-CN)Phe-Leu (5 min) (meta-CN)Phe-Leu (20 min)
1i (NO$_2$)	28.8	16.8–55.8	Gly-Gly-(meta-NO$_2$)Phe-Leu (5 min) (meta- NO$_2$)Phe-Leu (20 min)
1j (2-pyr)	26.8	15.4–53.7	(2-pyridyl)Ala-Leu (5 min) Gly-Gly-(2-pyridyl)Ala-Leu (30 min)
1k (3-pyr)	54.0	29.0–127.0	(3-pyridyl)Ala-Leu (10 min) Gly-Gly-(3-pyridyl)Ala-Leu (20 min)
1l (4-pyr)	78.1	47.5–165.4	(4-pyridyl)Ala-Leu (10 min) Gly-Gly-(4-pyridyl)Ala-Leu (30 min)

3. Methods

3.1. Synthetic Chemistry-General Considerations

Unless specified, all chemicals were purchased from commercial sources and used without further purification. All solvents used for synthesis were of analytical grade and used without further purification. Proton nuclear magnetic resonance (^{1}H-NMR) spectra, and carbon nuclear magnetic resonance (^{13}C-NMR) spectra were recorded on a Bruker AVIII 500 AVANCE spectrometer with a CPDUL cryoprobe (500 and 126 MHz, respectively) or a Bruker DRX 500 spectrometer (500 and 126 MHz, respectively). Fluorine nuclear magnetic resonance (^{19}F-NMR) spectra were recorded on a Bruker AVIII 500 AVANCE spectrometer with a CPDUL BBFO cryoprobe (376 MHz) or a Bruker DRX 500 spectrometer (376 MHz). Chemical shifts (δ) for protons are reported in parts per million (ppm) downfield from tetramethylsilane, and are referenced to proton resonance of solvent residual peak in the NMR solvent (MeOD-d_4: δ = 4.87 ppm or DMSO-d_6: δ = 2.50 ppm). Chemical shifts (δ) for carbon are reported in ppm downfield from tetramethylsilane, and are referenced to the carbon resonances of the solvent residual peak (MeOD-d_4: δ = 49.1 ppm or DMSO-d_6: δ = 39.52 ppm). ^{19}F-NMR chemical shifts (δ) are reported in ppm with respect to added internal standard: PhCF$_3$ (δ = −63.72 ppm). NMR data are represented as follows: chemical shift (ppm), multiplicity (s = singlet, d = doublet, dd = doublet of doublets, t = triplet, q = quartet, sept = septet, m = multiplet), coupling constant in Hertz (Hz), and integration. Exact mass determinations were obtained by using electrospray ionization using a time of flight mass analyzer (Waters LCT Premiere).

Peptides were synthesized using an Aapptec Focus XC automated peptide synthesizer coupled with a heating system using a solid phase peptide synthesis protocol using Fmoc chemistry. Preparative RP-HPLC was performed using an appropriate column and solvent system (described below) and final purity of peptides was determined by UV area % from UPLC analysis. Peptides were purified by Teledyne ISCO EZ Prep system on RediSep® C18 Prep column (30 × 250 mm, 100 Å). Purity analysis of final peptides was carried out using a Waters UPLC Aquity system equipped with a PDA eλ detector (200 to 400 nm) and a HSS T3 C18 column, (1.8 μM, 2.1 × 50 mm column), using one of two methods. Protocol A: gradient elution of 2% MeCN with 0.1% formic acid in H$_2$O to 98% MeCN over 2.5 min, then holding at 98% MeCN for 3 min at a flow rate of 0.6 mL/min. Protocol B: gradient elution of 2% MeCN with 0.1% formic acid in H$_2$O to 98% MeCN over 2.5 min, then holding at 98% MeCN for 1 min at a flow rate of 0.7 mL/min at 40 °C. Plasma stability was also assessed using the above UPLC column and solvent gradient program using a Waters H class Plus Acquity UPLC system coupled with a QDa detector using protocol B.

3.2. Synthesis of Peptides

Peptides were synthesized using a solid phase peptide synthesis protocol using an Aapptec Focus XC automated peptide synthesizer coupled with a heating system using the Fmoc chemistry and Wang resin as solid support [34]. To prepare the resin for synthesis, a reaction vessel equipped with a sintered glass bottom was charged with Fmoc-Leu-Wang resin (0.2 mM), and swelled in a mixture of dichloromethane and DMF (1:1) for 15 min. The resin was then transferred to a peptide synthesizer reaction vessel. The resin was deprotected twice using 20% piperidine in DMF for 5 min at 70 °C. Subsequently, an Fmoc-protected amino acid was double coupled with the Leucine-wang resin by treating with N,N'-diisopropylcarbodiimide (3.0 equiv., 0.2 M in DMF) and Oxyma (3.0 equiv., 0.2 M in DMF) at 70 °C for 8 min. Completion of coupling reactions was monitored by a Kaiser's test for the initial peptide [40]. Each coupling was followed by removal of the Fmoc group using 20% piperidine in DMF at 70 °C for 5 min and repeated once. The cycle of the Fmoc removal and coupling was repeated with subsequent Fmoc-protected amino acids to generate the desired resin-bound peptide. Cleavage of the peptide from resin and concomitant deprotection of the side chain protecting groups was carried out by shaking in TFA/triisopropylsilane/H$_2$0 (95/2.5/2.5; 5 mL), at ambient temperature for 3 h. Subsequent filtration afforded the peptide in the filtrate and the volume was reduced to 0.2 mL.

Then, the crude peptides were precipitated by adding cold diethyl ether, and the crude peptides were then purified by RP-HPLC. Synthesized peptides were characterized by NMR, and the high-resolution mass spectroscopy.

3.3. Materials Used in the Cellular Signaling Assays

Leu^5-enkephalin and forskolin, were purchased from Sigma-Aldrich (St. Louis, MO USA). (D-Ala^2, N-MePhe^4, Gly-ol) enkephalin (DAMGO) was purchased from Tocris Bioscience (Minneapolis, MN, USA). Radiolabels were from Perkin Elmer (Waltham, MA, USA).

3.4. Cell Culture and Biased Signaling Assays

cAMP inhibition and β-arrestin 2 recruitment assays were performed as previously described [12]. In brief, for cAMP inhibition assays HEK 293 (Life Technologies, Grand Island, NY, USA) cells were transiently transfected in a 1:3 ratio with FLAG-mouse δOR, or HA-mouse μOR and pGloSensor22F-cAMP plasmids (Promega, Madison, WI, USA) using Xtremegene9 (Sigma). Two days post-transfection cells (20,000 cells/well, 7.5 μL) were seeded in low volume Greiner 384-well plates (#82051-458, VWR, Batavia, IL, USA) and were incubated with Glosensor reagent (Promega, 7.5 μL, 2% final concentration) for 90 min at room temperature. Cells were stimulated with 5 μL drug solution for 20 min at room temperature prior to stimulation with 5 μL forskolin (final concentration 30 μM) for an additional 15 min at room temperature. For β-arrestin recruitment assays, CHO-human μOR PathHunter β-arrestin 2 cells or CHO-human δOR PathHunter β-arrestin 2 cells (DiscoverX, Fremont, CA, USA) were plated (2,500 cells/well, 10 μL) one day prior to stimulation with 2.5 μL drug solution for 90 min at 37 °C/5% CO$_2$, after which cells were incubated with 6 μL cell PathHunter assay buffer (DiscoverX) for 60 min at room temperature as per the manufacturer's protocol. Luminescence for each of these assays was measured using a FlexStation3 plate reader (Molecular Devices, Sunnyvale, CA, USA).

3.5. Radioligand Binding Assay

For the binding assay 50 μL of a dilution series of peptide was added to 50 μL of 3.3 nM [3H]DPDPE (K_d = 3.87 nM) or 2.35 nM of [3H]DAMGO (K_d = 1.07 nM) in a clear 96 well plate. Next, 100 μL of membrane suspension containing 7 μg protein was added to the agonist wells and incubated for 90 min at room temperature. The reaction mixture was then filtered over a GF-B filter plate (Perkin Elmer) followed by four quick washes with ice-cold 50 mM Tris HCl. The plate was dried overnight, after which 50 μL scintillation fluid (Ultimagold uLLT) was added and radioactivity was counted on a Packard TopCount NXT scintillation counter. All working solutions were prepared in a radioligand assay buffer containing 50 mM Tris HCl, 10 mM MgCl$_2$, and 1 mM ethylenediaminetetraacetic acid at pH 7.4.

3.6. Calculation of Bias Factor

Bias factors were calculated using the operational model equation in Prism 8 to calculate Log R (τ/KA) (Table S2) as previously described [12]. Subsequently, bias factors were calculated using Leu^5-enkephalin as reference compound for δOR and using either DAMGO or Leu^5-enkephalin as reference compound for μOR, respectively. Leu^5-enkephalin and DAMGO were more potent in the cAMP (G protein) assay than in the β-Arrestin 2 recruitment assay, and thus were not unbiased, but rather G protein-biased to begin with. A bias factor > 1 meant that the agonist was more G protein-biased than the reference compound; A bias factor < 1 meant that the agonist was less G protein-biased than the reference compound.

3.7. Data and Statistical Analysis

All data are presented as means ± standard error of the mean, and analysis was performed using GraphPad Prism 8 software (GraphPad Software, La Jolla, CA). For in vitro assays, nonlinear regression was conducted to determine pIC_{50} (cAMP) or pEC_{50} (β-arrestin 2 recruitment). Technical replicates were used to ensure the reliability of single values, specifically each data point for binding and β-arrestin recruitment was run in duplicate, and for the cAMP assay in triplicate. The averages of each independent run were counted as a single experiment and combined to provide a composite curve in favor of providing a 'representative' curve. In each experimental run, a positive control/reference compound was utilized to allow the data to be normalized and to calculate the log bias value. A minimum of three independent values were obtained for each compound in each of the cellular assays.

3.8. Assessment of Plasma Stability

Sprague Dawley rat plasma containing K_2-ethylenediaminetetraacetic acid (Innovative Research, MI, USA) was transferred into 300 μL aliquots and stored at −20 °C until use. The plasma stabilities of Leu^5-enkephalin and its synthesized analogs were determined in plasma diluted to 50% with saline (isotonic sodium chloride solution; 0.9% w/v) [41]. An aliquot of the resulting solution (25 μL) was incubated at 37 °C for 15 min before the addition of a solution of a Leu^5-enkephalin analog (25 μL of a 100 μM isotonic NaCl solution; 0.9% w/v). After adding analog, an aliquot of the mixture was removed at each indicated time point (0, 5, 10, 15, 20, 30, 60, 120, 240 min) and immediately quenched with 100 μL of a methanol solution containing 20 μM Fmoc-Leu-OH as an internal standard. The resulting peptide solutions were centrifuged at 13,000 rpm for 15 min at 4 °C on tubes equipped with 2000 MW filtrate tubes (Sartorius, USA). Then, the filtrate was transferred into vials and a 5 μL sample of the resulting solution was analyzed on an UPLC system coupled with a QDa detector. For quantitative determination, area-under-the-curve for the peaks corresponding to the UV chromatogram was measured for both the Leu^5-enkephalin analog and the internal standard. Determination of half-life ($t_{1/2}$) was carried out by using the GraphPad Prism one-phase decay method.

4. Conclusions

Meta-substitutions of Phe^4 of Leu^5-enkephalin were generally well tolerated and certain substitutions improved affinity, potency, δOR selectivity and stability of this endogenous opioid. The generated pharmacological data herein may aid computational modeling efforts to reveal ligand-receptor interactions at δOR and μOR that will guide the development of novel peptides with tuned selectivity and signaling profiles. The novel Leu^5-enkephalin analogs have superior δOR selectivity over μOR relative to DADLE, the gold-standard peptide for studying the role of δOR in cardiac ischemia. Additionally, the analogs generally have lower β-arrestin recruitment efficacy at μOR, which could further reduce potential adverse in vivo effects. Finally, relative to **DADLE**, the meta-substituents tune the bias profile at δOR (either more or less biased towards G-protein signaling), and the resulting tool compounds should be useful for investigating the importance of δOR mediated β-arrestin signaling in the peptides cardioprotective effects.

Supplementary Materials: The following are available online, Specifically, for compounds **1a–l**: Additional pharmacological characterization, stability data, NMR spectra and characterization data for peptides, UPLC traces for determining purity. Table S1: Efficacy of cAMP inhibition of Meta-substituted Phe^4 Analogs of Leu^5-enkephalin at δOR and μOR. Table S2: LogR values for Meta-substituted Phe^4 Analogs of Leu-enkephalin at δOR and μOR in the cAMP and β-arrestin 2 (β-arr2) assays. 95% confidence intervals are presented between parentheses.

Author Contributions: R.J.C. data acquisition and analysis, supervision and original draft preparation. K.K.S. design, synthesis, and analysis of analogs, original draft preparation. H.S. data acquisition and analysis. B.R.C. data acquisition and analysis. H.C. data acquisition and analysis. K.L.M. data acquisition and analysis. A.T.B. data acquisition and analysis. R.A.A. design and conceptualization, data analysis, original draft preparation, funding acquisition and supervision. R.M.v.R.: design and conceptualization, data analysis, original draft preparation, funding acquisition and supervision. All authors proofread and approved the final draft.

Funding: This research was funded by the National Institute on Alcohol Abuse and Alcoholism grants AA025368, AA026949, AA026675 (R.M.v.R.) and the National Institute on Drug Abuse grants DA045897 (R.M.v.R.) and DA036730 (R.A.A.) of the National Institutes of Health, and funds provided by the Purdue Institute for Drug Discovery and the Purdue University Department of Medicinal Chemistry and Molecular Pharmacology. NMR Instrumentation was provided by NIH Shared Instrumentation Grants (S10OD016360 and S10RR024664), NSF Major Research Instrumentation Grants (9977422 and 0320648), and an NIH Center Grant (P20GM103418). The APC was funded by DA036730 (R.A.A.).

Conflicts of Interest: All authors declare no biomedical financial interests or potential conflicts of interests.

References

1. Hughes, J.; Smith, T.W.; Kosterlitz, H.W.; Fothergill, L.A.; Morgan, B.A.; Morris, H.R. Identification of two related pentapeptides from the brain with potent opiate agonist activity. *Nature* **1975**, *258*, 577–580. [CrossRef]
2. Comb, M.; Seeburg, P.H.; Adelman, J.; Eiden, L.; Herbert, E. Primary structure of the human Met- and Leu-enkephalin precursor and its mRNA. *Nature* **1982**, *295*, 663–666. [CrossRef]
3. Ikeda, Y.; Nakao, K.; Yoshimasa, T.; Yanaihara, N.; Numa, S.; Imura, H. Existence of Met-enkephalin-Arg6-Gly7-Leu8 with Met-enkephalin, Leu-enkephalin and Met-enkephalin-Arg6-Phe7 in the brain of guinea pig, rat and golden hamster. *Biochem. Biophys. Res. Commun.* **1982**, *107*, 656–662. [CrossRef]
4. Simantov, R.; Kuhar, M.J.; Pasternak, G.W.; Snyder, S.H. The regional distribution of a morphine-like factors enkephalin in monkey brain. *Brain Res.* **1976**, *106*, 189–197. [CrossRef]
5. Akil, H.; Owens, C.; Gutstein, H.; Taylor, L.; Curran, E.; Watson, S. Endogenous opioids: Overview and current issues. *Drug Alcohol Depend.* **1998**, *51*, 127–140. [CrossRef]
6. Raynor, K.; Kong, H.; Chen, Y.; Yasuda, K.; Yu, L.; Bell, G.I.; Reisine, T. Pharmacological characterization of the cloned kappa-, delta-, and mu-opioid receptors. *Mol. Pharmacol.* **1994**, *45*, 330–334.
7. Belluzzi, J.D.; Grant, N.; Garsky, V.; Sarantakis, D.; Wise, C.D.; Stein, L. Analgesia induced in vivo by central administration of enkephalin in rat. *Nature* **1976**, *260*, 625–626. [CrossRef]
8. Schaz, K.; Stock, G.; Simon, W.; Schlor, K.H.; Unger, T.; Rockhold, R.; Ganten, D. Enkephalin effects on blood pressure, heart rate, and baroreceptor reflex. *Hypertens. (Dallas, Tex. 1979)* **1980**, *2*, 395–407. [CrossRef]
9. Violin, J.D.; Crombie, A.L.; Soergel, D.G.; Lark, M.W. Biased ligands at G-protein-coupled receptors: Promise and progress. *Trends Pharmacol. Sci.* **2014**, *35*, 308–316. [CrossRef]
10. Vicente-Sanchez, A.; Dripps, I.J.; Tipton, A.F.; Akbari, H.; Akbari, A.; Jutkiewicz, E.M.; Pradhan, A.A. Tolerance to high-internalizing delta opioid receptor agonist is critically mediated by arrestin 2. *Br. J. Pharmacol.* **2018**, *175*, 3050–3059. [CrossRef]
11. Robins, M.T.; Chiang, T.; Mores, K.L.; Alongkronrusmee, D.; van Rijn, R.M. Critical Role for Gi/o-Protein Activity in the Dorsal Striatum in the Reduction of Voluntary Alcohol Intake in C57Bl/6 Mice. *Front. Psychiatry* **2018**, *9*, 112. [CrossRef]
12. Chiang, T.; Sansuk, K.; Van Rijn, R.M. β-Arrestin 2 dependence of δ opioid receptor agonists is correlated with alcohol intake. *Br. J. Pharmacol.* **2016**, *173*, 332–343. [CrossRef]
13. Remesic, M.; Lee, Y.S.; Hruby, V.J. Cyclic Opioid Peptides. *Curr. Med. Chem.* **2016**, *23*, 1288–1303. [CrossRef]
14. Zhang, J.; Ferguson, S.S.G.; Barak, L.S.; Bodduluri, S.R.; Laporte, S.A.; Law, P.-Y.; Caron, M.G. Role for G protein-coupled receptor kinase in agonist-specific regulation of -opioid receptor responsiveness. *Proc. Natl. Acad. Sci.* **1998**, *95*, 7157–7162. [CrossRef]
15. Borlongan, C.V. Delta opioid peptide (D-ALA 2, D-LEU 5) enkephalin: Linking hibernation and neuroprotection. *Front. Biosci.* **2004**, *9*, 3392. [CrossRef]
16. Wolf, A.; Lusczek, E.R.; Beilman, G.J. Hibernation-Based Approaches in the Treatment of Hemorrhagic Shock. *SHOCK* **2018**, *50*, 14–23. [CrossRef]
17. Uchiyama, T.; Kotani, A.; Kishida, T.; Tatsumi, H.; Okamoto, A.; Fujita, T.; Murakami, M.; Muranishi, S.; Yamamoto, A. Effects of various protease inhibitors on the stability and permeability of [D-Ala2,D-Leu5]enkephalin in the rat intestine: Comparison with leucine enkephalin. *J. Pharm. Sci.* **1998**, *87*, 448–452. [CrossRef]

18. Beddell, C.R.; Clark, R.B.; Lowe, L.A.; Wilkinson, S.; Chang, K.J.; Cuatrecasas, P.; Miller, R. A conformational analysis for leucine-enkephalin using activity and binding data of synthetic analogues. *Br. J. Pharmacol.* **1977**, *61*, 351–356. [CrossRef]
19. Kovoor, A.; Nappey, V.; Kieffer, B.L.; Chavkin, C. μ and δ Opioid Receptors Are Differentially Desensitized by the Coexpression of β-Adrenergic Receptor Kinase 2 and β-Arrestin 2 in Xenopus Oocytes. *J. Biol. Chem.* **1997**, *272*, 27605–27611. [CrossRef]
20. Bohn, L.M.; Lefkowitz, R.J.; Gainetdinov, R.R.; Peppel, K.; Caron, M.G.; Lin, F.T. Enhanced morphine analgesia in mice lacking beta-arrestin 2. *Science* **1999**, *286*, 2495–2498. [CrossRef]
21. Whistler, J.L.; Chuang, H.; Chu, P.; Jan, L.Y.; von Zastrow, M. Functional Dissociation of μ Opioid Receptor Signaling and Endocytosis. *Neuron* **1999**, *23*, 737–746. [CrossRef]
22. Cassell, R.J.; Mores, K.L.; Zerfas, B.L.; Mahmoud, A.H.; Lill, M.A.; Trader, D.J.; van Rijn, R.M. Rubiscolins are naturally occurring G protein-biased delta opioid receptor peptides. *Eur. Neuropsychopharmacol.* **2019**, *29*, 450–456. [CrossRef]
23. Bella Ndong, D.; Blais, V.; Holleran, B.J.; Proteau-Gagné, A.; Cantin-Savoie, I.; Robert, W.; Nadon, J.-F.; Beauchemin, S.; Leduc, R.; Piñeyro, G.; et al. Exploration of the fifth position of leu-enkephalin and its role in binding and activating delta (DOP) and mu (MOP) opioid receptors. *Pept. Sci.* **2018**, *111*, e24070. [CrossRef]
24. Vezzi, V.; Onaran, H.O.; Molinari, P.; Guerrini, R.; Balboni, G.; Calo, G.; Costa, T.; Calò, G.; Costa, T. Ligands raise the constraint that limits constitutive activation in G protein-coupled opioid receptors. *J. Biol. Chem.* **2013**, *288*, 23964–23978. [CrossRef]
25. Aguila, B.; Coulbault, L.; Boulouard, M.; Leveille, F.; Davis, A.; Toth, G.; Borsodi, A.; Balboni, G.; Salvadori, S.; Jauzac, P.; et al. In vitro and in vivo pharmacological profile of UFP-512, a novel selective delta-opioid receptor agonist; correlations between desensitization and tolerance. *Br. J. Pharmacol.* **2007**, *152*, 1312–1324. [CrossRef]
26. Raehal, K.M.; Walker, J.K.L.; Bohn, L.M. Morphine Side Effects in β-Arrestin 2 Knockout Mice. *J. Pharmacol. Exp. Ther.* **2005**, *314*, 1195–1201. [CrossRef]
27. Soergel, D.G.; Subach, R.A.; Burnham, N.; Lark, M.W.; James, I.E.; Sadler, B.M.; Skobieranda, F.; Violin, J.D.; Webster, L.R. Biased agonism of the μ-opioid receptor by TRV130 increases analgesia and reduces on-target adverse effects versus morphine: A randomized, double-blind, placebo-controlled, crossover study in healthy volunteers. *Pain* **2014**, *155*, 1829–1835. [CrossRef]
28. Rosa, M.; Caltabiano, G.; Barreto-Valer, K.; Gonzalez-Nunez, V.; Gómez-Tamayo, J.C.; Ardá, A.; Jiménez-Barbero, J.; Pardo, L.; Rodríguez, R.E.; Arsequell, G.; et al. Modulation of the Interaction between a Peptide Ligand and a G Protein-Coupled Receptor by Halogen Atoms. *ACS Med. Chem. Lett.* **2015**, *6*, 872–876. [CrossRef]
29. Toth, G.; Kramer, T.H.; Knapp, R.; Lui, G.; Davis, P.; Burks, T.F.; Yamamura, H.I.; Hruby, V.J. [D-Pen2,D-Pen5]enkephalin analogues with increased affinity and selectivity for delta opioid receptors. *J. Med. Chem.* **1990**, *33*, 249–253. [CrossRef]
30. Weber, S.J.; Greene, D.L.; Sharma, S.D.; Yamamura, H.I.; Kramer, T.H.; Burks, T.F.; Hruby, V.J.; Hersh, L.B.; Davis, T.P. Distribution and analgesia of [3H][D-Pen2, D-Pen5]enkephalin and two halogenated analogs after intravenous administration. *J. Pharmacol. Exp. Ther.* **1991**, *259*, 1109–1117.
31. Weber, S.J.; Greene, D.L.; Hruby, V.J.; Yamamura, H.I.; Porreca, F.; Davis, T.P. Whole body and brain distribution of [3H]cyclic [D-Pen2,D-Pen5] enkephalin after intraperitoneal, intravenous, oral and subcutaneous administration. *J. Pharmacol. Exp. Ther.* **1992**, *263*, 1308–1316. [PubMed]
32. Grant Liska, M.; Crowley, M.G.; Lippert, T.; Corey, S.; Borlongan, C.V. Delta Opioid Receptor and Peptide: A Dynamic Therapy for Stroke and Other Neurological Disorders. In *Handbook of Experimental Pharmacology*, 1st ed.; Emily, J., Ed.; Springer: Cham, Switzerland, 2017; pp. 277–299.
33. He, X.; Sandhu, H.K.; Yang, Y.; Hua, F.; Belser, N.; Kim, D.H.; Xia, Y. Neuroprotection against hypoxia/ischemia: δ-opioid receptor-mediated cellular/molecular events. *Cell. Mol. Life Sci.* **2013**, *70*, 2291–2303. [CrossRef]
34. Shenmar, K.; Sharma, K.K.; Wangoo, N.; Maurya, I.K.; Kumar, V.; Khan, S.I.; Jacob, M.R.; Tikoo, K.; Jain, R. Synthesis, stability and mechanistic studies of potent anticryptococcal hexapeptides. *Eur. J. Med. Chem.* **2017**, *132*, 192–203. [CrossRef]
35. Mahindra, A.; Sharma, K.K.; Jain, R. Rapid microwave-assisted solution-phase peptide synthesis. *Tetrahedron Lett.* **2012**, *53*, 6931–6935. [CrossRef]
36. Bondi, A. van der Waals Volumes and Radii. *J. Phys. Chem.* **1964**, *68*, 441–451. [CrossRef]

37. Weinberger, S.B.; Martinez, J.L.J. Characterization of Hydrolysis of [Leu] enkephalin in Rat Plasma. *J. Pharmacol. Exp. Ther.* **1988**, *247*, 129–135.
38. Roques, B.; Noble, F. Dual inhibitors of enkephalin-degrading enzymes (neutral endopeptidase 24.11 and aminopeptidase N) as potential new medications in the management of pain and opioid addiction. *NIDA Res. Monogr.* **1995**, *147*, 104–145.
39. Suzanne, E.T.; Kenneth, L.A. Leucine-Enkephalin Metabolism in Brain Microvessel Endothelial Cells. *Peptides* **1994**, *15*, 109–116.
40. Sarin, V.K.; Kent, S.B.; Tam, J.P.; Merrifield, R.B. Quantitative monitoring of solid-phase peptide synthesis by the ninhydrin reaction. *Anal. Biochem.* **1981**, *117*, 147–157. [CrossRef]
41. Beaudeau, J.L.; Blais, V.; Holleran, B.J.; Bergeron, A.; Pineyro, G.; Guérin, B.; Gendron, L.; Dory, Y.L. N-Guanidyl and C-Tetrazole Leu-Enkephalin Derivatives: Efficient Mu and Delta Opioid Receptor Agonists with Improved Pharmacological Properties. *ACS Chem. Neurosci.* **2019**, *10*, 1615–1626. [CrossRef]

Sample Availability: Upon reasonable request and based on material in hand, compounds **1a–1l** can be distributed in a timely fashion by Dr. Altman. However, as supplies are finite, we cannot guarantee every request can be accommodated.

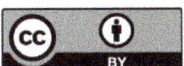

© 2019 by the authors. Licensee MDPI, Basel, Switzerland. This article is an open access article distributed under the terms and conditions of the Creative Commons Attribution (CC BY) license (http://creativecommons.org/licenses/by/4.0/).

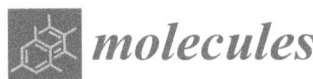

Article

Phenylalanine Stereoisomers of CJ-15,208 and [D-Trp]CJ-15,208 Exhibit Distinctly Different Opioid Activity Profiles

Ariana C. Brice-Tutt [1], Sanjeewa N. Senadheera [2], Michelle L. Ganno [3], Shainnel O. Eans [1], Tanvir Khaliq [4], Thomas F. Murray [5], Jay P. McLaughlin [1,*] and Jane V. Aldrich [4,*]

[1] Department of Pharmacodynamics, The University of Florida, Gainesville, FL 32610, USA; ariana.brice@ufl.edu (A.C.B.-T.); shaieans@cop.ufl.edu (S.O.E.)
[2] Department of Medicinal Chemistry, The University of Kansas, Lawrence, KS 66045, USA; nilendrasns@yahoo.com
[3] Torrey Pines Institute for Molecular Studies, Port St. Lucie, FL 34987, USA; condor1082@aol.com
[4] Department of Medicinal Chemistry, The University of Florida, Gainesville, FL 32610, USA; tanvirkhaliq@cop.ufl.edu
[5] Department of Pharmacology and Neuroscience, School of Medicine, Creighton University, Omaha, NE 68178, USA; tfmurray@creighton.edu
* Correspondence: jmclaughlin@cop.ufl.edu (J.P.M.); janealdrich@ufl.edu (J.V.A.); Tel.: +1-352-273-7207 (J.P.M.); +1-352-273-8708 (J.V.A.)

Academic Editor: Mariana Spetea
Received: 31 July 2020; Accepted: 31 August 2020; Published: 2 September 2020

Abstract: The macrocyclic tetrapeptide *cyclo*[Phe-D-Pro-Phe-Trp] (CJ-15,208) and its stereoisomer *cyclo*[Phe-D-Pro-Phe-D-Trp] exhibit different opioid activity profiles in vivo. The present study evaluated the influence of the Phe residues' stereochemistry on the peptides' opioid activity. Five stereoisomers were synthesized by a combination of solid-phase peptide synthesis and cyclization in solution. The analogs were evaluated in vitro for opioid receptor affinity in radioligand competition binding assays, and for opioid activity and selectivity in vivo in the mouse 55 °C warm-water tail-withdrawal assay. Potential liabilities of locomotor impairment, respiratory depression, acute tolerance development, and place conditioning were also assessed in vivo. All of the stereoisomers exhibited antinociception following either intracerebroventricular or oral administration differentially mediated by multiple opioid receptors, with kappa opioid receptor (KOR) activity contributing for all of the peptides. However, unlike the parent peptides, KOR antagonism was exhibited by only one stereoisomer, while another isomer produced DOR antagonism. The stereoisomers of CJ-15,208 lacked significant respiratory effects, while the [D-Trp]CJ-15,208 stereoisomers did not elicit antinociceptive tolerance. Two isomers, *cyclo*[D-Phe-D-Pro-D-Phe-Trp] (3) and *cyclo*[Phe-D-Pro-D-Phe-D-Trp] (5), did not elicit either preference or aversion in a conditioned place preference assay. Collectively, these stereoisomers represent new lead compounds for further investigation in the development of safer opioid analgesics.

Keywords: opioid peptide; macrocyclic tetrapeptide; multifunctional ligands; structure-activity relationships; kappa opioid receptor; delta opioid receptor; analgesics; opioid liabilities

1. Introduction

The endogenous opioid system is a valuable therapeutic target for the treatment of pain as it is extensively involved in pain perception and experience [1]. The majority of opioid ligands used clinically for the treatment of pain are mu-opioid receptor (MOR) agonists, although agonists of kappa (KOR) and delta (DOR) receptors also produce analgesia. However, opioid-selective agonists also produce a number of undesirable opioid-related side effects that complicate their therapeutic utility. MOR-selective agonists are reinforcing, and produce analgesic tolerance and respiratory depression [2]. In contrast, KOR selective agonists produce dysphoria, sedation, and psychotomimetic effects [3], while DOR-selective agonists can induce seizure activity [4].

Multifunctional opioids, ligands with mixed agonist and/or antagonist activity at one or more opioid receptor, have demonstrated potent antinociception, possibly due to synergistic effects [5]. Co-administration of either KOR [6,7] or DOR [8] agonists enhanced the antinociceptive effects of MOR-selective agonists. Some multifunctional opioids also produce reduced side effects [9], a profile attributed to simultaneous modulation of more than one opioid receptor that may counter their individual adverse effects [10]. For example, KOR agonism offsets MOR-mediated reinforcement [11] and respiratory depression [12], while DOR antagonism may slow the development of MOR agonist analgesic tolerance [13,14].

Multifunctional opioid activity has been observed for the structurally distinct macrocyclic tetrapeptide natural product CJ-15,208 (*cyclo*[Phe-D-Pro-Phe-Trp], Figure 1). Originally isolated from the fungus *Ctenomyces serratus*, initial testing found this peptide preferentially bound to KOR and antagonized this receptor in the electrically stimulated rabbit vas deferens [15]. When originally isolated the stereochemistry of the tryptophan residue was not determined, prompting us to synthesize both the L- and D-Trp stereoisomers [16,17]; the optical rotation of the L-Trp isomer was consistent with that reported for the natural product. The two isomeric peptides exhibited similar affinity for opioid receptors (see Table 1) and antagonized KOR in the GTPγS assay in vitro [16–19]. However, the peptides exhibited distinctly different opioid activity profiles when evaluated in vivo [19]. The D-Trp isomer primarily exhibited KOR antagonism with modest antinociception only at elevated doses, while the L-Trp-containing peptide exhibited mixed, multifunctional activity, with robust antinociception mediated by both KOR and MOR, followed by KOR-selective antagonism lasting several hours after the dissipation of antinociception. Both of these macrocyclic tetrapeptides are active after oral administration [20,21], increasing their potential as leads for drug discovery.

Therefore, we explored the influence of the stereochemistry of the two phenylalanine residues in CJ-15,208 and [D-Trp]CJ-15,208 (*cyclo*[Phe-D-Pro-Phe-D-Trp]) on opioid activity. All of the stereoisomers retained significant antinociception with reduced liabilities, while the different stereochemistries of the aromatic residues in the five analogs resulted in significant variation in their multifunctional opioid activity.

2. Results

2.1. Synthesis

The stereoisomers of CJ-15,208 and its D-Trp isomer (Figure 1) were synthesized by a combination of solid phase synthesis of the linear precursors followed by cyclization in solution using modifications to our original strategy [20,22] to improve the yields of the macrocyclic peptides.

The linear sequences chosen contained the turn inducing D-Pro residue in the middle of the peptide to facilitate cyclization [17], and the use of the 2-chlorotrityl chloride resin minimized the potential for diketopiperazine formation. The peptides were purified by silica gel flash chromatography, which permitted the facile purification of larger quantities of the macrocyclic peptides for in vivo pharmacological evaluation following oral administration. The purified peptides were analyzed by electrospray ionization mass spectrometry, thin layer chromatography, and in two analytical HPLC systems. All of the stereoisomers were obtained in high purity and reasonable yields (34–50% from the linear precursors) after purification.

	Amino acid stereochemistry		
	Phe1	Phe3	Trp4
CJ-15,208	L	L	L
[D-Trp4]CJ-15,208	L	L	D
1, D-Phe1	D	L	L
2, D-Phe3	L	D	L
3, D-Phe1,3	D	D	L
4, D-Phe1,D-Trp4	D	L	D
5, D-Phe3,D-Trp4	L	D	D

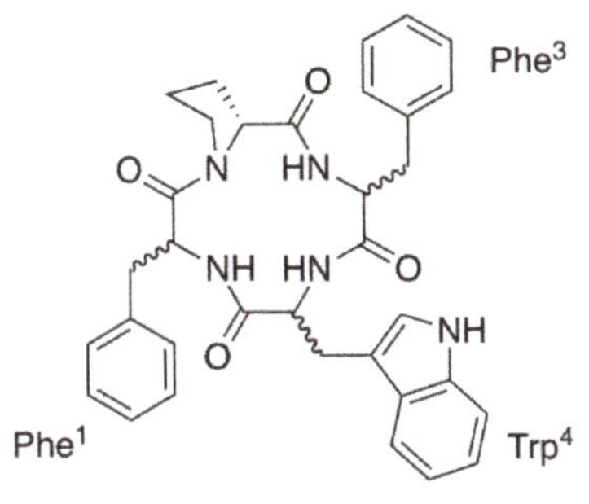

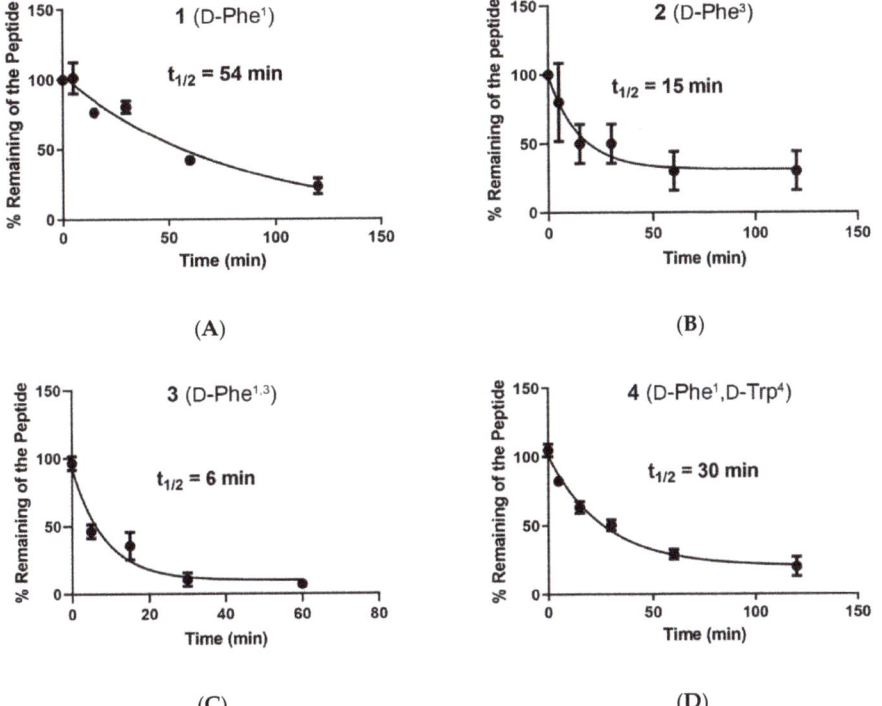

Figure 1. Structures of stereoisomers of CJ-15,208 and [D-Trp]CJ-15,208.

2.2. Metabolic Stability

We evaluated the metabolic stability of the stereoisomers in mouse liver microsomes. While macrocyclic peptides are stable to proteases, they can be metabolized by cytochrome P450 enzymes [23,24]. In all cases the peptides were stable in incubations lacking NADPH, but disappeared from the incubations containing NADPH, consistent with cytochrome P450 enzyme metabolism. The half-lives of the stereoisomers in the mouse liver microsomes were ≤30 min for all of the stereoisomers except for **1**, which displayed a half-life more than twice that of most of the other stereoisomers (Figure 2). The short half-lives of most of the stereoisomers are consistent with that of [D-Trp]CJ-15,208 (11 min), while the longer half-life of stereoisomer **1** is similar to that of CJ-15,208 (49 min) (Khaliq et al., manuscript in preparation).

Figure 2. *Cont.*

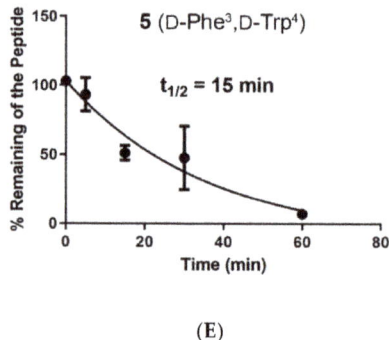

(E)

Figure 2. Metabolic stability in mouse liver microsomes of the stereoisomers: (**A**) **1**, (**B**) **2**, (**C**) **3**, (**D**) **4** and (**E**) **5**.

2.3. In Vitro Pharmacological Evaluation

In radioligand equilibrium competition binding assays the D-Phe stereoisomers of CJ-15,208 and [D-Trp]CJ-15,208 generally exhibited greatly reduced affinity for KOR and MOR compared to the two parent peptides (Table 1). Only the D-Phe^3 analogs (see Figure 1 for residue numbering) exhibited sub-micromolar affinity for any of the opioid receptors (K_i = ~350 nM for KOR). Similar to CJ-15,208 and [D-Trp]CJ-15,208 [19], the stereoisomers all exhibited negligible affinity for DOR. Also consistent with the results for CJ-15,208 and [D-Trp]CJ-15,208, none of the analogs exhibited appreciable efficacy at either KOR or MOR at 10 µM in [^{35}S]GTPγS assays.

Table 1. Opioid receptor affinities of the stereoisomers of CJ-15,208 and [D-Trp]CJ-15,208 [a,b].

Stereoisomer	K_i (nM ± SEM)		Selectivity
	KOR	MOR	K_i (MOR) / K_i (KOR)
1 (D-Phe^1)	5120 ± 690	>10,000	<2
2 (D-Phe^3)	362 ± 51	3920 ± 200	11
3 (D-Phe^{1,3})	2560 ± 480	7780 ± 410	3
CJ-15,208	27.4 ± 4.6	451 ± 114	16.5
4 (D-Phe^1, D-Trp^4)	>10,000	>10,000	-
5 (D-Phe^3, D-Trp^4)	353 ± 19	5800 ± 1450	16
[D-Trp^4]CJ-15,208	21.8 ± 4.8	259 ± 29	12

[a] Data are the mean K_i values ± SEM from at least three experiments. [b] None of the stereoisomers at 10 µM exhibited appreciable affinity for DOR (<30% inhibition of [^{3}H]cyclo[D-Pen^2,D-Pen^5]enkephalin (DPDPE) binding).

2.4. In Vivo Pharmacological Evaluation

The stereoisomers were initially evaluated for their antinociceptive activity in the 55 °C warm-water tail-withdrawal assay in C57BL/6J mice following i.c.v. administration (Figure 3A and Figure S1). All of the D-Phe stereoisomers produced significant time- and dose-dependent antinociception ($p < 0.05$, two-way RM ANOVA). Peak antinociception was produced 20 min after i.c.v administration for stereoisomers **1**, **3**, and **4** and at 30 min for isomers **2** and **5** (Figure S1). The duration of significant antinociception ($p < 0.05$; Dunnett's *post hoc* test) varied from 45 min (isomers **3** and **4**) to 90 min (isomers **2** and **5**), with isomer **1** exhibiting an intermediate duration. All of the isomers exhibited full and potent antinociception except for **2** (Figure 3A), which produced approximately 70% antinociception at the highest dose tested (100 nmol); the potencies of stereoisomers **1** and **3**–**5** were comparable to that of CJ-15,208 (Table 2). The maximal antinociception found for the stereoisomers **4** and **5** of [D-Trp]CJ-15,208 is in contrast to the parent peptide, which exhibits minimal antinociceptive activity [19].

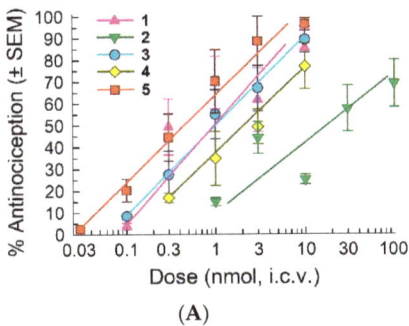
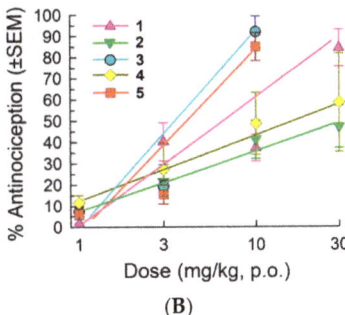

Figure 3. Antinociceptive activity in the 55 °C warm-water tail-withdrawal assay following (**A**) i.c.v. administration and (**B**) oral administration in C57BL/6J mice. All points represent antinociception at peak response, which occurred 20–30 min after administration. Points represent average % antinociception ± SEM from 4–16 mice for each set presented.

The D-Phe stereoisomers of CJ-15,208 and of [D-Trp]CJ-15,208 also exhibited significant antinociceptive effects following oral (p.o.) administration ($p < 0.05$, two-way RM ANOVA; Figure 3B and Figure S2). Isomers **1**, **3**, and **5** produced full antinociception with comparable potency to CJ-15,208 (Table 2) that peaked between 20-30 min, while isomers **2** and **4** produced only 45-60% antinociception at the highest oral dose tested (30 mg/kg, p.o.). The duration of significant antinociception ($p < 0.05$, Dunnett's *post hoc* test) was 50–60 min for all stereoisomers except **4** (30–40 min). While isomer **2** exhibited low antinociceptive efficacy by both routes of administration, isomer **4** exhibited decreased efficacy only following oral administration.

Table 2. Summary of in vivo opioid antinociceptive activity of the stereoisomers [a].

Stereoisomer	ED_{50} (and 95% Confidence Interval (C.I.)) Values		
	i.c.v. (nmol)	p.o. (mg/kg)	Receptors Involved
1	0.75 (0.36–1.44)	7.62 (5.12–12.2)	KOR, MOR, DOR
2	20.4 (10–58.7)	~	KOR, MOR
3	1.00 (0.64–1.60)	4.12 (3.30–5.31)	KOR, DOR
CJ-15,208 [b,c]	1.74 (0.62–4.82)	3.49 (1.98–5.73)	KOR, MOR
4	2.39 (1.40–4.56)	~	DOR, KOR
5	0.56 (0.38–0.91)	4.72 (3.70–6.39)	KOR, MOR, DOR
[D-Trp⁴]CJ-15,208 [b,d]	~	~	-

[a] In addition, isomer **1** exhibited antagonist activity at KOR, and isomer **5** exhibited antagonist activity at DOR.
[b] Ref. [19]; [c] Ref. [20]; [d] Ref. [21]. ~ Maximum antinociception not achieved, precluding calculation of an ED_{50} value.

2.4.1. Opioid Receptor Selectivity of Stereoisomer Antinociception

Pretreatment of mice with an opioid antagonist was used to assess receptor contribution to the observed antinociception, Naloxone (30 mg/kg., s.c.) pretreatment (20 min) significantly reduced the antinociceptive effects of all five analogs ($F_{(4,61)} = 2.68$, $p < 0.05$, two-way ANOVA with Sidak's *post hoc* test; Figure 4A), consistent with opioid receptors mediating the antinociception. The individual receptor contributions to the observed antinociception were then determined by pretreating the mice with the selective MOR, KOR and DOR antagonists β-FNA (10 mg/kg, i.p., −24 h), nor-BNI (10 mg/kg, i.p., −24 h), or naltrindole (20 mg/kg., i.p., −20 min), respectively, prior to administration of the macrocyclic tetrapeptide (isomers **1**, **3**, **4** and **5** at 10 nmol, and isomer **2** at 100 nmol, i.c.v; Figure 4B). Treatment with these antagonists significantly affected antinociception produced by the stereoisomers ($F_{(12,159)} = 11.2$, $p < 0.05$, two-way ANOVA). β-FNA, nor-BNI, and naltrindole all significantly antagonized the antinociception of stereoisomers **1** and **5** ($p < 0.05$, Tukey's *post hoc* test), suggesting that all three opioid receptors contributed to the antinociception produced by these stereoisomers. In contrast, isomer **2** demonstrated KOR- and MOR-mediated antinociception, whereas the antinociception produced by **3** and **4** was KOR- and DOR-mediated ($p < 0.05$, Tukey's *post hoc* test).

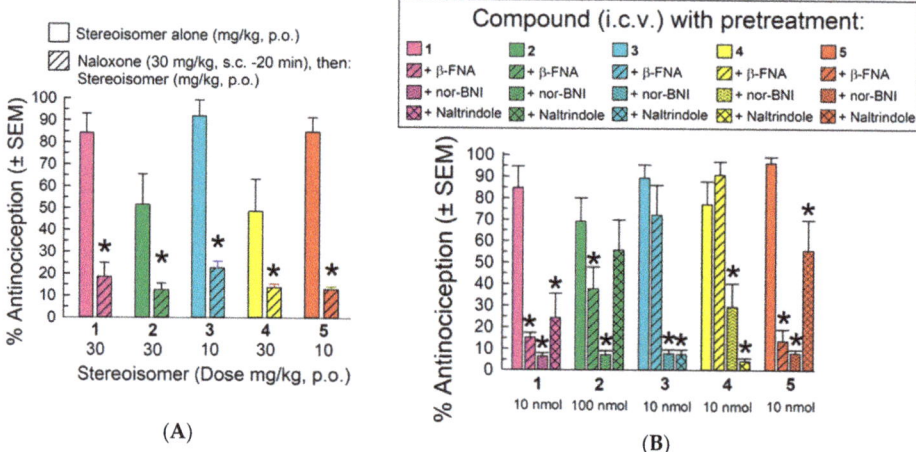

Figure 4. Evaluation of opioid receptor involvement in the antinociceptive activity of the stereoisomers in the 55 °C warm-water tail-withdrawal assay 20 min after (**A**) p.o. administration in mice pretreated with the non-selective opioid receptor antagonist naloxone (30 mg/kg., s.c., −20 min), or (**B**) 20 min after i.c.v. administration in mice pretreated with the selective MOR antagonist β-FNA (10 mg/kg, i.p., −24 h), the selective KOR antagonist nor-BNI (10 mg/kg, i.p., −24 h), or the selective DOR antagonist naltrindole (20 mg/kg, i.p., −20 min). Points represent average % antinociception ± SEM from 8–16 mice for each bar. * significantly different from response of stereoisomer alone ($p < 0.05$. ** two significant bars adjacent to each other.; two-way ANOVA with (**A**) Sidak's or (**B**) Tukey's multiple comparisons *post hoc* test).

2.4.2. Determination of Stereoisomer Opioid-Receptor Mediated Selective Antagonist Activity

Following dissipation of the antinociception, the stereoisomers were evaluated for antagonist activity against the KOR-selective agonist U50,488 (10 mg/kg., i.p.), the MOR-preferring agonist morphine (10 mg/kg, i.p.), and the DOR-selective agonist SNC-80 (100 nmol, i.c.v.; Figure 5). Only isomer **1** (30 nmol, i.c.v.) exhibited significant antagonism of U50,488 ($F_{(5,55)} = 5.81$, $p < 0.05$, one-way ANOVA with Sidak's *post hoc* test; Figure 5A). Interestingly, stereoisomer **5** (100 nmol, i.c.v) significantly antagonized SNC-80 ($F_{(5,55)} = 7.71$, $p < 0.05$, one-way ANOVA with Sidak's *post hoc* test; Figure 5C), while none of the peptides demonstrated antagonism against morphine (Figure 5B).

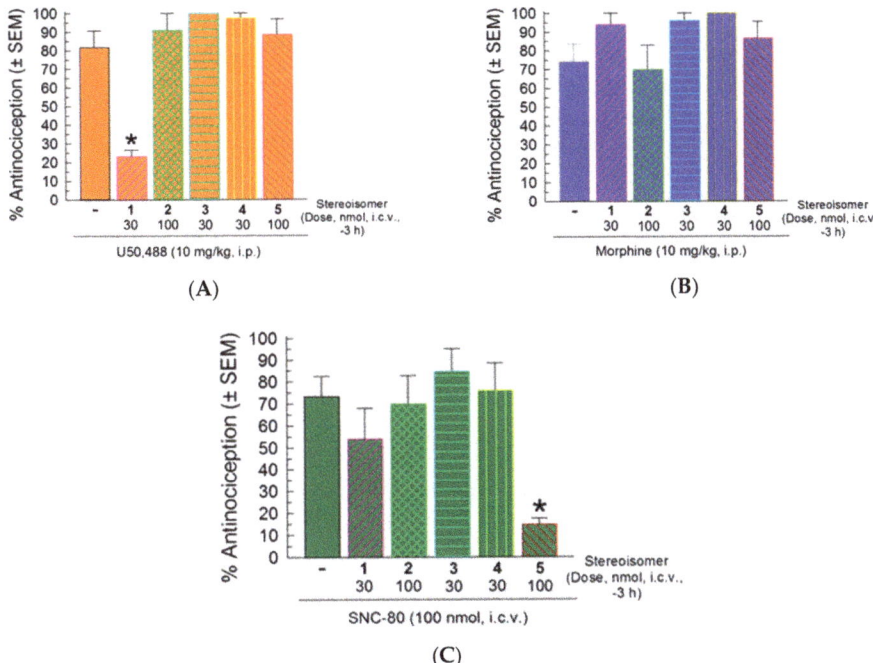

Figure 5. Opioid antagonist activity of the stereoisomers in the 55 °C warm-water tail-withdrawal assay. Mice were pretreated with a stereoisomer (30 or 100 nmol., i.c.v.) 3 h prior to the administration of (**A**) the KOR selective agonist U50,488 (10 mg/kg., i.p.), (**B**) the MOR preferring agonist morphine (10 mg/kg., i.p.), or (**C**) the DOR selective agonist SNC-30 (100 nmol, i.c.v.) to assess their ability to significantly reduce the antinociceptive effect of the opioid agonist. Mean % antinociception ± SEM from 8 mice for each bar. * significantly different from response of agonist alone ($p < 0.05$); one-way ANOVA with Sidak's multiple comparison *post hoc* test.

2.5. *In Vivo Assessment of Opioid Related Liabilities*

The five stereoisomers were then assessed for several potential liabilities produced by opioid agonists, specifically impairment of locomotor coordination, respiratory depression, hyperlocomotion and analgesic tolerance.

2.5.1. Assessment of Effects on Coordinated Locomotor Activity

Treatment with the stereoisomers (10 mg/kg, p.o.) or the KOR-selective agonist U50,488 (10 mg/kg, i.p.) had a significant effect on coordinated locomotor performance in the mouse rotarod assay ($F_{(6,49)} = 7.91$; $p < 0.05$, two-way RM ANOVA) over time ($F_{(6,294)} = 13.7$; $p < 0.05$, two-way RM ANOVA; Figure 6).

Whereas U50,488 significantly impaired coordinated locomotor activity after the first 10 min compared to vehicle ($p < 0.05$, Dunnett's *post hoc* test), the stereoisomers **2**, **3** and **5** lacked any significant effect, and isomers **1** (at 20, 40 and 50 min) and **4** (at 40 min) displayed limited impairment of performance ($p < 0.05$, Dunnett's *post hoc* test).

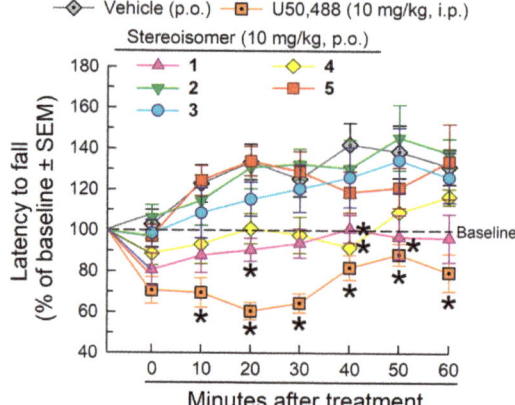

Figure 6. Effect of the stereoisomers on locomotor coordination after p.o. administration to C57BL/6J mice in the rotarod assay. Mice received the macrocyclic tetrapeptide (10 mg/kg, p.o.), vehicle (10% Solutol in saline, p.o.), or U50,488 (10 mg/kg, i.p.) and were tested on the rotarod apparatus with repeated measurements over time. Latencies to fall are given as the mean % change from baseline (100%) performance ± SEM. n = 8 mice per treatment. * significantly different from response of vehicle alone ($p < 0.05$); two-way RM ANOVA with Dunnett's multiple comparison *post hoc* test.

2.5.2. Evaluation of Respiratory and Spontaneous Locomotor Effects

The five stereoisomers (10 mg/kg, p.o.) were then assessed for their effect on spontaneous respiration rates and locomotor activity over a 1 h period using the Comprehensive Laboratory Animal Monitoring System (CLAMS) (Figure 7). As expected, the positive control morphine produced significant, time-dependent respiratory depression compared to vehicle (10–30 min; $F_{(10,165)} = 2.48$, $p < 0.05$, two-way RM ANOVA with Dunnett's multiple comparison *post hoc* test; Figure S2), while treatment with U50,488 resulted in significant, time-dependent increases in respiration rates (20–40 and 50–60 min; $p < 0.05$, Dunnett's *post hoc* test; Figure S2). Stereoisomers **1–3** of CJ-15,208 did not have any significant effect on respiration compared to vehicle (Figure 7A). Conversely, [D-Trp]CJ-15,208's isomers **4** and **5** produced significant decreases in respiration rates for the duration of the 60 min testing period ($F_{(5,50)} = 12.9$, $p < 0.05$, two-way RM ANOVA with Dunnett's multiple comparison *post hoc* test; Figure 7A). Among the D-Phe stereoisomers, only **3** had a significant effect on ambulation compared to vehicle, demonstrating elevated ambulations at several time-points (20–40 and 50–60 min; $F_{(5,47)} = 6.20$, $p < 0.05$, two-way RM ANOVA with Dunnett's multiple comparison *post hoc* test; Figure 7B). The positive control morphine produced robust, significant increases in ambulation over the last 40 min of testing ($F_{(10,215)} = 27.2$, $p < 0.05$, two-way RM ANOVA with Dunnett's multiple comparison *post hoc* test; Figure S2).

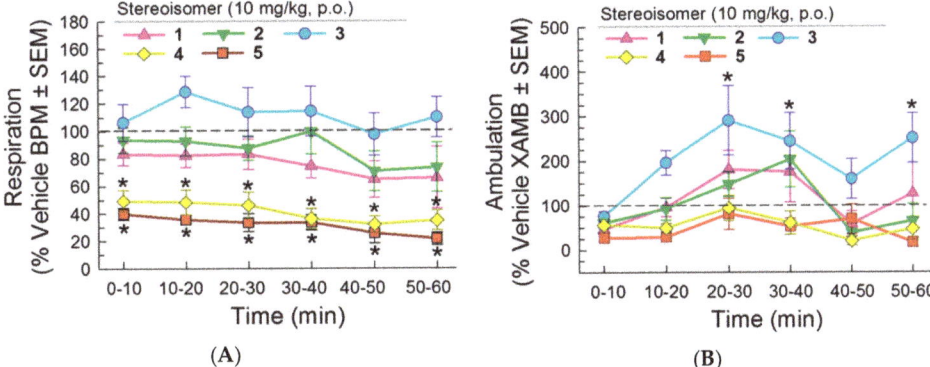

Figure 7. Effects of the stereoisomers on (**A**) respiration and (**B**) ambulation in C57BL/6J mice tested in the CLAMS/Oxymax system. Respiration and ambulation were monitored after administration of stereoisomer (10 mg/kg, p.o.) or vehicle using the CLAMS/Oxymax system. Data from 8–16 mice presented as % vehicle response ± SEM; breaths per minute, BPM (**A**) or ambulation, XAMB (**B**). * significantly different from vehicle control response ($p < 0.05$); two-way RM ANOVA with Dunnett's multiple comparison *post hoc* test.

2.5.3. Assessment of Acute Antinociceptive Tolerance Development

The stereoisomers were also tested in a model of acute antinociceptive tolerance [25] with repeated dosing (at 0 and 8 h, 0.1–300 nmol, i.c.v.) of morphine, CJ-15,208 or one of the five analogs. The development of acute antinociceptive tolerance was assessed by pretreating with the ED_{50} i.c.v. dose of the test compound, followed 8 h later by treatment with one of a range of graded doses; antinociceptive tolerance was indicated by a significant increase in the ED_{50} value compared to the value observed in naïve animals. As expected, morphine demonstrated acute antinociceptive tolerance, with a significant 7.63-fold rightward shift in the dose-response curve of the second dose administered ($F_{(1,4)} = 26.2$, $p < 0.05$; non-linear regression analysis; Table 3; see also Figure S3). Neither stereoisomer **4** or **5** demonstrated any significant changes in the ED_{50} values collected at 8 h vs. 0 h (Table 3). Both stereoisomers **1** and **3** demonstrated greater acute antinociceptive tolerance than CJ-15,208, with significant rightward shifts in their second dose-response curves (31.2-fold ($F_{(1,5)} = 39.9$ $p < 0.05$) and 5.19-fold ($F_{(1,5)} = 27.3$, $p < 0.05$), respectively; non-linear regression analysis). While isomer **2** demonstrated a 6.13-fold increase in its ED_{50} value after pretreatment, the increase was not statistically significant ($F_{(1,4)} = 2.99$, $p = 0.16$.)

Table 3. Comparison of ED_{50} (and 95% C.I.) values in naïve subjects and after again 8 h after a treatment of an ED_{50} dose of the respective compound [a].

Stereoisomer	Naïve ED_{50} (95% C.I.)	ED_{50} (95% C.I.) Pretreated Mice	Fold-Shift, Naïve ED_{50} vs. Second ED_{50}
1	0.65 (0.31–1.31)	20.3 * (11.1–41.7)	31.2
2	20.4 (10–58.7)	125 (89.9–224)	6.13
3	1.00 (0.64–1.60)	5.19 * (2.57–11)	5.19
4	2.39 (1.40–4.56)	1.28 (0.96–1.66)	0.54
5	0.45 (0.28–0.70)	0.49 (0.09–1.36)	1.09
CJ-15,208	1.82 (1.22–2.74)	5.23 (4.23–6.48)	2.87
Morphine	2.91 (2.48–3.41)	22.2 * (14.0–55.3)	7.63

[a] Data are ED_{50} values (nmol) from C57BL/6J mice tested with one of several doses (i.c.v.) of compound in the 55 °C warm-water tail-withdrawal assay in either naïve animals or mice who were pretreated with the ED_{50} dose of the respective compound, followed by administration of varying doses 8 h later. * significantly different from ED_{50} value in naïve mice ($p < 0.05$), non-linear regression analysis. n = 8–16 mice/dose tested.

2.5.4. Evaluation of Potential Reinforcing or Aversive Properties

Analogs **3** and **5** were further evaluated in a conditioned place-preference assay (Figure 8). Following a two-day place conditioning paradigm, mice conditioned with morphine (10 mg/kg, i.p.) demonstrated a significant place-preference for the morphine-paired chamber, whereas mice conditioned with U50,488 (10 mg/kg, i.p.) demonstrated a significant conditioned place avoidance ($F_{(3,53)} = 5.38$, $p < 0.05$; two-way ANOVA with Sidak's multiple comparison *post hoc* test; Figure 8).

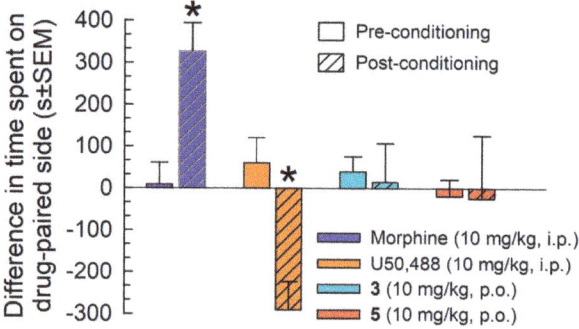

Figure 8. Evaluation of potential rewarding or aversive properties of isomer **3** and **5**. After determination of initial preconditioning preferences, C57BL/6J mice were place conditioned daily for two days with morphine (10 mg/kg, i.p.), U50,488 (10 mg/kg, i.p.), or stereoisomer (10 mg/kg, p.o.) using a counterbalanced design. Data is presented as mean difference in time spent on the drug-paired side ± SEM, with positive and negative values indicating a preference for and avoidance of the drug-paired chamber, respectively. * significantly different from matching preconditioning preference ($p < 0.05$), two-way ANOVA. n = 14–28 mice/compound.

However, mice place conditioned with either analog **3** or **5** (10 mg/kg, p.o.) demonstrated no significant preference or aversion for their respective drug-paired chamber.

3. Discussion

The macrocyclic tetrapeptide CJ-15,208 is structurally distinct from the endogenous opioid peptides, representing a novel lead compound for the development of new ligands for KOR. Its structure is particularly appealing for modification because its small macrocyclic structure imparts stability to degradation by proteases and facilitates penetration of biological barriers, including both the intestinal and blood-brain barriers [20,21] (Khaliq et al., manuscript in preparation), facilitating systemic, even oral, administration.

Changes in stereochemistry had differential effects on the contributions of the three opioid receptors to antinociception in vivo. While all three aromatic residues of CJ,15-208 were previously found to be important for KOR agonist activity [26], all of the stereoisomers, including the isomers of [D-Trp]CJ-15,208, exhibited KOR agonist activity in vivo regardless of residue stereochemistry. In contrast, only stereoisomer **1** retained KOR antagonist activity. Unlike the parent compounds, all of the stereoisomers except **2** demonstrated antinociception also mediated in part by DOR. This is in contrast to the in vitro results, where the stereoisomers all lacked affinity for DOR in radioligand binding assays; such discrepancies between in vitro and in vivo activity have been found for other CJ-15,208 analogs [26–28]. D-Phenylalanine in position 1 appears to favor DOR agonist activity; of the four isomers where DOR contributes to the observed antinociception only **5** does not contain D-Phe[1], and DOR appears to contribute less to the antinociception of this isomer than for the other isomers (Figure 4B). MOR contributes to the antinociception of three of the stereoisomers, but not to antinociception produced by isomers **3** and **4**. The lack of MOR contribution in these peptides cannot be attributed to the change in stereochemistry of any specific residue; it may instead be related to differences in peptide backbone conformation and the resulting effect on the orientation of one or more of the aromatic residues. Thus only isomer **2** retained the mixed MOR/KOR agonism of CJ-15,208, but this isomer did not exhibit maximum antinociception nor KOR antagonist activity.

All of the stereoisomers retained antinociceptive activity following oral administration, despite the rapid metabolism of most of these peptides by liver microsomes. Such hydrophobic peptides, including the parent peptides (Khaliq et al., manuscript in preparation), generally have high plasma protein binding which can protect compounds from metabolism and clearance, and thereby extend the duration of their activity in vivo. Only in the case of isomer **4** was there a difference in the maximum antinociception following oral vs. central administration. The decreased maximum response and shorter duration following oral administration for this isomer are likely due to its pharmacokinetic properties (metabolism, clearance and/or intestinal absorption).

The stereoisomers exhibited different potential liabilities of use. While KOR agonism contributed to the antinociception of all of the stereoisomers, in the rotarod assay only isomer **5** exhibited significantly decreased locomotor coordination at multiple time points, suggesting that activity at multiple opioid receptors mitigated this known side effect of KOR agonists. The lack of significant decreases in respiratory rates for all three CJ-15,208 isomers was very promising. We have previously shown that the multifunctional macrocyclic tetrapeptide *cyclo*[Pro-Sar-Phe-D-Phe] exhibits reduced liabilities, particularly respiratory effects, and that the peptide's KOR agonist activity appears to offset respiratory depression mediated by MOR [9]. In contrast, treatment with [D-Trp]CJ-15,208 isomers **4** and **5** decreased respiratory rates; this effect of **4** was surprising, given the lack of MOR agonist activity by this isomer. While not significant, there was a trend towards decreased ambulation following treatment with **4** and **5**, so it is possible that the decreased respiration rates could be due in part to decreased movement by these mice. In contrast to their effects on respiration rates, neither of the [D-Trp]CJ-15,208 stereoisomers exhibited evidence of acute tolerance, while, unlike the parent peptide, the CJ-15,208 isomers exhibited rightward shifts of the dose-response curves to varying degrees. Thus there was a dichotomy between the liabilities observed for the CJ-15,208 stereoisomers, which lacked respiratory depression but exhibited variable acute tolerance, and the [D-Trp]CJ-15,208 isomers, that exhibited the opposite pattern of decreased respiratory rates, but without significant acute tolerance.

Two isomers, **3** and **5**, were selected for testing in the conditioned place-preference assay for reinforcing (conditioned place preference, CPP) or aversive (conditioned place aversion, CPA) effects. Among the CJ-15,208 isomers, **3** demonstrated the most promising activity, producing full antinociception without locomotor impairment or respiratory effects, while the [D-Trp]CJ-15,208 isomer **5** produced full antinociception without acute antinociceptive tolerance. Mice place conditioned with either isomer demonstrated no significant preference or aversion for their respective drug-paired chamber. These results are consistent with earlier tests of multifunctional macrocyclic tetrapeptides [9,19] and could reflect the counteracting effects of agonism at multiple opioid receptors such as MOR and KOR [9,10]. In contrast to **5**, isomer **3** did not demonstrate significant MOR-mediated agonism, but rather KOR- and DOR-mediated antinociception. Mixed action DOR/MOR agonists such as MMP-2200 reportedly do not produce CPP and exhibit limited reinforcing effects [29]. Isomer **5** also displayed DOR antagonism which has been shown to prevent the conditioned place preference of MOR agonists in studies of bivalent ligands [30] and peptidomimetics [31]. To the best of our knowledge, no one has examined the effect of combined KOR agonists/DOR agonists or antagonists. Additional testing of higher doses of **3** and **5** are required to confirm the absence of the place conditioning demonstrated here.

The liabilities of the different stereoisomers did not correlate with the receptor involvement determined in the antinociceptive assay. The antinociception of both the CJ-15,208 stereoisomer **3** and the [D-Trp]CJ-15,208 isomer **4** were mediated by DOR and KOR, without significant contribution from MOR, but these peptides had opposite liability profiles. The same was true for stereoisomers **1** and **5**, where agonist activity mediated by all three opioid receptors contribute to the observed antinociception.

Additional studies will be necessary to explore potential mechanisms for the observed agonist (and in two cases antagonist) activity of these stereoisomers and to better understand receptor contributions to the observed side effects. Such studies are currently ongoing in our laboratories.

The stereoisomer [D-Phe^{1,3}]CJ-15,208 (3) is a very promising new lead compound for further exploration. Its potent antinociception after oral administration and lack of respiratory depression or locomotor impairment holds significant promise for the identification of safer analgesics.

4. Materials and Methods

4.1. Chemicals

The sources of the reagents, amino acids, solid phase resin and solvents for peptide synthesis are the same as reported previously [17,26,27]. Amino acids are the L-isomer unless otherwise specified, and abbreviations for amino acids follow the IUPAC-IUB joint commission of biochemical nomenclature (*Eur. J. Biochem.* **1984**, *138*, 9–37). All other chemicals were obtained from Sigma-Aldrich (St. Louis, MO, USA). Thin layer chromatography was performed on glass backed precoated silica gel plates (Sorbent Technologies, Atlanta, GA, USA, or Whatman, aluminum backed, 250 μm layer, Fisher Scientific, Pittsburg, PA, USA), and flash chromatography was performed on standard grade (32–63 μm) silica gel (Sorbent Technologies). HPLC analysis was performed on a Vydac 218TP C18 reversed phase column (Grace Davison, Columbia, MD, USA, 4.6 × 50 mm, 5 μm).

4.2. Instruments

Electrospray ionization mass spectra were acquired on a LCT Premier time of flight mass spectrometer (Waters Corp., Milford MA, USA) at the University of Kansas. HPLC analysis was performed using an Agilent 1200 HPLC system (Agilent, Santa Clara, CA, USA).

4.3. Peptide Synthesis and Purification

The linear peptide precursors (based on the parent sequences L-/D-Trp-Phe-D-Pro-Phe-OH) were synthesized on a 2-chlorotrityl chloride resin by Fmoc (fluorenylmethoxycarbonyl) peptide synthesis, and the peptides cleaved from the resin with 1% trifluoroacetic acid (TFA) in dichloromethane as described previously [17,26,27]. The crude linear peptides were cyclized using the following general procedure [20,22,27]: The crude linear peptide (0.5 equiv, 21 mM in *N,N*-dimethylformamide, DMF) was added dropwise at a rate of 1.0 mL/h (using a KD Scientific single infusion syringe pump) to a dilute solution of HATU (2-(1H-7-azabenzotriazol-1-yl)-1,1,3,3-tetramethyluronium hexafluorophosphate, 0.75 equiv, 1.2 mM) and *N,N*-diisopropylethylamine (DIEA, 4 equiv, 5 mM) in DMF. After 15 h additional HATU (0.75 equiv) was then added to the reaction in one portion, and additional linear peptide (0.5 equiv, 21 mM in DMF) was added dropwise at a rate of 1.0 mL/h as described above to give a final concentration of the linear tetrapeptide of 2.5 mM. The reaction was then stirred for 6 h at room temperature, followed by an additional 24 h at 37 °C. The solvent was evaporated under reduced pressure, and the crude macrocyclic tetrapeptides isolated as previously described [17,20,26].

The crude peptides were purified by silica gel chromatography using a step gradient of 60–90% EtOAc in hexane (with EtOAc increased in 10% increments), followed by 0–10% MeOH in EtOAc (with MeOH increased in 1% increments). The purified peptides were dissolved in aqueous acetonitrile (water:MeCN, 4:1) and then lyophilized to give the pure peptides as white solids. The purified peptides were analyzed by electrospray ionization mass spectrometry, thin layer chromatography, and in two analytical HPLC systems (see Table 4). The peptides were all >98% pure in both HPLC systems except for **4** which exhibited slightly lower purity. HPLC chromatograms are included in the Supplementary Materials.

Table 4. Analytical data for stereoisomers of CJ-15,208 and [D-Trp]CJ-15,208.

Isomer	Observed ES-MS, m/z [a]	R_f [b]	TLC System A [c]	HPLC, t (min) System B [d]
1	600.2568	0.70	18.4	23.0
2	600.2565	0.10	18.9	–
3	600.2578	0.67	22.4	22.6
4	600.2584	0.49	18.6 [e]	21.9 [e]
5	600.2605	0.53	21.1	23.8

[a] M + Na+, calculated m/z 600.2587; [b] EtOAc: MeOH, 9:1; [c] 15–55% MeCN over 40 min with 0.1% TFA, detection at 214 nm; [d] 30–70% MeOH over 45 min with 0.1% TFA, detection at 230 nm. [e] 94% and 96% pure in systems A and B, respectively.

4.3.1. [D-Phe¹]CJ-15,208 (1)

Cyclization of the linear peptide (600 mg) according to the general procedure yielded stereoisomer **1** as a white solid (193 mg, 34% yield).

4.3.2. [D-Phe³]CJ-15,208 (2)

The linear peptide (400 mg) was cyclized according to the general procedure, except that the second addition of peptide was added at a rate of 0.8 mL/h and the final concentration of the linear peptide in the reaction mixture was 4.5 mM. The peptide was purified starting at 60% EtOAc in hexane as described above, followed by 0–30% MeOH in EtOAc (with MeOH increased in 3% increments) to yield stereoisomer **2** as a white solid (167 mg, 43% yield).

4.3.3. [D-Phe¹,³]CJ-15,208 (3)

Cyclization of the linear peptide (600 mg) was performed according to the general procedure above. The purification was performed starting at 50% EtOAc in hexane (with EtOAc increased in 10% increments), followed by 0–5% MeOH in EtOAc (with MeOH increased in 1% increments) to yield **3** as a white solid (294 mg, 50% yield).

4.3.4. [D-Phe¹,D-Trp⁴]CJ-15,208 (4)

The linear peptide (400 mg) was cyclized according to the general procedure above, except that the first addition of peptide was added at a rate of 1.2 mL/h and the final concentration of the linear peptide in the reaction mixture was 1.5 mM. The purification was performed starting at 30% EtOAc in hexane (with EtOAc increased in 10% increments), followed by 0–3% MeOH in EtOAc (with MeOH increased in 1% increments) to yield **4** as a white solid (174 mg, 45% yield).

4.3.5. [D-Phe³,D-Trp⁴]CJ-15,208 (5)

The linear peptide (430 mg) was cyclized according to the general procedure, except that the second addition of peptide was added at a rate of 0.8 mL/h and the final concentration of the linear peptide in the reaction mixture was 3.6 mM. The peptide was purified starting at 60% EtOAc in hexane as described above, followed by 0–5% MeOH in EtOAc (with MeOH increased in 5% increments) to yield stereoisomer **5** as a white solid (200 mg, 48% yield).

4.4. Metabolism by Mouse Liver Microsomes

The macrocyclic tetrapeptide (5 μM) in 1% acetonitrile was incubated with mouse liver microsomes (0.25 mg/mL protein, Xenotech, Lenexa, KS, USA) at 37 °C in the presence or absence of co-factor NADPH RapidStart System (1 mM, Xenotech) or NADPH solution (Sigma, St. Louis, MO, USA) in potassium phosphate buffer (50 mM, pH 7.4). Aliquots (100 μL) taken at 0, 5, 15, 30, 60 and 120 min were quenched with ice-cold acetonitrile (1 vol) containing internal standard ([D-NMeAla²]CJ-15,208 [26], 5 μM) to precipitate the proteins. The lack of endogenous interference with the analysis of the stereoisomer or internal standard was confirmed by analyzing samples lacking the macrocyclic tetrapeptide.

Following centrifugation at 10,000× g rpm for 10 min, the supernatant (50 µL) was diluted with water (75 µL), stored overnight at −20 °C and analyzed by LC-MS/MS using methodology similar to that described for [D-Trp]CJ-15,208 [32]. Liquid chromatography was performed on a Hypersil BDS C_8 column (50 mm × 2.1 mm, 3 µm) with a flow rate of 0.2 mL/min and an injection volume of 20 µL using an Acquity UPLC system (Waters, Milford, MA, USA). The peptides were separated using a gradient of aqueous acetonitrile containing 0.08% formic acid of 20% B (0–2 min), 20–50% B (2–3 min), 50–80% B (3–6 min), 80% B (6–7 min), 80–20% B (7–8 min) and 20% B (8–10 min).

ESI-MS/MS was performed on a Waters Quatro triple quadrupole instrument operating in the positive ion multiple reaction monitoring mode. Data acquisition was carried out with Mass Lynx 4.1 software with the following settings: capillary voltage, 2500 V; cone voltage, 30 V; source temperature, 100 °C; desolvation temperature, 250 °C; cone gas flow, 279 L/h; desolvation gas flow, 1157 L/h; LM 1 resolution, 14; HM 1 resolution, 14; ion energy 1, 1.0; MS/MS mode entrance, -1; MS/MS collision energy, 35 eV; MS/MS mode exit, 2; LM 2 resolution, 13.0; HM 2 resolution, 13.0; ion energy 2, 1.5; multiplier, 650; collision cell pressure, 1.63×10^{-3} mbar; collision gas, argon. The transition m/z 578.2 ($[M + H]^+$) → 217.2 was monitored to determine the peak area counts of the stereoisomers, and m/z 566.2 ($[M + H]^+$) → 232.9 was monitored to determine the peak area counts of the internal standard (collision energy 22 eV) with the following settings: dwell time, 0.3 s; delay, 0.05 s.

4.5. In Vitro Pharmacological Evaluation

Opioid receptor affinities were determined by equilibrium radioligand binding assays as previously described [19,26,33] with membranes from Chinese hamster ovary (CHO) cells stably expressing rat KOR, rat MOR or mouse DOR using the radioligands [^{3}H]diprenorphine, [^{3}H][D-Ala^2,N-MePhe^4,glyol]enkephalin (DAMGO) and [^{3}H]DPDPE, respectively. Following determination of IC$_{50}$ values by nonlinear regression using Prism software (GraphPad Software Co., La Jolla, CA, USA) K$_i$ values were calculated using the Chen and Prusoff equation [34]. The results are presented as the mean ± SEM from at least three separate experiments each performed in triplicate.

Agonist stimulation of [^{35}S]GTPγS binding to membranes from CHO cells stably expressing KOR or MOR was assayed as described previously [19,26,35]. The macrocyclic tetrapeptides were screened at 10 µM for efficacy compared to the reference full agonists dynorphin A-(1-13) amide for KOR and DAMGO for MOR. The stereoisomers all exhibited negligible stimulation of GTPγS binding at both KOR and MOR.

4.6. In Vivo Testing

4.6.1. Animals and Drug Administration

Adult male wild-type C57BL/6J mice weighing 20–25 g were obtained from Jackson Labs (Bar Harbor, ME, USA). Food pellets and distilled water were available ad libitum. All mice were kept on a 12 h light-dark cycle and were housed and cared for in accordance with the National Institute of Health Guide for the Care and Use of Laboratory Animals. All results of animal testing are reported in accordance with ARRIVE guidelines [36].

For intracerebroventricular (i.c.v.) administration the macrocyclic tetrapeptides were dissolved in dimethyl sulfoxide (DMSO), followed by addition of sterile saline (0.9%) so that the final vehicle was 50% DMSO and 50% saline, and the i.c.v. injections performed as described previously [26]. This concentration of DMSO was not observed to have antinociceptive or behavioral effects in previous use [9,19,21]. For *per os* (p.o.) administration the macrocyclic tetrapeptides were administered in 10% Solutol in 0.9% saline. All solutions for animal administration were prepared fresh daily.

4.6.2. Antinociceptive Testing

The 55 °C warm-water tail-withdrawal assay was performed in mice as previously described [37], with the latency of the mouse to withdraw its tail from the water taken as the endpoint (a cut-off time of 15 sec was used in this assay). Antinociception was calculated according to the following formula: % antinociception = 100 × (test latency − control latency)/(15 − control latency). Tail-withdrawal data points are the means of 8–16 mice, unless otherwise indicated, with SEM shown by error bars.

The opioid receptor involvement in the agonist activity of the macrocyclic peptides was determined by pretreating mice with a single dose of β-funaltrexamine (β-FNA, 10 mg/kg, i.p.) or nor-BNI (10 mg/kg, i.p.) 24 h in advance of administration of a dose of a macrocyclic tetrapeptide. Additional mice were pretreated with a single dose of naloxone (30 mg/kg, s.c.) or naltrindole (20 mg/kg, i.p.) 20 min in advance of administration of the macrocyclic tetrapeptide.

To determine antagonist activity, mice were pretreated with the macrocyclic tetrapeptide 140 min prior to the administration of the MOR-preferring agonist morphine (10 mg/kg, i.p.), KOR-selective agonist U50,488 (10 mg/kg, i.p.) or DOR-selective agonist SNC-80 (100 nmol, i.c.v.); at this time the antinociceptive activity of the stereoisomers had dissipated. Antinociception produced by these established agonists was then measured 40 min after their administration.

4.6.3. Acute Antinociceptive Tolerance Determination

A standardized state of tolerance was induced by administration of morphine or test compound at times 0 and 8 h [25,38,39] to quantitatively evaluate development of acute opioid tolerance. This assay was used to efficiently measure the potential of compounds to cause tolerance using a minimum amount of compound while yielding reliable results. Mice were administered an ED_{50} dose (i.c.v.) of test compound in the morning (time = 0) and a second dose (varying between 0.1–300 nmol, i.c.v.) 8 h later. The degree of tolerance was calculated from the shift in ED_{50} value from the singly- to repeatedly-treated condition [40]. All compounds were administered i.c.v., with antinociception assessed 30 min after injection of morphine or at the time of peak antinociceptive effect of the macrocyclic tetrapeptides, as determined in their initial antinociceptive characterization.

4.6.4. Coordinated Locomotor Activity

The stereoisomers were tested for their possible impairment of locomotor coordination in the rotarod assay as described previously [9,21]. Locomotor activity was recorded using an automated, computer-controlled rotarod apparatus (San Diego Instruments, San Diego, CA, USA). Mice were first habituated to the rotarod over seven trials, with the last trial serving as the baseline response. Mice so habituated were then administered a 10 mg/kg dose of a stereoisomer (p.o.), U50,488 (i.p.), or vehicle 15 min prior to assessment in accelerated speed trials (180 s max latency at 0–20 rpm) performed every 10 min over a 60 min period. Mice were thus tested a total of 14 trials (seven habituation trials prior to treatment + seven drug trials). Decreased latencies to fall in the rotarod test indicate impaired motor coordination/sedation.

4.6.5. Respiration and Ambulation

Respiration rates (in breaths per minute) and animal locomotive activity (as ambulations) were assessed using the Oxymax/CLAMS system (Columbus Instruments, Columbus, OH, USA) as described previously [9,25]. Mice were habituated to their individual sealed housing chambers for 60 min before testing. Mice were administered stereoisomer (10 mg/kg, p.o.), morphine (10 mg/kg, i.p.), U50,488 (10 mg/kg, i.p.), or vehicle, as indicated, and five min later confined to the CLAMS testing chambers. Pressure monitoring within the sealed chambers measured frequency of respiration. Infrared beams located in the floor measured locomotion as number of beam breaks. Respiration and locomotive data were averaged over 10 min periods for 60 min post-injection of the test compound. Data is presentenced as % vehicle response ± SEM, ambulation or breaths per minute.

4.6.6. Evaluation of Potential Conditioned Place Preference and Conditioned Place Aversion

An automated, balanced three-compartment place conditioning apparatus (San Diego Instruments, San Diego, CA, USA) and a 2-day counterbalanced place conditioning design was used similar to methods previously described [21]. The amount of time subjects spent in each of the three compartments was measured over a 30 min testing period. Prior to place conditioning an initial preference test was performed in which the animals could freely explore all open compartments; the animals did not demonstrate significant differences in their time spent exploring the outer left versus right compartments ($p > 0.05$, Student's t-test). For place conditioning mice were administered 0.9% saline (i.p.) and consistently confined in a randomly assigned outer compartment: half of each group in the right chamber, and half in the left chamber. Four hours later, mice were administered test compound and confined to the opposite compartment for 40 min. To determine if **3** or **5** (10 mg/kg, p.o.) produced CPP or CPA, mice were place conditioned in this way for two days, with a final preference test taken on the fourth day, as this has been shown to produce dependable morphine CPP and U50,488-induced CPA [41]. Additional groups of mice were placed conditions with morphine or U50,488 (10 mg/kg, i.p.) as positive controls.

4.7. Statistical Analysis

All dose-response lines were analyzed by regression, and ED_{50} (effective dose producing 50% antinociception) values and 95% confidence intervals (C.I.) determined using individual data points from graded dose-response curves with Prism 8.0 software (GraphPad, La Jolla, CA, USA). Percent antinociception was used to determine within group effects and to allow comparison to baseline latency in tail-withdrawal experiments. The statistical significance of differences between ED_{50} values was determined by evaluation of the ED_{50} value shift via nonlinear regression modeling with Prism software. Significant differences in behavioral data were analyzed by ANOVA (one-way or two-way with repeated measures (RM), as appropriate). Significant results were further analyzed with Sidak's, Tukey's, or Dunnett's multiple comparison *post hoc* tests, as appropriate. Data for conditioned place preference experiments were analyzed by two-way RM ANOVA, with analyses examining the main effect of conditioned place preference phase (e.g., pre- or post-conditioning) and the interaction of drug pretreatment. Significant effects were further analyzed using Sidak's HSD *post hoc* testing. All data are presented as mean ± SEM, with significance set at $p < 0.05$.

5. Patents

J.V. Aldrich and S. Senadheera, Cyclic Tetrapeptide Stereoisomers, U.S. Patent 10,259,843 B2, 2019, and European patent EP3,166,625, 23019.

Supplementary Materials: The following are available online, Figure S1: Time-course of antinociceptive activity in the 55 °C warm-water tail-withdrawal assay following (A) i.c.v. administration and (B) oral administration in C57Bl/6J mice of a maximally efficacious dose. Points represent average % antinociception ± SEM from 4–16 mice for each set presented, Figure S2. Effects of the U50,488 or morphine on (A) respiration and (B) ambulation in C57BL76J mice. Respiration and ambulation were monitored after administration of U50,488 or morphine (10 mg/kg, i.p.) using the CLAMS/Oxymax system. Data from 9–18 mice presented as % vehicle response ± SEM; breaths per minute, BPM (A) or ambulation, XAMB (B). * significantly different from response of saline alone ($p < 0.05$); two-way RM ANOVA with Dunnett's multiple comparison post hoc test., Figure S3. Evaluation of acute antinociceptive tolerance in the 55 °C warm-water tail-withdrawal assay following i.c.v. administration of morphine, (A) CJ-15,208, (B) **1**, (C) **2**, (D) **3**, (E) **4** or (F) **5**. All points represent antinociception at peak response in naïve mice (Time 0 h) and mice that were previously administered an ED_{50} dose of test compound (as listed) prior to additional administration of a graded dose of test compound eight hours later (Time 8 h). Points represent average % antinociception ± SEM from 8–16 mice for each set presented, Figure S4. HPLC chromatograms of the peptides in 15–55% MeCN over 40 min with 0.1% TFA, detection at 214 nm, (A) **1**, (B) **2**, (C) **3**, (D) **4** and (E) **5**, Figure S5. HPLC chromatograms of the peptides in 30–70% MeOH over 40 min with 0.1% TFA, detection at 230 nm, (A) **1**, (B) **3**, (C) **4** and (D) **5**.

Author Contributions: Conceptualization, S.N.S., J.P.M. and J.V.A.; methodology, S.N.S., M.L.G., S.O.E., T.K., T.F.M., J.P.M. and J.V.A.; validation, J.P.M. and J.V.A.; formal analysis, A.C.B.-T., T.F.M., J.P.M., and J.V.A.; investigation, A.C.B.-T., S.N.S., M.L.G., S.O.E., T.K., T.F.M., J.P.M. and J.V.A.; resources, S.N.S., T.F.M., J.P.M.

and J.V.A.; data curation, A.C.B.-T., S.N.S., M.L.G., S.O.E., T.K., T.F.M., J.P.M. and J.V.A.; writing—original draft preparation, A.C.B.-T. and J.V.A.; writing—review and editing, A.C.B.-T., J.P.M., and J.V.A.; visualization, J.P.M. and J.V.A.; supervision, J.P.M. and J.V.A.; project administration, J.P.M. and J.V.A.; funding acquisition, J.P.M. and J.V.A. All authors have read and agreed to the published version of the manuscript.

Funding: This research was funded by the National Institute on Drug Abuse, grants R01 DA18832 and R01 DA032928.

Acknowledgments: We thank Bridget Sefranek and Stacey Sigmon for their assistance with the in vitro pharmacological assays.

Conflicts of Interest: The authors declare no conflict of interest. The funders had no role in the design of the study; in the collection, analyses, or interpretation of data; in the writing of the manuscript, or in the decision to publish the results.

References

1. Corder, G.; Castro, D.C.; Bruchas, M.R.; Scherrer, G. Endogenous and Exogenous Opioids in Pain. *Annu. Rev. Neurosci.* **2018**, *41*, 453–473. [CrossRef] [PubMed]
2. Volkow, N.D.; McLellan, A.T. Opioid Abuse in Chronic Pain—Misconceptions and Mitigation Strategies. *N. Engl. J. Med.* **2016**, *374*, 1253–1263. [CrossRef] [PubMed]
3. Pfeiffer, A.; Brantl, V.; Herz, A.; Emrich, H.M. Psychotomimesis mediated by κ opiate receptors. *Science* **1986**, *233*, 774–776. [CrossRef] [PubMed]
4. Jutkiewicz, E.M.; Baladi, M.G.; Folk, J.E.; Rice, K.C.; Woods, J.H. The Convulsive and Electroencephalographic Changes Produced by Nonpeptidic δ-Opioid Agonists in Rats: Comparison with Pentylenetetrazol. *J. Pharmacol. Exp. Ther.* **2006**, *317*, 1337–1348. [CrossRef] [PubMed]
5. Schiller, P.W. Bi- or multifunctional opioid peptide drugs. *Life Sci.* **2010**, *86*, 598–603. [CrossRef]
6. Ko, M.; Husbands, S.M. Effects of atypical kappa-opioid receptor agonists on intrathecal morphine-induced itch and analgesia in primates. *J. Pharmacol. Exp. Ther.* **2008**, *328*, 193–200. [CrossRef] [PubMed]
7. Negus, S.S.; Schrode, K.; Stevenson, G.W.; Schrode, K.K. Mu/kappa opioid interactions in rhesus monkeys: Implications for analgesia and abuse liability. *Exp. Clin. Psychopharmacol.* **2008**, *16*, 386–399. [CrossRef]
8. Stevenson, G.W.; Folk, J.E.; Linsenmayer, D.C.; Rice, K.C.; Negus, S.S.; Litman, T.; Skovsgaard, T.; Stein, W.D. Opioid Interactions in Rhesus Monkeys: Effects of δ + µ and δ + κ Agonists on Schedule-Controlled Responding and Thermal Nociception. *J. Pharmacol. Exp. Ther.* **2003**, *307*, 1054–1064. [CrossRef]
9. Brice-Tutt, A.C.; Wilson, L.L.; Eans, S.O.; Stacy, H.M.; Simons, C.A.; Simpson, G.G.; Coleman, J.S.; Ferracane, M.J.; Aldrich, J.V.; McLaughlin, J.P. Multifunctional opioid receptor agonism and antagonism by a novel macrocyclic tetrapeptide prevents reinstatement of morphine-seeking behaviour. *Br. J. Pharmacol.* **2020**, *177*, 4209–4222. [CrossRef]
10. Anand, J.P.; Montgomery, D. Multifunctional Opioid Ligands. *Handb. Exp. Pharmacol.* **2018**, *247*, 21–51. [CrossRef]
11. Bolaños, C.A.; Garmsen, G.M.; Clair, M.A.; McDougall, S.A. Effects of the κ-opioid receptor agonist U-50,488 on morphine-induced place preference conditioning in the developing rat. *Eur. J. Pharmacol.* **1996**, *317*, 1–8. [CrossRef]
12. Dosaka-Akita, K.; Tortella, F.C.; Holaday, J.W.; Long, J.B. The Kappa Opioid Agonist U-50, 488H Antagonizes Respiratory Effects of Mu Opioid Receptor Agonists in Conscious. *Rats* **1993**, *264*, 631–637. [CrossRef]
13. Hepburn, M.J.; Little, P.J.; Gingras, J.; Kuhn, C.M. Differential effects of naltrindole on morphine-induced tolerance and physical dependence in rats. *J. Pharmacol. Exp. Ther.* **1997**, *281*, 1350–1356.
14. Daniels, D.J.; Kulkarni, A.; Xie, Z.; Bhushan, R.G.; Portoghese, P.S. A bivalent ligand (KDAN-18) containing delta-antagonist and kappa-agonist pharmacophores bridges delta2 and kappa1 opioid receptor phenotypes. *J. Med. Chem.* **2005**, *48*, 1713–1716. [CrossRef] [PubMed]
15. Saito, T.; Hirai, H.; Kim, Y.-J.; Kojima, Y.; Matsunaga, Y.; Nishida, H.; Sakakibara, T.; Suga, O.; Sujaku, T.; Kojima, N. CJ-15,208, a novel kappa opioid receptor antagonist from a fungus, Ctenomyces serratus ATCC15502. *J. Antibiot.* **2002**, *55*, 847–854. [CrossRef] [PubMed]
16. Kulkarni, S.S.; Ross, N.C.; McLaughlin, J.P.; Aldrich, J.V. Synthesis of cyclic tetrapeptide CJ 15,208: A novel kappa opioid receptor antagonist. *Adv. Exp. Med. Biol.* **2009**, *611*, 269–270. [CrossRef] [PubMed]
17. Ross, N.C.; Kulkarni, S.S.; McLaughlin, J.P.; Aldrich, J.V. Synthesis of CJ-15,208, a novel κ-opioid receptor antagonist. *Tetrahedron Lett.* **2010**, *51*, 5020–5023. [CrossRef]

18. Dolle, R.E.; Michaut, M.; Martinez-Teipel, B.; Seida, P.R.; Ajello, C.W.; Muller, A.L.; DeHaven, R.N.; Carroll, P.J. Nascent structure–activity relationship study of a diastereomeric series of kappa opioid receptor antagonists derived from CJ-15,208. *Bioorg. Med. Chem. Lett.* **2009**, *19*, 3647–3650. [CrossRef]
19. Ross, N.C.; Reilley, K.J.; Murray, T.F.; Aldrich, J.V.; McLaughlin, J.P. Novel opioid cyclic tetrapeptides: Trp isomers of CJ-15,208 exhibit distinct opioid receptor agonism and short-acting κ opioid receptor antagonism. *Br. J. Pharmacol.* **2012**, *165*, 1097–1108. [CrossRef]
20. Aldrich, J.V.; Senadheera, S.N.; Ross, N.C.; Ganno, M.L.; Eans, S.O.; McLaughlin, J.P. The Macrocyclic Peptide Natural Product CJ-15,208 Is Orally Active and Prevents Reinstatement of Extinguished Cocaine-Seeking Behavior. *J. Nat. Prod.* **2013**, *76*, 433–438. [CrossRef]
21. Eans, S.; Ganno, M.L.; Reilley, K.J.; A Patkar, K.; Senadheera, S.N.; Aldrich, J.V.; McLaughlin, J.P. The macrocyclic tetrapeptide [D-Trp]CJ-15,208 produces short-acting κ opioid receptor antagonism in the CNS after oral administration. *Br. J. Pharmacol.* **2013**, *169*, 426–436. [CrossRef] [PubMed]
22. Senadheera, S.N.; Kulkarni, S.S.; McLaughlin, J.P.; Aldrich, J.V. Improved Synthesis of CJ-15,208 Isomers and Their Pharmacological Activity at Opioid Receptors. In *Peptides: Building Bridges*; Lebl, M., Ed.; American Peptide Society: San Diego, CA, USA, 2011; pp. 346–347.
23. Christians, U.; Sewing, K.-F. Cyclosporin metabolism in transplant patients. *Pharmacol. Ther.* **1993**, *57*, 291–345. [CrossRef]
24. Delaforge, M.; André, F.; Jaouen, M.; Dolgos, H.; Benech, H.; Gomis, J.-M.; Noel, J.-P.; Cavelier, F.; Verducci, J.; Aubagnac, J.-L.; et al. Metabolism of Tentoxin by Hepatic Cytochrome P-450 3A Isozymes. *JBIC J. Boil. Inorg. Chem.* **1997**, *250*, 150–157. [CrossRef] [PubMed]
25. Hoot, M.R.; Sypek, E.I.; Reilley, K.J.; Carey, A.N.; Bidlack, J.M.; McLaughlin, J.P. Inhibition of G??-subunit signaling potentiates morphine-induced antinociception but not respiratory depression, constipation, locomotion, and reward. *Behav. Pharmacol.* **2013**, *24*, 144–152. [CrossRef] [PubMed]
26. Aldrich, J.V.; Kulkarni, S.S.; Senadheera, S.N.; Ross, N.C.; Reilley, K.J.; Eans, S.O.; Ganno, M.L.; Murray, T.F.; McLaughlin, J.P. Unexpected Opioid Activity Profiles of Analogues of the Novel Peptide Kappa Opioid Receptor Ligand CJ-15,208. *ChemMedChem* **2011**, *6*, 1739–1745. [CrossRef] [PubMed]
27. Aldrich, J.V.; Senadheera, S.N.; Ross, N.C.; A Reilley, K.; Ganno, M.L.; E Eans, S.; Murray, T.F.; McLaughlin, J.P. Alanine analogues of [D-Trp]CJ-15,208: Novel opioid activity profiles and prevention of drug- and stress-induced reinstatement of cocaine-seeking behaviour. *Br. J. Pharmacol.* **2014**, *171*, 3212–3222. [CrossRef] [PubMed]
28. Ferracane, M.J.; Brice-Tutt, A.C.; Coleman, J.S.; Simpson, G.G.; Wilson, L.L.; Eans, S.O.; Stacy, H.M.; Murray, T.F.; McLaughlin, J.P.; Aldrich, J.V. Design, Synthesis, and Characterization of the Macrocyclic Tetrapeptide cyclo[Pro-Sar-Phe-D-Phe]: A Mixed Opioid Receptor Agonist–Antagonist Following Oral Administration. *ACS Chem. Neurosci.* **2020**, *11*, 1324–1336. [CrossRef] [PubMed]
29. Stevenson, G.W.; Luginbuhl, A.; Dunbar, C.; Lavigne, J.; Dutra, J.; Atherton, P.; Bell, B.; Cone, K.; Giuvelis, D.; Polt, R.; et al. The mixed-action delta/mu opioid agonist MMP-2200 does not produce conditioned place preference but does maintain drug self-administration in rats, and induces in vitro markers of tolerance and dependence. *Pharmacol. Biochem. Behav.* **2015**, *132*, 49–55. [CrossRef]
30. Lenard, N.R.; Daniels, D.J.; Portoghese, P.S.; Roerig, S.C. Absence of conditioned place preference or reinstatement with bivalent ligands containing mu-opioid receptor agonist and delta-opioid receptor antagonist pharmacophores. *Eur. J. Pharmacol.* **2007**, *566*, 75–82. [CrossRef]
31. Anand, J.P.; E Kochan, K.; Nastase, A.F.; Montgomery, D.; Griggs, N.W.; Traynor, J.R.; I Mosberg, H.; Jutkiewicz, E.M. In vivo effects of µ-opioid receptor agonist/δ-opioid receptor antagonist peptidomimetics following acute and repeated administration. *Br. J. Pharmacol.* **2018**, *175*, 2013–2027. [CrossRef]
32. Khaliq, T.; Williams, T.D.; Senadheera, S.N.; Aldrich, J.V. Development of a robust, sensitive and selective liquid chromatography-tandem mass spectrometry assay for the quantification of the novel macrocyclic peptide kappa opioid receptor antagonist [D-Trp]CJ-15,208 in plasma and application to an initial pharmacokinetic study. *J. Chromatogr. B* **2016**, *1028*, 11–15. [CrossRef]
33. Arttamangkul, S.; Ishmael, J.E.; Murray, T.F.; Grandy, D.K.; DeLander, G.E.; Kieffer, B.L.; Aldrich, J.V. Synthesis and Opioid Activity of Conformationally Constrained Dynorphin A Analogues. 2.1Conformational Constraint in the "Address" Sequence. *J. Med. Chem.* **1997**, *40*, 1211–1218. [CrossRef] [PubMed]

34. Cheng, Y.C.; Prusoff, W.H. Relationship between the inhibition constant (Ki) and the concentration of inhibitor which causes 50 percent inhibition (IC50) of an enzymatic reaction. *Biochem. Pharmacol.* **1973**, *22*, 3099–3108. [PubMed]
35. Siebenaller, J.F.; Murray, T.F. Hydrostatic Pressure Alters the Time Course of GTP[S] Binding to G Proteins in Brain Membranes from Two Congeneric Marine Fishes. *Boil. Bull.* **1999**, *197*, 388–394. [CrossRef]
36. McGrath, J.; Drummond, G.; McLachlan, E.M.; Kilkenny, C.; Wainwright, C.L. Guidelines for reporting experiments involving animals: The ARRIVE guidelines. *Br. J. Pharmacol.* **2010**, *160*, 1573–1576. [CrossRef]
37. McLaughlin, J.P.; Hill, K.P.; Jiang, Q.; Sebastian, A.; Archer, S.; Bidlack, J.M. Nitrocinnamoyl and chlorocinnamoyl derivatives of dihydrocodeinone: In vivo and in vitro characterization of mu-selective agonist and antagonist activity. *J. Pharmacol. Exp. Ther.* **1999**, *289*, 304–311.
38. Jiang, Q.; Seyed-Mozaffari, A.; Sebastian, A.; Archer, S.; Bidlack, J.M. Preventing morphine antinociceptive tolerance by irreversible mu opioid antagonists before the onset of their antagonism. *J. Pharmacol. Exp. Ther.* **1995**, *273*, 680–688. [CrossRef]
39. Mathews, J.L.; Smrcka, A.V.; Bidlack, J.M. A novel Gbetagamma-subunit inhibitor selectively modulates mu-opioid-dependent antinociception and attenuates acute morphine-induced antinociceptive tolerance and dependence. *J. Neurosci.* **2008**, *28*, 12183–12189. [CrossRef]
40. Way, E.L.; Loh, H.H.; Shen, F.H. Simultaneous quantitative assessment of morphine tolerance and physical dependence. *J. Pharmacol. Exp. Ther.* **1969**, *167*, 1–8.
41. Spetea, M.; O Eans, S.; Ganno, M.L.; Lantero, A.; Mairegger, M.; Toll, L.; Schmidhammer, H.; McLaughlin, J.P. Selective κ receptor partial agonist HS666 produces potent antinociception without inducing aversion after i.c.v. administration in mice. *Br. J. Pharmacol.* **2017**, *174*, 2444–2456. [CrossRef]

Sample Availability: Samples of the compounds *cyclo*[D-Phe-D-Pro-Phe-Trp] (**1**), *cyclo*[Phe-D-Pro- D-Phe-Trp] (**2**), *cyclo*[D-Phe-D-Pro- D-Phe-Trp] (**3**), *cyclo*[D-Phe-D-Pro-Phe-D-Trp] (**4**) and *cyclo*[Phe-D-Pro- D-Phe-D-Trp] (**5**) are available from the authors.

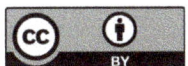

© 2020 by the authors. Licensee MDPI, Basel, Switzerland. This article is an open access article distributed under the terms and conditions of the Creative Commons Attribution (CC BY) license (http://creativecommons.org/licenses/by/4.0/).

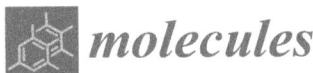

Article

Zerumbone-Induced Analgesia Modulated via Potassium Channels and Opioid Receptors in Chronic Constriction Injury-Induced Neuropathic Pain

Banulata Gopalsamy [1], Jasmine Siew Min Chia [2], Ahmad Akira Omar Farouk [1], Mohd Roslan Sulaiman [1] and Enoch Kumar Perimal [1,3,*]

[1] Department of Biomedical Sciences, Faculty of Medicine and Health Sciences, Universiti Putra Malaysia, Serdang 43400, Selangor, Malaysia; banulata@upm.edu.my (B.G.); ahmadakira@upm.edu.my (A.A.O.F.); mrs@upm.edu.my (M.R.S.)
[2] Centre for Community Health Studies, Faculty of Health Sciences, Universiti Kebangsaan Malaysia, Kuala Lumpur 50300, Malaysia; jasminecsm@ukm.edu.my
[3] Australian Research Council Centre of Excellence for Nanoscale BioPhotonics, University of Adelaide, Adelaide 5000, Australia
* Correspondence: enoch@upm.edu.my; Tel./Fax: +61-603-8947-2774

Academic Editors: Mariana Spetea and Aleksandra Misicka-Kesik
Received: 1 July 2020; Accepted: 3 August 2020; Published: 26 August 2020

Abstract: Zerumbone, a monocyclic sesquiterpene from the wild ginger plant *Zingiber zerumbet* (L.) Smith, attenuates allodynia and hyperalgesia. Currently, its mechanisms of action in neuropathic pain conditions remain unclear. This study examines the involvement of potassium channels and opioid receptors in zerumbone-induced analgesia in a chronic constriction injury (CCI) neuropathic pain mice model. Male Institute of Cancer Research (ICR) mice were subjected to CCI and behavioral responses were tested on day 14. Responses toward mechanical allodynia and thermal hyperalgesia were tested with von Frey's filament and Hargreaves' tests, respectively. Symptoms of neuropathic pain were significantly alleviated following treatment with zerumbone (10 mg/kg; intraperitoneal, i.p.). However, when the voltage-dependent K^+ channel blocker tetraethylammonium (TEA, 4 mg/kg; i.p.), ATP-sensitive K^+ channel blocker, glibenclamide (GLIB, 10 mg/kg; i.p.); small-conductance Ca^{2+}-activated K^+ channel inhibitor apamin (APA, 0.04 mg/kg; i.p.), or large-conductance Ca^{2+}-activated K^+ channel inhibitor charybdotoxin (CHAR, 0.02 mg/kg; i.p.) was administered prior to zerumbone (10 mg/kg; i.p.), the antiallodynic and antihyperalgesic effects of zerumbone were significantly reversed. Additionally, non-specific opioid receptors antagonist, naloxone (NAL, 10 mg/kg; i.p.), selective µ-, δ- and κ-opioid receptor antagonists; β-funaltrexamine (β-FN, 40 mg/kg; i.p.), naltrindole (20 mg/kg; s.c.), nor-binaltorphamine (10 mg/kg; s.c.) respectively attenuated the antiallodynic and antihyperalgesic effects of zerumbone. This outcome clearly demonstrates the participation of potassium channels and opioid receptors in the antineuropathic properties of zerumbone. As various clinically used neuropathic pain drugs also share this similar mechanism, this compound is, therefore, a highly potential substitute to these therapeutic options.

Keywords: zerumbone; chronic constriction injury (CCI); allodynia; hyperalgesia; potassium channels; opioid receptors

1. Introduction

Neuropathic pain occurs following a disease or injury to the peripheral and central nervous system. This chronic pain condition remains a therapeutic challenge in clinical settings, as modern therapies are only partially effective. Various biochemical and pathophysiological changes occur following neural damage, which leads to a morphological and functional adaptation of the nervous system to external stimuli. This adaptation plays an essential role in the commencement and maintenance of pain symptoms. Even though this chronic pain state is mediated by both peripheral and central mechanisms, the pathological overexcitability of nociceptive afferents is often the trigger. Factors that lead to peripheral sensitization include sprouting of sympathetic nerves [1], inflammatory mechanisms [2], and altered activity or expression of various proteins that are related to neuronal excitability [3].

One common and consistent feature of neuropathic remodeling that occurs within the degenerating peripheral nociceptors and occasionally in the non-nociceptive afferents is the downregulation of the pool of K^+ channels. Suppression in K^+ channel pools is present not only in neuropathic pain conditions, but also in inflammatory and cancer pain [4]. Injured axons undergo Wallerian degeneration and demyelination of myelinated axons, whereby their functions are immediately disrupted. The distal axonal segments gradually degenerate and slowly become unexcitable. Following demyelination, Schwann cells produce new myelin sheaths as a repairing process in the peripheral nervous system. However, the architecture of these re-myelinated nerve fibers is different than normal nerve fibers [5]. Ion channels are differentially expressed due to an upsurge in the nodes number per unit length, as the number of myelin lamella is decreased. The regions that were initially internodal, having a lower density of ion channels, then have new nodes of Ranvier with denser ion channels; this density is essential for saltatory conduction [6]. Furthermore, the irregular re-myelination process may mask, block, or hide paranodal K^+ channels, leading to the suppression of the channel function and at the same time making them resistant to drugs.

The downregulation of K^+ channel pools has also been successfully modelled across various animal models of neuropathic pain [7,8]. Therapeutic strategies aim to activate K^+ currents in neurons, as they are able to provide an antiexcitatory effect with no regard for the source that causes overexcitation. Considering that K^+ channels are essential in normal nerve conductivity, a potent drug should be able to "reset" afferent excitability to a higher threshold and restore normal sensitivity. Pharmacologically, enhancement of K^+ channels by the use of openers or enhancers has been recently identified and optimized to validate the potential of this approach as a pain treatment [9].

First-line treatments for neuropathic pain comprise tricyclic antidepressants and antiepileptics. Controlled-release opioid analgesics are often regarded as the second- or third-line treatments for moderate to severe pain and will only be prescribed if the first-line analgesic options have been exhausted [10]. Nevertheless, opioids are also prescribed as first-line treatments in certain circumstances. This is due to the effectiveness reported in some randomized clinical trials involving patients with different types of neuropathic pain [11]. Recommendations for the treatments are individualized based on the drugs' efficacy, accessibility, side-effect profile, as well as cost-effectiveness. Opioids such as tramadol, morphine [12], methadone, and oxycodone [12,13] are the usual treatments for neuropathic pain in clinical settings.

There are a few drawbacks to the use of opioids—mainly that they often involve health complications such as sedation, dependence, dizziness, vomiting, nausea, constipation, and respiratory depression [14]. In addition, repeated or prolonged opioid administration leads to tolerance to a particular dose, resulting in a higher dosage being required to achieve the same pain relief effect [15]. Long-term opioid usage could also cause addiction, triggering compulsive drug-seeking behavior. Moreover, the discontinuation of opioid therapy results in severe withdrawal effects, which usually occur in patients who have developed tolerance [16]. Therefore, drugs derived from natural products that are able to provide substantial pain relief with fewer side effects might be preferred.

Zerumbone is an active compound isolated from the wild ginger plant, *Zingiber zerumbet* (L.) Smith. This plant is native to Southeast Asia and mainly grows in tropical and subtropical regions [17]. Ginger plants have been reported for their vast medicinal properties and have been used since earlier times as folkloric medicine [18] to treat minor diseases and ailments, such as indigestion, stomach upset, colic, cramp, morning sickness, fever, congestion, sore throat, nausea, asthma, toothache, fracture, swelling, diabetes, rheumatism, and arthritis [19–21]. Therefore, active compounds of this plant have been isolated and studied for their properties in recent years. Scientific testing of the possible pain relief effects of zerumbone have proved that it effectively inhibited pain in models of nociception [22,23] and inflammation [24]. Interestingly, zerumbone also attenuated allodynia and hyperalgesia in a mice model of neuropathic pain [25–28].

Zerumbone (2,6,9,9-tetramethyl-[2E,6E,10E]-cycloundeca-2,6,10-trien-1-one) is a monocyclic sesquiterpene with three double bonds (two conjugated and one isolated) and a conjugated carbonyl group in an 11-membered ring structure [29]. A wide array of molecular targets have been reported in existing literature on this the α,β-unsaturated, carbonyl-based compound, which has great potential for cancer and nociceptive treatments [30,31]. Recently, Hwang et al. [32] reported on the pharmacokinetic properties of zerumbone, which possesses good water solubility with blood–brain barrier and central nervous system (CNS) permeability values using absorption, distribution, metabolism, excretion, toxicity (ADMET) simulation. Using in silico methods, zerumbone has shown binding capacity to several proteins and receptor sites [33,34]. Despite the vast amount of literature on zerumbone's characteristics, interactions of this compound with potassium channels and opioid receptors remain unknown. Based on docking analysis, the α,β-unsaturated carbonyl scaffold is the main force responsible for zerumbone's therapeutic effects [32,35,36].

To further understand the exact underlying mechanism of this compound, we aimed to investigate if zerumbone's actions involve potassium channels and opioid receptors in a chronic constriction injury (CCI)-induced mice model of neuropathic pain.

2. Results

2.1. Involvement of Voltage-Dependent K^+ Channels in Zerumbone's Antiallodynic and Antihyperalgesic Effects

The involvement of voltage-dependent K^+ channels in the antineuropathic properties of zerumbone was investigated by blocking the channels with a voltage-dependent K^+ channel blocker, tetraethylammonium (TEA). Pre-treatment the animals (n = 8) with TEA (4 mg/kg; i.p.) prior to zerumbone significantly reversed the antiallodynic effect of zerumbone (10 mg/kg; i.p.) ($p \leq 0.05$) (Figure 1A). Similarly, pre-treatment with TEA (n = 8, 4 mg/kg; i.p.) also reversed the antihyperalgesic effect of zerumbone (10 mg/kg; i.p.) ($p \leq 0.05$) (Figure 1B). Treatment with TEA alone (n = 8) did not elicit any effect on the withdrawal threshold or latency in either test.

2.2. Involvement of ATP-Sensitive K^+ Channels in Zerumbone's Antiallodynic and Antihyperalgesic Effects

The involvement of ATP-sensitive K^+ channels in the ability of zerumbone to induce analgesia was investigated by pre-treating the animals with an ATP-sensitive K^+ channel antagonist, glibenclamide (GLIB). GLIB (10 mg/kg; i.p.) significantly reversed the antiallodynic effect (n = 8) (Figure 2A) and antihyperalgesic (n = 8) (Figure 2B) effects of zerumbone (10 mg/kg; i.p.) ($p \leq 0.05$). Administration of the antagonist alone did not elicit any effect on this mice model.

2.3. Involvement of Small- and Large-Conductance Ca^{2+}-Activated K^+ Channels in Zerumbone-Induced Antiallodynia and Antihyperalgesia

The involvement of small-conductance Ca^{2+}-activated K^+ channels in the antineuropathic properties of zerumbone was investigated using a selective small-conductance Ca^{2+}-activated K^+ channel inhibitor, apamin (APA). APA (0.04 mg/kg; i.p.) was administered prior to zerumbone treatment, while the antiallodynic (n = 8) (Figure 3A) and antihyperalgesic (n = 8) (Figure 3B) effects of zerumbone (10 mg/kg; i.p.) ($p \leq 0.05$) were absent. Treatment with APA (0.04 mg/kg; i.p.) alone did not elicit any effect on the animal's behavioral responses.

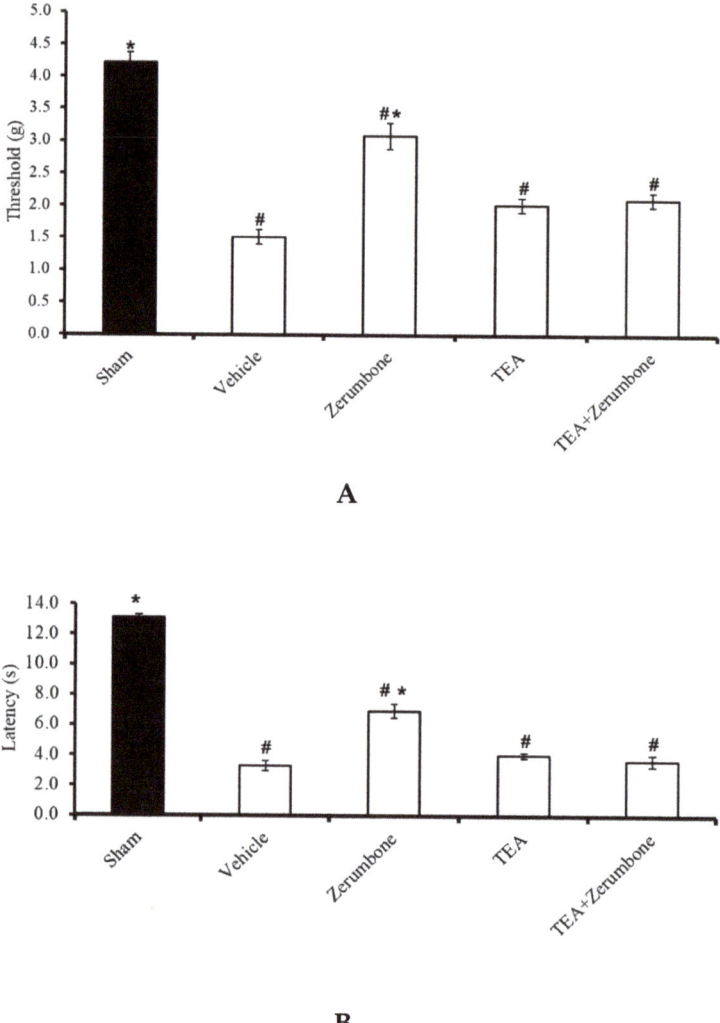

A

B

Figure 1. Effect of zerumbone (10 mg/kg; i.p.) and pre-treatment with a voltage-dependent K^+ channel blocker (tetraethylammonium, TEA; 4 mg/kg; i.p.) on the responses toward (**A**) mechanical allodynia and (**B**) thermal hyperalgesia on chronic constriction injury (CCI)-induced neuropathic pain in mice. Each column represents the mean ± SEM; n = 8 mice per group. Note: [#] significantly different ($p \leq 0.05$) than sham group; * significantly different ($p \leq 0.05$) than vehicle group (one-way ANOVA followed by Tukey's post hoc test).

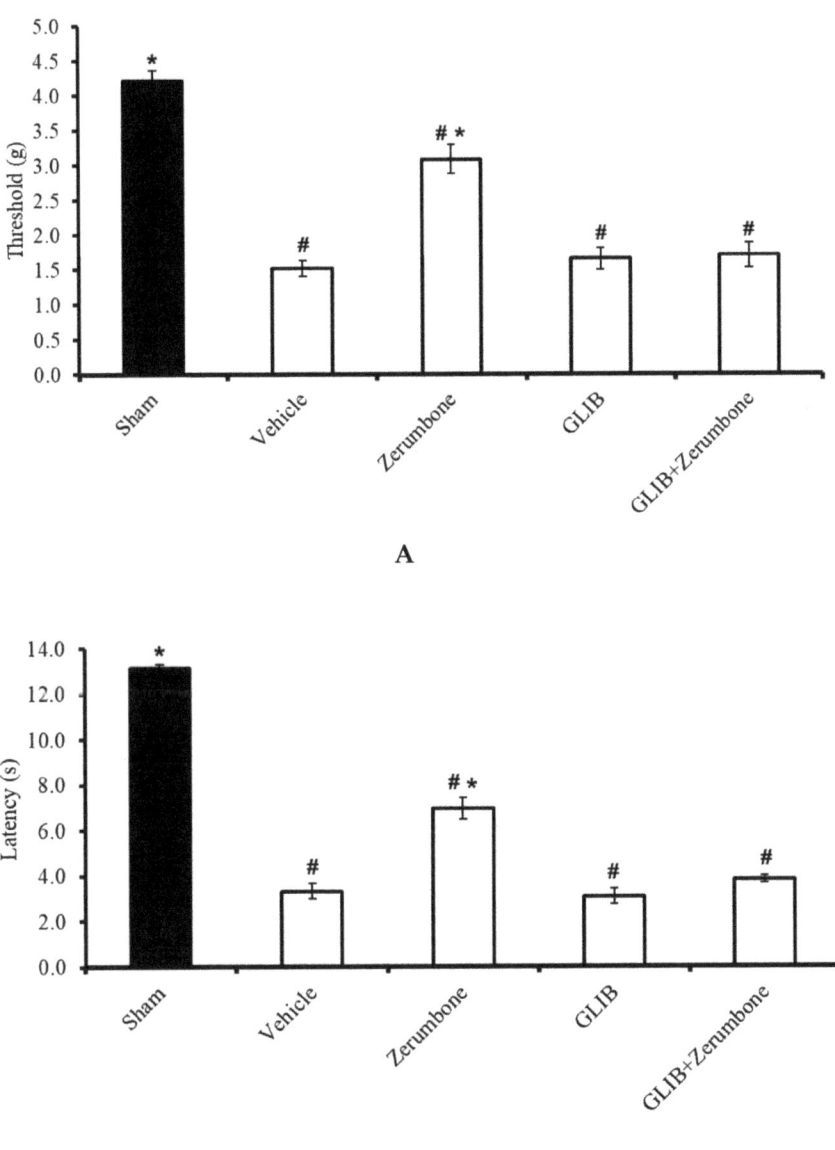

Figure 2. Effect of zerumbone (10 mg/kg; i.p.) and pre-treatment with an ATP-sensitive K$^+$ channel blocker (glibenclamide, GLIB; 10 mg/kg; i.p.) on the responses toward (**A**) mechanical allodynia and (**B**) thermal hyperalgesia on CCI-induced neuropathic pain in mice. Each column represents the mean ± SEM; n = 8 mice per group. Note: $^{\#}$ significantly different ($p \leq 0.05$) than sham group; * significantly different ($p \leq 0.05$) than vehicle group (one-way ANOVA followed by Tukey's post hoc test).

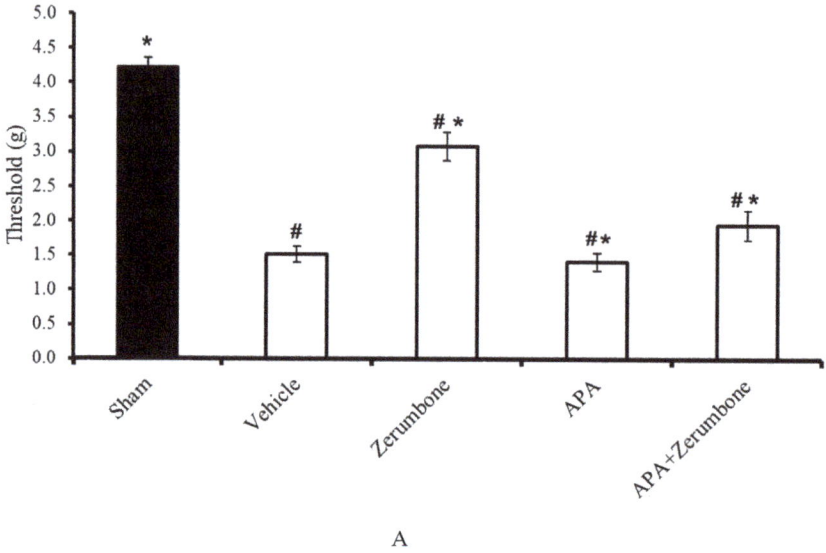

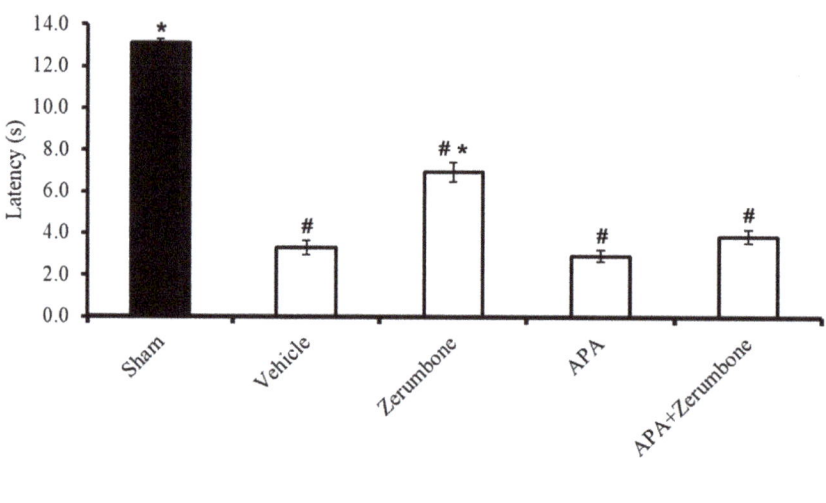

Figure 3. Effect of zerumbone (10 mg/kg; i.p.) and pre-treatment with a small-conductance Ca^{2+}-activated K^+ channel inhibitor (apamine, APA; 0.04 mg/kg; i.p.) on the responses toward (**A**) mechanical allodynia and (**B**) thermal hyperalgesia on CCI-induced neuropathic pain in mice. Each column represents the mean ± SEM; n = 8 mice per group. Note: # significantly different ($p \leq 0.05$) than sham group; * significantly different ($p \leq 0.05$) than vehicle group (one-way ANOVA followed by Tukey's post hoc test).

The large-conductance Ca^{2+}-activated K^+ channel inhibitor charybdotoxin (CHAR; 0.02 mg/kg; i.p.) was administered prior to zerumbone (10 mg/kg; i.p.) to investigate whether the action of zerumbone is carried out via large-conductance Ca^{2+}-activated K^+ channels. The results show significant ($p \leq 0.05$) reversal of the antiallodynic (n = 8) (Figure 4A) and antihyperalgesic (n = 8) (Figure 4B) effect elicited by zerumbone alone, demonstrating the role of large-conductance Ca^{2+}-activated K^+ channels in zerumbone's properties of attenuating neuropathic pain symptoms.

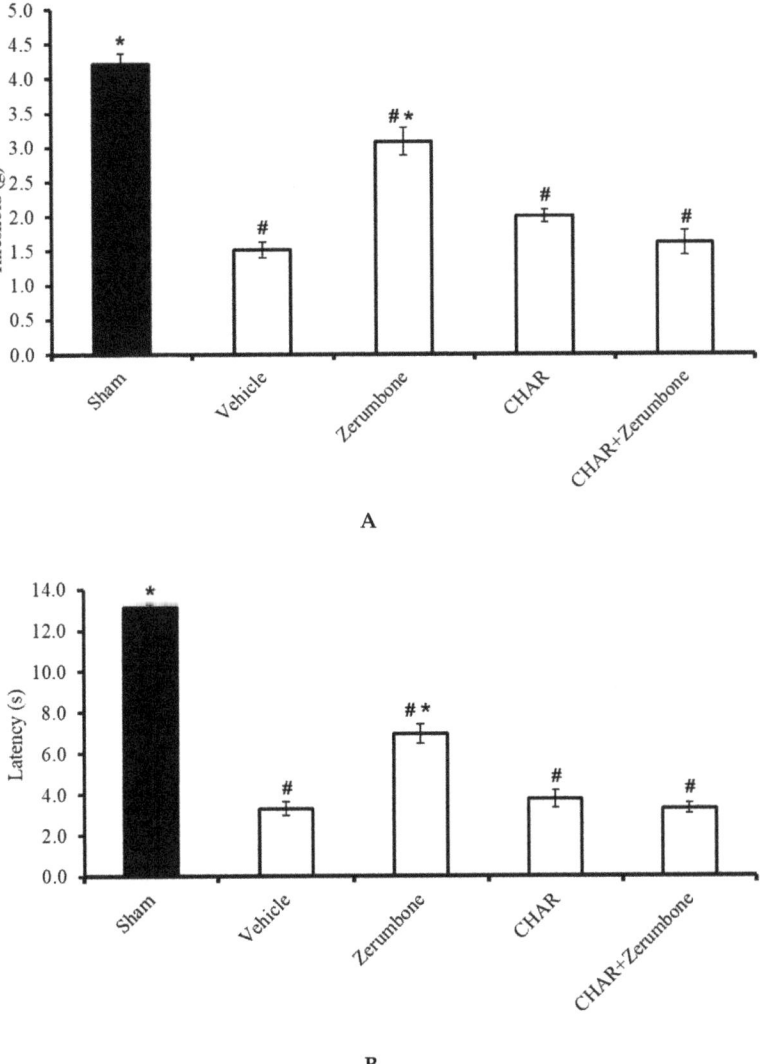

Figure 4. Effect of zerumbone (10 mg/kg; i.p.) and pre-treatment with a large-conductance Ca^{2+}-activated K^+ channel inhibitor (charybdotoxin, CHAR; 0.02 mg/kg; i.p.) on the responses toward (**A**) mechanical allodynia and (**B**) thermal hyperalgesia on CCI-induced neuropathic pain in mice. Each column represents the mean ± SEM; n = 8 mice per group. Note: # significantly different ($p \leq 0.05$) than sham group; * significantly different ($p \leq 0.05$) than vehicle group (one-way ANOVA followed by Tukey's post hoc test).

2.4. Involvement of Non-Selective Opioid Receptors

The antiallodynic effects observed in the zerumbone (10 mg/kg; i.p.)-treated group was absent when the animals were pre-treated with naloxone (NAL; 10 mg/kg; i.p.) before administering zerumbone (10 mg/kg; i.p.) ($p \leq 0.05$) (Figure 5A). Similarly, the outcome of the Hargreaves' test shows that the administration of NAL (10 mg/kg; i.p.) before zerumbone (10 mg/kg; i.p.) treatment caused a complete reversal ($p \leq 0.05$) of zerumbone's antihyperalgesic effect (Figure 5B). It is important to note that NAL (10 mg/kg; i.p.) alone does not exhibit any significant ($p > 0.05$) effect on CCI mice. In both tests, the antiallodynic and antihyperalgesic effects of morphine in CCI-induced mice were also reversed by pre-treatment of the non-selective opioid receptor blocker.

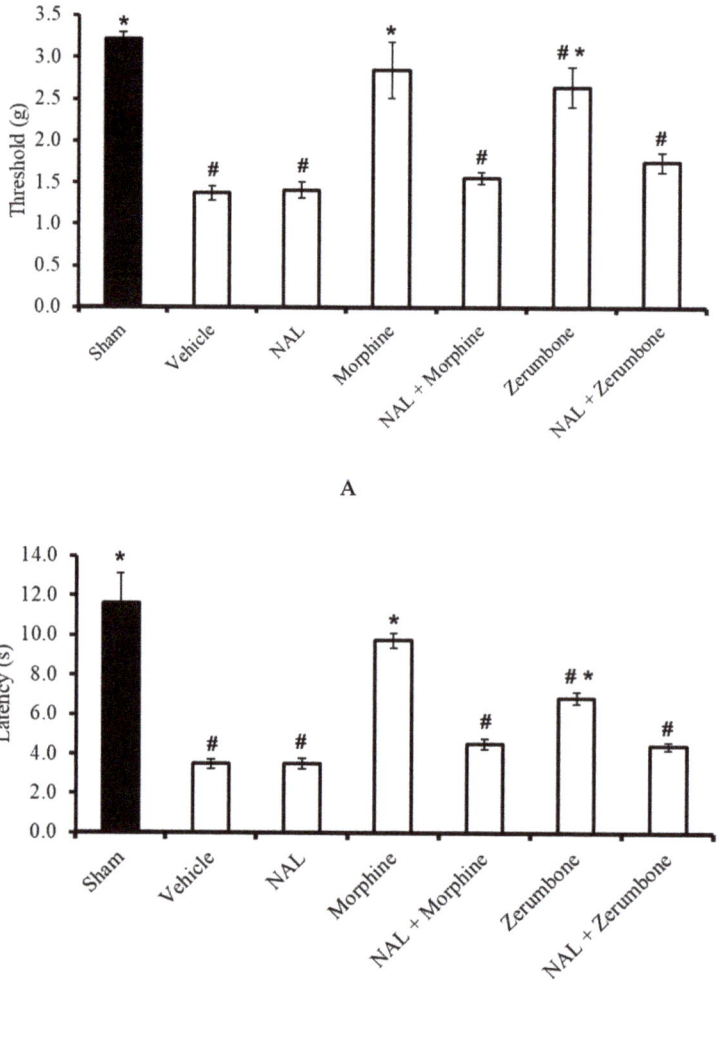

Figure 5. Effects of zerumbone (10 mg/kg; i.p.) and morphine (10 mg/kg; i.p.) and pre-treatment with a non-selective opioid receptor antagonist (naloxone, NAL; 10 mg/kg; i.p.) on the responses toward (**A**) mechanical allodynia and (**B**) thermal hyperalgesia on CCI-induced neuropathic pain in mice. Each column represents the mean ± SEM; n = 8 mice per group. Note: # significantly different ($p \leq 0.05$) than sham group; * significantly different ($p \leq 0.05$) than vehicle group (one-way ANOVA followed by Tukey's post hoc test).

2.5. Involvement of Selective μ-Opioid Receptors

The participation of μ-opioid receptor subtypes was investigated by blocking the receptors with a selective μ-opioid antagonist, β-funaltrexamine (β-FN). Pre-treatment with β-FN (40 mg/kg; subcutaneous, s.c.) prior to zerumbone significantly reversed the antiallodynic effect of zerumbone (10 mg/kg; i.p.) ($p \leq 0.05$) (Figure 6A). Similarly, pre-treatment with β-FN (40 mg/kg; s.c.) also reversed the antihyperalgesic effect of zerumbone (10 mg/kg; i.p.) ($p \leq 0.05$) (Figure 6B).

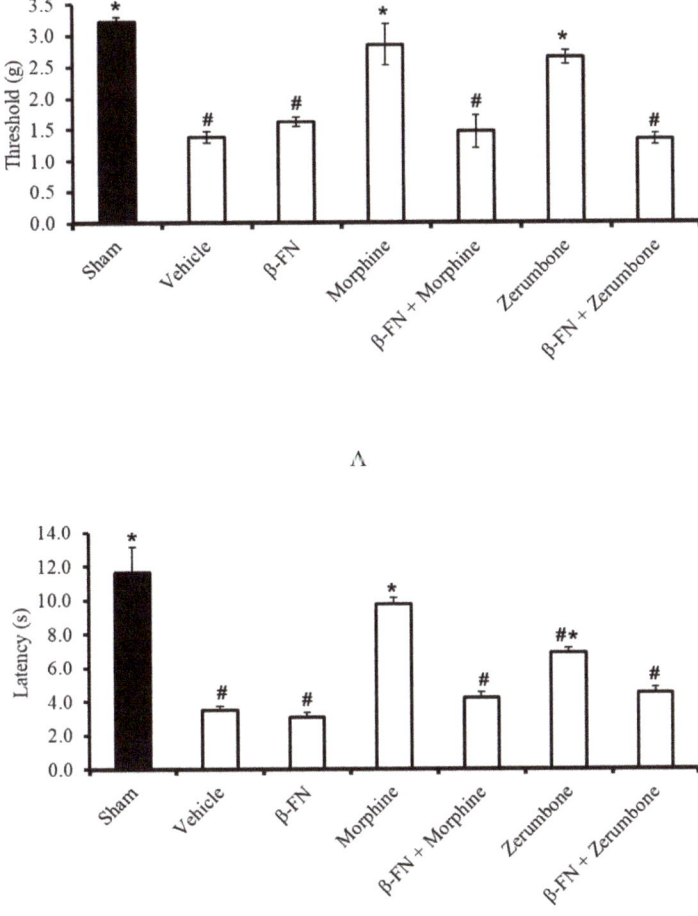

Figure 6. Effect of zerumbone (10 mg/kg; i.p.) and pre-treatment with a selective μ-opioid receptor antagonist (β-funaltrexamine, β-FN; 40 mg/kg; s.c.) on the responses toward (**A**) mechanical allodynia and (**B**) thermal hyperalgesia on CCI-induced neuropathic pain in mice. Each column represents the mean ± SEM; n = 8 mice per group. Note: # significantly different ($p \leq 0.05$) than sham group; * significantly different ($p \leq 0.05$) than vehicle group (one-way ANOVA followed by Tukey's post hoc test).

2.6. Involvement of Selective δ-Opioid Receptors

The involvement of δ-opioid receptors in the action of zerumbone was investigated by pre-treating the animals with a selective δ-opioid subtype antagonist, naltrindole (NTI). Pre-treatment with NTI (20 mg/kg; s.c.) prior to zerumbone significantly reversed the antiallodynic (Figure 7A) and antihyperalgesic (Figure 7B) effects of zerumbone (10 mg/kg; i.p.) ($p \leq 0.05$).

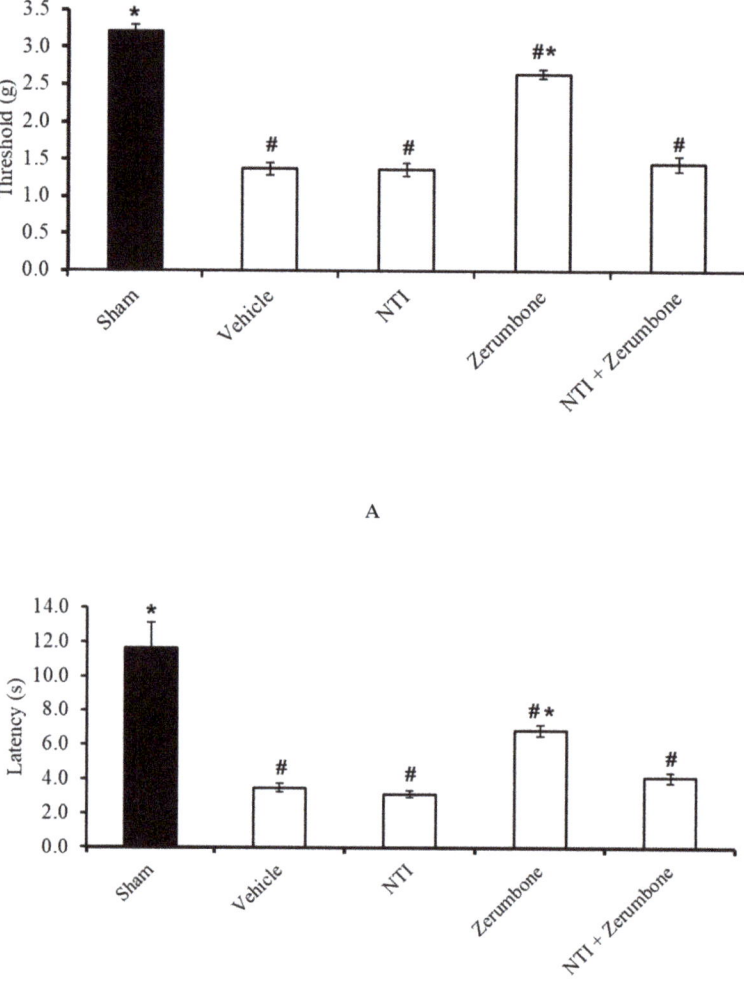

A

B

Figure 7. Effect of zerumbone (10 mg/kg; i.p.) and pre-treatment with a selective δ-opioid receptor antagonist (naltrindole, NTI; 20 mg/kg; s.c.) on the responses toward (**A**) mechanical allodynia and (**B**) thermal hyperalgesia on CCI-induced neuropathic pain in mice. Each column represents the mean ± SEM; n = 8 mice per group. Note: # significantly different ($p \leq 0.05$) than sham group; * significantly different ($p \leq 0.05$) than vehicle group (one-way ANOVA followed by Tukey's post hoc test).

2.7. Involvement of Selective κ-Opioid Receptors

The involvement of κ-opioid receptors in the antineuropathic properties of zerumbone were investigated using a selective κ-opioid subtype antagonist, nor-binaltorphimine (nor-BNI; 10 mg/kg; s.c.). The nor-BNI was administered prior to zerumbone treatment and the antiallodynic (Figure 8A) and antihyperalgesic (Figure 8B) effects of zerumbone (10 mg/kg; i.p.) ($p \leq 0.05$) were absent. Treatment with nor-BNI (10 mg/kg; s.c.) alone did not elicit any effect on the animal's behavioral responses.

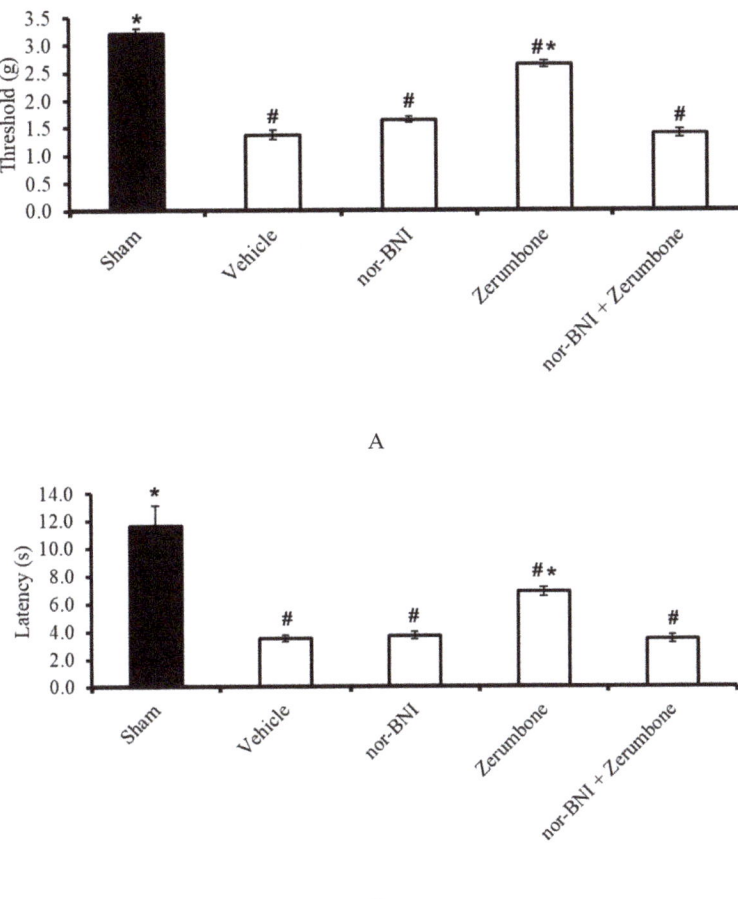

Figure 8. Effect of zerumbone (10 mg/kg; i.p.) and pre-treatment with a selective κ-opioid receptor antagonist (nor-binaltorphamine, nor-BNI; 10 mg/kg; s.c.) on the responses toward (**A**) mechanical allodynia and (**B**) thermal hyperalgesia on CCI-induced neuropathic pain in mice. Each column represents the mean ± SEM; n = 8 mice per group. Note: [#] significantly different ($p \leq 0.05$) than sham group; * significantly different ($p \leq 0.05$) than vehicle group (one-way ANOVA followed by Tukey's post hoc test).

2.8. Rota Rod Assay

All the mice in the sham, zerumbone (10 mg/kg; i.p.), TEA (4 mg/kg; i.p.), GLIB (10 mg/kg; i.p.), APA (0.04 mg/kg; i.p.), CHAR (0.02 mg/kg; i.p.), NAL (10 mg/kg; i.p.), β-FN (40 mg/kg; i.p.),

NAL (20 mg/kg; s.c.), nor-BNI (10 mg/kg; s.c.), and morphine (10 mg/kg; i.p.) groups were able to survive on the rota rods throughout the period of three minutes (n = 8) (Figure 9).

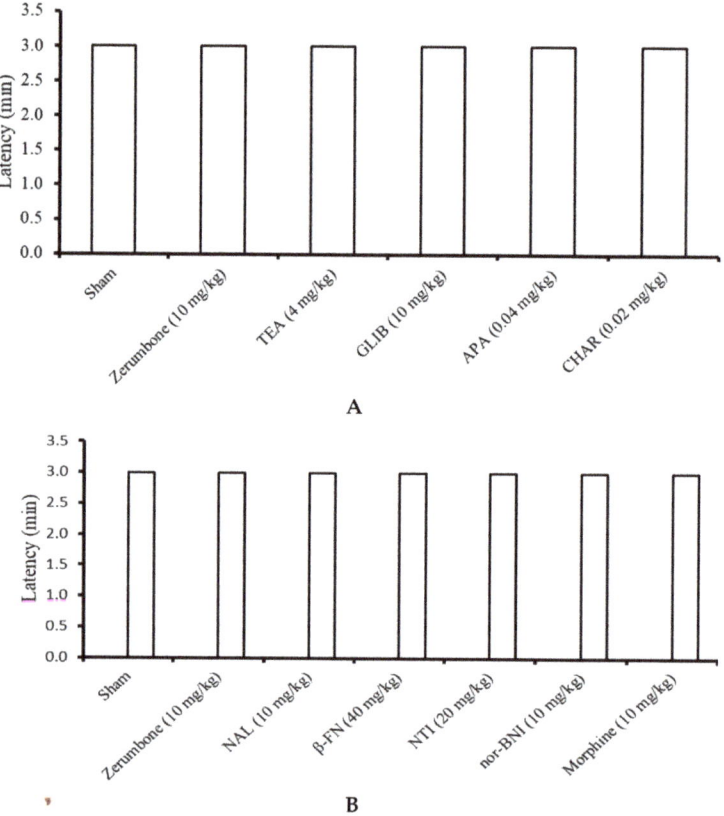

Figure 9. Effects of the treatments on the rota rod performance in mice following treatment with zerumbone, (**A**) potassium channel antagonists, and (**B**) opioid receptor antagonists. (TEA: Tetraethylammonium; GLIB: Glibeclamide; APA: Apamine; CHAR: Charybdotoxin; NAL: Naloxone; β-FNI: β-funaltrexamine; NTI: Naltrindole; nor-BNI: nor-binaltorphamine). Values represent the means ± SEM; n = 8 mice per group (one-way ANOVA followed by Tukey's post hoc test).

3. Discussion

The involvement of K^+ channels, specifically the K_V, K_{ATP}, SK_{Ca}, and BK_{Ca} channels, were demonstrated in zerumbone's action of inducing analgesia in the CCI model of neuropathic pain. This is due to the reversal of the antiallodynic and antihyperalgesic effects exhibited by zerumbone (10 mg/kg; i.p.) following pre-treatment with channel blockers or inhibitors. The respective inhibitors specifically deterred zerumbone's action on those channels, meaning zerumbone failed to lower the pain threshold or latency values. The rota rod assay ensured that the outcome was entirely a behavioral response and not a consequence of impaired motor function, a possible sedative effect of the treatments, or a suppression of general behavior [37,38], as all mice were able to survive on the rota rod for the entire three minutes without falling or rolling over.

Voltage-gated potassium channels (K_V) channels in myelinated axons are present in the paranodal, internodal, and even the juxtaparanodal regions. However, they are generally absent in the nodal regions in mammalian nerves [39]. K_V channels are also present in unmyelinated axons, as well as in distinct populations of dorsal root ganglion (DRG) neurons, which influence neuronal excitability following pharmacological blockade [40]. In the case of nerve injury, myelin sheaths will be disrupted or removed, leading to conduction blockage. The blockage is due to an increase in membrane capacitance and decline in membrane resistance. K$^+$ channels at juxtaparanodes are usually electrically isolated but are exposed or appear uncovered during demyelination, reducing neuronal excitability. Therefore, pharmacological compounds that block K$_V$ channels improve conduction in those demyelinated axons [39].

The opening of K$_V$ channels could be blocked by TEA, a small ion that binds to the inner and outer sites of the channels. Blockade at the internal mouth of the channel pores is voltage-dependent but blockade at the outer mouth is almost voltage independent [41]. In this study, intraperitoneal administration of TEA alone at 4 mg/kg had no effect on the behavioral response. However, zerumbone's antiallodynic and antihyperalgesic effects were absent following pre-treatment of TEA, clearly indicating the involvement of K$_V$ channels in zerumbone-induced analgesia.

There are various mechanisms for drugs to carry out their functions. Drug molecules can reside in the pockets in the inner mouth of channel pores, where typical blockers reside when they interact with other molecules. These drugs displace the blockers, preventing them from acting on the channels [42]. Another interesting mechanism is when drug molecules attach themselves to the "gating hinges", disrupting the normal function of the channel gates. Retigabine, a K$_V$7 activator, uses this mechanism in its action [43]. Furthermore, drugs can also act as disinactivators and interrupt the association between α- and β-subunits, thus altering the channel behavior [44].

Many drugs and analgesics share similar mechanisms by acting as K$_V$ channel openers or activators. Triaminopyridines such as flupiritne and retigabine are analgesics, which act by enhancing maximum steady-state K$^+$ conductance at saturating voltages. Thermal hyperalgesia in neuropathic rats was alleviated when flupitine was injected at neuroma sites [45]. Retigabine on the other hand reduces bradykinin-induced pain [46] and carrageenan-induced hyperalgesia [47]. Fampridine, a non-selective K$_V$ channel modulator, has already been established as being able to treat multiple sclerosis [48].

K$_{ATP}$ channels can be selectively blocked by glibenclamide [49]. In this study, the involvement of K$_{ATP}$ channels in zerumbone's antiallodynic and antihyperalgesic effects was clearly demonstrated. Likewise, Perimal et al. [23] reported that zerumbone exhibited marked inhibition of pain against chemical models of nociception in mice, with the possible opening of K$_{ATP}$ channels.

Clinically available drugs such as clonidine [50], 5-HT$_1$ agonists [51], and morphine [52] are analgesics that are specifically mediated by K$_{ATP}$ channels. Other blockers of potassium channels do not alter the analgesic effects of these drugs but are only reversed following pre-treatment with a selective K$_{ATP}$ antagonist. Other drugs such as cromakalim, pinacidil [53], minoxidil [54], and nicorandil [55] have also been reported to mediate their analgesic effects via K$_{ATP}$ channels.

A high expression of BK$_{Ca}$ channels in the trigeminal ganglion [56], superficial dorsal horn [57], and dorsal root ganglion, DRG [58] induces antihyperalgesic effects in neuropathic pain models. However, the expression of BK$_{Ca}$ channels was suppressed in DRG neurons following L4–L5 nerve ligation injury [58] and in the superficial dorsal horn in a partial sciatic nerve ligation model [57].

The involvement of BK$_{Ca}$ channels in the antiallodynic and antihyperalgesic effects of zerumbone was also observed in this study, as the effects were reversed when mice were pre-treated with CHAR (0.02 mg/kg; i.p.), a selective BK$_{Ca}$ channel inhibitor. The opening of BK$_{Ca}$ channels in DRG neurons reduces the depolarization-evoked firing of action potentials [59]. BK$_{Ca}$ channels are ideal cell excitability feedback regulators. This is due to BK$_{Ca}$ channels having high conductance, whereby the duration of action potentials is shortened by BK$_{Ca}$ channel activation. This consequently increases the rate of repolarization and reduces depolarization, leading to rapid post-polarization effects [59].

The stimulation of BK$_{Ca}$ is subject to dual control, where it is either activated by a rise in the cytosolic Ca^{2+} concentration or by membrane depolarization. The induction of BK$_{Ca}$ openings can be caused by intracellular free calcium alone while the domains of voltage sensors remain activated [60].

Furthermore, the induction of these channels can also be due to voltage alone, indicating that the dual control of these channels could function either synergistically or via independent mechanisms [61].

The large-conductance BK_{Ca} channels are rather weakly sensitive to voltage [62]. When cytoplasmic Ca^{2+} concentrations are at resting levels, the BK_{Ca} channels can only be opened by the presence of very positive voltages. However, the voltage-dependent activation takes a leftward shift along the voltage axis towards a more negative membrane potential. An increase in the free Ca^{2+} concentration shifts the activity of these channels in the physiologic membrane potential range [61]. Membranes remain hyperpolarized when BK_{Ca} channels are in an open state during neuronal firing. This further causes an inhibitory feedback, limiting the influx of Ca^{2+} and excitability. Therefore, these channels are powerful regulators of synaptic transmission at nerve terminals [63]. Due to maladaptive pain signaling and abnormal excitability of the somatosensory system in chronic pain conditions, the role of these channels is vital, and drug targeting of these channels and their actions might be more effective.

Small-conductance SK_{Ca} channels were also involved in the antiallodynic and antihyperalgesic effects of zerumbone in this study, as the compound's effects were reversed when mice were pre-treated with apamin (APA; 0.04 mg/kg; i.p.), a selective SK_{Ca} channel inhibitor. This outcome suggests that zerumbone enhances SK_{Ca} channel activity, leading to a substantial reduction in the sensory input. Compound (E)-2-(4,6-difluoro-1-indanylidene) acetamide and drugs such as chloroxazone [64] and riluzole [65] are enhancers of SK_{Ca} channel activity and are potent analgesics. The effects of resveratrol, a drug that exhibits peripheral antinociceptive activity, were reversed in the presence of APA [66].

Zerumbone also used the opioidergic pathway to elicit its analgesic effects on the neuropathic pain models. This is because the antiallodynic and antihyperalgesic effects exerted by zerumbone (10 mg/kg; i.p.) were reversed when mice were pre-treated with a non-selective opioid receptor antagonist, NAL. NAL showed no effect when administered alone. Similarly, morphine (positive control), an opiate known for its analgesic action, specifically via the μ-opioid receptor, also showed a complete reversal of its action when treated with NAL.

The opioidergic pathway plays a role in pain modulation, whereby activation of opioid receptors is implicated with pain regulation, neuroendocrine modulation, reinforcement and reward behavior, and changes in neurotransmitter release. Numerous endogenous opioid peptides such as dynorphin-A, met-enkeplin, and β-endorphin are produced by the body's innate response to pain [67]. Opioid-mediated analgesia includes both the ascending and descending pain pathways and exerts both centrally and peripherally mediated effects [67]. Opioids act as agonists of either one or more of the three classic opioid receptors subtypes (μ, κ, and δ) to activate the pathway [68].

Activation of opioid receptors induces the pain inhibitory modulation via three main events, which are activation of the inwardly rectifying K^+ channels, inhibition of the voltage sensitive Ca^{2+} channels, and reduction of the cyclic adenosine monophosphate (cAMP) production following the inhibition of adenylyl cyclase [69]. Conversely, opioid receptors utilize other intermediate messenger systems to activate the cascade of mitogen-activated protein kinase, phospholipase C, and large-conductance Ca^{2+}-activated K^+ channels [70]. This series of events, especially the modulation of K^+ and Ca^{2+} channels, lowers neuronal excitability, decreases the rate of neuronal firing, and inhibits neurotransmitter release [67,71].

Opioid receptors are widely distributed in the brain [72–74]. Two important brain centers involved in opioid-produced antinociception are the rostral ventromedial medulla (RVM) and periaqueductal gray (PAG) of the midbrain. These centers are critical targets for both endogenous opioids and opioid pharmaceuticals. Spinally projecting neurons in the RVM are activated by cells in the PAG, which then inhibit nociceptive cells in the spinal cord [75,76]. Furthermore, high densities of opioid receptors can also be found in the hypothalamus, hippocampus [77], habenula, nucleus raphe magnus, caudate nucleus, and the spinal cord [74]. It is important to note that opioid receptors are also found in peripheral neurons, which also play a role in antinociception [67]. However, from this experimental design we could not speculate on the exact site of zerumbone's action, as the compound was employed via the intraperitoneal route and was present systemically.

Zerumbone's ability to attenuate thermal hyperalgesia was reversed when the mice were pre-treated with β-FN, the μ-opioid receptor antagonist. This indicates that zerumbone possibly acts as the μ-opioid receptors' agonist and modulates pain by activating these receptors. It was reported earlier that the functional involvement of different opioid receptor subtypes and neuronal pathways differentially is influenced by the modalities of the noxious stimuli [78]. A thermal noxious stimulus responds more effectively to μ-type agonists [79], further supporting the effectiveness of zerumbone in attenuating thermal hyperalgesia. Morphine, whose analgesic effect is modulated by μ-opioid receptors, is a drug that is prescribed for the management of moderate to severe pain [80]. The clear benefits of μ-agonists in pain treatments have been reported for over 1000 years [80].

The antiallodynic and antihyperalgesic effects of zerumbone were reversed when δ-opioid receptors were blocked with a specific δ-opioid receptor antagonist, naltrindole. This clearly indicates the involvement of these receptors in zerumbone-induced analgesia. The function of δ-opioid receptors in the pain pathway was evident when δ-receptor knockout mice amplified inflammatory [81] and neuropathic [82] pain conditions. This demonstrates the presence of endogenous δ-opioid receptors' activity in effectively reducing chronic and persistent pain. Therefore, systemically active δ-opioid receptor agonists are useful targets for chronic pain [83]. Various novel δ-agonists have been developed as preclinical model analgesics. They include NIH 11,082 [84], DL5859 [85], KNT-127 [86], and compound 8e [87].

Zerumbone when administered alone reduced the pain response towards mechanical allodynia and thermal hyperalgesia. However, when mice were pre-treated with nor-binaltorphamine, a κ-opioid receptor antagonist, the effects of zerumbone were reversed. This indicates that zerumbone also acts as a κ-opioid receptor agonist to carry out pain modulation. Nociception caused by pressure has also been reported to preferentially respond to κ-opioid receptor agonists [79], providing evidence of the properties of zerumbone, which shows a lowered response towards mechanical hyperalgesia.

Although κ-opioid agonists' maximum effect has been reported to be weaker than μ-opioids such as morphine, researchers were still very interested in developing κ-opioid agonists. This is because κ-opioid agonists can be used for pain-relief without activating the reward pathways, which are stimulated by μ-opioids. However, κ-opioid agonists can cause problems, such as constipation, dysphoria, and diuresis [88]. Therefore, if zerumbone was able to act in the same way as κ-opioid agonists in providing analgesia without the presence of adverse effects, perhaps it would be a better option to be considered as a treatment for pain relief.

Furthermore, the activation of κ-opioid receptors directly closes Na^+ channels [89]. This is an important feature of any drug for the treatment of neuropathic pain, as the pathophysiology of neuropathic pain shows the increased density and expression of abnormal of Na^+ channels along the primary afferent neurons. The increased spontaneous membrane potential oscillation and alterations to the conductance of those channels reduce the firing threshold, resulting in the spontaneous activity of sensory neurons [90]. Drugs such as lidocaine, which act as sodium channel blockers, are currently used as treatments for neuropathic pain [90].

Overall, we found that zerumbone utilizes the opioidergic pathway. Natural products are known to utilize multiple receptors of varying mechanisms to exhibit their actions. Similarly, we hypothesize that zerumbone acts through multiple receptors to attenuate allodynia and hyperalgesia in neuropathic pain models. Previously, zerumbone was shown to utilize the serotonergic pathway in CCI-induced allodynia and hyperalgesia [27]. Activation of serotonergic receptors stimulates the release of opioids and gamma-aminobutyric acid, GABA, thus inhibiting transmission of nociceptive signals [91]. Therefore, we postulate that serotonin and its receptors may correlate with the opioidergic pathway for zerumbone to exhibit its antineuropathic effects.

In the study by Zulazmi et al. [26], the antiallodynic and antihyperalgesic effects of zerumbone in a neuropathic pain mouse model was postulated to act through L-arginine-nitric oxide-cGMP-K^+ ATP channels. The NO-cGMP pathway activation and K$^+$ channels have been shown to correlate [92,93]. In a recent report by the research team, the antiallodynic and antihyperalgesic effects of zerumbone were shown to interact with the noradrenergic system, TRPV1, and NMDA receptors [94]. The noradrenergic system has been shown to act synergistically with the opioidergic pathway at both spinal and supraspinal sites [95–97]. TRPV and NMDA receptors are primarily involved in excitatory nociceptive processing. The nociceptive action of these receptors is modulated by calcium ions [98,99]. As mentioned earlier, the opioidergic pathway reduces neuronal activity by modulating calcium and potassium channels. Therefore, current literature on the mechanisms of action of zerumbone support our current observations regarding opioid receptors.

The antagonists of potassium channels TEA, GLIB, APA, and CHAR; and opioid receptors NAL and NTI were administered 15 min prior to zerumbone treatment, but β-FN and nor-BNI were administered 24 h prior to zerumbone treatment. This is because different drugs and blockers have different targets, binding affinities, and efficacies, which take different durations to exhibit their effects [100]. The mode of drug administration also differs between groups. Drug administration via the intraperitoneal mode causes faster absorption into the blood stream compared to subcutaneous administration. Drugs are administered subcutaneously if a slower release of the drug into the vasculature is required, whereby fast administration might produce adverse effect such as respiratory depression [100]. The antagonist's modes of administration, dose, and duration of effect were pre-tested to ensure they did not increase pain or sensitivity in the animals prior to testing on the actual experimental animals. This protocol was reported by Ming-Tatt et al. [92] and Zakaria et al. [101].

The pathophysiological changes that occur after nerve injury include altered expression and efficacy of potassium channels and opioid receptors at various sites of the pain pathway. The changes can occur in the peripheral nerves, dorsal root ganglion, spinal cord, along the ascending and descending pathways, as well as in the brain [9,102,103]. In this study, we administered zerumbone systemically to test the involvement of potassium channels and opioid receptors. However, the exact target site of zerumbone could not be determined in this study design, which is a limitation of this study. In this study, evidence was provided of the involvement of potassium and opioid receptors in zerumbone's action solely on the behavioral outcome. However, we did not screen for the effect of zerumbone on the receptor and receptor subtype's molecular expression along the pain pathway, which is another limitation of this study. Therefore, future studies should evaluate the underlying molecular mechanisms and narrow down the specific sites of zerumbone's action to allow translational research into targeted forms of therapy.

The expression of opioid receptors and potassium channels was altered in CCI animals. The effects of each antagonist were confirmed by having groups treated by zerumbone alone and antagonists alone to confirm the partial contribution of each as a standard protocol for these experiments. A study by Le Guen et al. [104] reported that when opioid receptor antagonists were administered into naïve rats, behavioral changes occurred, indicating tonic activity in the endogenous opioid peptides acting on mu opioid receptors. NAL or β-FN triggered Fos-like immunoreactivity in the nucleus of the solitary tract, area postrema, rostral ventrolateral medulla, supramammillary nucleus, central nucleus of the amygdala, and the Kölliker–Fuse nucleus of the central nervous system [104,105]. NTI and nor-BNI showed no effect on naïve rats [104].

On the other hand, potassium channel blockers (TEA, APA, CHAR) reduce the mouse immobility time of intensity in forced swimming tests, an animal model for depression. These blockers produce an antidepressant-like effect by preventing hyperpolarization, leading to a higher excitatory response [106]. Hyperalgesia and antinociception also do not occur in mice when GLIB is administered alone [106,107].

When a particular drug that uses a single receptor or channel type provides a good level of analgesia, it is presumed that the summation effect of zerumbone (i.e., using all μ-, κ-, and δ-opioid receptors, as well as K_V, KATP, BKCa, and SKCa channels) should provide better pain relief. However, this was not reflected in our outcome, as the pain threshold and latency were lower than the levels in the sham control group and in the animals that received morphine. Achieving 100% analgesia is almost unachievable, unless it is accompanied by severe sedative and nervous suppression. The pharmacodynamics of zerumbone is not fully understood, but it is known to interact with multiple pathways without causing any adverse effects. We are unable to provide a summation analysis of the individual effects of zerumbone through these experiments, as the antagonists were administered on different groups of animals. Therefore, we suggest that future studies could aim to characterize the binding properties of zerumbone in opioid receptors and potassium channels.

4. Materials and Methods

4.1. Preparation of Zerumbone

Zerumbone was extracted from the rhizomes of *Zingiber zerumbet* as outlined by Perimal et al. [23]. Rhizomes of *Z. zerumbet* were obtained from the Chow Kit wet market in Kuala Lumpur. Mr. Shamsul Khamis, a resident botanist at Institute of Bioscience, Universiti Putra Malaysia, identified and confirmed the plant species, then a sample specimen was inserted at the herbarium of the Laboratory of Natural Products, Institute of Bioscience, Universiti Putra Malaysia, with the voucher number of SK622/07.

Freshly purchased rhizomes were washed, sliced into small pieces, and allowed to air-dry overnight. The rhizome pieces were then ground in a commercial food processor (Cgoldenwall, Hangzou, China) into powder. Then, the powder was dissolved with hexane and water before the solution was repetitively subjected to hydrodistillation. Soluble oil was collected and water was removed. Crude essential oil was collected after the solvent had evaporated by using a rotary evaporator (Heidolph, Schwabach, Germany).

The crude essential oil was refrigerated at 4 °C for 48 h. Pure crystals that were formed were subjected to column chromatography (LiChro CART, Darmstadt, Germany). The purity of the eluate was determined by thin-layer chromatography (Merck, New York, NY, USA). Following repetitive recrystallization, zerumbone was stored at −80 °C until further use. High-performance liquid chromatography (HPLC) (Waters 2695, Pliening, Germany) analysis carried out on a sample of this batch of zerumbone showed 96.2% purity. Dimethyl sulfoxide (DMSO), Tween 20, and 0.9% NaCl at a ratio of 5:5:90 were used to dissolve zerumbone prior to treatment administration.

4.2. Drugs and Chemicals

Tetraethylammonium, glibenclamide, apamin, and charybdotoxin were purchased from Tocris (Bristol, UK). DMSO and Tween 20 were purchased from Sigma-Aldrich (St. Louis, MO, USA). Naloxone hydrochloride, β-funaltrexamine, naltrindole, nor-binaltorphimine, DMSO, and Tween 20 were bought from Sigma-Aldrich (St. Louis, MO, USA). Morphine sulphate was purchased from Lipomed (Cambridge, MA, USA). All drugs were dissolved in 0.9% NaCl. The vehicle consisted of DMSO, Tween 20, and 0.9% NaCl at a ratio of 5:5:90. All treatments were administered either intraperitoneally or subcutaneously at a volume of 10 mL/kg of body weight. Intraperitoneal injection was administered in the intraperitoneal cavity and subcutaneous administrations were made into the loose skin over the interscapular area.

4.3. Animals

Male ICR mice aged seven to eight weeks old (>25 g) were used in this study. Animals were randomly housed eight mice (n = 8) per cage for each treatment group at room temperature (24 ± 2 °C) and under standard environmental conditions of 12 h light and 12 h dark cycles. An acclimatization period of one week was allowed before the animals were subjected to tests. Standard laboratory feed and tap water was available ad libitum. All experimental procedures were evaluated and approved by the Institutional Animal Care and Use Committee (IACUC) of Universiti Putra Malaysia (reference number UPM/IACUC/AUP-R060/2013). All efforts to minimize the use of animals and pain caused to the animals were taken.

4.4. Induction of Neuropathic Pain

Neuropathic pain was induced by making constrictions to the sciatic nerve as previously described by Bennett and Xie [108], with slight modifications [109]. The entire surgical procedure was carried out under sterile conditions. First, the mice were anaesthetized with an intraperitoneal (i.p.) injection of tribromoethanol (250 mg/kg). The mid-thigh region of the hind limb was shaved before a small incision of approximately 5 mm was made to the skin. The biceps femoris muscle was separated by blunt dissection to expose the sciatic nerve. Three loose ligatures spaced 1 mm apart were made around the nerve proximal to the trifurcation using 4/0 silk sutures. Then, the incision to the skin was closed using a non-absorbable suture. Animals allocated in the sham group underwent the entire surgical procedure, however the sciatic nerves were not ligated. Povidone iodine was applied to the wound and animals were allowed to recover on flat paper bedding before they were returned to their home cages.

4.5. Experimental Design

On day 14 post-surgery, CCI-induced mice were pre-administered with either tetraethylammonium (a voltage-dependent K^+ channel blocker, 4 mg/kg; i.p.), glibenclamide (an ATP-sensitive K^+ channel blocker, 10 mg/kg; i.p.), apamin (a small-conductance Ca^{2+}-activated K^+ channel inhibitor, 0.04 mg/kg; i.p.), or charybdotoxin (a large-conductance Ca^{2+}-activated K^+ channel inhibitor 0.02 mg/kg; i.p.) 15 min prior to zerumbone (10 mg/kg; i.p.) treatment to determine the involvement of potassium channels in zerumbone-induced analgesia.

To determine the involvement of opioid receptors in zerumbone's action, CCI-induced mice were pre-treated with NAL (a non-specific opioid receptor antagonist 10 mg/kg; i.p.) or NTI (a selective δ-opioid receptor antagonist, 20 mg/kg; s.c.), then 15 min before zerumbone (10 mg/kg; i.p.) treatment β-FN (a selective μ-opioid receptor antagonist; 40 mg/kg; s.c.) or nor-BNI (a selective κ-opioid receptor antagonist; 10 mg/kg; s.c.), was administered 24 h prior to zerumbone (10 mg/kg; i.p.) treatment. Morphine (10 mg/kg; i.p.) was used as the positive control in the NAL and β-FN groups [92].

Sham, vehicle, and zerumbone-only groups were administered treatments accordingly. The mice were subjected to nociceptive assays 30 min later.

4.6. Nociceptive Assays

Nociceptive assays were carried out via von Frey's filament test followed by the Hargreaves test to evaluate the responses towards mechanical allodynia and thermal hyperalgesia. An interval of 5 min was allowed between assays

4.6.1. VON Frey's Filament Test

The treatment effects on the response towards mechanical allodynia were evaluated by von Frey's filament test as described by Martinov et al. [110]. Briefly, the mice were allowed to acclimatize after they were placed in a Plexiglass chamber on an elevated wire mesh grid. Electronic von Frey's anesthesiometer filaments (IITC Life Science Inc., Los Angeles, CA, USA) were applied to the middle dorsum of the ipsilateral paw of the mice when the animals were on all four limbs. The pressure at which the animals withdrew their paws from the filament was read from the automated reader. The mean of three readings was recorded as the withdrawal threshold. The cut-off point was set at 5 g within 20 s.

4.6.2. Hargreaves Test

The treatment effects on the response towards thermal hyperalgesia were evaluated by the Hargreaves test as described by Hargreaves et al. [111]. Mice were allowed to acclimatize in a Plexiglass chamber placed on top of an elevated clear platform. Then, a radiant heat source from a Hargreaves apparatus (37370, UgoBasile, CA, USA) was directed to the mid-plantar surface of the ipsilateral paw when the animals were on all four limbs. The time taken for the mice to remove its paw from the heat source was recorded as the withdrawal latency. A cut off latency was set at 20 s, after which the heat was removed to prevent injury to the paws.

4.7. Rota Rod Test

In order to ensure that the behavioral responses exhibited by the animals were not due to the possible sedative effects of the treatments, the rota rod test was carried out. On day 14 post-CCI, the rota rod test was performed after 30 min in the zerumbone group and at the respective time points where nociceptive assays were carried out in the other groups. Each mouse was placed on a rota rod bar (UgoBasile, Gemonio, Italy) rotating at 20 rpm. The time each mouse spent on the rotating bar throughout a period of 3 min was recorded [26,28].

4.8. Statistical Analysis

Data are expressed as mean ± SEM. Statistical analysis was carried out using Statistical Analysis for Social Science (SPSS) version 16.0. Comparisons between groups were made with one-way ANOVA followed by Tukey's post hoc test, where *p*-values of less than 0.05 were considered as significant.

5. Conclusions

We conclude that zerumbone's antiallodynic and antihyperalgesic effects exhibited in the CCI-induced mice model of neuropathic pain involve K^+ channels, specifically the K_V, K_{ATP}, BK_{Ca}, and SK_{Ca} channels. Furthermore, zerumbone also involves the μ-, δ-, and κ-opioid receptor subtypes in its neuropathic pain modulation. Future research studies aiming to further investigate the other possible mechanisms of action are warranted in order to fully characterize the antineuropathic properties of zerumbone.

Author Contributions: Conceptualization, B.G. and E.K.P.; methodology, B.G.; software, B.G.; validation, B.G., J.S.M.C., and E.K.P.; formal analysis, B.G.; investigation, B.G.; resources, E.K.P.; data curation, B.G.; writing—original draft preparation, B.G.; writing—review and editing, J.S.M.C., E.K.P., A.A.O.F., and M.R.S.; visualization, B.G., J.S.M.C., A.A.O.F., M.R.S., and E.K.P.; supervision, E.K.P.; project administration, E.K.P.; funding acquisition, E.K.P. All authors have read and agreed to the published version of the manuscript.

Funding: This research was supported by Universiti Putra Malaysia under the Ministry of Science, Technology, and Innovation, Science Fund Scheme (grant 5450778).

Acknowledgments: The authors thank the Faculty of Medicine and Health Sciences, Universiti Putra Malaysia, and the Physiology Laboratory for providing the necessary support for the study.

Conflicts of Interest: The authors declare no conflict of interest.

References

1. Chung, K.; Lee, B.H.; Yoon, Y.W.; Chung, J.M. Sympathetic sprouting in the dorsal root ganglia of the injured peripheral nerve in a rat neuropathic pain model. *J. Comp. Neurol.* **1996**, *376*, 241–252. [CrossRef]
2. Ren, K.; Dubner, R. Inflammatory Models of Pain and Hyperalgesia. *ILAR J.* **1999**, *40*, 111–118. [CrossRef] [PubMed]
3. Campbell, J.N.; Meyer, R.A. Mechanisms of neuropathic pain. *Neuron* **2006**, *52*, 77–92. [CrossRef] [PubMed]
4. Zheng, Q.; Fang, N.; Liu, M.; Cai, J.; Wan, Y.; Han, J.-S.; Xing, G.-G. Suppression of KCNQ/M (Kv7) potassium channels in dorsal root ganglion neurons contributes to the development of bone cancer pain in a rat model. *Pain* **2013**, *154*, 434–448. [CrossRef] [PubMed]
5. Mi, H.; Deerinck, T.; Ellisman, M.; Schwarz, T. Differential distribution of closely related potassium channels in rat Schwann cells. *J. Neurosci.* **1995**, *15*, 3761–3774. [CrossRef]
6. Arroyo, E.J.; Scherer, S.S. On the molecular architecture of myelinated fibers. *Histochem. Cell Boil.* **2000**, *113*, 1–18. [CrossRef]

7. Kim, D.S.; Choi, J.O.; Rim, H.D.; Cho, H.J. Downregulation of voltage-gated potassium channel α gene expression in dorsal root ganglia following chronic constriction injury of the rat sciatic nerve. *Mol. Brain Res.* **2002**, *105*, 146–152. [CrossRef]
8. Sarantopoulos, C.; McCallum, J.B.; Rigaud, M.; Fuchs, A.; Kwok, W.-M.; Hogan, Q.H. Opposing effects of spinal nerve ligation on calcium-activated potassium currents in axotomized and adjacent mammalian primary afferent neurons. *Brain Res.* **2007**, *1132*, 84–99. [CrossRef]
9. Busserolles, J.; Tsantoulas, C.; Eschalier, A.; García, J.A.L. Potassium channels in neuropathic pain. *Pain* **2016**, *157*, S7–S14. [CrossRef]
10. Moulin, D.E.; Clark, A.J.; Gilron, I.; A Ware, M.; Watson, C.P.N.; Sessle, B.J.; Coderre, T.; Morley-Forster, P.K.; Stinson, J.; Boulanger, A.; et al. Pharmacological management of chronic neuropathic pain—Consensus statement and guidelines from the Canadian Pain Society. *Pain Res. Manag.* **2007**, *12*, 13–21. [CrossRef]
11. Dworkin, R.H.; O'Connor, A.B.; Audette, J.; Baron, R.; Gourlay, G.K.; Haanpää, M.L.; Kent, J.L.; Krane, E.J.; Lebel, A.A.; Levy, R.M.; et al. Recommendations for the Pharmacological Management of Neuropathic Pain: An Overview and Literature Update. *Mayo Clin. Proc.* **2010**, *85*, S3–S14. [CrossRef] [PubMed]
12. Raja, S.N.; Haythornthwaite, J.A.; Pappagallo, M.; Clark, M.R.; Travison, T.G.; Sabeen, S.; Royall, R.M.; Max, M.B. Opioids versus antidepressants in postherpetic neuralgia: A randomized, placebo-controlled trial. *Neurology* **2002**, *59*, 1015–1021. [CrossRef] [PubMed]
13. Moulin, D.E.; Palma, D.; Watling, C.; Schulz, V. Methadone in the Management of Intractable Neuropathic Noncancer Pain. *Can. J. Neurol. Sci.* **2005**, *32*, 340–343. [CrossRef] [PubMed]
14. Benyamin, R.; Trescot, A.M.; Datta, S.; Buenaventura, R.; Adlaka, R.; Sehgal, N.; E Glaser, S.; Vallejo, R. Opioid complications and side effects. *Pain Phys.* **2008**, *11*, 105–120.
15. Dumas, E.O.; Pollack, G.M. Opioid Tolerance Development: A Pharmacokinetic/Pharmacodynamic Perspective. *AAPS J.* **2008**, *10*, 537–551. [CrossRef]
16. Kosten, T.R.; George, T.P. The Neurobiology of Opioid Dependence: Implications for Treatment. *Sci. Pr. Perspect.* **2002**, *1*, 13–20. [CrossRef]
17. Baby, S.; Dan, M.; Thaha, A.R.M.; Johnson, A.J.; Kurup, R.; Balakrishnapillai, P.; Lim, C.K. High content of zerumbone in volatile oils of Zingiber zerumbet from southern India and Malaysia. *Flavour Fragr. J.* **2009**, *24*, 301–308. [CrossRef]
18. Koga, A.Y.; Beltrame, F.L.; Pereira, A.V. Several aspects of Zingiber zerumbet: A review. *Rev. Bras. de Farm.* **2016**, *26*, 385–391. [CrossRef]
19. Butt, M.S.; Sultan, M.T. Ginger and its Health Claims: Molecular Aspects. *Crit. Rev. Food Sci. Nutr.* **2011**, *51*, 383–393. [CrossRef]
20. Sahebkar, A. Potential efficacy of ginger as a natural supplement for nonalcoholic fatty liver disease. *World J. Gastroenterol.* **2011**, *17*, 271–272. [CrossRef]
21. Sultana, S.; Ripa, F.; Hamid, K. Comparative antioxidant activity study of some commonly used spices in Bangladesh. *Pak. J. Boil. Sci.* **2010**, *13*, 340–343. [CrossRef] [PubMed]
22. Sulaiman, M.; Perimal, E.; Zakaria, Z.; Mokhtar, F.; Akhtar, M.; Lajis, N.; Israf, D. Preliminary analysis of the antinociceptive activity of zerumbone. *Fitoterapia* **2009**, *80*, 230–232. [CrossRef] [PubMed]
23. Perimal, E.K.; Akhtar, M.N.; Mohamad, A.S.; Khalid, M.H.; Ming, O.H.; Khalid, S.; Tatt, L.M.; Kamaldin, M.N.; Zakaria, Z.A.; Israf, D.A.; et al. Zerumbone-Induced Antinociception: Involvement of the l-Arginine-Nitric Oxide-cGMP -PKC-K+ATP Channel Pathways. *Basic Clin. Pharmacol. Toxicol.* **2010**, *108*, 155–162. [CrossRef] [PubMed]
24. Sulaiman, M.R.; Perimal, E.; Akhtar, M.; Mohamad, A.; Khalid, M.; Tasrip, N.; Mokhtar, F.; Zakaria, Z.; Lajis, N.; Israf, D. Anti-inflammatory effect of zerumbone on acute and chronic inflammation models in mice. *Fitoterapia* **2010**, *81*, 855–858. [CrossRef]
25. Zulazmi, N.A.; Gopalsamy, B.; Farouk, A.A.O.; Sulaiman, M.R.; Bharatham, B.H.; Perimal, E.K. Antiallodynic and antihyperalgesic effects of zerumbone on a mouse model of chronic constriction injury-induced neuropathic pain. *Fitoterapia* **2015**, *105*, 215–221. [CrossRef]
26. Zulazmi, N.A.; Gopalsamy, B.; Min, J.C.S.; Akira, A.; Sulaiman, M.R.; Bharatham, B.H.; Perimal, E.K. Zerumbone Alleviates Neuropathic Pain through the Involvement of l-Arginine-Nitric Oxide-cGMP-K+ ATP Channel Pathways in Chronic Constriction Injury in Mice Model. *Molecules* **2017**, *22*, 555. [CrossRef] [PubMed]

27. Chia, J.S.M.; Farouk, A.A.O.; Mohamad, A.S.; Sulaiman, M.R.; Perimal, E.K. Zerumbone alleviates chronic constriction injury-induced allodynia and hyperalgesia through serotonin 5-HT receptors. *Biomed. Pharm.* **2016**, *83*, 1303–1310. [CrossRef] [PubMed]
28. Gopalsamy, B.; Farouk, A.A.O.; Tengku Mohamad, T.A.S.; Sulaiman, M.R.; Perimal, E.K. Antiallodynic and antihyperalgesic activities of zerumbone via the suppression of IL-1beta, IL-6, and TNF-alpha in a mouse model of neuropathic pain. *J Pain Res.* **2017**, *10*, 2605–2619. [CrossRef] [PubMed]
29. Kitayama, T.; Okamoto, T.; Hill, R.K.; Kawai, Y.; Takahashi, S.; Yonemori, S.; Yamamoto, Y.; Ohe, K.; Uemura, S.; Sawada, S. Chemistry of Zerumbone. 1. Simplified Isolation, Conjugate Addition Reactions, and a Unique Ring Contracting Transannular Reaction of Its Dibromide. *J. Org. Chem.* **1999**, *64*, 2667–2672. [CrossRef]
30. Maimone, T.J.; Baran, P.S. Modern synthetic efforts toward biologically active terpenes. *Nat. Chem. Biol.* **2007**, *3*, 396–407. [CrossRef] [PubMed]
31. Haque, A.; Jantan, I.; Arshad, L.; Bukhari, S.N.A. Exploring the immunomodulatory and anticancer properties of zerumbone. *Food Funct.* **2017**, *8*, 3410–3431. [CrossRef] [PubMed]
32. Hwang, J.; Youn, K.; Ji, Y.; Lee, S.; Lim, G.; Lee, J.; Ho, C.-T.; Leem, S.-H.; Jun, M. Biological and Computational Studies for Dual Cholinesterases Inhibitory Effect of Zerumbone. *Nutrients* **2020**, *12*, 1215. [CrossRef] [PubMed]
33. Fatima, A.; Abdul, B.; Abdullah, R.; Karjiban, R.; Lee, V. Docking studies reveal zerumbone targets β-catenin of the Wnt-β-catenin pathway in breast cancer. *J. Serbian Chem. Soc.* **2018**, *83*, 575–591. [CrossRef]
34. Eid, E.E.M.; Azam, F.; Hassan, M.; Taban, I.M.; Halim, M.A. Zerumbone binding to estrogen receptors: An in-silico investigation. *J. Recept. Signal Transduct.* **2018**, *38*, 342–351. [CrossRef] [PubMed]
35. Murakami, A.; Takahashi, D.; Kinoshita, T.; Koshimizu, K.; Kim, H.W.; Yoshihiro, A.; Nakamura, Y.; Jiwajinda, S.; Terao, J.; Ohigashi, H. Zerumbone, a Southeast Asian ginger sesquiterpene, markedly suppresses free radical generation, proinflammatory protein production, and cancer cell proliferation accompanied by apoptosis. The alpha,beta unsaturated carbonyl group is a prerequisite. *Carcinogenesis* **2002**, *23*, 795–802. [CrossRef]
36. Singh, S.P.; Nongalleima, K.; Singh, N.I.; Doley, P.; Singh, C.B.; Singh, T.R.; Sahoo, D. Zerumbone reduces proliferation of HCT116 colon cancer cells by inhibition of TNF-alpha. *Sci. Rep.* **2018**, *8*, 1–11. [CrossRef]
37. Chen, L.; Chen, W.; Qian, X.; Fang, Y.; Zhu, N. Liquiritigenin alleviates mechanical and cold hyperalgesia in a rat neuropathic pain model. *Sci. Rep.* **2014**, *4*, 5676. [CrossRef]
38. Deacon, R. Measuring motor coordination in mice. *J. Vis. Exp.* **2013**, *75*, e2609. [CrossRef]
39. Rasband, M.N.; Trimmer, J.S.; Schwarz, T.L.; Levinson, S.R.; Ellisman, M.H.; Schachner, M.; Shrager, P. Potassium Channel Distribution, Clustering, and Function in Remyelinating Rat Axons. *J. Neurosci.* **1998**, *18*, 36–47. [CrossRef]
40. McKeown, L.; Swanton, L.; Robinson, P.; Jones, O.T. Surface expression and distribution of voltage-gated potassium channels in neurons (Review). *Mol. Membr. Boil.* **2008**, *25*, 332–343. [CrossRef]
41. Taglialatela, M.; Vandongen, A.M.; A Drewe, J.; Joho, R.H.; Brown, A.M.; E Kirsch, G. Patterns of internal and external tetraethylammonium block in four homologous K+ channels. *Mol. Pharmacol.* **1991**, *40*, 299–307.
42. Del Camino, D.; Holmgren, M.; Liu, Y.; Yellen, G. Blocker protection in the pore of a voltage-gated K+ channel and its structural implications. *Nature* **2000**, *403*, 321–325. [CrossRef]
43. Wuttke, T.V.; Seebohm, G.; Bail, S.; Maljevic, S.; Lerche, H. The New Anticonvulsant Retigabine Favors Voltage-Dependent Opening of the Kv7.2 (KCNQ2) Channel by Binding to Its Activation Gate. *Mol. Pharmacol.* **2005**, *67*, 1009–1017. [CrossRef]
44. Lü, Q.; Peevey, J.; Jow, F.; Monaghan, M.M.; Mendoza, G.; Zhang, H.; Wu, J.; Kim, C.Y.; Bicksler, J.; Greenblatt, L.; et al. Disruption of Kv1.1 N-type inactivation by novel small molecule inhibitors (disinactivators). *Bioorganic Med. Chem.* **2008**, *16*, 3067–3075. [CrossRef]
45. Rose, K.; Ooi, L.; Dalle, C.; Robertson, B.; Wood, I.C.; Gamper, N. Transcriptional repression of the M channel subunit Kv7.2 in chronic nerve injury. *Pain* **2011**, *152*, 742–754. [CrossRef]
46. Liu, B.; Linley, J.E.; Du, X.; Zhang, X.; Ooi, L.; Zhang, H.; Gamper, N. The acute nociceptive signals induced by bradykinin in rat sensory neurons are mediated by inhibition of M-type K+ channels and activation of Ca2+-activated Cl- channels. *J. Clin. Investig.* **2010**, *120*, 1240–1252. [CrossRef]

47. Passmore, G.M.; Selyanko, A.A.; Mistry, M.; Al-Qatari, M.; Marsh, S.J.; Matthews, E.A.; Dickenson, A.H.; Brown, T.A.; Burbidge, S.A.; Main, M.; et al. KCNQ/M Currents in Sensory Neurons: Significance for Pain Therapy. *J. Neurosci.* **2003**, *23*, 7227–7236. [CrossRef]
48. Wulff, H.; Castle, N.A.; Pardo, L.A. Voltage-gated potassium channels as therapeutic targets. *Nat. Rev. Drug Discov.* **2009**, *8*, 982–1001. [CrossRef]
49. Gribble, F.M.; Reimann, F. Sulphonylurea action revisited: The post-cloning era. *Diabetologia* **2003**, *46*, 875–891. [CrossRef]
50. Ocaña, M.; Baeyens, J.M. Differential effects of K^+ channel blockers on antinociception induced by alpha 2-adrenoceptor, GABAB and kappa-opioid receptor agonists. *Br. J. Pharmacol.* **1993**, *110*, 1049–1054.
51. Robles, L.-I.; Barrios, M.; Del Pozo, E.; Dordal, A.; Baeyens, J. Effects of K+ channel blockers and openers on antinociception induced by agonists of 5-HT1A receptors. *Eur. J. Pharmacol.* **1996**, *295*, 181–188. [CrossRef]
52. Ocaña, M.; Del Pozo, E.; Barrios, M.; Robles, L.I.; Baeyens, J. An ATP-dependent potassium channel blocker antagonizes morphine analgesia. *Eur. J. Pharmacol.* **1990**, *186*, 377–378. [CrossRef]
53. Zushida, K.; Onodera, K.; Kamei, J. Effect of diabetes on pinacidil-induced antinociception in mice. *Eur. J. Pharmacol.* **2002**, *453*, 209–215. [CrossRef]
54. Campbell, V.C.; Welch, S.P. The role of minoxidil on endogenous opioid peptides in the spinal cord: A putative co-agonist relationship between K-ATP openers and opioids. *Eur. J. Pharmacol.* **2001**, *417*, 91–98. [CrossRef]
55. Sun, H.-S.; Feng, Z.-P. Neuroprotective role of ATP-sensitive potassium channels in cerebral ischemia. *Acta Pharmacol. Sin.* **2012**, *34*, 24–32. [CrossRef]
56. Wulf-Johansson, H.; Hay-Schmidt, A.; Poulsen, A.N.; Klaerke, D.A.; Olesen, J.; Jansen, I. Expression of BKCa channels and the modulatory β-subunits in the rat and porcine trigeminal ganglion. *Brain Res.* **2009**, *1292*, 1–13. [CrossRef]
57. Furukawa, N.; Takasusuki, T.; Fukushima, T.; Hori, Y. Presynaptic large-conductance calcium-activated potassium channels control synaptic transmission in the superficial dorsal horn of the mouse. *Neurosci. Lett.* **2008**, *444*, 79–82. [CrossRef]
58. Chen, S.-R.; Cai, Y.-Q.; Pan, H.-L. Plasticity and emerging role of BKCa channels in nociceptive control in neuropathic pain. *J. Neurochem.* **2009**, *110*, 352–362. [CrossRef]
59. Liu, C.-Y.; Lu, Z.-Y.; Li, N.; Yu, L.-H.; Zhao, Y.-F.; Ma, B. The role of large-conductance, calcium-activated potassium channels in a rat model of trigeminal neuropathic pain. *Cephalalgia* **2014**, *35*, 16–35. [CrossRef]
60. Horrigan, F.T.; Cui, J.; Aldrich, R.W. Allosteric Voltage Gating of Potassium Channels I. *J. Gen. Physiol.* **1999**, *114*, 277–304. [CrossRef]
61. Hill, M.A.; Yang, Y.; Ella, S.R.; Davis, M.J.; Braun, A.P. Large conductance, Ca2+-activated K+ channels (BKCa) and arteriolar myogenic signaling. *FEBS Lett.* **2010**, *584*, 2033–2042. [CrossRef]
62. Cui, J.; Yang, H.; Lee, U.S. Molecular mechanisms of BK channel activation. *Cell. Mol. Life Sci.* **2008**, *66*, 852–875. [CrossRef]
63. Ocaña, M.; Cendán, C.M.; Cobos, E.J.; Entrena, J.M.; Baeyens, J.M. Potassium channels and pain: Present realities and future opportunities. *Eur. J. Pharmacol.* **2004**, *500*, 203–219. [CrossRef]
64. Cao, Y.; Dreixler, J.C.; Roizen, J.D.; Roberts, M.T.; Houamed, K.M. Modulation of recombinant small-conductance Ca(2+)-activated K(+) channels by the muscle relaxant chlorzoxazone and structurally related compounds. *J. Pharmacol. Exp. Ther.* **2001**, *296*, 683–689.
65. Thompson, J.M.; Ji, G.; Neugebauer, V. Small-conductance calcium-activated potassium (SK) channels in the amygdala mediate pain-inhibiting effects of clinically available riluzole in a rat model of arthritis pain. *Mol. Pain* **2015**, *11*, 51. [CrossRef]
66. Granados-Soto, V.; Argüelles, C.F.; Ortiz, M.I. The peripheral antinociceptive effect of resveratrol is associated with activation of potassium channels. *Neuropharmacology* **2002**, *43*, 917–923. [CrossRef]
67. Kapitzke, D.; Vetter, I.; Cabot, P.J. Endogenous opioid analgesia in peripheral tissues and the clinical implications for pain control. *Ther. Clin. Risk Manag.* **2005**, *1*, 279–297.
68. Chang, K.J.; Cuatrecasas, P. Multiple opiate receptors. Enkephalins and morphine bind to receptors of different specificity. *J. Boil. Chem.* **1979**, *254*, 2610–2618.
69. Stoeber, M.; Jullié, D.; Li, J.; Chakraborty, S.; Majumdar, S.; Lambert, N.A.; Manglik, A.; Von Zastrow, M. Agonist-selective recruitment of engineered protein probes and of GRK2 by opioid receptors in living cells. *eLife* **2020**, *9*, e54208. [CrossRef]

70. Al-Hasani, R.; Bruchas, M.R. Molecular Mechanisms of Opioid Receptor-dependent Signaling and Behavior. *Anesthesiology* **2011**, *115*, 1363–1381. [CrossRef]
71. Ossipov, M.H.; Morimura, K.; Porreca, F. Descending pain modulation and chronification of pain. *Curr. Opin. Support Palliat Care* **2014**, *8*, 143–151.
72. Pradhan, A.A.; Clarke, P.B. Comparison between delta-opioid receptor functional response and autoradiographic labeling in rat brain and spinal cord. *J. Comp. Neurol.* **2005**, *481*, 416–426. [CrossRef]
73. Poulin, J.-F.; Chevalier, B.; Laforest, S.; Drolet, G. Enkephalinergic afferents of the centromedial amygdala in the rat. *J. Comp. Neurol.* **2006**, *496*, 859–876. [CrossRef]
74. Le Merrer, J.; Becker, J.A.J.; Befort, K.; Kieffer, B.L. Reward processing by the opioid system in the brain. *Physiol. Rev.* **2009**, *89*, 1379–1412. [CrossRef]
75. Basbaum, A.I.; Fields, H.L. Endogenous pain control mechanisms: Review and hypothesis. *Ann. Neurol.* **1978**, *4*, 451–462. [CrossRef]
76. Basbaum, A.I.; Fields, H.L. Endogenous pain control systems: Brainstem spinal pathways and endorphin circuitry. *Annu. Rev. Neurosci.* **1984**, *7*, 309–338. [CrossRef]
77. Drake, C.T.; Chavkin, C.; Milner, T.A. Opioid systems in the dentate gyrus. *Prog. Brain Res.* **2007**, *163*, 245–814. [CrossRef]
78. Upton, N.; Sewell, R.D.; Spencer, P.S. Analgesic actions of mu- and kappa-opiate agonists in rats. *Arch. Int. de Pharmacodyn. et de Ther.* **1983**, *262*, 199–207.
79. Tyers, M.B. A classification of opiate receptors that mediate antinociception in animals. *Br. J. Pharmacol.* **1980**, *69*, 503–512. [CrossRef]
80. Goodman, A.J.; Le Bourdonnec, B.; Dolle, R.E. Mu Opioid Receptor Antagonists: Recent Developments. *Chem. Med. Chem.* **2007**, *2*, 1552–1570. [CrossRef]
81. Gaveriaux-Ruff, C.; Karchewski, L.A.; Hever, X.; Matifas, A.; Kieffer, B.L. Inflammatory pain is enhanced in delta opioid receptor-knockout mice. *Eur. J. Neurosci.* **2008**, *27*, 2558–2567. [CrossRef] [PubMed]
82. Nadal, X.; Banos, J.E.; Kieffer, B.L.; Maldonado, R. Neuropathic pain is enhanced in delta-opioid receptor knockout mice. *Eur. J. Neurosci.* **2006**, *23*, 830–834. [CrossRef] [PubMed]
83. Vanderah, T.W. Delta and Kappa Opioid Receptors as Suitable Drug Targets for Pain. *Clin. J. Pain* **2010**, *26*, S10–S15. [CrossRef] [PubMed]
84. Aceto, M.D.; May, E.L.; Harris, L.S.; Bowman, E.R.; Cook, C.D. Pharmacological studies with a nonpeptidic, delta-opioid (−)-(1R,5R,9R)-5,9-dimethyl-2′-hydroxy-2-(6-hydroxyhexyl)-6,7-benzomorphan hydrochloride ((−)-NIH 11082). *Eur. J. Pharmacol.* **2007**, *566*, 88–93. [CrossRef] [PubMed]
85. Le Bourdonnec, B.; Windh, R.T.; Ajello, C.W.; Leister, L.K.; Gu, M.; Chu, G.-H.; Tuthill, P.A.; Barker, W.M.; Koblish, M.; Wiant, D.D.; et al. Potent, Orally Bioavailable Delta Opioid Receptor Agonists for the Treatment of Pain: Discovery of N,N-Diethyl-4-(5-hydroxyspiro[chromene-2,4′-piperidine]-4-yl)benzamide (ADL5859). *J. Med. Chem.* **2008**, *51*, 5893–5896. [CrossRef]
86. Saitoh, A.; Sugiyama, A.; Nemoto, T.; Fujii, H.; Wada, K.; Oka, J.-I.; Nagase, H.; Yamada, M. The novel δ opioid receptor agonist KNT-127 produces antidepressant-like and antinociceptive effects in mice without producing convulsions. *Behav. Brain Res.* **2011**, *223*, 271–279. [CrossRef]
87. Jones, P.; Griffin, A.M.; Gawell, L.; Lavoie, R.; Delorme, D.; Roberts, E.; Brown, W.; Walpole, C.; Xiao, W.; Boulet, J.; et al. N,N-Diethyl-4-[(3-hydroxyphenyl)(piperidin-4-yl)amino] benzamide derivatives: The development of diaryl amino piperidines as potent delta opioid receptor agonists with in vivo anti-anociceptive activity in rodent models. *Bioorganic Med. Chem. Lett.* **2009**, *19*, 5994–5998.
88. Chavkin, C. The Therapeutic Potential of [kappa]-Opioids for Treatment of Pain and Addiction. *Neuropsychopharmacology* **2011**, *36*, 369–370. [CrossRef]
89. Su, X.; Castle, N.A.; Antonio, B.; Roeloffs, R.; Thomas, J.B.; Krafte, D.S.; Chapman, M.L. The effect of kappa-opioid receptor agonists on tetrodotoxin-resistant sodium channels in primary sensory neurons. *Anesth. Analg.* **2009**, *109*, 632–640. [CrossRef]
90. Amir, R.; Michaelis, M.; Devor, M. Membrane Potential Oscillations in Dorsal Root Ganglion Neurons: Role in Normal Electrogenesis and Neuropathic Pain. *J. Neurosci.* **1999**, *19*, 8589–8596. [CrossRef]
91. Giordano, J.; Schultea, T. Serotonin 5-HT (3) receptor mediation of pain and anti-anociception: Implications for clinical therapeutics. *Pain Physician* **2004**, *7*, 141–147. [PubMed]

92. Ming-Tatt, L.; Khalivulla, S.I.; Akhtar, M.N.; Lajis, N.; Perimal, E.K.; Akira, A.; Ali, D.I.; Sulaiman, M.R. Anti-hyperalgesic effect of a benzilidine-cyclohexanone analogue on a mouse model of chronic constriction injury-induced neuropathic pain: Participation of the κ-opioid receptor and KATP. *Pharmacol. Biochem. Behav.* **2013**, *114*, 58–63. [CrossRef] [PubMed]
93. Gutierrez, V.P.; Zambelli, V.O.; Picolo, G.; Chacur, M.; Sampaio, S.C.; Brigatte, P.; Konno, K.; Cury, Y. The peripheral L-arginine–nitric oxide–cyclic GMP pathway and ATP-sensitive K$^+$ channels are involved in the antinociceptive effect of crotalphine on neuropathic pain in rats. *Behav. Pharmacol.* **2012**, *23*, 14–24. [CrossRef] [PubMed]
94. Chia, J.S.M.; Izham, N.A.M.; Farouk, A.A.O.; Sulaiman, M.R.; Mustafa, S.; Hutchinson, M.R.; Perimal, E.K. Zerumbone Modulates α2A-Adrenergic, TRPV1, and NMDA NR2B Receptors Plasticity in CCI-Induced Neuropathic Pain In Vivo and LPS-Induced SH-SY5Y Neuroblastoma In Vitro Models. *Front. Pharmacol.* **2020**, *11*, 92. [CrossRef] [PubMed]
95. Stone, L.S.; Macmillan, L.B.; Kitto, K.F.; Limbird, L.E.; Wilcox, G.L. The α2a Adrenergic Receptor Subtype Mediates Spinal Analgesia Evoked by α2 Agonists and Is Necessary for Spinal Adrenergic–Opioid Synergy. *J. Neurosci.* **1997**, *17*, 7157–7165. [CrossRef]
96. Fairbanks, C.A.; Stone, L.S.; Kitto, K.F.; Nguyen, H.O.; Posthumus, I.J.; Wilcox, G.L. α2C-Adrenergic Receptors Mediate Spinal Analgesia and Adrenergic-Opioid Synergy. *J. Pharmacol. Exp. Ther.* **2002**, *300*, 282–290. [CrossRef]
97. Ossipov, M.H.; Lopez, Y.; Bian, D.; Nichols, M.L.; Porreca, F. Synergistic Antinociceptive Interactions of Morphine and Clonidine in Rats with Nerve-ligation Injury. *Anesthesiology* **1997**, *86*, 196–204. [CrossRef]
98. Caterina, M.J.; Schumacher, M.A.; Tominaga, M.; Rosen, T.A.; Levine, J.D.; Julius, D. The capsaicin receptor: A heat-activated ion channel in the pain pathway. *Nature* **1997**, *389*, 816–824. [CrossRef]
99. Fundytus, M.E. Glutamate Receptors and Nociception. *CNS Drugs* **2001**, *15*, 29–58. [CrossRef]
100. Trivedi, M.; Shaikh, S.; Gwinnut, C. Pharmacology of opioids. *Anaesthesia* **2011**, 118–124.
101. Zakaria, Z.; Rahim, M.H.A.; Roosli, R.A.J.; Sani, M.H.M.; Marmaya, N.H.; Omar, M.H.; Teh, L.K.; Salleh, M.Z. Antinociceptive Activity of Petroleum Ether Fraction of Clinacanthus nutans Leaves Methanolic Extract: Roles of Nonopioid Pain Modulatory Systems and Potassium Channels. *BioMed. Res. Int.* **2019**, *2019*, 6593125. [CrossRef] [PubMed]
102. Klein, A.H.; Mohammad, H.K.; Ali, R.; Peper, B.; Wilson, S.P.; Raja, S.N.; Ringkamp, M.; Sweitzer, S. Overexpression of µ-Opioid Receptors in Peripheral Afferents, but Not in Combination with Enkephalin, Decreases Neuropathic Pain Behavior and Enhances Opioid Analgesia in Mouse. *Anesthesiology* **2018**, *128*, 967–983. [CrossRef] [PubMed]
103. Thompson, S.J.; Pitcher, M.H.; Stone, L.S.; Tarum, F.; Niu, G.; Chen, X.; Kiesewetter, D.O.; Schweinhardt, P.; Bushnell, M.C. Chronic neuropathic pain reduces opioid receptor availability with associated anhedonia in rat. *Pain* **2018**, *159*, 1856–1866. [CrossRef] [PubMed]
104. Le Guen, S.; Gestreau, C.; Besson, J.-M. Morphine withdrawal precipitated by specific mu, delta or kappa opioid receptor antagonists: A c-Fos protein study in the rat central nervous system. *Eur. J. Neurosci.* **2003**, *17*, 2425–2437. [CrossRef] [PubMed]
105. Gestreau, C.; Besson, J.-M. Is there tonic activity in the endogenous opioid systems? A c-Fos study in the rat central nervous system after intravenous injection of naloxone or naloxone-methiodide. *J. Comp. Neurol.* **2000**, *427*, 285–301. [CrossRef]
106. Galeotti, N.; Ghelardini, C.; Caldari, B.; Bartolini, A. Effect of potassium channel modulators in mouse forced swimming test. *Br. J. Pharmacol.* **1999**, *126*, 1653–1659. [CrossRef]
107. Welch, S.P.; Dunlow, L.D. Antinociceptive activity of intrathecally administered potassium channel openers and opioid agonists: A common mechanism of action? *J. Pharmacol. Exp. Ther.* **1993**, *267*, 390–399.
108. Bennett, G.J.; Xie, Y.-K. A peripheral mononeuropathy in rat that produces disorders of pain sensation like those seen in man. *Pain* **1988**, *33*, 87–107. [CrossRef]
109. Gopalsamy, B.; Sambasevam, Y.; Zulazmi, N.A.; Chia, J.S.M.; Farouk, A.A.O.; Sulaiman, M.R.; Mohamad, T.A.S.T.; Perimal, E.K. Experimental Characterization of the Chronic Constriction Injury-Induced Neuropathic Pain Model in Mice. *Neurochem. Res.* **2019**, *44*, 2123–2138. [CrossRef]

110. Martinov, T.; Mack, M.R.; Sykes, A.; Chatterjea, D. Measuring changes in tactile sensitivity in the hind paw of mice using an electronic von Frey apparatus. *J. Vis. Exp.* **2013**, *82*, e51212. [CrossRef]
111. Hargreaves, K.; Dubner, R.; Brown, F.; Flores, C.; Joris, J. A new and sensitive method for measuring thermal nociception in cutaneous hyperalgesia. *Pain* **1988**, *32*, 77–88. [CrossRef]

Sample Availability: Samples of zerumbone are available from the authors.

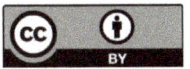 © 2020 by the authors. Licensee MDPI, Basel, Switzerland. This article is an open access article distributed under the terms and conditions of the Creative Commons Attribution (CC BY) license (http://creativecommons.org/licenses/by/4.0/).

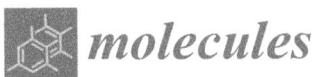

Article

Comparisons of In Vivo and In Vitro Opioid Effects of Newly Synthesized 14-Methoxycodeine-6-*O*-sulfate and Codeine-6-*O*-sulfate

Ferenc Zádor [1,2], Amir Mohammadzadeh [1], Mihály Balogh [1], Zoltán S. Zádori [1], Kornél Király [1], Szilvia Barsi [1], Anna Rita Galambos [1], Szilvia B. László [1], Barbara Hutka [1], András Váradi [3], Sándor Hosztafi [3], Pál Riba [1], Sándor Benyhe [2], Susanna Fürst [1] and Mahmoud Al-Khrasani [1,*]

1. Department of Pharmacology and Pharmacotherapy, Faculty of Medicine, Semmelweis University, Nagyvárad tér 4, P.O. Box 370, H-1445 Budapest, Hungary; zador.ferenc@pharma.semmelweis-univ.hu (F.Z.); mohammadzadeh.amir@med.semmelweis-univ.hu (A.M.); baloghmisi90@gmail.com (M.B.); zadori.zoltan@med.semmelweis-univ.hu (Z.S.Z.); kiraly.kornel@med.semmelweis-univ.hu (K.K.); szilvi.barsi@gmail.com (S.B.); galambos.anna@pharma.semmelweis-univ.hu (A.R.G.); laszlo.szilvia@med.semmelweis-univ.hu (S.B.L.); hutka.barbara@semmelweis-univ.hu (B.H.); riba.pal@med.semmelweis-univ.hu (P.R.); furst.zsuzsanna@med.semmelweis-univ.hu (S.F.)
2. Institute of Biochemistry, Biological Research Center of the Hungarian Academy of Sciences, Temesvári krt. 62., H-6726 Szeged, Hungary; benyhe.sandor@brc.hu
3. Department of Pharmaceutical Chemistry, Semmelweis University, Hőgyes Endre u., 9. H-1092 Budapest, Hungary; uvamortifera@gmail.com (A.V.); hosztafi.sandor@pharma.semmelweis-univ.hu (S.H.)
* Correspondence: al-khrasani.mahmoud@med.semmelweis-univ.hu; Tel.: +36-1-2104-416

Received: 15 February 2020; Accepted: 15 March 2020; Published: 17 March 2020

Abstract: The present work represents the in vitro (potency, affinity, efficacy) and in vivo (antinociception, constipation) opioid pharmacology of the novel compound 14-methoxycodeine-6-*O*-sulfate (14-OMeC6SU), compared to the reference compounds codeine-6-*O*-sulfate (C6SU), codeine and morphine. Based on in vitro tests (mouse and rat vas deferens, receptor binding and [^{35}S]GTPγS activation assays), 14-OMeC6SU has µ-opioid receptor-mediated activity, displaying higher affinity, potency and efficacy than the parent compounds. In rats, 14-OMeC6SU showed stronger antinociceptive effect in the tail-flick assay than codeine and was equipotent to morphine, whereas C6SU was less efficacious after subcutaneous (s.c.) administration. Following intracerebroventricular injection, 14-OMeC6SU was more potent than morphine. In the Complete Freund's Adjuvant-induced inflammatory hyperalgesia, 14-OMeC6SU and C6SU in s.c. doses up to 6.1 and 13.2 µmol/kg, respectively, showed peripheral antihyperalgesic effect, because co-administered naloxone methiodide, a peripherally acting opioid receptor antagonist antagonized the measured antihyperalgesia. In addition, s.c. C6SU showed less pronounced inhibitory effect on the gastrointestinal transit than 14-OMeC6SU, codeine and morphine. This study provides first evidence that 14-OMeC6SU is more effective than codeine or C6SU in vitro and in vivo. Furthermore, despite C6SU peripheral antihyperalgesic effects with less gastrointestinal side effects the superiority of 14-OMeC6SU was obvious throughout the present study.

Keywords: peripheral antinociception; 14-methoxycodeine-6-*O*-sulfate; codeine-6-*O*-sulfate

1. Introduction

Natural, semisynthetic and synthetic µ type opioid receptor (MOR) agonists are essential and the most efficient medicines to relieve moderate to severe pain in the clinical practice. MORs, together with δ and κ type opioid receptors (abbreviated as DOR and KOR, respectively), are $G_{i/o}$-type G-protein coupled receptors, which reduce cAMP levels, inhibit calcium channels (N/P) and open potassium channels, overall resulting in the inhibition of neurotransmitter release from the presynaptic membrane [1,2] and hyperpolarizing the post synaptic membrane [3]. From a general point of view, opioids produce analgesia by full or partial activation of opioid receptors, in particular MOR types at the spinal and supraspinal levels. In addition, pharmacological evidence has shown that opioids are also capable to produce antinociception by the activation of opioid receptors reside outside the central nervous system [4–10]. Indeed, opioid agonists that have been reported to induce peripheral antinociception display a prerequisite physiochemical property, a limited central nervous system (CNS) penetration [4,5,7]. Thus, over the last four decades many opioid research groups have undertaken the task of synthesis and pharmacological characterization of opioid compounds with limited CNS penetration and thereby inducing antinociception by activating opioid receptors at the periphery. It is worth noting that quaternization of nitrogen on morphine-based structure derivatives has been reported to have negative impact on both the affinity and agonist activity of generated analogs [11]. To overcome this issue, medicinal chemists have been seeking for other ways to develop opioid agonists with limited CNS penetration, meanwhile retaining or even increasing the pharmacological profile, when compared to the parent molecules [12].

One of the most successful chemical approaches to improve the safety (limited CNS penetration) profile and the efficacy of morphine and other morphinans, is the synthesis of zwitterionic structures. This chemical structure modification was carried out by the introduction of ionizable groups into the C-6 position such as sulfate, amino acids or guanido groups as described previously [6,13–21]. Such compounds have been demonstrated to have reduced central side effects as well [5,21]. Extreme increase in the affinity, efficacy and analgesic activity was measured for 14-methoxy analogs of morphine or oxymorphone compared to the parent compounds [4,6,20,22,23].

A study by Zuckerman and co-workers has shown that codeine-6-O-sulfate (C6SU) displayed exclusive affinity for MOR, yet it was found that intracerebroventricularly administered C6SU produced weak analgesia at lower doses and increasing the dose of C6SU evoked convulsion and death that hampered the assessment of its analgesia [17]. Indeed, convulsion following intracerebroventricular (i.c.v.) injection of codeine has also been reported, though systemic codeine is used as an analgesic for mild to moderate pain and the World Health Organization approves its usage as the second step of the analgesic ladder for cancer pain [24]. To the best of our knowledge, no data have been reported on the systemic analgesic effect of C6SU.

Compared to morphine, codeine has a weaker affinity for opioid receptors and preferably binds to the MOR [25–28]. As with all opioids, codeine also produces central adverse effects such as addiction and respiratory depression [26,29–31], as well as peripheral ones such as constipation [30,31]. These are mainly mediated through the MOR [32,33]. It is therefore imperative to increase the analgesic efficacy of C6SU by the above mentioned strategy and underline again the analgesic properties of C6SU and codeine after both central and peripheral administrations.

The aims of the present work were to synthesize and characterize 14-methoxycodeine-6-O-sulfate (14-OMeC6SU) and to compare the structure-activity relationship of the novel compound to the already characterized C6SU [14,17], to the parent compound codeine (for structures see Figure 1) and to morphine, a prototypical opioid analgesic. During pharmacological characterization we analyzed its receptor preference (selectivity and affinity) by biochemical (equilibrium radioligand competition binding) and by biological assays (MVD, mouse vas deferens; RVD, rat vas deferens). A further objective was to measure the analgesic effect of the novel compound and compare to C6SU, codeine and morphine in rat tail-flick test. We have also characterized the antinociceptive effects of 14-OMeC6SU and C6SU on hyperalgesia induced by Complete Freund's Adjuvant (CFA) in order to draw a conclusion on the possible peripheral antinociception. Additionally, constipation, one of the most common side effects of codeine was also investigated, by analyzing the changes in gastrointestinal transit with the charcoal meal assay in the presence of the test compound.

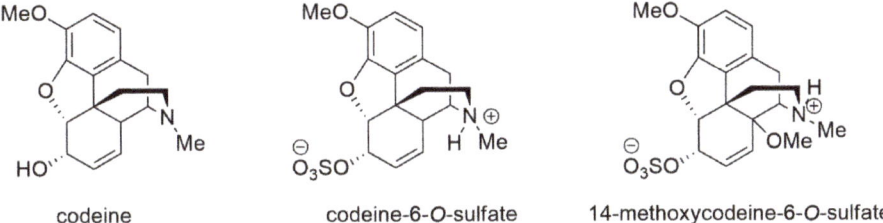

Figure 1. The structure of codeine, codeine-6-O-sulfate and 14-methoxycodeine-6-O-sulfate.

2. Results

2.1. Receptor Binding Assays

2.1.1. 14-OMeC6SU Displayed High Affinity and MOR Selectivity in Radioligand Competition Binding Assay

The novel codeine analog 14-OMeC6SU, CS6U and the parent compound codeine were tested for opioid receptor binding affinity and selectivity in in vitro radioligand competition binding assays using prototypic selective radioligands for MOR and DOR in rat brain membrane homogenates, or for KOR in guinea pig brain membrane homogenates. The prototypic opioid ligands displayed high affinity as expected and are in accordance with previous data [20,23].

14-OMeC6SU showed higher affinity for MOR 28 and 217 times when compared to C6SU and codeine, respectively (Figure 2A, Table 1). In addition, it displayed affinity for DOR and KOR but the affinity was 101 and 72 fold, respectively, lower than that for MOR, (Figure 2B, Table 1). Although 14-OMeC6SU displayed relevant KOR affinity, the displacement was only 51.34% (±11.53) compared to total specific binding (Figure 2C, Table 1). Compared to codeine, C6SU showed significantly higher MOR affinity and endowed a micromolar affinity to the DOR, however, C6SU did not displace the DOR radioligand completely to the non-specific binding level at the highest concentration (26.45 ± 6.02%, Figure 2B). Furthermore, in contrast to 14-OMeC6SU, C6SU did not show significant KOR affinity (Figure 2C, Table 1). The parent compound codeine showed poor affinity for MOR and none for DOR and KOR (Figure 2 and Table 1).

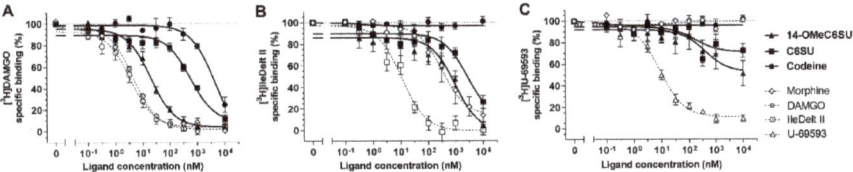

Figure 2. Dose-response curves featuring binding affinity of 14-methoxycodeine-6-O-sulfate (14-OMeC6SU) and codeine-6-O-sulfate (C6SU) to μ-opioid receptor (**A**), δ-opioid receptor (**B**) and κ-opioid receptor (**C**) compared to codeine and morphine in competition binding experiments performed in rat (**A** and **B**) and guinea pig (**C**) brain membrane homogenate. For control the unlabeled form of the applied radioligands are also indicated. All figures represent the specific binding of the corresponding radioligand (**A**: [^{3}H]DAMGO, **B**: [^{3}H]Ile^{5,6}-deltorphin II [IleDelt II], **C**: [^{3}H]U-69593) in percentage (means ± S.E.M.) normalized to total specific binding (100%) in the presence of increasing concentrations (0.1 nM–10 μM) of the indicated unlabeled ligands. Total specific binding was determined in the absence of the indicated unlabeled ligands and indicated with a dotted line. The K_i ± S.E.M. values are presented in Table 1.

Table 1. Inhibitory constant values ($K_i \pm$ S.E.M.) and selectivity ratios of codeine-6-O-*sulfate* (C6SU) and 14-methoxycodeine-6-O-sulfate (14-OMeC6SU) compared to codeine in competition binding assays with [^{3}H]DAMGO, [^{3}H]IleDelt II and [^{3}H]U-69593, which are μ type opioid receptor (MOR), δ type opioid receptor (DOR) and κ type opioid receptor (KOR) specific radioligands, respectively performed in rat or guinea pig brain membrane homogenates. The unlabeled form of the radioligands are also indicated for control and for further comparison.

Compounds	$K_i \pm$ S.E.M. (nM)			Selectivity Ratio		
	[^{3}H]DAMGO (μ) [1]	[^{3}H]IleDelt II (δ) [1]	[^{3}H]U-69593 (κ) [2]	δ/μ	κ/μ	δ/κ
14-OMeC6SU	3.37 ± 0.48 ** (n = 6)	345.52 ± 132.52 (n = 5)	245.57 ± 215.01 (n = 5)	102.5	72.9	1.4
C6SU	96.91 ± 20.3 * (n = 5)	968.28 ± 471.38 (n = 6)	N.D.[3] (n = 5)	9.9	-	-
Codeine	736.74 ± 319.63 (n = 4)	N.D.[4] (n = 4)	N.D.[4] (n = 4)	-	-	-
Morphine [5]	0.76 ± 0.08 (n = 7)	114.21 ± 44.83 (n = 6)	N.D.[4] (n = 4)	150.3	-	-
Homologous ligand[6]	0.59 ± 0.12 (n = 5)	3.81 ± 0.88 (n = 6)	5.51 ± 0.97 (n = 5)	-	-	-

[1] performed in rat brain membrane homogenates; [2] performed in guinea pig brain membrane homogenates; [3] the compound did not inhibit total specific radioligand binding (100%) to 50%, thus the K_i value cannot be interpreted (N.D. not determined); [4] the compound did not alter significantly (One-sample t test) the total specific radioligand binding (100%), thus the K_i value cannot be interpreted (N.D. not determined); [5] adopted from [23]; [6] indicates the unlabeled form of the radioligands and represent a control for the assay (μ: DAMGO δ: IleDelt II, κ: U-69593); * compared to codeine (One-way ANOVA, with Sidak's multiple comparison test; ** $P < 0.01$, *** $P < 0.001$).

2.1.2. 14-OMeC6SU Shows Strong Agonist Activity in [^{35}S]GTPγS Binding Assay

The agonist activity of 14-OMeC6SU was analyzed in [^{35}S]GTPγS G-protein activity assay and compared to C6SU, codeine and the prototypical opioid receptor selective agonists for μ, δ and κ opioid receptors (DAMGO, deltorphin II and U-69593, respectively) (Figure 3 and Table 2). Similar to competition binding experiments, rat and guinea pig brain tissues were used to measure the agonist potency and efficacy of the test compounds. In addition, 14-OMeC6SU was also measured in rat spinal cord and compared to MOR and DOR selective agonists. The agonist properties (EC$_{50}$, E$_{max}$,) of the reference compounds were as expected and as reported previously [20,23]. Additionally, in rat brain tissues we aimed to demonstrate whether U-69593 can produce measurable KOR activity. In accordance with previous work [34] the KOR agonist did not show significant agonist activity (Figure 3A, Table 2) in contrast to guinea pig brain (Figure 3B, Table 2).

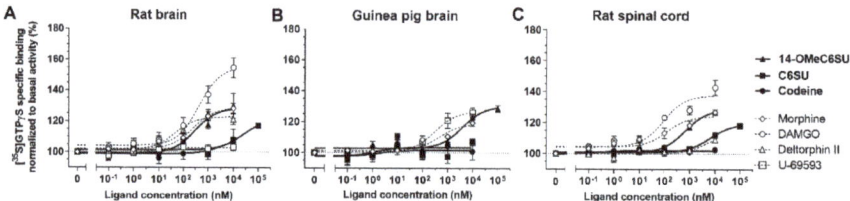

Figure 3. 14-methoxycodeine-6-O-sulfate (14-OMeC6SU) compared to codeine-6-O-sulfate (C6SU) and codeine in [^{35}S]GTPγS binding assays performed in rat (**A**) and guinea pig (**B**) brain and rat spinal cord (**C**) membrane homogenates. For comparison standard μ-, δ- and κ-opioid receptor selective agonists, DAMGO, deltorphin II (Delt II) and U-69593, respectively are also presented. Figures represent the specific binding of [^{35}S]GTPγS in percentage (means ± S.E.M.) in the presence of increasing concentrations (0.1 nM–100 μM) of the indicated ligands. "Total" on the x-axis indicates the basal activity of the monitored G-protein (defined as 100%, its level is presented as a dotted line), which is measured in the absence of the compounds and also represents the total specific binding of [^{35}S]GTPγS. E$_{max}$ and EC$_{50}$ ± S.E.M. values are presented in Table 2.

Table 2. Maximum G-protein efficacy (E_{max}) and potency (EC_{50}) of 14-methoxycodeine-6-O-sulfate (14-OMeC6SU) compared to codeine-6-O-sulfate (C6SU) and codeine in [^{35}S]GTPγS binding assays in rat or guinea pig brain and rat spinal cord membrane homogenates. The table also indicates the μ-, δ- and κ-opioid receptor specific agonists DAMGO, deltorphin II (Delt II) and U-69593, respectively.

Compounds	Tissue Samples (n)	E_{max} ± S.E.M. (%)	EC_{50} ± S.E.M. (nM)
14-OMeC6SU	Rat brain (7)	128.6 ± 3.69	301.1 ± 196.6
	Guinea pig brain (6)	130.2 ± 2.72	>1000
	Rat spinal cord (5)	128.8 ± 1.51	674.2 ± 157.9
C6SU	Rat brain (5)	121 ± 7.27	>10000
	Guinea pig brain (5)	101.7 ± 1.97	N.D.[1]
	Rat spinal cord (5)	119.3 ± 1.81	>1000
Codeine	Rat brain (5)	109.7 ± 11.48	N.D.[1]
	Guinea pig brain (5)	103.6 ± 2.04	N.D.[1]
	Rat spinal cord (4)	102.1 ± 0.49	N.D.[1]
Morphine	Rat brain (7) [2]	128.8 ± 2.66	250 ± 131.7
	Guinea pig brain (5) [3]	119 ± 1.99	461.6 ± 250.1
	Rat spinal cord (7) [2]	124.4 ± 2.09	126 ± 72.37
DAMGO (μ)	Rat brain (7)	155.3 ± 4.98	427 ± 201.9
	Rat spinal cord (5)	137.8 ± 2.65	90.14 ± 40.61
Delt II (δ)	Rat brain (7)	122.9 ± 1.77	44.39 ± 23.51
	Rat spinal cord (3)	113 ± 3.32	>1000
U-69593 (κ)	Rat brain (4)	103 ± 0.84	N.D.[1]
	Guinea pig brain (7)	126.8 ± 3.05	298.3 ± 176.2

[1] not determined, the compound did not alter significantly the basal activity (100%) of the G-protein, thus the EC_{50} value cannot be interpreted (One sample t test, hypothetical value 100%; [2] adopted from [35]; [3] adopted from [23]; * compared to data obtained from guinea pig brain membranes (One-way ANOVA, with Sidak's multiple comparison test, $P < 0.05$)

14-OMeC6SU and DAMGO showed comparable agonist potencies, but 14-OMeC6SU displayed lower E_{max} value than DAMGO (Figure 3, Table 2). On the other hand, 14-OMeC6SU displayed similar agonist efficacy (E_{max}) in rat and guinea pig brain or rat spinal cord tissues, but the potency of the compound was significantly weaker in guinea pig brain membranes (Figure 3, Table 2). C6SU showed partial agonist activity in rat brain or spinal cord and failed to produce agonist effect in guinea pig brain (Figure 3, Table 2). Codeine did not alter G-protein basal activity, thus it did not show agonist activity in any of the investigated samples (Figure 3, Table 2).

14-OMeC6SU showed naloxone reversible effect in rat brain or guinea pig brain, indicating that the test compound produces its effect through the opioid receptors (Table 3).

Table 3. Examining the opioid receptor mediation in G-protein activity ([^{35}S]GTPγS specific binding normalized to basal activity) of 14-OMeC6SU in the presence or absence of 10 μM naloxone in [^{35}S]GTPγS binding assays performed in rat and guinea pig brain membrane homogenates. 14-OMeC6SU was added in 10 and 100 μM in rat and guinea pig brain membranes, respectively.

Compounds	[^{35}S]GTPγS Specific Binding ± S.E.M. (%)	
	Rat Brain	Guinea Pig Brain
14-OMeC6SU	130.1 ± 7.99 (n = 7)	128.7 ± 2.08 (n = 5)
+10 μM naloxone	96.24 ± 4.51 ** (n = 5)	95.84 ± 1.34 *** (n = 5)

* compared to C6SU (unpaired t test, two-tailed P-value, **: $P < 0.01$; ***$P < 0.001$).

2.2. 14-OMeC6SU Is a Full Agonist in MVD and RVD

14-OMeC6SU in a concentration dependent manner, inhibited the mouse vas deferens smooth muscle contractions (Figure 4A). The measured E_{max} (efficacy) was similar to that of DAMGO, however DAMGO was 2 times more potent than 14-OMeC6SU (Table 4, Figure 4A). 14-OMeC6SU showed significant efficacy compared to C6SU, codeine or morphine in inhibition of the contraction of MVD (Table 4, Figure 4A). C6SU, similar to morphine, showed concentration-response curves reaching a ceiling effect in a submaximal range (Table 4, Figure 4A). The EC_{50} of test compounds are presented in Table 4.

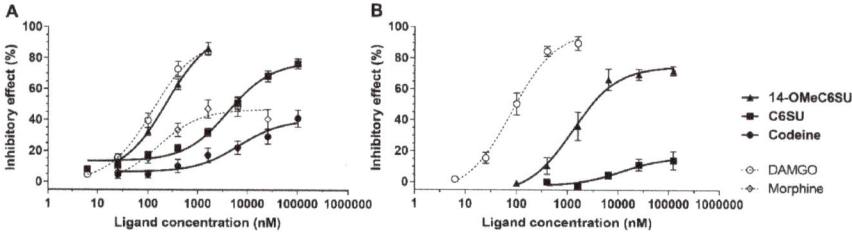

Figure 4. The inhibitory effect of 14-OMeC6SU on electrically evoked contractions of MVD (panel **A**) or RVD (panel **B**) compared to C6SU, codeine, morphine or DAMGO. Data are presented as mean ± S.E.M. The E_{max} and EC_{50} values are presented in Table 4.

Table 4. The agonist activity of 14-OMeC6SU described by maximum efficacy (E_{max}) and ligand potency (EC_{50}) to inhibit electrically evoked mouse vas deferens contractions and rat vas deferens contractions (MVD and RVD, respectively). Results were compared to C6SU, codeine or to prototypic opioid agonists, morphine and DAMGO.

Compounds (n)	E_{max} ± S.E.M. (%)		EC_{50} ± S.E.M. (nM)	
	MVD	RVD	MVD	RVD
14-OMeC6SU (13; 6)	98.31 ± 0.52 ***/###/+++	74.81 ± 2.74 ***/×××/$$$	239.2 ± 6.15 ***/###	>1000
C6SU (10; 5)	77.81 ± 3.11 ###/+++	16.15 ± 3.25 ×××	>1000 ##/+++/×××	>10000
Codeine (5; 4)	40.33 ± 4.69	No effect	>1000	N.D. [2]
Morphine (8; 6) [1]	46.91 ± 3.23	No effect	154.5 ± 93.36	N.D. [2]
DAMGO (8; 5)	91.91 ± 2.97	97.57 ± 4.52	122.4 ± 19.55	79.81 ± 19.61

* compared to C6SU (One-way ANOVA, with Sidak's multiple comparison test, *** $P < 0.001$); # compared to codeine (One-way ANOVA, with Sidak's multiple comparison test, ### $P < 0.001$; ## $P < 0.01$); + compared to morphine (One-way ANOVA, with Sidak's multiple comparison test, +++ $P < 0.001$); × compared to DAMGO (One-way ANOVA, with Sidak's multiple comparison test, ××× $P < 0.001$; ×× $P < 0.01$); $ compared to 14-OMeC6SU in MVD (unpaired t-test, two tailed P value; $$$ $P < 0.001$); [1] adopted from [23]; [2] not determined, since the compounds did not show inhibitory effect.

The opioid receptor type preference of 14-OMeC6SU was assessed in the MVD assay in the presence of naloxone as non-selective opioid antagonist. Furthermore, 14-OMeC6SU receptor preference was also examined in the presence of naltrindole or nor-BNI, selective antagonist for DOR or KOR, respectively. For comparison, the prototype agonists, DAMGO, DPDPE and U-69593 for MOR, DOR and KOR, respectively were also used. The K_e values of the antagonists are presented in Table 5. The obtained K_e values of naloxone against 14-OMeC6SU, C6SU or DAMGO were not significantly different from one another, indicating that the test compounds act on MOR.

In RVD, 14-OMeC6SU produced 74.81 ± 2.74% maximum effect (efficacy), which is significantly less than in MVD bioassay (98.31 ± 0.52%). Statistical analysis revealed that the efficacy of the novel compound significantly decreased compared to DAMGO (E_{max}: 97.57 ± 4.52%), though the fall in the values did not exceed 25% indicating that the novel compound produced substantial efficacy in this organ. On the other hand, the E_{max} of C6SU did not exceed 20%, showing that there was a pronounced drop in the efficacy compared to the novel compound or DAMGO (Table 4, Figure 3B). Morphine and codeine failed to produce any inhibitory effect in RVD. The K_e values of naloxone against 14-OMeC6SU and DAMGO did not differ significantly from each other (Table 5), indicating a MOR-mediated effect.

Table 5. The opioid receptor selectivity of 14-OMeC6SU in electrically evoked contractions of MVD and RVD bioassays compared to C6SU, indicated by the K_e value of selective opioid antagonists. Reference opioid agonists were also measured for control.

	$K_e \pm$ S.E.M. (nM)			
	Naloxone (μ)		Naltrindole (δ)	nor-BNI (κ)
Compounds	MVD	RVD	MVD	MVD
14-OMeC6SU	2.08 ± 0.16 (n = 11)	2.59 ± 0.53 (n = 4)	4.01 ± 1.06 (n = 4)	5.31 ± 1.09 (n = 4)
C6SU	3.25 ± 0.77 (n = 10)	N.D.[1]	2.69 ± 0.93 (n = 4)	3.05 ± 0.89 (n = 6)
DAMGO (μ)	1.8 ± 0.32 (n = 5)	1.87 ± 0.4 (n = 5)	N.D.[1]	N.D.[1]
DPDPE (δ)	N.D.[1]	N.D.[1]	0.63 ± 0.33 (n = 6)	N.D.[1]
U-69593 (κ)	N.D.[1]	N.D.[1]	N.D.[1]	0.33 ± 0.14 (n = 3)

[1] not determined.

2.3. 14-OMeC6SU Produces Antinociceptive Effect in Rat Tail-flick Assay

Following the in vitro characterization, rat tail-flick test as an in vivo thermal pain model was applied to examine the acute antinociceptive effect of 14-OMeC6SU, and to compare it that of C6SU, codeine or morphine. After s.c. administration 14-OMeC6SU showed antinociceptive effect equipotent to morphine and stronger than codeine (Table 6, Figure 5A). The test compounds achieved peak effect at 30 min. C6SU showed weak antinociception displaying a ceiling effect, which did not reach 20% (19.91 ± 2.67 at 26.35 μmol/kg; Figure 5A). ED_{50} values (μmol/kg) of 14-OMeC6SU, codeine and morphine were 5.33, 54.01 and 6.87, respectively (Table 6). Additionally, the antinociceptive effect of 12.21 μmol/kg 14-OMeC6SU (76.42% ± 9.08; n = 10) was completely blocked by co-administered 3.06 μmol/kg naloxone (0.01% ± 5.91; n = 5).

After i.c.v. administration the peak effects of 14-OMeC6SU and morphine were achieved at 10 and 30 min, respectively (Table 7, Figure 5B). Of note, in accordance with previous studies [17], i.c.v. C6SU caused convulsions which hampered the assessment of its antinociception. The ED_{50} values (μmol/animal) of 14-OMeC6SU and morphine were 0.017 and 0.039, respectively (Table 7).

Table 6. Antinociceptive potencies (ED_{50}) of 14-OMeC6SU and codeine against radiant heat induced nociception in rat tail-flick test after 30 and 60 min of s.c. administration. As a reference compound morphine was also indicated.

	ED_{50} (95% Confidence Limit) (μmol/kg)	
	Time After s.c. Administration (min)	
Compounds	30	60
14-OMeC6SU	5.34 [a] (3.14–9.06)	9.88 (7.47–13.06)
Codeine	54.01 [a] (33.97–85.88)	89.86 (61.54–131.2)
Morphine [1]	6.87 [a] (4.59–10.27)	14.17 (10.24–19.62)

[1] [23]; [a] Peak of effect.

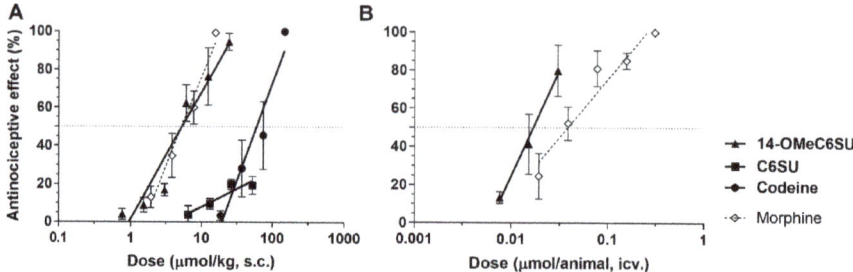

Figure 5. The antinociceptive effect (see Tables 3 and 4) of 14-OMeC6SU, compared to C6SU codeine and morphine in rat tail-flick test after s.c. (**A**) and i.c.v. (**B**) administration. Data represent means ± S.E.M.

Table 7. Antinociceptive potencies (ED_{50}) of 14-OMeC6SU against radiant heat induced nociception in rat tail-flick test after 10, 20 and 30 min of i.c.v. administration. As a reference compound morphine was also indicated. The calculated s.c./i.c.v. ratio of ED_{50} values from Table 6 are also indicated.

	ED_{50} (95% Confidence Limit) (µmol/animal)			
	Time after i.c.v. Administration (min)			ED_{50} s.c./i.c.v. Ratio
Compounds	10	20	30	
14-OMeC6SU	0.017 [a] (0.011–0.026)	0.018 (0.012–0.028)	-	314.12
Morphine	-	0.055[2] (0.032–0.095)	0.039 [a,2] (0.022–0.068)	176.15

[2] [22]; [a] Peak of effect.

2.4. 14-OMeC6SU (in Certain Doses) and C6SU Possess Peripheral Antinociceptive Effects after Systemic Administration in Rats with CFA-Induced Inflammatory Pain

The antinociceptive effect of 14-OMeC6SU was further investigated in CFA-induced inflammatory pain, using Randall-Selitto paw pressure test. The paw pressure threshold (PPT) was reduced in the inflamed right paw by 54.38 ± 1.75 (n = 21) after the 4th day and by 61.59 ± 2.11 (n = 21) after 7th day following CFA treatment. The antinociceptive effect of 14-OMeC6SU was measured in doses of 0.76, 1.52, 3.05, 6.1 and 12.2 µmol/kg, 30 and 60 min after s.c. treatment both in inflamed and noninflamed paws (Figure 6A). 14-OMeC6SU in dose of 6.1 µmol/kg abolished hyperalgesia in the inflamed paws and having no effect on the noninflamed paws, indicating that the effect was localized to the inflamed one (Figure 6A). Furthermore, the antihyperalgesic effect of this dose was abolished by co-administered naloxone methiodide (NAL-M; 10.65 µmol/kg), the peripheral restricted opioid antagonist (Figure 7A). In the applied dose NAL-M failed to affect the pain thresholds of either the inflamed or noninflamed paws (Figure 7A). Higher dose of 14-OMeC6SU (12.2 µmol/kg) produced significant increase in the pain threshold of both inflamed and noninflamed paws after 30 min (Figure 6A), and this effect was partially affected by NAL-M in the inflamed paw (Figure 7A). Since C6SU produced weak antinociception but free of CNS effects such as convulsion in rat tail-flick test after s.c. administration, it was also further investigated in a similar setup. The test doses of s.c. C6SU were 3.3, 6.6 and 13.2 µmol/kg. Similar to 14-OMeC6SU, C6SU reached antinociceptive peak effect after 30 minutes. C6SU in doses of 6.6 and 13.2 µmol/kg produced significant antihyperalgesic action in the inflamed paw and failed to affect the noninflamed paws (Figure 6B). In contrast to 14-OMeC6SU, C6SU at higher doses produced an effect only in the inflamed paw. In addition, the impact of the highest dose of C6SU was reversed by 10.65 µmol/kg NAL-M (Figure 7B). Vehicle failed to affect either the inflamed or noninflamed paws.

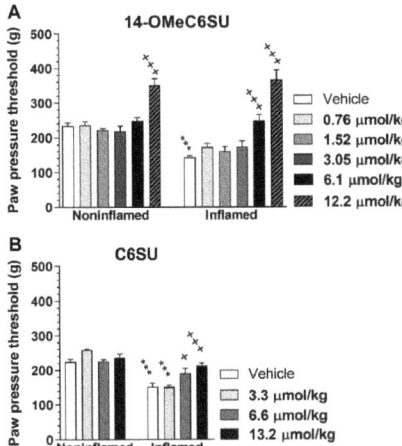

Figure 6. The peak antinociceptive effects of subcutaneously administered 14-OMeC6SU (**A**) and C6SU (**B**) in Complete Freund's Adjuvant (CFA)-induced inflammatory pain. Figures indicate the paw pressure threshold in g-s in the presence of 14-OMeC6SU or C6SU in the indicated dosages 30 min after the injection of the tests compounds. Data represent means ± S.E.M. (n = 5–11 per group). * significant difference between inflamed and noninflamed paw within the corresponding treated group (two-way ANOVA, Sidak's multiple comparisons test). + significant difference compared to inflamed paw of vehicle treated group or compared to vehicle and 14-OMeC6SU 6.1 µmol/kg in the noninflamed (two way ANOVA, Tukey's multiple comparisons test) ***/+++ $P < 0.001$; + $P < 0.05$.

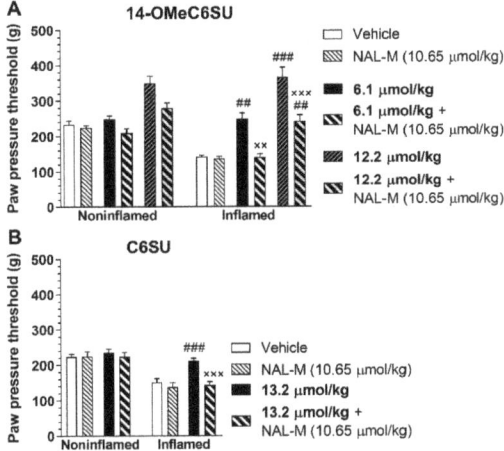

Figure 7. Antagonist action of co-administered naloxone methiodide (NAL-M) on the antinociceptive effect of 14-OMeC6SU (**A**) and C6SU (**B**) in CFA-induced inflammatory pain 30 min after the injection of the compounds. Figures indicate the paw pressure threshold in g-s in the presence of 14-OMeC6SU, C6SU and NAL-M, and in the presence of NAL-M co-administered with 14-OMeC6SU or C6SU in the indicated dosages. Data represent means ± S.E.M. (n = 5–11 per group). # significant difference within the inflamed paw compared to vehicle, NAL-M and to 6.1 µmol/kg 14-OMeC6SU + NAL-M in panel A (two-way ANOVA, Tukey's multiple comparisons test). × significant difference within the inflamed paw compared to the correspondent test compound alone in the appropriate dose (two-way ANOVA, Tukey's multiple comparisons test). ××/## $P < 0.01$; ×××/### $P < 0.001$.

2.5. Inhibitory Effect of Systemic 14-OMeC6SU on Gastrointestinal Transit in Rats

After s.c. administration, 14-OMeC6SU up to 12.2 µmol/kg induced mild, but statistically significant inhibition of the gastrointestinal transit, whereas at higher dose (24.4 µmol/kg) it evoked a marked (~68%) inhibition compared to vehicle (Figure 8A). C6SU displayed significant inhibitory effect only in higher, 52.7 µmol/kg, which effect was comparable to that of 14-OMeC6SU and morphine in 12.2 and 15.54 µmol/kg dose, respectively (Figure 8B). C6SU at a higher, 105.4 µmol/kg dose further inhibited gastrointestinal transit, although the effect was not as strong as seen with 14-OMeC6SU with the highest applied dose (Figure 8A and B). Codeine, similar to C6SU was examined in higher doses, however it showed a more pronounced effect, than C6SU (Figure 8C and B). On the other hand, 148.88 µmol/kg codeine showed a similar level of inhibitory effect with 24.4 µmol/kg 14-OMeC6SU, which is more than a 6-fold difference in the doses (Figure 8C and A). As expected, 31.08 µmol/kg morphine induced pronounced inhibition of the gastrointestinal transit (Figure 8D).

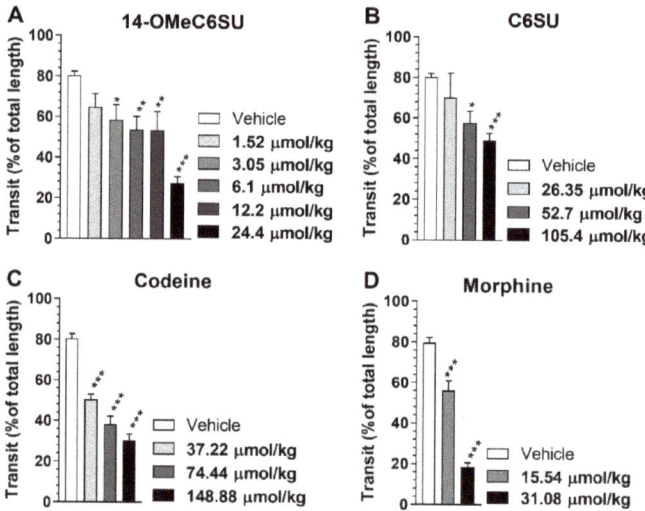

Figure 8. The effect of 14-OMeC6SU (**A**) on rat gastrointestinal transit compared to C6SU (**B**), codeine (**C**) and morphine (**D**). The figure represents the inhibition of gastrointestinal transit in percentage (means ± S.E.M.) of total length compared to vehicle treated group in the presence of 14-OMeC6SU, C6SU and morphine in the indicated dosages. * indicates the significant difference compared to control (One-way ANOVA, Tukey's multiple comparisons post hoc test, $P < 0.001$). * $P < 0.05$; ** $P < 0.01$; *** $P < 0.001$.

3. Discussion

In this study for the first time we present the in vitro and the in vivo pharmacological properties of 14-OMeC6SU applying biochemical, biological (isolated organs), acute and sub chronic pain model assays. We also studied the acute effect of 14-OMeC6SU compared to C6SU or the clinically established analgesic compound, morphine on rat intestinal transit. The in vitro results (affinity, potency and efficacy) are alongside with the superiority of the novel compound, 14-OMeC6SU over C6SU or codeine. Interestingly, results of in vivo studies for C6SU, particularly which obtained in inflammatory pain model or in gastrointestinal transit assay, are of potential benefit in clinical practice: peripheral analgesia and lower gastrointestinal adverse effect compared to 14-OMeC6SU. However, in terms of analgesic potency 14-OMeC6SU was more potent than the C6SU in the applied pain models (thermal and inflammatory pain) under the present experimental circumstances.

In vitro assays were applied to assess the affinity, agonist potency, efficacy and receptor preference (selectivity) of 14-OMeC6SU compared to that of parent or reference compounds. The consequence of the chemical modification, the introduction of methoxy group into the C-14 of C6SU resulted in a significant increase in the efficacy. Taking a backward step, the chemical modification carried on codeine by Zuckerman [17], namely the introduction of -OSO$_3$ into C-6 of codeine has improved both the affinity and the potency, yet limited the CNS access following systemic administration. Nonetheless, both compounds, C6SU and codeine showed very low affinity for DOR (C6SU) and had no measurable affinity for KOR. On the other hand, 14-OMeC6SU beside its affinity for MOR displayed also measurable affinity for DOR and KOR. These results are reflected by the dose ratios produced by naloxone, naltrindole and nor-BNI against 14-OMeC6SU, which were 9, 4 and 5, respectively. Accordingly, 14-OMeC6SU showed the highest affinity for MOR compared to C6SU or codeine and displayed similar binding properties as described in earlier studies, together with codeine [14,17,27]. Our results correspond well with previous data and confirm that the 14-O-methylation of the morphinan structure significantly enhances not only the affinity for MOR, but also for DOR and KOR [4,6,20,22,23]. Other research groups have reported that 14-O-methyl analogs of oxymorphone have improved affinity, agonist activity and antinociceptive potency compared to their parent compound, oxymorphone [36]. Indeed, a positive tremendous impact on the affinity and efficacy of morphine has been achieved following introduction of -OSO$_3$ and O-methyl into C-6 and C-14, respectively [22].

The analgesic efficacy of opioid agonists against acute and subchronic inflammatory pain has been established in broad panel of human studies and rodent pain models. However, the achieved analgesia following systemic administration of currently available opioids in clinical practice is a CNS-mediated action, though a large number of studies carried out on humans and rodents has demonstrated the presence of functionally active peripheral opioid receptors [6,16,37,38]. As a result, substantial research has been undertaken to synthesize a new generation of peripheral opioid receptor agonists free of central adverse effects (respiratory depression, addiction, tolerance, etc.), since the opioid overdose related deaths are stemmed from such mechanisms, particularly respiratory depression. Therefore, it is an unmet medical need that require new inventive tools to solve the current opioid overdose crisis. It can be speculated that opioid ligands with limited CNS penetration may produce analgesia through the activation of opioid receptors reside outside the CNS, namely on sensory neurons at the periphery. Previously, Schmidhammer and Spetea and their coworkers have developed several 14-alkyloxymorphinan and 14-O-methyloxymorphone analogs to improve the pharmacology and safety profile of such compounds [36,39]. A similar strategy was carried out for the synthesis of 14-O-methylmorphin-6-O-sulfate by our group [22] and here for the novel codeine analog, 14-OMeC6SU. Herein, we found that 14-OMeC6SU, codeine and morphine produced dose-dependent antinociception in acute thermal pain model. On the other hand, C6SU showed antinociceptive dose-response curve of ceiling effect (maximum effect was 20%). We can hypothesize that this is due to both the pharmacodynamic and pharmacokinetic properties of C6SU. The former feature reflects the efficacy of C6SU, meaning that it activates the peripheral opioid receptors which can produce only submaximal analgesia. The observed weak antinociceptive response for C6SU is supported by data obtained from experiments carried out in [^{35}S]GTPγS binding assays as well as in the MVD or RVD. For example, in RVD C6SU showed E$_{max}$ (efficacy) that could not exceed 20 percent of response achieved by DAMGO, a highly selective MOR agonist with high efficacy demonstrated in in vitro and in vivo animal experiments [37,40,41].

The latter feature (pharmacokinetic) indicates that the possible access of C6SU into the brain is limited, because the injection of C6SU directly into the brain evoked convulsion observed in our present experiments and also reported by Zuckerman et al. [17]. At the present, we speculate that in the rat tail-flick test, which is an acute thermal pain model and MORs are not undertaken to substantial changes related to their number, the peripheral MOR reserve is not large enough for C6SU to produce stronger analgesic effect. Therefore, based on the above, we further extended our studies to examine the effect of 14-OMeC6SU compared to C6SU in animal pain model whereas the MORs reserve is significantly up-regulated [7,42,43]. Thus, CFA-induced inflammatory pain model suits the prerequisite condition for partial agonists—like C6SU in the present work—because ours and other research groups have reported on increased peripheral MOR expression in the inflamed paw in this model [37]. It is well known, that partial agonists show lower agonist activity than the higher efficacy opioid agonists when the MOR reserve is decreased [40]. Additionally, this pain model is widely used in opioid research to assess the contribution of the peripheral opioid receptors to antinociception [5,44]. Here we found that systemic administration of both 14-OMeC6SU and C6SU abolished the reduced pain threshold of the inflamed paws, indicating the antihyperalgesic effects of the test compounds. Of note, the antihyperalgesic effect of 14-OMeC6SU which is limited to inflamed paw was achieved by two times smaller dose than that achieved by C6SU. This result indicates that the introduction of 14-methoxy in C6SU enhanced the antinociceptive effect in accordance with our and results obtained by Schmidhammer and co-workers [36]. To examine whether this effect is peripherally related, we applied systemic naloxone methiodide, a peripherally acting opioid antagonist [45–47]. Accordingly, 14-OMeC6SU only in 6.1 µmol/kg dose produced naloxone methiodide reversible antihyperalgesic effect. However, co-administered NAL-M failed to antagonize the antihyperalgesic effect of 12.2 µmol/kg 14-OMeC6SU, indicating the involvement of MORs within the CNS. We have paid attention to the chosen dose of NAL-M when we designed the experiments. The 10.65 µmol/kg NAL-M dose was chosen based on results published by Fürst and Schmidhammer groups as well as by Lackó et al. [5,6]. In the work by Fürst et al., the applied NAL-M dose was five times less than we used here and ten times less than used by Lackó et al. [5]. Keeping in mind that the HS-731, a MOR agonist of high efficacy with limited CNS penetration, was proved to be 209 times more potent analgesic agent than morphine after s.c. administration. In the present study applying a similar animal pain model, 14-OMeC6SU produced equivalent analgesia with morphine following s.c. administration. NAL-M at five times lower dose than in the present study as mentioned above, was able to antagonized the effect of the highly potent opioid agonist, HS-731. It therefore is unlikely that the applied NAL-M dose in our study was unable to fully antagonize the higher dose (12.2 µmol/kg) of 14-OMeC6SU, rather than the penetration of 14-OMeC6SU to the CNS [6]. Herein, C6SU in doses of 6.6 µmol/kg and 13.2 µmol/kg reversed the developed hyperalgesia in the inflamed paws and showed no significant impact on the noninflamed paws. Moreover, this effect was sensitive to the co-administered naloxone methiodide, indicating the peripheral mediated effect. In addition, no convulsive effect was observed in agreement with data obtained in the tail-flick test and in contrast to the convulsive effect reported by Zuckerman following i.c.v injection [17]. Of note, C6SU in s.c. dose of 13.2 µmol/kg abolished the CFA-induced hyperalgesia, whereas 105.4 µmol/kg produced weak antinociception (see tail-flick assay). It means that the dose of C6SU that peripherally abolishes hyperalgesia is 8 fold less than the highest dose applied in thermal pain model.

Furthermore, the possible impact of 14-OMeC6SU and C6SU on gastrointestinal transit was also investigated, since the activation of gut opioid receptors is the crucial mechanism involved in the development of constipation [48]. Opioid-induced constipation is a main issue in discontinuing treatment with opioids, though antagonists for reversal of opioid-induced constipation such as methylnaltrexone have been approved [49]. Indeed, peripherally acting opioids of lower inhibitory effect on gastrointestinal transit are a new generation of pain treatment [50]. According to our results, 14-OMeC6SU inhibited gastrointestinal transit more pronounced than C6SU or codeine and it was similar to that of morphine. In fact, among the investigated compounds, C6SU was the least effective in this test, displaying similar gastrointestinal transit inhibition at 9- and 3-fold higher dose compared to that of 14-OMeC6SU and codeine, respectively. In other words, C6SU showed less gastrointestinal side-effect than 14-OMeC6SU, codeine and morphine in terms of opioid-induced constipation following systemic administration and no CNS symptoms—such as convulsion—which have been reported earlier for C6SU following a direct administration to CNS [17]. Nevertheless, opioid agonists of high efficacy such as 14-OMeC6SU and others with limited CNS penetration might offer stronger peripheral analgesia when we are considering different pain types, including those where the peripheral opioid receptor reserve is not altered. Actually, future studies are needed to elucidate whether or not the peripheral analgesic tolerance is developed following chronic administration of high and low efficacy compounds such as 14-OMeC6SU and C6SU, respectively in inflammatory pain. Though according to the researcher's standpoints, high efficacy opioids are favored in terms of tolerance. In general 14-OMeC6SU produced higher agonist efficacy and stronger antinociceptive effect than C6SU. However, C6SU showed less gastrointestinal side-effect.

4. Materials and Methods

4.1. Animals

For mouse vas deferens (MVD) experiments male NMRI mice (35–45 g, 6–10 weeks of age) were used. Further studies were carried out on male Wistar rats weighing 140-240 g (4–7 weeks of age; tail-flick test) and 160–260 g (5–8 weeks of age; rat vas deferens (RVD), CFA and gastrointestinal charcoal meal tests). Mice and rats were obtained from Toxi-Coop Zrt. (Budapest, Hungary) and the Animal House of Semmelweis University (Budapest, Hungary), respectively. Animals were housed in the local animal house of the Department of Pharmacology and Pharmacotherapy, Semmelweis University (Budapest, Hungary).

For in vitro receptor binding assays, male Wistar rats (250–300 g body weight; 6–10 weeks of age) and male guinea pigs (~400–700 g body weight, 4–8 weeks of age; LAL/HA/BR strain) were used. Rats were purchased from and housed in the local animal house of the Biological Research Centre (Szeged, Hungary), guinea pigs were obtained from and housed in LAB-ÁLL Bt. (Budapest, Hungary).

The animals were kept in a temperature controlled room (21–24 °C) under a 12:12 light and dark cycle and were provided with water and food ad libitum. All housing and experiments were handled in accordance with the European Communities Council Directives (2010/63/EU), the Hungarian Act for the Protection of Animals in Research (XXVIII.tv. 32.§) and local animal care committee (PEI/001/276-4/2013). All efforts were made to minimize the number of animals and their suffering.

4.2. Chemicals

Codeine-6-O-sulfate (C6SU) and 14-methoxycodeine-6-O-sulfate (14-OMeC6SU) were synthesized as described under Section 4.3. Tris-HCl, EGTA, NaCl, $MgCl_2 \times 6H_2O$, Na-HCO_3, KCl, KH_2PO_4, glucose, 11.0; $CaCl_2$, GDP, the GTP analog GTPγS, naloxone methiodide and the KOR agonist U-69593 were purchased from Sigma-Aldrich (Budapest, Hungary). The MOR selective agonist enkephalin analog Tyr-D-Ala-Gly-(NMe)Phe-Gly-ol (DAMGO) and the DOR selective agonist deltorphin II (Delt II) were obtained from Bachem Holding AG (Bubendorf, Switzerland). The selective DOR agonist Ile^{5,6}-deltorphin II (IleDelt II) was synthesized in the Laboratory of Chemical Biology group of the Biological Research Centre of the Hungarian Academy of Sciences (Szeged, Hungary). The non-selective opioid receptor antagonist naloxone was kindly provided by the company Endo Laboratories DuPont de Nemours (Wilmington, DE, USA). Morphine and codeine hydrochloride were obtained from Alkaloida-ICN (Tiszavasvári, Hungary). Complete Freund's Adjuvant (CFA), a water-in-oil emulsion of killed mycobacterium, was purchased from Calbiochem (San Diego, CA). For in vitro tests, all ligands were dissolved in water and were stored in 1 mM stock solution at 20 °C. Ligands used for in vivo assays were dissolved in saline prior to the experiments.

The radiolabeled GTP analog, [^{35}S]GTPγS (specific activity: 1250 Ci/mmol) was purchased from PerkinElmer (through Per-form kft., Budapest, Hungary). [^{3}H]DAMGO (specific activity: 38.8 Ci/mmol), [^{3}H]IleDelt II (specific activity: 19,6 Ci/mmol) were radiolabeled by the Laboratory of Chemical Biology group in BRC (Szeged, Hungary). [^{3}H]U-69593 (specific activity: 43,6 Ci/mmol) were purchased from PerkinElmer (through Per-Form Hungária Kft., Budapest, Hungary). The UltimaGold™ MV aqueous scintillation cocktail was purchased from PerkinElmer (through Per-Form Hungária Kft., Budapest, Hungary).

4.3. Chemistry

4.3.1. Synthesis of the Studied Compounds

The preparation of 14-methoxycodeinone was accomplished by the procedure of Kobylecki et al. [51]. 14-hydroxycodeinone was O-alkylated with dimethyl sulfate or methyl iodide in the presence of sodium hydride. The reduction of 14-methoxycodeinone with sodium borohydride in methanol yielded 14-methoxycodeine. It was documented that the sodium borohydride reduction of codeinone or 14-hydroxy-codeinone always proceeds streospecifically resulting in only the 6α-hydroxy derivative of codeine or 14-hydroxy-codeine but never the 6β-isomers. The hydride ion cannot attack from the α-side of the codeinone molecule because of the steric hindrance of ring E (dihydrofuran) oxygen. With the ring E is open, the reduction of 4-hydroxy-7,8-didehydro-morphinan-6-one affords the C-6 epimer secondary alcohols in equal amounts [52,53].

The preparation of 14-methoxycodeine-6-O-sulfate ester was accomplished by our reported method, the sulfation was performed with sulfur trioxide-pyridine complex in pyridine solvent. The structures of codeine-6-O-sulfate and 14-methoxycodeine-6-O-sulfate were elucidated by NMR spectroscopy. It is noteworthy that the influence of C-6 sulfate ester group is significant in the NMR spectrum. For example, the chemical shifts of H-1 and H-2 aromatic protons separate remarkably comparing with the chemical shifts of the parent compounds. In the case of H-5, H-6 and H-7, the resonances of the sulfate esters were deshielded, resulting in a 0.5–1.0 ppm shift compared with the corresponding values of codeine and 14-methoxycodeine. The lower field chemical shifts of the H-5, H-6 and H-7 protons are explained by the electron withdrawing effect of sulfate group [54].

4.3.2. Codeine-6-O-sulfate

Codeine-6-O-sulfate was synthesized using our previously reported method [54]. Codeine (0.90 g, 3.00 mmol) was dissolved in 10 mL anhydrous pyridine. To this solution, pyridine-SO$_3$ complex (1.43 g, 3 equiv.) was added in small portions and the slurry was stirred for 3.5 hours at 60 °C (Figure 9). The crude product precipitated during the reaction as a white powder. Cold water (10 mL) and chloroform (10 mL) were added to the suspension and was kept in the freezer overnight. The precipitate was collected by filtration, washed twice with cold water and crystallized from boiling water to give pure codeine-6-O-sulfate (colorless crystals, 37% crystallized yield). Mass spectra were recorded on Agilent 6410 Triple Quad instrument using electrospray ionization (ESI) and negative polarity. The purity of the samples was determined on HPLC system acetonitril–acetate buffer (0.02 mol, pH = 4.75, 30/70 *v/v*). The purity of codein-6-O-sulfate was > 97%. M.p.: 239–241 °C decomp. (water) $C_{18}H_{21}NO_6S$ ESI MS: 379.

^{1}H-NMR (600 MHz, dmso) δ 9.68 (s, 1H, N-H), 6.74 (d, *J* = 8.2 Hz, 1H, H-2), 6.58 (d, *J* = 8.2 Hz, 1H, H-1), 5.76 (d, *J* = 9.8 Hz, 1H, H-7), 5.32–5.27 (m, 1H, H-8), 4.99 (d, *J* = 6.0 Hz, 1H, H-5), 4.62 (br d, *J* = 2.0 Hz, 1H, H-6), 4.17 (s, 1H, H-9), 3.72 (s, 3H, O-CH$_3$), 3.31 (m, 2H, H-10b, H-16b), 2.92 (s, 3H, N-CH$_3$), 2.86 (s, 1H, H-14), 2.86 (m, 1H, H-16a), 2.78 (m, 1H, H-10a), 2.24 (s, 1H, H-15b), 1.96 (s, 1H, H-15a). ^{13}C-NMR (150 MHz, DMSO-d$_6$): δ = 147.3, 141.9, 132.6, 128.9, 125.5, 123.9, 119.3, 114.0, 89.5, 70.4, 59.5, 56.0, 46.4, 41.6, 40.6, 38.2, 32.6, 20.9.

4.3.3. 14-Methoxycodeine-6-O-sulfate

14-OH-codeinone (3.00 g, 9.10 mmol) was dissolved in anhydrous DMF (15 mL), NaH (0.75 g, 3.5 equiv.) was added in small batches and the resulting slurry was stirred for 1h at rt (Figure 9). Then it was placed on an ice bath and dimethyl sulfate (1.2 mL, ~1.4 equiv.) was added dropwise after which the mixture was stirred for 4h at rt. Water (10 mL) and 25% NH$_4$OH (5 mL) was added, then solvent was evaporated under vacuum. The residue was dissolved in chloroform (100 mL), rinsed with brine, dried over anhydrous Na$_2$SO$_4$ (Figure 9), which was followed by the evaporation of the solvent to yield 14-O-methylcodeinone as a dark red oil. A portion of this crude product (2.15 g, 6.50 mmol) was dissolved in methanol (50 mL) and was placed on an ice bath while NaBH$_4$ (1.5 g, ~6 equiv.) was added in small portions (Figure 9). Then, the resulting mixture was stirred for 2 h at rt. The mixture was made alkaline (pH = 9) by adding K$_2$CO$_3$, then the solvent was evaporated and the residue was taken up in water (50 mL) and extracted with chloroform (3 × 30 mL), rinsed with brine and dried over anhydrous Na$_2$SO$_4$. Removal of the solvent yielded 14-methoxycodeine as a pale yellow oil. This was dissolved in dry pyridine and esterified as described for the synthesis of codeine-6-O-sulfate (Figure 9). The purity of 14-methoxycodein-6-sulfate ester was > 97%. Crude 14-methoxycodeine-6-O-sulfate was crystallized from boiling water to yield 1.5 g pure product (colourless crystals, 59% crystallized yield). M.p. > 285 °C decomp. (water) C$_{19}$H$_{23}$NO$_7$S ESI MS: 409

^{1}H-NMR (600 MHz, DMSO-d6) δ 9.06 (s, 1H, N-H), 6.76 (d, *J* = 8.3 Hz, 1H, H-2), 6.60 (d, *J* = 8.2 Hz, 1H, H-1), 6.07 (dt, *J* = 10.0, 1.7 Hz, 1H, H-7), 5.57 (dd, *J* = 10.0, 3.3 Hz, 1H, H-8), 4.92 (dd, *J* = 6.2, 1.3 Hz, 1H, H-5), 4.86 (ddd, *J* = 5.9, 3.2, 2.1 Hz, 1H, H-6), 4.34 (d, *J* = 6.5 Hz, 1H, H-9), 3.74 (s, 3H, O-CH$_3$), 3.50 (d, *J* = 19.9 Hz, 1H, H-10b), 3.20 (s, 3H, O-CH$_3$), 3.19 (d, *J* = 4.6 Hz, 1H, H-16b), 2.93 (d, *J* = 4.4 Hz, 3H, N-CH$_3$), 2.91–2.81 (m, 2H, H-10a, H-16a), 2.47 (td, *J* = 13.6, 4.9 Hz, 1H, H-15b), 1.86 (dd, *J* = 13.4, 3.7 Hz, 1H, H-15a). ^{13}C-NMR (150 MHz, DMSO-d$_6$): δ = 143.4, 137.4, 136.6, 131.6, 127.7, 125.1, 118.3, 115.9, 89.0, 73.7, 64.8, 56.1, 55.9, 46.4, 44.7, 42.0, 29.3, 28.6, 21.3 ppm.

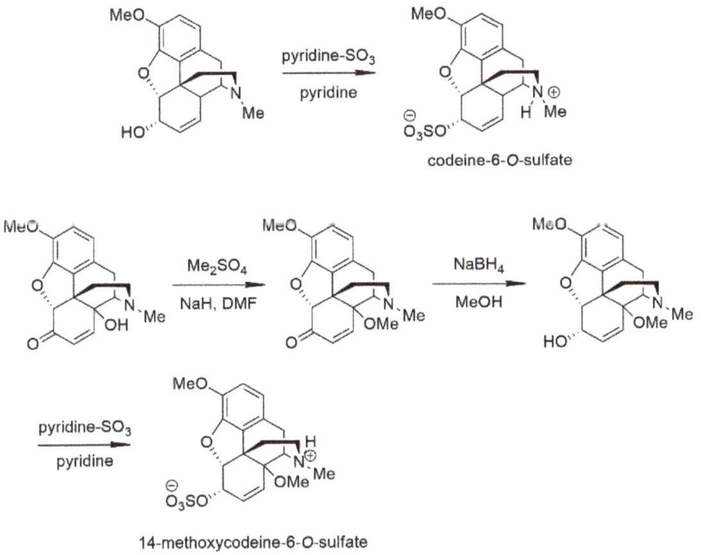

Figure 9. The synthesis of codeine-6-O-sulfate and 14-methoxycodeine-6-O-sulfate. For further details, see Section 4.3.

4.4. Receptor Binding Assays

4.4.1. Membrane Preparations

Animals were decapitated and their brains and spinal cords (from rats only) were quickly removed. The tissue samples were prepared for membrane preparation according to Benyhe and co-workers [55]. Membrane fractions were prepared for competition and [^{35}S]GTPγS binding assays according to Zádor and co-workers [56]. Spinal cord membranes were only used for [^{35}S]GTPγS binding assays. In brief, samples were homogenized and then centrifuged in ice-cold 50 mM Tris-HCl (pH 7.4) buffer and incubated at 37 °C for 30 min in a shaking water-bath. After incubation, the centrifugation was repeated and the final pellet was suspended in 50 mM Tris-HCl pH 7.4 buffer, containing 0.32 M sucrose and stored at −80 °C for further use. For the [^{35}S]GTPγS binding experiments the final pellet of rat/guinea pig brain or spinal cord membrane fractions were suspended in ice-cold TEM (Tris-HCl, EGTA, MgCl$_2$) buffer and stored at −80 °C for further use.

4.4.2. Radioligand Competition Binding Assays

In competition binding assays the affinity of an unlabeled compound is analyzed by measuring radioligand specific binding in the presence of increasing concentrations of the unlabeled test compound [57].

Aliquots of frozen rat and guinea pig brain membrane homogenates were centrifuged (40,000 g, 20 min, 4°C) to remove sucrose and the pellets were suspended in 50 mM Tris-HCl buffer (pH 7.4). Brain membranes homogenates containing 0.3-0.5 mg/mL of protein were incubated in the presence of increasing concentrations (0.1 nM-10 μM) of C6SU, 14-OMeC6SU, codeine or with the equivalent homologues of the radioligands (DAMGO, Ile^{5,6}-deltorphin II and U-69593 for control) with ~ 1-3 nM concentrations of the given radioligand. The incubation temperature and time were based on the correspondent radioligand and were the following: [^{3}H]DAMGO and [^{3}H]Ile^{5,6}-deltorphin II in 35 °C for 45 min, [^{3}H]U-69593 in 30°C for 30 min. Experiments with [^{3}H]U-69593 were performed in guinea pig brain membrane homogenates, since the guinea pig brain has significantly more KORs than the rat brain, while the rest of the radioligands ([^{3}H]DAMGO and [^{3}H]Ile^{5,6}-deltorphin II) were incubated together with rat brain membrane homogenates. Non-specific and total binding was determined in the presence of 10 μM unlabeled naloxone and in the absence of unlabeled compounds, respectively. The reaction was terminated by rapid filtration under vacuum (Brandel M24R Cell Harvester), and washed three times with 5 mL ice-cold 50 mM Tris-HCl through Whatman GF/C ([^{3}H]DAMGO, [^{3}H]Ile^{5,6}-deltorphin II or GF/B ([^{3}H]U-69593) glass fibers (GE Healthcare Life Sciences through Izinta Kft., Budapest, Hungary). The radioactivity of the filters was detected in UltimaGold^{TM} MV aqueous scintillation cocktail with Packard Tricarb 2300TR liquid scintillation counter. The competition binding assays were performed in duplicate and repeated at least three times.

4.4.3. Functional [^{35}S]GTPγS Binding Assays

In [^{35}S]GTPγS binding experiments we measure the GDP→GTP exchange of the G$_{\alpha i/o}$ protein in the presence of the test compound in increasing concentrations to measure ligand potency and the maximal effect (efficacy) of receptors G-protein [58]. The nucleotide exchange is monitored by a radioactive, non-hydrolysable GTP analog, [^{35}S]GTPγS.

The functional [^{35}S]GTPγS binding experiments were performed as previously described [59,60], with modifications. Briefly, the rat or guinea pig brain or rat spinal cord membrane homogenates containing ~10 μg/mL protein were incubated at 30 °C for 60 min in Tris-EGTA buffer (pH 7.4) composed of 50 mM Tris-HCl, 1 mM EGTA, 3 mM MgCl$_2$, 100 mM NaCl. The incubation mixture also contained 0.05 nM [^{35}S]GTPγS and increasing concentrations (0.1 nM-10 μM) of C6SU, 14-OMeC6SU, codeine, morphine, DAMGO, deltorphin II or U-69593 and excess GDP (30 μM) in a final volume of 1 mL. Experiments examining KOR activity were performed only with guinea pig brain membrane homogenates. To demonstrate the low reserve of KORs in rat brain, U-69593 was measured in these samples in the same experimental set up as described above. Finally, specific binding of [^{35}S]GTPγS was also measured in the combination of 10 or 100 μM of 14-OMeC6SU in rat, or guinea pig brains, respectively with 10 μM naloxone.

Total binding was measured in the absence of test compounds, while non-specific binding was determined in the presence of 10 μM unlabeled GTPγS. The bound and unbound [^{35}S]GTPγS were separated as described in previous section through Whatmann GF/B glass fibers (GE Healthcare Life Sciences through Izinta Kft., Budapest, Hungary). The radioactivity of the filters was also detected as described in the previous section. [^{35}S]GTPγS binding experiments were performed in triplicates and repeated at least three times.

4.5. Isolated Organs

4.5.1. Mouse vas Deferens (MVD)

Vasa deferentia were taken out from male mice. The preparation and the experimental procedures were done as described previously [61]. Briefly, *vasa deferentia* were cleaned out from tissues and suspended between two electrodes in organ baths of 5mL volume with 0.1g initial tension. The upper and the lower electrodes have ring and straight form, respectively. The organ baths were filled with Mg^{2+} free Krebs solution, of the following composition (mM/L): NaCl, 118.0; $Na-HCO_3$, 25.0; KCl, 4.7; KH_2PO_4, 1.2; glucose, 11.0; $CaCl_2$, 2.5 aerated with carbogen (95% O_2 + 5% CO_2) and kept at 31°C. The stimulation parameters were as follows: field stimulation, pairs (100 ms pulse distance) of rectangular impulses (1 ms pulse width, 9V/cm i.e., supramaximal intensity) were repeated by 10 s. The muscle contractions were monitored by LabChart 6.0 software.

4.5.2. Rat vas Deferens (RVD)

Vasa deferentia were removed from Wistar male rats and the experimental procedure was as described for MVD, with the following modifications: use of Krebs solution with Mg^{2+}, 0.5 g initial tension and the electrical field stimulation (pulse width,1 ms; intensity, 9 V/cm) was delivered at 0.1 Hz frequency.

4.5.3. Experimental Paradigms of MVD and RVD

The experimental paradigm was similar as described previously [22]. Briefly, after the equilibration time (30-40 min and 90-120 min for MVD and RVD, respectively) the first dose of agonist was added and the concentration-effect curves were constructed in a cumulative manner. After that the preparations were washed and allowed to regain their pre-drug twitch height. Then *vasa deferentia* were equilibrated with antagonist for 20 min, and without washing a single concentration of agonist was added. In some experiments antagonists were added cumulatively followed by 20 min equilibration time. To determine dissociation constants of the antagonist, dose ratio (DR) values were obtained by the single-dose method described by Kosterlitz and Watt [62].

4.6. Thermal Acute Pain Model (Tail-flick Test)

The rat tail-flick test was performed in order to analyze the acute antinociceptive effect of 14-OMeC6SU and C6SU. The test compounds were dissolved in saline and administered subcutaneously (s.c.) or intracerebroventricularly (i.c.v.) as previously described [6]. Drugs or saline delivered in a volume of 2.5 mL/kg for s.c. administration (under skin over the neck), 10 µL/rat for i.c.v. injections. The experiments were carried out as described earlier [63]. Briefly, a beam of light was focused onto the dorsum of the lower third of the rat tail. Then, the time latencies until the rats flick their tails were determined before (baseline) and after injection of the test compounds. Eight seconds was used as a cut off time in order to avoid tissue damage. The antinociceptive activity was assessed 30 and 60 min after s.c. drug administration and 10, 20 and 30 min after i.c.v. administration.

4.7. Inflammatory Pain Model (CFA-Evoked Hyperalgesia)

For inducing inflammation, rats were injected intraplantarly (i.pl.) on the right hind paw under brief isoflurane (Sigma-Aldrich, Budapest, Hungary) anaesthesia with 150 µL CFA as described previously [5]. This treatment consistently produces localized inflammation of the inoculated paw, characterized by an increase in paw volume, paw temperature and infiltration with various types of immune cells [64]. Following the 4th and 7th day after the i.pl. CFA injection, baseline (to pretest compound) paw pressure thresholds (PPTs) of the inflamed and noninflamed paws were determined by paw pressure algesiometry (modified Randall–Selitto test; Ugo Basile, Comerio, Italy) as described in detail previously [37,65]. PPTs were then re-evaluated at 30 and 60 min after s.c. drug administration in the indicated dosages, using an arbitrary cut-off weight of twice the control and expressed in grams. Additionally, the peak effect dosage of the given test compound was blocked by the peripheral restricted naloxone methiodide to assert the peripheral opioid receptor mediation.

4.8. Determination the Effect of Test Compounds on Gastrointestinal Transit

In order to determine the effect of 14-OMeC6SU and C6SU on the gastrointestinal transit and to compare to that of codeine and morphine, the charcoal meal test was applied in rats, as described before [23]. Briefly, male Wistar rats were fasted 18 h prior to the experiments, with free access to water. After the fasting period, a charcoal suspension (10% charcoal in 5% gum arabic) was given in a volume of 2 mL/animal by an oral gavage. A total of 30 min later the rats were euthanized, their entire small intestines were removed and the distance travelled by the charcoal suspension was measured and compared to the total length of small intestine. 14-OMeC6SU, C6SU, codeine and morphine were given s.c. at various doses, in a volume of 0.25 mL/100 g, 30 min before the application of the charcoal suspension and 60 min before the assessment of distance of the charcoal travel. The applied doses were based on those used in the rat tail-flick test and considering the time-lag.

4.9. Data Analysis

4.9.1. Receptor Binding Assays

The specific binding of the radiolabeled compound ([^{3}H]ligand, [^{35}S]GTPγS) was calculated by the subtraction the level of non-specific binding from the level of total binding and was given in percentage. Data were normalized to total specific binding, settled 100%, which in case of [^{35}S]GTPγS also represents the level of basal activity of the G-protein. The means ± S.E.M. of data sets were plotted in the function of the applied ligand concentration range in logarithm form and were fitted with the professional curve fitting program, GraphPad Prism 5.0 (GraphPad Prism Software Inc., San Diego, CA), using non-linear regression. In the radioligand competition binding assays the 'Dose-response - Inhibition' equation was applied to determine IC_{50} (unlabeled ligand affinity) and to further calculate the inhibitory constant (K_i) value according to the Cheng-Prusoff equation [66]. Selectivity ratios were calculated based on the K_i values. In case of [^{35}S]GTPγS binding assays the 'Dose-response - Stimulation' equation was applied to obtain the maximum G-protein efficacy (E_{max}) and ligand potency (EC_{50}), respectively.

For two data sets unpaired Student's t test with two-tailed P value for more than two data sets One-way ANOVA, with Holm-Sidak's multiple comparison test was used. One sample t-test with a hypothetical value of 100% was applied when given specific binding values were compared to total specific binding (100%) in receptor binding assays. Statistical analysis was performed with GraphPad Prism 5.0 program; significance was accepted at $P < 0.05$ level.

4.9.2. MVD and RVD Bioassays

The means ± S.E.M. of data sets were plotted in the function of the applied ligand concentration range in logarithm form and were fitted with non-linear regression in GraphPad Prism 5.0 (GraphPad Prism Software Inc., San Diego, CA), using 'Dose-response-Stimulation' equation. From the concentration-response curves the 50% effective concentration (EC_{50}) and maximal effect (E_{max}) were determined. In MVD, the equilibrium dissociation constant of naloxone (K_e) of opioid receptor selective antagonist, naloxone (MOR), naltrindole (DOR) and nor-BNI (KOR) were also calculated in the presence of the test compounds with the single-dose method as described previously [62]. Antagonist affinities (K_e) were calculated as follows: Ke = [antagonist concentration]/[dose ratio]-1.

4.9.3. Rat Tail-flick Test, Gastrointestinal Transit and CFA-Evoked Hyperalgesia Tests

In RTF test, after the dose-response curves were constructed the dose necessary to produce a 50% effect (ED_{50}) and 95% confidence limits were calculated by the Litchfield–Wilcoxon method [67].

In case of gastrointestinal transit test the distance travelled by the charcoal suspension was expressed as a percentage of total small intestine length. Significance was determined by One-way ANOVA with Tukey's multiple comparisons test. In CFA-evoked hyperalgesia test results between and within noninflamed-inflamed group were compared with two-way ANOVA using Sidak's or Tukey's multiple comparisons test, respectively. Statistical analysis for the described experiments here were performed with GraphPad Prism 5.0 program, while the significance level was accepted at $P < 0.05$.

5. Conclusions

14-OMeC6SU proved to be a MOR agonist of higher antinociceptive potency and efficacy, than the parent compound C6SU or codeine. Systemic C6SU has an antinociceptive effect of ceiling pattern in thermal pain model. 14-OMeC6SU in certain doses showed peripheral antihyperalgesic effect in the inflammatory pain model. Despite the analgesic ceiling effect of systemic C6SU compared to 14-OMeC6SU, codeine or morphine in thermal pain model under present experimental conditions, C6SU showed peripheral antihyperalgesic effect with fewer gastrointestinal side effects.

Author Contributions: Conceptualization, M.A.-K., Z.S.Z., K.K., M.B., F.Z.; methodology, M.A-K., K.K., Z.S.Z., M.B., F.Z., S.H.; validation, M.A.-K., Z.S.Z., M.B., K.K., F.Z.; formal analysis, F.Z., M.B., S.B. (Szilvia Barsi), Z.S.Z., B.H., S.B.L.; investigation, S.B. (Szilvia Barsi), A.R.G., F.Z., M.B., A.M., S.B.L., B.H., A.V., M.A.-K.; resources, A.R.G., A.M., F.Z., B.H., S.B.L.; writing—original draft preparation, M.A.-K., F.Z., Z.S.Z.; writing—review and editing, M.A.-K., F.Z., Z.S.Z., K.K., M.B., P.R., S.B. (Sándor Benyh), S.F., A.V., S.H.; visualization, F.Z., M.A.-K.; supervision, M.A.-K., K.K.,Z.S.Z.; project administration, M.A.-K., Z.S.Z., F.Z.; funding acquisition, M.A.-K., Z.S.Z., S.B. (Sándor Benyh). All authors have read and agreed to the published version of the manuscript.

Funding: This work was supported by Higher Education Institutional Excellence Programme of the Ministry of Human Capacities in Hungary, within the framework of the Neurology Thematic Programme of Semmelweis University (FIKP, 2018) and by the National Research, Development and Innovation Office of Hungary (NKFI FK 124878) and by the Economic Development and Innovation Operational Programme (GINOP 2.3.2-15-2016-00034).

Acknowledgments: The authors would like to acknowledge the assistance of lab manager Veronika Pol-Maruzs.

Conflicts of Interest: The authors declare no conflict of interest.

References

1. Burford, N.; Wang, D.; Sadee, W. G-protein coupling of mu-opioid receptors (OP3): Elevated basal signalling activity. *Biochem. J.* **2000**, *537*, 531–537. [CrossRef]
2. Koneru, A.; Satyanarayana, S.; Rizwan, S. Endogenous opioids: Their physiological role and receptors. *Glob. J Pharmacol.* **2009**, *3*, 149–153.
3. Perret, D.; Luo, Z. Targeting voltage-gated calcium channels for neuropathic pain management. *Neurotherapeutics* **2009**, *6*, 679–692. [CrossRef]
4. Khalefa, B.I.; Mousa, S.A.; Shaqura, M.; Lackó, E.; Hosztafi, S.; Riba, P.; Schäfer, M.; Ferdinandy, P.; Fürst, S.; Al-Khrasani, M. Peripheral antinociceptive efficacy and potency of a novel opioid compound 14-O-MeM6SU in comparison to known peptide and non-peptide opioid agonists in a rat model of inflammatory pain. *Eur. J. Pharmacol.* **2013**, *713*, 54–57. [CrossRef]
5. Lackó, E.; Riba, P.; Giricz, Z.; Váradi, A.; Cornic, L.; Balogh, M.; Király, K.; Csekő, K.; Mousa, S.A.; Hosztafi, S.; et al. New Morphine Analogs Produce Peripheral Antinociception within a Certain Dose Range of Their Systemic Administration. *J. Pharmacol. Exp. Ther.* **2016**, *359*, 171–181. [CrossRef]
6. Fürst, S.; Riba, P.; Friedmann, T.; Tímár, J.; Al-Khrasani, M.; Obara, I.; Makuch, W.; Spetea, M.; Schütz, J.; Przewlocki, R.; et al. Peripheral versus central antinociceptive actions of 6-amino acid-substituted derivatives of 14-O-methyloxymorphone in acute and inflammatory pain in the rat. *J. Pharmacol. Exp. Ther.* **2005**, *312*, 609–618. [CrossRef]
7. Balogh, M.; Zádori, Z.S.; Lázár, B.; Karádi, D.; László, S.; Mousa, S.A.; Hosztafi, S.; Zádor, F.; Riba, P.; Schäfer, M.; et al. The Peripheral Versus Central Antinociception of a Novel Opioid Agonist: Acute Inflammatory Pain in Rats. *Neurochem. Res.* **2018**, *43*, 1250–1257. [CrossRef]
8. Joris, J.L.; Dubner, R.; Hargreaves, K.M. Opioid analgesia at peripheral sites: A target for opioids released during stress and inflammation? *Anesth. Analg.* **1987**, *66*, 1277–1281. [CrossRef]

9. Ferreira, S.H.; Nakamura, M. II - Prostaglandin hyperalgesia: The peripheral analgesic activity of morphine, enkephalins and opioid antagonists. *Prostaglandins* **1979**, *18*, 191–200. [CrossRef]
10. McDougall, J.J. Peripheral analgesia: Hitting pain where it hurts. *Biochim. Biophys. Acta Mol. Basis Dis.* **2011**, *1812*, 459–467. [CrossRef]
11. Kosterlitz, H.W.; Waterfield, A.A. In Vitro Models in the Study of Structure-Activity Relationships of Narcotic Analgesics. *Annu. Rev. Pharmacol.* **1975**, *15*, 29–47. [CrossRef]
12. Mazak, K.; Noszal, B.; Hosztafi, S. Physicochemical and Pharmacological Characterization of Permanently Charged Opioids. *Curr. Med. Chem.* **2017**, *24*, 3633–3648. [CrossRef]
13. Preechagoon, D.; Brereton, I.; Staatz, C.; Prankerd, R. Ester prodrugs of a potent analgesic, morphine-6-sulfate: Syntheses, spectroscopic and physicochemical properties. *Int. J. Pharm.* **1998**, *163*, 177–190. [CrossRef]
14. Crooks, P.A.; Kottayil, S.G.; Al-Ghananeem, A.M.; Byrn, S.R.; Allan Butterfield, D. Opiate receptor binding properties of morphine-, dihydromorphine-, and codeine 6-O-sulfate ester congeners. *Bioorg. Med. Chem. Lett.* **2006**, *16*, 4291–4295. [CrossRef]
15. Schmidhammer, H.; Spetea, M.; Windisch, P.; Schütz, J.; Riba, P.; Al-Khrasani, M.; Furst, S. Functionalization of the Carbonyl Group in Position 6 of Morphinan-6-ones. Development of Novel 6-Amino and 6-Guanidino Substituted 14-Alkoxymorphinans. *Curr. Pharm. Des.* **2014**, *19*, 7391–7399. [CrossRef]
16. Al-Khrasani, M.; Spetea, M.; Friedmann, T.; Riba, P.; Király, K.; Schmidhammer, H.; Furst, S. DAMGO and 6β-glycine substituted 14-O-methyloxymorphone but not morphine show peripheral, preemptive antinociception after systemic administration in a mouse visceral pain model and high intrinsic efficacy in the isolated rat vas deferens. *Brain Res. Bull.* **2007**, *74*, 369–375. [CrossRef]
17. Zuckerman, A.; Bolan, E.; de Paulis, T.; Schmidt, D.; Spector, S.; Pasternak, G.W. Pharmacological characterization of morphine-6-sulfate and codeine-6-sulfate. *Brain Res.* **1999**, *842*, 1–5. [CrossRef]
18. Brown, C.E.; Roerig, S.C.; Burger, V.T.; Cody, R.B.; Fujimoto, J.M. Analgesic Potencies of Morphine 3- and 6-Sulfates After Intracerebroventricular Administration in Mice: Relationship to Structural Characteristics Defined by Mass Spectrometry and Nuclear Magnetic Resonance. *J. Pharm. Sci.* **1985**, *74*, 821–824. [CrossRef]
19. Mori, M.; Oguri, K.; Yoshimura, H.; Shimomura, K.; Kamata, O.; Ueki, S. Chemical synthesis and analgesic effect of morphine ethereal sulfates. *Life Sci. I.* **1972**, *11*, 525–533. [CrossRef]
20. Spetea, M.; Friedmann, T.; Riba, P.; Schütz, J.; Wunder, G.; Langer, T.; Schmidhammer, H.; Fürst, S. In vitro opioid activity profiles of 6-amino acid substituted derivatives of 14-O-methyloxymorphone. *Eur. J. Pharmacol.* **2004**, *483*, 301–308. [CrossRef]
21. Holtman, J.R.; Crooks, P.A.; Johnson-Hardy, J.; Wala, E.P. Antinociceptive effects and toxicity of morphine-6-O-sulfate sodium salt in rat models of pain. *Eur. J. Pharmacol.* **2010**, *648*, 87–94. [CrossRef]
22. Lacko, E.; Varadi, A.; Rapavi, R.; Zador, F.; Riba, P.; Benyhe, S.; Borsodi, A.; Hosztafi, S.; Timar, J.; Noszal, B.; et al. A novel μ-opioid receptor ligand with high in vitro and in vivo agonist efficacy. *Curr Med Chem* **2012**, *19*, 4699–4707. [CrossRef]
23. Zádor, F.; Balogh, M.; Váradi, A.; Zádori, Z.S.; Király, K.; Szűcs, E.; Varga, B.; Lázár, B.; Hosztafi, S.; Riba, P.; et al. 14-O-Methylmorphine: A Novel Selective Mu-Opioid Receptor Agonist with High Efficacy and Affinity. *Eur. J. Pharmacol.* **2017**, *814*, 264–273. [CrossRef]
24. Chidambaran, V.; Sadhasivam, S.; Mahmoud, M. Codeine and opioid metabolism: Implications and alternatives for pediatric pain management. *Curr. Opin. Anaesthesiol.* **2017**, *30*, 349–356. [CrossRef]
25. Hennies, H.H.; Friderichs, E.; Schneider, J. Receptor binding, analgesic and antitussive potency of tramadol and other selected opioids. *Arzneimittelforschung.* **1988**, *38*, 877–880.
26. Neil, A. Affinities of some common opioid analgesics towards four binding sites in mouse brain. *Naunyn. Schmiedebergs. Arch. Pharmacol.* **1984**, *328*, 24–29. [CrossRef]
27. Mignat, C.; Wille, U.; Ziegler, A. Affinity profiles of morphine, codeine, dihydrocodeine and their glucuronides at opioid receptor subtypes. *Life Sci.* **1995**, *56*, 793–799. [CrossRef]
28. Chen, Z.R.; Irvine, R.J.; Somogyi, A.A.; Bochner, F. Mu receptor binding of some commonly used opioids and their metabolites. *Life Sci.* **1991**, *48*, 2165–2171. [CrossRef]
29. Peechakara, B.V.; Gupta, M. *Codeine*; StatPearls Publishing: Treasure Island, FL, USA, 2019. Available online: https://www.ncbi.nlm.nih.gov/books/NBK526029/ (accessed on 17 March 2020).
30. Nielsen, S.; MacDonald, T.; Johnson, J.L. Identifying and treating codeine dependence: A systematic review. *Med. J. Aust.* **2018**, *208*, 451–461. [CrossRef]

31. Moore, R.A.; McQuay, H.J. Prevalence of opioid adverse events in chronic non-malignant pain: Systematic review of randomised trials of oral opioids. *Arthritis Res. Ther.* **2005**, *7*, R1046–R1051. [CrossRef]
32. Benyamin, R.; Trescot, A.M.; Datta, S.; Buenaventura, R.; Adlaka, R.; Sehgal, N.; Glaser, S.E.; Vallejo, R. Opioid complications and side effects. *Pain Physician.* **2008**, *11*, S105–S120.
33. Vowles, K.E.; McEntee, M.L.; Julnes, P.S.; Frohe, T.; Ney, J.P.; van der Goes, D.N. Rates of opioid misuse, abuse, and addiction in chronic pain. *Pain* **2015**, *156*, 569–576. [CrossRef]
34. Thomasy, S.M.; Moeller, B.C.; Stanley, S.D. Comparison of opioid receptor binding in horse, guinea pig, and rat cerebral cortex and cerebellum. *Vet. Anaesth. Analg.* **2007**, *34*, 351–358. [CrossRef]
35. Balogh, M.; Zádor, F.; Zádori, Z.S.; Shaqura, M.; Király, K.; Mohammadzadeh, A.; Varga, B.; Lázár, B.; Mousa, S.A.; Hosztafi, S.; et al. Efficacy-Based Perspective to Overcome Reduced Opioid Analgesia of Advanced Painful Diabetic Neuropathy in Rats. *Front. Pharmacol.* **2019**, *10*, 347. [CrossRef]
36. Schmidhammer, H.; Aeppli, L.; Atwell, L.; Fritsch, F.; Jacobson, A.E.; Nebuchla, M.; Sperk, G. Synthesis and biological evaluation of 14-alkoxymorphinans. 1. Highly potent opioid agonists in the series of (-)-14-methoxy-N-methylmorphinan-6-ones. *J. Med. Chem.* **1984**, *27*, 1575–1579. [CrossRef]
37. Khalefa, B.I.; Shaqura, M.; Al-Khrasani, M.; Fürst, S.; Mousa, S.A.; Schäfer, M. Relative contributions of peripheral versus supraspinal or spinal opioid receptors to the antinociception of systemic opioids. *Eur. J. Pain* **2012**, *16*, 690–705. [CrossRef]
38. Stein, C. Targeting pain and inflammation by peripherally acting opioids. *Front. Pharmacol.* **2013**, *4*, 123. [CrossRef]
39. Spetea, M.; Schmidhammer, H. Recent advances in the development of 14-alkoxy substituted morphinans as potent and safer opioid analgesics. *Curr. Med. Chem.* **2012**, *19*, 2442–2457. [CrossRef]
40. Al-Khrasani, M.; Orosz, G.; Kocsis, L.; Farkas, V.; Magyar, A.; Lengyel, I.; Benyhe, S.; Borsodi, A.; Rónai, A.Z. Receptor constants for endomorphin-1 and endomorphin-1-ol indicate differences in efficacy and receptor occupancy. *Eur. J. Pharmacol.* **2001**, *421*, 61–67. [CrossRef]
41. Koch, T.; Widera, A.; Bartzsch, K.; Schulz, S.; Brandenburg, L.O.; Wundrack, N.; Beyer, A.; Grecksch, G.; Höllt, V. Receptor Endocytosis Counteracts the Development of Opioid Tolerance. *Mol. Pharmacol.* **2005**, *67*, 280–287. [CrossRef]
42. Stein, C.; Machelska, H.; Binder, W.; Schäfer, M. Peripheral opioid analgesia. *Curr. Opin. Pharmacol.* **2001**, *1*, 62–65. [CrossRef]
43. Stein, C.; Lang, L.J. Peripheral mechanisms of opioid analgesia. *Curr. Opin. Pharmacol.* **2009**, *9*, 3–8. [CrossRef]
44. Schäfer, M.; Imai, Y.; Uhl, G.R.; Stein, C. Inflammation enhances peripheral μ-opioid receptor-mediated analgesia, but not μ-opioid receptor transcription in dorsal root ganglia. *Eur. J. Pharmacol.* **1995**, *279*, 165–169. [CrossRef]
45. Bianchi, G.; Fiocchi, R.; Tavani, A.; Manara, L. Quaternary narcotic antagonists' relative ability to prevent antinociception and gastrointestinal transit inhibition in morphine-treated rats as an index of peripheral selectivity. *Life Sci.* **1982**, *30*, 1875–1883. [CrossRef]
46. Lewanowitsch, T.; Irvine, R.J. Naloxone methiodide reverses opioid-induced respiratory depression and analgesia without withdrawal. *Eur. J. Pharmacol.* **2002**, *445*, 61–67. [CrossRef]
47. Riba, P.; Ben, Y.; Nguyen, T.M.-D.; Furst, S.; Schiller, P.W.; Lee, N.M. [Dmt(1)]DALDA is highly selective and potent at mu opioid receptors, but is not cross-tolerant with systemic morphine. *Curr. Med. Chem.* **2002**, *9*, 31–39. [CrossRef]
48. Holzer, P. Opioid receptors in the gastrointestinal tract. *Regul. Pept.* **2009**, *155*, 11–17. [CrossRef]
49. Mehta, N.; O'Connell, K.; Giambrone, G.; Baqai, A.; Diwan, S. Efficacy of Methylnaltrexone for the Treatment of Opiod-Induced Constipation: A Meta-Analysis and Systematic Review. *Postgrad. Med.* **2016**, *128*, 282–289. [CrossRef]
50. Pergolizzi, J.V.; Raffa, R.B.; Pappagallo, M.; Fleischer, C.; Pergolizzi, J.; Zampogna, G.; Duval, E.; Hishmeh, J.; LeQuang, J.A.; Taylor, R.; et al. Peripherally acting μ-opioid receptor antagonists as treatment options for constipation in noncancer pain patients on chronic opioid therapy. *Patient Prefer. Adherence* **2017**, *11*, 107–119. [CrossRef]
51. Kobylecki, R.J.; Carling, R.W.; Lord, J.A.; Smith, C.F.; Lane, A.C. Common anionic receptor site hypothesis: Its relevance to the antagonist action of naloxone. *J. Med. Chem.* **1982**, *25*, 116–120. [CrossRef]

52. Currie, A.C.; Gillon, J.; Newbold, G.T.; Spring, F.S. 157. Some reactions of 14-hydroxycodeine. *J. Chem. Soc.* **1960**, 773–781. [CrossRef]
53. Sawa, Y.K.; Horiuchi, M.; Tanaka, K. Elimination of the 4-hydroxyl group of the alkaloids related to morphine—IX: Synthesis of 3-methoxy-n-methylisomorphinan derivatives. *Tetrahedron* **1968**, *24*, 255–260. [CrossRef]
54. Váradi, A.; Gergely, A.; Béni, S.; Jankovics, P.; Noszál, B.; Hosztafi, S. Sulfate esters of morphine derivatives: Synthesis and characterization. *Eur. J. Pharm. Sci.* **2011**, *42*, 65–72. [CrossRef]
55. Benyhe, S.; Farkas, J.; Tóth, G.; Wollemann, M. Met5-enkephalin-Arg6-Phe7, an endogenous neuropeptide, binds to multiple opioid and nonopioid sites in rat brain. *J. Neurosci. Res.* **1997**, *48*, 249–258. [CrossRef]
56. Zádor, F.; Kocsis, D.; Borsodi, A.; Benyhe, S. Micromolar concentrations of rimonabant directly inhibits delta opioid receptor specific ligand binding and agonist-induced G-protein activity. *Neurochem. Int.* **2014**, *67*, 14–22. [CrossRef]
57. Frey, K.A.; Albin, R.L. Receptor Binding Techniques. *Curr. Protoc. Neurosci.* **1997**, *1*, 1–4. [CrossRef]
58. Strange, P.G. Use of the GTPγS ([35S]GTPγS and Eu-GTPγS) binding assay for analysis of ligand potency and efficacy at G protein-coupled receptors. *Br. J. Pharmacol.* **2010**, *161*, 1238–1249. [CrossRef]
59. Selley, D.E.; Sim, L.J.; Xiao, R.; Liu, Q.; Childers, S.R. mu-Opioid receptor-stimulated guanosine-5'-O-(gamma-thio)-triphosphate binding in rat thalamus and cultured cell lines: Signal transduction mechanisms underlying agonist efficacy. *Mol. Pharmacol.* **1997**, *51*, 87–96. [CrossRef]
60. Traynor, J.; Nahorski, S. Modulation by mu-opioid agonists of guanosine-5'-O-(3-[^{35}S]thio)triphosphate binding to membranes from human neuroblastoma SH-SY5Y cells. *Mol. Pharmacol.* **1995**, *47*, 848–854.
61. Rónai, A.Z.; Gráf, L.; Székely, J.I.; Dunai-Kovács, Z.; Bajusz, S. Differential behaviour of LPH-(61-91)-peptide in different model systems: Comparison of the opioid activities of LPH-(61-91)-peptide and its fragments. *FEBS Lett.* **1977**, *74*, 182–184. [CrossRef]
62. Kosterlitz, H.W.; Watt, A.J. Kinetic parameters of narcotic agonists and antagonists, with particular reference to N-allylnoroxymorphone (naloxone). *Br. J. Pharmacol. Chemother.* **1968**, *33*, 266–276. [CrossRef]
63. Fürst, Z.; Búzás, B.; Friedmann, T.; Schmidhammer, H.; Borsodi, A. Highly potent novel opioid receptor agonist in the 14-alkoxymetopon series. *Eur. J. Pharmacol.* **1993**, *236*, 209–215. [CrossRef]
64. Rittner, H.L.; Brack, A.; Machelska, H.; Mousa, S.A.; Bauer, M.; Schäfer, M.; Stein, C. Opioid Peptide–expressing Leukocytes. *Anesthesiology* **2001**, *95*, 500–508. [CrossRef]
65. Mousa, S.A.; Cheppudira, B.P.; Shaqura, M.; Fischer, O.; Hofmann, J.; Hellweg, R.; Schafer, M. Nerve growth factor governs the enhanced ability of opioids to suppress inflammatory pain. *Brain* **2007**, *130*, 502–513. [CrossRef]
66. Cheng, Y.; Prusoff, W.H. Relationship between the inhibition constant (K1) and the concentration of inhibitor which causes 50 per cent inhibition (I50) of an enzymatic reaction. *Biochem. Pharmacol.* **1973**, *22*, 3099–3108.
67. Litchfield, J.; Wilcoxon, F. A simplified method of evaluating dose-effectexperiments. *J. Pharmacol. Exp. Ther.* **1949**, *96*, 99–113.

Sample Availability: Upon reasonable request and considering the amount of material in hand, 14-methoxycodeine-6-O-sulfate and codeine-6-O-sulfate can be distributed in a timely fashion by Dr. Hosztafi. However, as supplies are finite, we cannot guarantee every request can be accommodated.

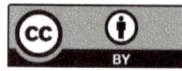

© 2020 by the authors. Licensee MDPI, Basel, Switzerland. This article is an open access article distributed under the terms and conditions of the Creative Commons Attribution (CC BY) license (http://creativecommons.org/licenses/by/4.0/).

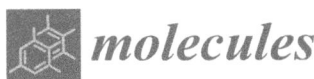

Review

On the Role of Peripheral Sensory and Gut Mu Opioid Receptors: Peripheral Analgesia and Tolerance

Susanna Fürst [1,*], Zoltán S. Zádori [1], Ferenc Zádor [1,2], Kornél Király [1], Mihály Balogh [1], Szilvia B. László [1], Barbara Hutka [1], Amir Mohammadzadeh [1], Chiara Calabrese [3], Anna Rita Galambos [1], Pál Riba [1], Patrizia Romualdi [3], Sándor Benyhe [2], Júlia Timár [1], Helmut Schmidhammer [4], Mariana Spetea [4] and Mahmoud Al-Khrasani [1]

[1] Department of Pharmacology and Pharmacotherapy, Faculty of Medicine, Semmelweis University, Nagyvárad tér 4, P.O. Box 370, H-1445 Budapest, Hungary; zadori.zoltan@med.semmelweis-univ.hu (Z.S.Z.); zador.ferenc@pharma.semmelweis-univ.hu (F.Z.); kiraly.kornel@med.semmelweis-univ.hu (K.K.); mbalogh@mdanderson.org (M.B.); laszlo.szilvia@med.semmelweis-univ.hu (S.B.L.); hutka.barbara@semmelweis-univ.hu (B.H.); mohammadzadeh.amir@med.semmelweis-univ.hu (A.M.); galambos.anna@pharma.semmelweis-univ.hu (A.R.G.); riba.pal@med.semmelweis-univ.hu (P.R.); timar.julia@med.semmelweis-univ.hu (J.T.); al-khrasani.mahmoud@med.semmelweis-univ.hu (M.A.-K.)

[2] Institute of Biochemistry, Biological Research Center, Temesvári krt. 62., H-6726 Szeged, Hungary; benyhe.sandor@brc.hu

[3] Department of Pharmacy and Biotechnology (FaBiT), Alma Mater Studiorum University of Bologna Via Irnerio 48, 40126 Bologna, Italy; chiara.calabrese2@studio.unibo.it (C.C.); patrizia.romualdi@unibo.it (P.R.)

[4] Department of Pharmaceutical Chemistry, Institut of Pharmacy and Center for Molecular Biosciences Innsbruck (CMBI), University of Innsbruck, Innrain 80-82, 6020 Innsbruck, Austria; helmut.schmidhammer@uibk.ac.at (H.S.); mariana.spetea@uibk.ac.at (M.S.)

* Correspondence: furst.zsuzsanna@med.semmelweis-univ.hu; Tel.: +36-1-2104416; Fax: +36-1-2104412

Received: 22 April 2020; Accepted: 24 May 2020; Published: 26 May 2020

Abstract: There is growing evidence on the role of peripheral μ-opioid receptors (MORs) in analgesia and analgesic tolerance. Opioid analgesics are the mainstay in the management of moderate to severe pain, and their efficacy in the alleviation of pain is well recognized. Unfortunately, chronic treatment with opioid analgesics induces central analgesic tolerance, thus limiting their clinical usefulness. Numerous molecular mechanisms, including receptor desensitization, G-protein decoupling, β-arrestin recruitment, and alterations in the expression of peripheral MORs and microbiota have been postulated to contribute to the development of opioid analgesic tolerance. However, these studies are largely focused on central opioid analgesia and tolerance. Accumulated literature supports that peripheral MORs mediate analgesia, but controversial results on the development of peripheral opioid receptors-mediated analgesic tolerance are reported. In this review, we offer evidence on the consequence of the activation of peripheral MORs in analgesia and analgesic tolerance, as well as approaches that enhance analgesic efficacy and decrease the development of tolerance to opioids at the peripheral sites. We have also addressed the advantages and drawbacks of the activation of peripheral MORs on the sensory neurons and gut (leading to dysbiosis) on the development of central and peripheral analgesic tolerance.

Keywords: peripheral μ-opioid receptors; analgesia; peripheral analgesic tolerance; dysbiosis

1. Introduction

The present consensus is that all opioid agonists used in clinical practice produce analgesia primarily mediated by μ-opioid receptors (MORs) located within the brain and spinal cord along the pain transmission pathways. On the other hand, the adverse effects of opioids are also mediated through the activation of opioid receptors (ORs), both in the central nervous system (CNS) and in the periphery [1–3]. There are four opioid receptor types named as MORs, δ-opioid receptors (DORs), κ-opioid receptors (KORs), and the nociceptin opioid receptor that have been cloned and extensively pharmacologically characterized [4–13]. ORs belong to the large family of G protein-coupled receptors (GPCRs) [14,15]. The binding of opioid agonists to central and peripheral ORs initiate signaling downstream events that lead to the activation of $G_{i/o}$ proteins, β-arrestin recruitment, opening of G protein-coupled inwardly rectifying potassium (GIRK) channels and the inhibition of voltage-gated Ca^{2+} channels [10,14,16,17]. Concurrently, besides receptor-type selectivity, the central versus peripheral distribution of opioid receptors and their functional relevance have gained increased attention in the opioid research. ORs are distributed on key points involved in the modulation of nociception along the ascending and descending pain pathways [3,18]. Unfortunately, the activation of ORs in the CNS and in the periphery results in the occurrence of undesirable side effects. Centrally mediated adverse effects of opioid analgesics include respiratory depression, sedation, nausea, and dizziness, while constipation predominantly results from the activation of intestinal opioid receptors. The development of analgesic tolerance, together with abuse potential, often limit the clinical utility of MOR analgesics leading to early discontinuation, under-dosing, and inadequate analgesia in pain patients.

At present, in the clinical setting, the only option available to overcome the development of analgesic tolerance is to increase the dose (escalation to higher dose) or to use other opioid analgesics to maintain analgesia (opioid rotation). The consequence of increasing opioid dose is exposing the patient to the risk of adverse events, including overdose as well as the misuse of and addiction potential to opioids [19]. It is well-known that opioid analgesic tolerance develops to all clinically used opioids; however, the degree and the rate of tolerance to the opioid side effects depends on the target that hosts the opioid receptors. For example, opioid tolerance develops more rapidly to the analgesic effects, whereas little tolerance manifests to constipation [20]. This phenomenon is described as differential tolerance development [21]. In a clinical setting, it means that analgesic tolerance is rapidly developed compared to the development of tolerance to gastrointestinal (GI) side effects (constipation, if it occurs at all). In addition, along the GI tract, there are regional differences in opioid tolerance development, namely in the upper GI tract tolerance can develop to the motility, whereas in the colon such is not the case, which is reflected by a persistent constipation following chronic treatment with opioids [22]. From these observations, it could be concluded that opioid tolerance development is the fastest and most profound for the analgesic actions, less for the respiratory depressant effects and least for GI motility [21–23].

Physicians' view on opioid euphoric tolerance is that drug abusers are seeking a higher opioid dose in order to maintain the euphoric effect. This dose escalation might lead to overdose deaths, which is the major cause contributing to the current opioid epidemic [24–27]. In humans addicted to morphine, tolerance reaches an extreme degree, with doses of 300–600 mg (30–60 times the normal dose) often being taken several times a day [20,28,29].

The magnitude of analgesic tolerance also depends on the pharmacological profiles of opioids; an important one is the agonist efficacy, but also the pharmacokinetic profiles such as the route of administration. Though in the latter case, it has been reported that in tolerant subjects, the pharmacokinetic parameters of morphine such as absorption, metabolism, and excretion were unaffected [30]. Nevertheless, the dosing, the intervals, and routes of administration, the applied methodologies, as well as the animal species have been reported to substantially affect the development of analgesic tolerance [28,29,31].

The putative target for opioid analgesics currently available in clinical practice is the CNS, which hosts many targets that mediate analgesia and other effects including analgesic tolerance, respiratory depression, and addiction liability. The growing evidence on the existence of functional peripheral ORs, particularly MORs has initiated research efforts to develop opioid analgesics with limited CNS penetration in order to gain analgesia free of the central unwanted side effects [2,26,32–39]. On the other hand, recent studies have also suggested that MORs that are distributed in the periphery on dorsal root ganglia (DRG) or GI tract are implicated in the development of analgesic tolerance [40,41].

In this review, we focus on the MORs-mediated peripheral analgesia in different animal pain models. Next, the contribution of MORs and drawbacks upon their activation to opioid-induced analgesic tolerance is discussed. The review also briefly discusses the following questions: (i) Besides peripheral analgesia, does the activation of MORs located on the sensory afferent neurons influence the central analgesic effect of opioids? (ii) What is the role of MORs' activation in the alteration of gut microbiota and whether or not these changes can contribute to the development of central analgesic tolerance? (iii) What is the current view on the role of microbiota alteration in the development of peripheral analgesic tolerance?

2. Contribution of Peripheral MORs to Opioid-Induced Analgesia and Analgesic Tolerance

There is substantial evidence demonstrating the involvement of peripheral ORs in MOR agonists-induced analgesia following systemic administration in acute thermal pain models in rat or mouse [34,42]. Research from our laboratory (Schmidhammer and Spetea's, Al-Khrasani and Fürst's and Benyhe's research teams) and others have reported on effective, peripheral analgesic effects of opioids following local or systemic administration applying various pharmacological approaches in rodent models of inflammatory and visceral pain [2,35–39,43–53]. On the other hand, in animal models of neuropathic pain, the peripheral analgesic effect of opioids is a question of debate [54–59]. Animal studies that examine peripheral analgesic effects following systemic administration of peripherally restricted MOR agonists and consideration of time-dependent changes of MORs reserve and analgesia peri-induction of neuropathic pain will reopen old avenues in this field of pain research.

In opioid research as well as other drug discovery areas, the limited access of substances to the CNS can be achieved by either quaternization of the molecule or the introduction of functional groups endowing the molecule to have a zwitterionic structure at body pH (Table 1) [34–37,47,60–65] The number of MOR agonists with limited CNS penetration and displaying peripheral analgesia have been increasing over the years, but they have not been proven so far to be of clinical value [43,52,66,67]. In addition, these results may initiate further studies to examine the development of peripheral analgesic tolerance, since most research has been focused on the evaluation of the central opioid analgesic tolerance. For examination of peripheral analgesia, studies have shed light on the peripheral analgesic tolerance [68,69]. Research on the development of the centrally mediated opioid analgesic tolerance and related mechanisms has been reviewed extensively elsewhere [20,23,70–72]. Available evidence related to peripheral analgesia and analgesic tolerance is summarized below. This section reviews the evidence related to peripheral analgesia and analgesic tolerance according to the animal pain models studied, namely (1) acute thermal, (2) acute and subchronic inflammatory, and (3) neuropathic.

Table 1. Examples of MOR agonists from the class of morphinans with limited CNS penetration and peripheral analgesic effect.

Structure	R_1	R_2	R_3	Compound	Ref.
	H	OSO_3^-	H	Morphine-6-O-sulfate	[73]
	OCH_3	OSO_3^-	H	14-O-methylmorphine-6-O-sulfate	[62]
	H	OSO_3^-	CH_3	Codeine-6-O-sulfate	[60]
	OCH_3	OSO_3^-	CH_3	14-O-methylcodeine-6-O-sulfate	[65]
	OCH_3	$HNCH_2COOH$	H	14-O-methyloxymorphone-6β-glycine (HS-731)	[34,35]

2.1. Peripheral Opioid Analgesia and Tolerance in Animal Models of Acute Thermal Pain

The group of G.W. Pasternak has reported on the analgesic effects of morphine, [D-Ala^2, N-Me-Phe^4,-Gly-ol^5]enkephalin (DAMGO), and morphine-6β-glucuronide (M6G) following local administration to the mouse tail in the tail-flick assay, which is an acute thermal pain model [74]. In this study, the intrathecal administration of antisense targeting exons 1 and 4 of MOR-1 blocked the local analgesic effect of morphine, indicating the involvement of the terminals of sensory neurons. Moreover, the repeated systemic administration of morphine or repeated daily exposure of the tail to morphine caused profound analgesic tolerance to the local analgesic effect of morphine [75]. Systemic or local but not intrathecal MK801, an N-methyl-D-aspartate (NMDA) receptor antagonist, abrogated morphine-induced peripheral analgesic tolerance when morphine was applied superficially in DMSO solution. One of the key observations of this study regarding the peripheral analgesic tolerance is that peripheral NMDA receptors are implicated in the development of analgesic tolerance to topically applied morphine. Notably, the same group also showed mixed results in terms of cross-tolerance, which occurred only between morphine and DAMGO, but not between morphine and M6G. Furthermore, M6G but not morphine or DAMGO produced 3-methoxynaltrexone sensitive local analgesic effect, indicating a unique mechanism of action of M6G. It has also been reported that beside MK-801, ketamine was able to suppress tolerance development. These data are in agreement with other studies where NMDA receptor antagonists inhibited the development of opioid analgesic tolerance, despite the fact that the sites of actions are different. In addition, the involvement of NMDA receptors in neural plasticity explains the effectiveness of NMDA receptor antagonists in the inhibition of central opioid analgesic tolerance, as described by many research groups [74–79]. Nevertheless, the existence of NMDA receptors on peripheral sensory neurons is well-documented [80–82], but the role of these receptors on peripheral opioid analgesic tolerance remains unclear.

DRG is the MORs' synthesis machinery of primary sensory neurons, and any changes in DRG-related MORs are able to alter the magnitude of analgesia evoked by peripherally administered opioid agonists. Meuser and coworkers [83] showed that systemic morphine treatment (4 days 2 × 10 mg/kg) caused naloxone reversible downregulation of MOR mRNA in the DRG of rats that developed morphine analgesic tolerance in the hot-plate test. The repeated treatments resulted in the decrease in the expression of MORs in the DRG, which might contribute to a reduction in peripheral analgesia. Aδ and C primary sensory afferent fibers convey the pain from the site of injury into the spinal cord, and the decrease in functional MORs can affect the pain intensity. In this work, the authors used an acute thermal pain model, where the MORs' reserve upon the induction of pain remains unchanged [83]. Sun and co-workers developed conditional knock-out (KO) mice, in which the expression of the MOR gene (Oprm1) was entirely abolished in DRGs and substantially decreased in the spinal cord [84]. In the Oprm1 conditional KO animals, systemic or intrathecal morphine treatment showed limited effect in acute thermal and mechanical pain. In addition, opioid-induced hyperalgesia (OIH) following chronic morphine treatment was completely absent in these animals. In addition, systemic morphine treatment showed weak analgesic effect in these conditional KO animals that hampered assessing analgesic tolerance as well.

Work carried out by the groups of Fürst, Spetea, and Schmidhammer has reported on the involvement of peripheral ORs in mediating the antinociceptive effect of systemically (subcutaneous, s.c.) administered 6β-glycine substituted 14-O-methyloxymorphone, HS-731 (Table 1), which is an MOR selective agonist with limited CNS penetration in a rat model of acute thermal (tail-flick test) pain [34]. The antinociceptive efficacy of HS-731 resulting from the activation of peripheral ORs was also demonstrated in rat models of inflammatory pain (formalin test and carrageenan-induced hyperalgesia) [34,35], in a mouse model of visceral pain (acetic acid-induced writhing assay) [37,51], and in the mouse eye-wiping trigeminal nociceptive test [36]. Other 6-amino acid- and 6-dipeptide-substituted derivatives of 14-O-methyloxymorphone derivatives were also reported to produce peripherally-mediated antinociception after systemic (s.c.) administration in rats and mice [37]. The effect of repeated systemic (s.c.) treatment of rats with HS-731 on the development of analgesic tolerance was measured in the tail-flick test. Daily treatment of rats for 14 days resulted in no analgesic tolerance for HS-731 (Figure 1) (Fürst and Spetea, unpublished data). This finding provides clear evidence that the selective activation of peripheral ORs leads to effective antinociceptive effects without resulting in analgesic tolerance following systemic opioid administration.

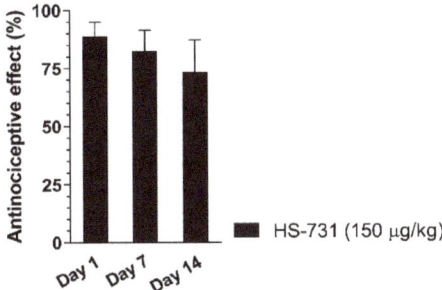

Figure 1. Effect of chronic treatment on the development of peripheral analgesic tolerance of HS-731 in the rat tail-flick test after systemic (s.c.) administration. Rats were s.c. administered daily for two weeks HS-731 (150 µg/kg). Antinociceptive effects were measured at days 1, 7, and 14, at 60 min after administration of HS-731. There was no significant effect day 7 vs. day 1 and day 14 vs. day 1. Statistical differences were determined with one-way ANOVA and Newman–Keuls multiple comparisons post-hoc test. Data represent means ± S.E.M (n = 7 per group). Experiments were performed and analyzed as described previously [62]. Tolerance protocol was developed by Fürst and Spetea.

In another study, 14-O-methylmorphine-6-O-sulfate (Table 1), a novel selective MOR agonist [62], proved to produce peripheral antinociceptive effects in rats in the tail-flick test following s.c. administration (Al-Khrasani et al., unpublished data, Figure 2). However, the peripheral effect of 14-O-methylmorphine-6-O-sulfate was measured only after administration of low doses, since at higher doses, a central analgesic effect was observed. In addition, it was proven that this molecule produced less analgesic tolerance than morphine in mice, although the applied doses in these experiments were high enough to produce a central effect [85]. No study on the peripheral analgesic tolerance of 14-O-methylmorphine-6-O-sulfate has been reported so far.

2.2. Peripheral Opioid Analgesia and Tolerance in Animal Acute and Subchronic Inflammatory Pain Models

Aley and coworkers [86] found that intradermal co-injection of the highly selective MOR agonist peptide DAMGO and the adenosine A1-receptor agonist, N6-cyclopenthyladenosin, into the rat hind paw can dose-dependently inhibit PGE2 induced hyperalgesia. Repeated administration of both compounds (3× hourly) caused a rapid and cross-tolerance development. In addition, either naloxone or the A1 receptor antagonist PACPX caused (cross) withdrawal hyperalgesia in pretreated animals. Co-treatment with the receptor antagonists mentioned above blocked the development of tolerance and agonist-induced hyperalgesia. The same group [76] reported that NO generation and protein kinase C (PKC) activation are contributing to the development of analgesic tolerance and withdrawal hyperalgesia, respectively.

Honoré and coworkers [87] investigated spinal c-Fos expression and pressure hyperalgesia following systemic (i.v.) or intraplantar (i.pl.) morphine treatment in a carrageenan-induced pain model. Morphine given systemically (i.v.) or locally (i.pl.) blocked carrageenan-induced increase in spinal c-Fos expression and the development of hyperalgesia, which was indicated by a decrease in paw pressure threshold. These behavioral effects were abolished when animals were subjected to three days pretreatment with s.c. morphine (80 mg/kg).

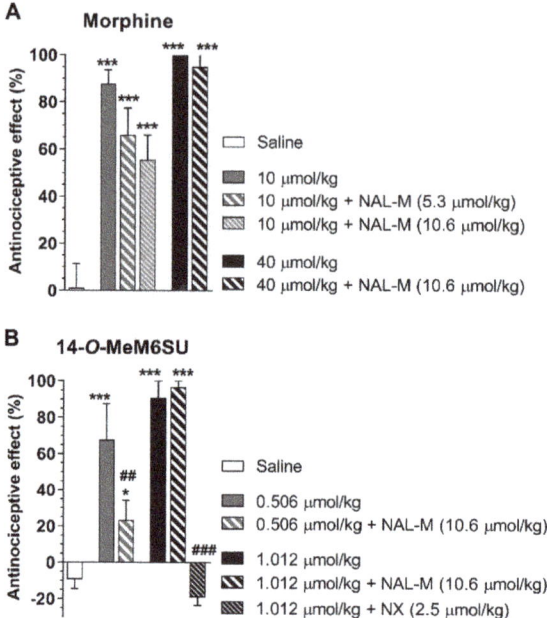

Figure 2. The analgesic effect of morphine (**A**) and 14-*O*-methylmorphine-6-*O*-sulfate (14-*O*-MeM6SU; **B**) in the rat tail-flick test at 30 and 60 min, respectively after s.c. administration. Their effects were assessed in the presence of naloxone methiodide (NAL-M), which is a peripherally acting OR antagonist. The analgesic effect of the highest dose 14-*O*-MeM6SU was abolished by the OR antagonist naloxone (NX). (*$p < 0.05$ and ***$p < 0.001$, compared to saline group; ##$p < 0.05$ and ###$p < 0.001$, compared to 14-O-MeM6SU alone). Statistical differences were determined with one-way ANOVA and Newman–Keuls multiple comparisons post-hoc test. Data represent means ± S.E.M (n = 3–9 per group). Experiments were performed and analyzed as described previously [62].

Among the most established chemical nociceptive stimuli, bradykinin has been reported to be an important mediator of pain [88]. The MOR agonist morphine showed a naloxone-reversible analgesic effect on bradykinin-induced pain in mice in a study carried out by Tokuyama and co-workers [89]. In addition, the effect of morphine was localized in the affected limb, since systemic or local administration to the contralateral limb failed to produce analgesia. In this work, the authors have proved that DAMGO and U-69,593, but not [D-Ser^2,-Leu^5,-Thr^6]-enkephalin (DSLET), which are selective agonists for MOR, KOR, and DOR, respectively, were effective in inducing peripheral analgesia [89]. Systemic pretreatment with morphine (5 days, 10 mg/kg) caused tolerance to analgesic effect of s.c. morphine measured by the tail-pinch test, but the effect of local morphine on the bradykinin-induced nociceptive flexion was unaffected. These findings were later confirmed by the same group [90]. On the other hand, they also reported that the repeated local treatment with morphine caused tolerance to its local effect [91]. This tolerance development was effectively blocked by PKC α and γ inhibitors, but less by PKC δ inhibitors.

In inflammatory conditions such as arthritis, peripheral ORs are upregulated [33,92–94]. This upregulation was demonstrated to contribute to peripheral opioid analgesia in animals as well as in humans [94–96]. The presence of inflammation leads to the release of endogenous mediators that can enhance levels of peripheral ORs' proteins and mRNA expression and also increased axonal transport and G protein coupling [92,93,97]. Additional changes related to peripheral ORs include increased ORs trafficking and opioid-related actions, such as cyclic adenosine monophosphate (cAMP) accumulation, the modulation of voltage-dependent cation channels etc., and the accessibility to the

ORs in the transperineurium of ORs is also enhanced [93,97]. Several studies have also demonstrated that opioid agonists produced pronounced peripheral analgesia in animal models of inflammatory pain [33,98]. Thus, the question is whether the inflammation evoked MORs expression has the ability to affect the development of peripheral analgesic tolerance following repeated peripheral opioid treatment.

Fernandez-Duenas and coworkers [99] investigated the analgesic effect of s.c. morphine in the plantar (Hargreaves test), Randall-Selitto and von Frey tests with or without complete Freund's adjuvant (CFA)-induced paw inflammation in naive and morphine pellet-exposed mice. They found that acute s.c. morphine treatment resulted in decreased antinociception in mice with CFA-induced paw inflammation compared to mice that were not subjected to CFA treatment. In the plantar test, the antinociceptive effect of morphine was mostly centrally mediated in control animals, but in the case of mice with inflammation, the peripheral analgesic component was increased. On the other hand, the antiallodynic effect of morphine was mainly centrally mediated independent of the presence or absence of inflammation. The potency of morphine was enhanced in mechanical and thermal inflammatory states. Pretreatment with a morphine pellet (3 days from 4 to 7 day after CFA) caused a rightward shift of dose–response curves and a decrease in maximum effect in all test methods [99]. Following chronic morphine treatment, the antinociceptive effect of morphine was the same in mice with or without inflammation, so the relative tolerance was higher in inflammatory conditions. In the paw pressure test, the same research group [100] has also reported the effects of different i.pl.-injected opioids (morphine, fentanyl, buprenorphine, [D-Pen^2,-D-Pen^5]enkephalin (DPDPE) and U50488H) and corticotrophin releasing factor (CRF), which is known to induce endogenous opioid release. They demonstrated that all compounds were ineffective in the absence of inflammation, yet in inflamed paws, they were able to increase the pain threshold, achieving a maximal effect of 88% for fentanyl and 48–64% for the rest of the compounds. In morphine-tolerant mice, locally administered morphine failed to produce analgesia, yet a significant decrease in analgesic effects of DPDPE, U50488H, and CRF were indicated by the rightward shift of dose–response curves. In addition, they showed a small decrease in the antinociceptive and maximal effects for fentanyl and no significant change in case of buprenorphine. They concluded that inflammation is required for the local action of opioids and chronic systemic exposure causes (cross) tolerance toward this effect. They investigated further β-arrestin1 and β-arrestin2 expressions in the absence and in the presence of inflammation upon morphine treatment. They found that CFA increases the level of both β-arrestins, which can decrease after acute and chronic morphine exposure, but morphine alone without inflammation caused no change in the expression levels of β-arrestins.

Other investigators [68] showed that the local analgesic effect of i.pl. fentanyl was not affected by 4 days pretreatment with s.c. morphine 10 mg/kg twice daily in CFA-induced inflammatory pain. Such studies raised the question of whether rats subjected to repeated morphine treatment and developed analgesic tolerance in an acute thermal pain model would also develop morphine analgesic tolerance in a subchronic inflammatory pain model. Our (Al-Khrasani's) research group performed behavioral studies assessing the development of analgesic tolerance in rats with CFA-induced hyperalgesia. The analgesic effect of s.c. morphine was determined using the thermal tail-flick assay and the Randall–Selitto paw pressure test. In these experiments, analgesic tolerance was developed in both non-inflamed and inflamed paws. In addition, there was no difference in non-inflamed and inflamed paw in the effect of morphine in tolerant rats in contrast to non-tolerant animals at higher dose (Figure 3) (Al-Khrasani et al., unpublished data).

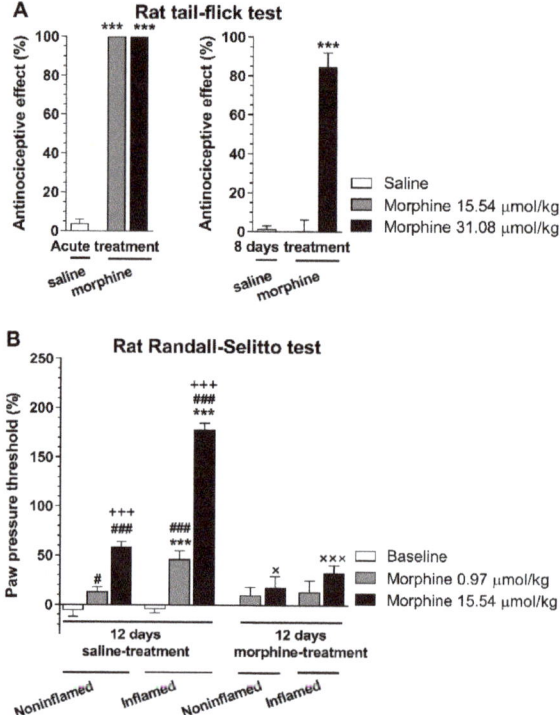

Figure 3. Analgesic effect of morphine in tolerant and non-tolerant rats in the rat tail-flick (**A**) and Randall–Selitto test (**B**). **A**: The analgesic effect in acute treatments was determined 30 min after morphine s.c. injection in the indicated doses. In chronic treatments, animals received 31.08 µmol/kg s.c. twice a day for 8 days. On the 8th day, the antinociceptive effect was determined 30 min after s.c. injection of morphine in the indicated doses (***$p < 0.001$, saline- vs. morphine-treated group). Statistical difference was determined with one-way ANOVA and Holm–Sidak's multiple comparison post-hoc test. **B**: Inflammatory pain was induced by complete Freund's adjuvant (CFA) injection in the hind paw. Animals were subjected to either saline or 31.08 µmol/kg s.c. twice a day for 12 days. On the 8th day, CFA was injected intraplantar (i.pl.) and on 12th day, paw pressure thresholds were determined prior to and 30 min after s.c. injection of morphine in the indicated doses. (***$p < 0.001$, non-inflamed vs. inflamed paw; #$p < 0.05$ and ###$p < 0.001$, saline vs. morphine treated group within non-inflamed or inflamed paw; +++$p < 0.001$, 0.97 µmol/kg vs. 15.54 µmol/kg morphine group; x$p < 0.05$ and xxx$p < 0.001$, 12 days saline vs. 12 days morphine within the corresponding groups). Statistical difference was determined with two-way ANOVA, with Holm–Sidak's multiple comparison post-hoc test. All data represent means ± S.E.M (n = 5–20 per group). Rat tail-flick and Randall–Selitto tests were performed and analyzed as previously described [65], tolerance protocol was developed based on Király et al. [85].

In another study carried out by Eidson and Murphy, morphine tolerance was investigated in a rat model of peripheral inflammation (CFA-induced) [101]. They reported that morphine tolerance is accompanied by increased glial cell activation within the ventrolateral periaqueductal gray (vlPAG). Interestingly, persistent peripheral inflammation inhibited the development of morphine tolerance, presumably via the inhibition vlPAG glial activation. This indicates that complex peripheral mechanisms influence the development of analgesic tolerance [33,65].

In a recent study, the combination of loperamide (a peripheral restricted MOR preferring opioid agonist) with the DOR agonist oxymorphindole caused peripheral synergistic analgesia in CFA-induced hyperalgesia in mice [102]. This approach sought to utilize the upregulation of MORs and DORs and their heterodimer formation during inflammation in sensory axons. According to these results, the loperamide–oxymorphindole combination was 150 times more potent systemically and 84 times more effective locally compared to single drug administration. They also concluded that the repeated topical administration of loperamide–oxymorphindole (twice daily for 3 days) did not induce analgesic tolerance in animals with inflammatory pain [102]. Data were assessed by the Hargreaves plantar assay and inflammation was induced by CFA. The majority of the discussed studies suggest the decrease in the peripheral analgesic effects of opioids, although the time lag of chronic treatments, the route of administration, and the efficacy of test compounds are different among these works.

2.3. Peripheral Opioid Analgesia and Tolerance in Animal Neuropathic Pain Models

Neuropathic pain management is a clinical challenge of great interest, because not all patients with neuropathic pain respond to the current available medications [103–105]. The background mechanisms related to the poor effectiveness of opioids in the treatment of neuropathic pain is still not clarified. One possible explanation is the loss of MORs following nerve injury, which implicates the appliance of higher dosage of opioids, therefore resulting in severe central side effects [56,106–109]. The functional role of peripheral MORs in peripheral opioid analgesia and analgesic tolerance following the peripheral administration of opioids has not been elucidated yet in neuropathic pain conditions. Early studies used rat peripheral mononeuropathic pain models to assess the analgesic effect of morphine following systemic administration (i.v.). Kayser and coworkers [110] found that low systemic morphine doses produced antiallodynic effect with a mechanism involving the participation of peripheral ORs. In another study, the same group showed that treatment with a higher dose of morphine 10 mg/kg s.c. (twice daily for 4 days) induced complete tolerance to the analgesic effect of low acute morphine doses (0.1–1.0 mg/kg i.v.). The development of analgesic tolerance to morphine was abolished by L-365,260, a selective cholecystokinin-B (CCKB) receptor antagonist [111].

He and coworkers [40] investigated the effect of systemic and local (i.pl.) loperamide on spinal nerve injury-induced allodynia in mice. They found that local and systemic loperamide inhibited allodynia assessed in the von Frey test. In this study, repeated treatments with different i.pl. doses of loperamide developed tolerance only to the local drug effect. On the other hand, systemic pretreatment caused local and systemic tolerance to loperamide; however, systemic morphine remained effective. Furthermore, they also measured the effect of local administration of DAMGO, which also induced analgesic tolerance. The development of tolerance to systemic loperamide was attenuated by naltrexone pretreatment but not by co-treatment with naloxone or naloxone-methiodide. The NMDA receptor antagonist MK-801 attenuated tolerance development to systemic loperamide, but it was not influenced by the glycine β-site antagonist MDL 105,519 [75]. Analgesic tolerance to local loperamide was not influenced by naloxone methiodide or MK-801. Additionally, they found a decrease in total MOR protein in L5 segment of the spinal cord after Seltzer nerve ligation (SNL), which was more pronounced in saline-treated animals than in morphine- or loperamide-treated groups. The Ser375 phosphorylation, which is important in desensitization and tolerance development, was also increased in the morphine-treated group but not in loperamide-treated group. In an in vitro model of loperamide tolerance—KCl-induced Ca^{2+} current in DRG neurons—they found that tolerance was developed after exposure to loperamide, which was attenuated by the DOR antagonist, naltrindole.

An interesting and promising approach to overcome the reduced levels of peripheral MOR expression during neuropathic pain is the viral vector delivery of the MOR via herpes simplex virus type 1 (HSV-1) [109]. Upon infection of mice with nerve injury, the immune reactivity of MORs significantly increased in epidermal nerve fibers in the plantar hind paw skin, in large and medium-diameter DRG cells and in lamina I–III of the dorsal lumbar spinal cord. Additionally, the properties of cutaneous afferents also changed upon infection. HSV-1 MOR inoculation in Aδ-fibers hindered the SNL-induced enhancement to suprathreshold stimulation, while the occurrence of C-fibers with spontaneous activity was reduced. Most importantly, HSV-1 MOR inoculation reversed mechanical allodynia and thermal hyperalgesia, and it also showed a leftward shift in loperamide- and morphine-induced analgesia in nerve-injured animals.

These findings raise important questions, such as: How does viral vector delivery of MOR in the periphery affect opioid-induced tolerance in the periphery or even in the CNS? Additionally, if the low MORs reserve in the periphery can be restored or further improved following nerve injury, the previously described peripherally acting opioid compounds with limited CNS penetration [34,47,60,62,65] might be able to achieve significant antinociception in neuropathic pain. Exploring these questions would be of interest to effectively treat neuropathic pain with opioids and to overcome opioid-induced analgesic tolerance (Table 2).

Table 2. Summary of evaluated compounds for peripheral opioid analgesic tolerance in different pain models.

Pain Model	Assay and Species	Test Compound	Route of Administration	Tolerance Induction	Main Findings	Ref.
Acute thermal	MTF	Morphine M6G	Tail injection	s.c. morphine	High grade tolerance	[74]
Acute thermal	MTF	Morphine M6G DAMGO	DMSO solution immersion	topical morphine	High grade tolerance	[75]
PGE2-induced pain	RS in rat	DAMGO	i.pl. injection	i.pl. injection DAMGO	Tolerance, withdrawal hyperalgesia	[76,86]
Bradykinin-induced flexion reflex	mouse	DAMGO U69,593 DESLET morphine	i.pl. infusion	s.c. morphine	No tolerance to local effect	[89,90]
Bradykinin-induced flexion reflex	mouse	Morphine	i.pl. infusion	i.pl. morphine	Tolerance to local effect	[91]
Carrageenan-induced inflammation	RS in rat, spinal c-Fos	Morphine	i.pl. (and i.v.) injection	s.c. morphine 3 days 2x	Tolerance to i.pl. or i.v.	[87]
CFA-induced inflammation	Plantar, RS, von Frey in mouse	Morphine	s.c.	morphine pellet 3 days	Higher grade tolerance on CFA treated paw than noninflamed	[99]
CFA-induced inflammation	RS in mouse	Morphine Fentanyl Bup. DPDPE U50488H CRF	i.pl.	morphine pellet 3 days	$E_{max}\downarrow$ in all case (exc. buprenorphine) and rightward shift (exc. buprenorphine and fentanyl)	[100]
CFA-induced inflammation	RS in rat	Fentanyl	i.pl.	s.c. morphine (4 days 2x)	Tolerance developed only in absence of inflammation	[68]
SNL	von Frey in mouse	Loperamide	i.pl./s.c.	i.pl./s.c. loperamide	i.pl. loperamide caused tolerance only on i.pl., caused both for i.pl. and s.c.; s.c. morphine remained effective	[40]
CFA-induced inflammation	Hargreaves assay in rat	Loperamide–oxymorphindole	topical (left hind paw)	twice a daily for 3 days	No tolerance to local effect	[102]

MTF: mouse tail-flick; Bup.: buprenorphine; RS: Randal–Selitto; SNL: spinal nerve ligation; i.pl.: intraplantar; s.c.: subcutaneous; i.v.: intravenous; CFA: complete Freund's adjuvant; CRF: corticotrophin releasing factor; DMSO: dimethyl sulfoxide.

3. Drawbacks of Peripheral MORs Activation Related to Opioid Analgesic Tolerance

3.1. The Consequence of MORs Activation on Primary Sensory Neurons

All desirable and unwanted opioid side effects largely stem from the activation of MORs that are distributed either in the CNS or in the periphery [97]. A general assumption was that central analgesic tolerance is the consequence of a decrease in the central MORs response to opioid analgesics; however, the involvement of peripheral MORs in the development of central analgesic tolerance has also gained attention recently [112,113].

Recent data from Corder and co-workers showed that the activation of peripheral MORs (expressed by primary afferent nociceptors) is involved in the development of central analgesic tolerance to MOR agonists [114]. In addition, these receptors also have a crucial role in OIH. Namely, the deletion of these peripheral receptors eliminated both morphine tolerance and OIH. This finding was further supported by the pharmacological inhibition of MORs at peripheral sites. Methylnaltrexone, a peripherally acting opioid antagonist, abrogated the analgesic tolerance when co-administered with morphine, without diminishing the analgesic effect of morphine, in different pain models (perioperative and chronic pain models). These results indicate that the systemic co-administration of peripherally acting opioid antagonists with opioid analgesics that readily penetrate into the CNS might be a new clinical approach for the prevention of central analgesic tolerance development [114]. Earlier studies by Danysz and co-workers found that the co-administration of naloxone methiodide inhibited the development of morphine tolerance [77]. They investigated the effects of morphine in morphine-tolerant mice in the tail-flick test in different subspecies of mice [77]. Another strategy for central analgesic tolerance prevention might be the activation of other peripheral ORs (DORs or KORs). In the late 1990s, Walker and co-workers found that peripherally acting KOR agonists successfully alleviated pain symptoms in morphine-tolerant rats in a sciatic nerve injury model [115]. Although this way seems promising, only few peripherally acting compounds reached clinical studies up to this date [116].

Upon the chronic use of centrally acting opioids, anti-opioid systems also actively contribute to the development of opioid analgesia. On the other hand, drugs that inhibit anti-opioid systems (NMDA, CCK) have been long reported to abrogate analgesic tolerance [117–120]. These systems appear to have a crucial role in the development of peripheral opioid analgesic tolerance, although few data are available. In 2005, Danysz and co-workers proved the role of peripheral NMDA receptors in analgesic tolerance development in the tail-flick test in different subspecies of mice [77]. They used peripherally acting NMDA receptor/glycine B site antagonists (MRZ 2/596 and MDL), after proving their lack of CNS effects. Their results indicated that the peripheral blockade of NMDA receptor/glycine B sites can attenuate morphine analgesic tolerance.

In this regard, under neuropathic pain conditions, the peripheral MORs have been reported to be also decreased [121–123], but it seems that this change does not alter the development of central opioid analgesic tolerance, although it has not been thoroughly investigated so far. According to the above studies, the correlation between the change in the MORs reserve in primary sensory neurons and the development of central and peripheral opioid analgesia may be worth investigating. In contrast, a recent study by Klein and co-workers [109] demonstrated that the herpes simplex virus (HSV) MOR inoculation increased the analgesic activity of loperamide or morphine following systemic administration.

The development of tolerance is a highly complex mechanism that is still not fully understood. This complicated mechanism involves several different pathways, not just centrally, but also peripherally. Among the strategies that might hinder the development of central opioid analgesic tolerance are those affecting the downstream targets of opioid receptors, such as ATP-sensitive potassium (K_{ATP}) channels. The activity of these channels can influence the efficacy of opioids and represent an important factor in tolerance development. Cole Fisher and co-workers demonstrated that the downregulation of SUR1 subtype K_{ATP} channels in the spinal cord and DRG potentiated the development of morphine tolerance and withdrawal syndrome in mice [124]. SUR1 agonists (diazoxide and NN-414) attenuated tolerance development. These results suggested that increasing neuronal K_{ATP} channel activity in the peripheral nervous system might be a viable option to alleviate central opioid analgesic tolerance and withdrawal syndrome. Several recent studies have outlined how peripheral MORs affect the central analgesic tolerance. Of importance is the consequence of the activation of peripheral MORs on the gut.

The above-mentioned strategies might potentially solve the development of central analgesic tolerance, but the addiction liability of centrally acting opioid analgesics remains unsolved.

3.2. The Role of MORs in the Gut Microbiota: Dysbiosis, Opioid Tolerance

In the past decades, a huge amount of data has been accumulated on the role of gut microbiota in the pathogenesis of various GI (irritable bowel syndrome, inflammatory bowel diseases, colorectal cancer), endocrine (obesity, diabetes), cardiovascular, and even neuropsychiatric diseases [125–127]. Based on recent findings [41,128–131], the development of opioid analgesic tolerance can also be added to the continuously increasing list of adverse events related to microbial alterations (dysbiosis) in the GI tract. This section provides a brief overview of opioid-induced dysbiosis and the data supporting the concept that microbial alterations contribute to analgesic tolerance. Notably, a detailed review by Mischel and co-workers [132] has been recently published, to which the reader is referred for further information and more extensive bibliography.

Regarding opioid-induced dysbiosis, to date, most of the data originate from preclinical studies, in which mice were exposed to morphine for different time periods [128,129,131,133–135]. However, in some experiments, other opioid agents were used, such as loperamide [136,137] or hydromorphone [138], and there are some common patterns in the microbial composition of animals irrespective of the type of opioid used, allowing to draw some general conclusions on the effect of opioids on microbiota. Moreover, some of these changes have also been observed in non-human primates [139], as well as in opioid user cirrhotic patients compared to those not on opioids [140], or in heroin addicts [141], further supporting the complexity and translational relevance of the results.

Although there are some variabilities between the findings of the different studies, which may also result from the various treatment protocols [135], the administration of opioids is in general accompanied by the expansion of *Staphylococcus* and *Enterococcus* genera within the *Firmicutes phylum* and by reduced abundance of the *Lactobacillus* genus. The decreased representation of the *Clostridia* class and in particular the contraction of the *Lachnospiraceae* and *Ruminococcaceae* families are also relatively consistent results. Another common finding in opioid-treated rodents is the expansion of the *Proteobacteria phylum* with increased abundances of *Enterobacteriales* and the genus *Sutterella*. In addition, various (and sometimes contradictory) changes within the *Bacteroidetes phylum* have been reported, from which the expansion of the *Porphyromonadaceae* and *Prevotellaceae* families appears in several reports. These effects depend on the activation of MORs, as morphine failed to induce dysbiosis in naltrexone-treated and MOR-KO animals [129,133,134].

It is noteworthy that several bacteria with increased abundance are considered to be potentially pathogenic, including *Enterococcus*, *Sutteralla*, and *Enterobacteriaceae* [142–144], whereas bacteria with decreased amount (*Lactobacillus*, *Lachnospiraceae*, *Ruminococcaceae*) have anti-inflammatory properties, and some *Lactobacillus* species are widely used probiotics [145,146]. Hence, opioid-induced microbial alterations can generate a pro-inflammatory milieu, which can compromise the gut epithelial barrier and allow luminal aggressive factors (bacteria, bile acids) to penetrate into the gut wall and trigger an immune response, further amplifying the initial inflammation. Gut inflammation in response to opioid administration is typically characterized by enhanced intestinal permeability, the activation of Toll-like receptor-2 (TLR-2), TLR-4, and elevated levels of various pro-inflammatory cytokines, including tumor necrosis factor-α (TNF-α), interleukin-1β (IL-1β), IL-6, IL-17) in the intestine, mesenteric lymph nodes, and remote organs [128,133,134,138].

Several lines of evidence suggest that opioid-induced dysbiosis contributes to the development of analgesic tolerance. Elimination of the gut microbiota, either by using germ-free mice or by treating conventionally raised animals with a broad-spectrum antibiotic cocktail, significantly attenuated tolerance development to chronic morphine in different in vivo assays [128,131]. By contrast, prolonged exposure to morphine induced tolerance in germ-free mice that had undergone fecal microbiota transplantation with samples obtained from conventionally raised mice [128]. Among tested antibiotics, vancomycin, a non-absorbable glycopeptide antibiotic that selectively eliminates Gram-positive bacteria, appeared to have the most prominent effect, as it was able to reduce morphine tolerance even alone, although not as effectively as in combination with other antibiotics [130,131]. Therefore, the expansion of distinct Gram-positive strains in response to opioid treatment may have a pivotal role in the development of analgesic tolerance. This concurs with the findings that the exposure of morphine promoted Gram-positive sepsis and the production of IL-17 in a TLR-2-dependent manner (which receptor recognizes components of the Gram-positive cell wall) [133,134]. Moreover, the genetic deletion of TLR-2 had a more pronounced inhibitory effect on the development of opioid tolerance than deletion of TLR-4 (which is primarily activated by the Gram-negative cell wall component lipopolysaccharide) [128]. Among the Gram-positive bacteria *Enterococcus* may be of particular relevance, as it blooms in the gut of opioid-treated animals [129,133,134,138] and can also be detected in the peritoneal organs of these animals due to impaired epithelial barrier and bacterial translocation [133]. Further evidence for the importance of this pathogen is that infection with *Enterococcus faecalis* augmented the development of morphine tolerance in mice [129].

The above-mentioned data provide clear evidence for the contribution of opioid-induced dysbiosis to the development of analgesic tolerance; however, research is still going on to identify the underlying mechanisms. In addition, dysbiosis following opioid treatment is typically characterized by the expansion of potentially pathogenic bacteria, which may trigger epithelial damage and intestinal inflammation. This inflammatory reaction is likely to be a key factor in tolerance development, and based on some evidence, it is effectively reduced by antibiotic treatment. For example, whereas the colonic mucosa of morphine-treated animals was characterized by histological damage and elevated levels of the pro-inflammatory cytokine IL-1β, these changes were largely prevented by an antibiotic cocktail [128]. Similar results were found by Zhang et al. [125,128], who reported reduced damage and lower tissue levels of TNF-α, IL-1β, and IL-6 in the ileum of mice treated with both morphine and antibiotics, compared to only morphine-treated animals.

However, it is still unclear exactly which sites of the pain pathway are affected primarily by the intestinal inflammation. Some studies point to the importance of inflammation-induced alteration in the excitability of DRG neurons. As mentioned before, the activation of MORs expressed by these neurons have been reported to contribute significantly to opioid tolerance via initiating multiple downstream events in pain conducting pathways [114]. In addition, it is well-established that inflammation of the GI tract induces hyperexcitability in nociceptive DRG neurons [147], and it was recently demonstrated that experimental colitis induced by 2,4,6-trinitro-benzene sulfonic acid (TNBS) enhanced the development of morphine tolerance in mice [148]. Therefore, it is plausible that opioid-induced dysbiosis, accompanied by epithelial injury and tissue inflammation, results in analgesic tolerance at least due in part to the altered activity of primary afferents. This assumption is supported by the findings that the inhibitory effect of antibiotic treatment on the development of opioid analgesic tolerance can also be demonstrated in DRG neurons [130,131]. Namely, in animals treated with both morphine and an antibiotic cocktail (or vancomycin), the inhibitory effect of an acute morphine challenge on the excitability of DRG neurons remained unaltered, in contrast to animals treated chronically only with morphine, where due to cellular tolerance development, acute morphine administration failed to affect the neuronal activity. Besides altering the functions of primary afferents, opioid-induced dysbiosis and systemic inflammation may induce tolerance in nociceptive circuits of the central nervous system as well. A growing body of evidence links enhanced central immune signaling and increased neuronal excitability to the development of opioid tolerance [149], and bacterial components and systemic inflammatory mediators originating in the gut may evoke central neuronal responses as well, especially if the blood–brain barrier is compromised due to chronic opioid exposure [150].

The question arises: Which MOR-mediated opioid effects are mainly responsible for the observed microbial alterations? Different opioids, including morphine, can suppress the activity of basically all cell types involved in innate and adaptive immunity [151]. Since the immune system is one of the major determinants of the microbiota composition [152], opioid-induced alterations in the intestinal immune functions may have a significant role in the pathogenesis of dysbiosis. Indeed, in the study of Banerjee and co-workers [134], morphine failed to induce dysbiosis in severely immunocompromised mice, indicating that the effects of morphine on the microbiome depend on immune modulation. The opioid-induced inhibition of GI motility is also likely to be involved in dysbiosis [41]. The bidirectional interaction between motility and microbiota is well-known [136,153], and as mentioned above, loperamide-induced dysbiosis resembles in some aspects that caused by morphine [136,137]. In addition, changes in bile acid metabolism due to opioids may also contribute to the consequence of dysbiosis [134,139].

The fact that opioid-induced dysbiosis has a significant role in the tolerance development to the analgesic effect of opioids has several important clinical implications. First of all, the modulation of the microbiota composition either directly (with probiotics or GI-restricted antibiotics) or indirectly (with dietary manipulation or promoting the GI peristalsis) may provide a novel approach to prevent or reduce opioid tolerance. Some of these manipulations have already been proven to be effective in animal experiments—for example, treatment with vancomycin (as mentioned before), administration of the probiotic VSL#3 [128], or oral treatment with butyrate (which has both anti-inflammatory and motility promoting effects) [41]. Certainly, clinical studies are warranted to confirm the tolerance-reducing property of these treatments in humans and to find the best strategies with the lowest risk–benefit ratio. On the other hand, the phenomenon of dysbiosis-related analgesic tolerance suggests that even peripherally restricted opioids may lose their analgesic properties in the case of chronic administration due to their GI effects. Whether and to which extent the peripherally restricted opioids that have been recently proved to produce peripheral analgesia can alter the gut microbiota, and whether this dysbiosis correlates with peripheral analgesic tolerance, are issues that warrant further investigation.

4. Summary and Conclusions

Many attempts have been made to minimize the development of opioid analgesic tolerance in order to avoid the consequence of opioid dose escalation. These studies focused largely on the central mechanisms underlying opioid analgesic tolerance. It is worth mentioning that the worldwide opioid crisis is the result of the use of centrally acting opioid analgesics for controlling pain. Targeting the functional peripheral ORs is an alternative strategy to provide adequate pain relief with less health risks that are related to the current opioid epidemic due to centrally acting opioids. A huge body of evidence indicates the development of central analgesic tolerance to all opioid analgesics. On the other hand, few studies have been published in relation to peripheral analgesic tolerance of opioids. Herein, the reviewed data suggest that the development of peripheral analgesic tolerance is largely dependent on the pain entity, animal pain models and the route of administration, locally versus systemically. Apparently, there is no consensus on the occurrence, magnitude, and the time course regarding the development of analgesic tolerance at peripheral sites in animal models of acute thermal, inflammatory, and neuropathic pains. There are promising approaches to avoid analgesic tolerance, such as designing opioid agonists with limited CNS penetration. However, evaluations of these compounds in relation to peripheral analgesic tolerance have not been fully carried out yet. In addition, the question can be raised as to whether these compounds produce significant peripheral analgesic effects upon long-term treatment. Opioid analgesic tolerance is developed as a consequence of the reduction in the number of available ORs for agonists on the cell surface in key points of pain pathways including the periphery. Consequently, novel opioids of high efficacy and limited CNS penetration might be of clinical value, because the risk of CNS-mediated side effects such as respiratory depression, addictive liability, and overdose incidence can be decreased. Despite the published data on the drawbacks of targeting peripheral MORs in the development of central analgesic tolerance, convincing pharmacological and genetic (the inclusion of peripheral MORs) approaches related to peripheral analgesia and tolerance support such claims. Additionally, restoring the opioid-induced dysbiosis might have an important potential in clinical practice. Finally, the success in developing opioid agonists devoid of central opioid side effects while inducing effective, peripherally mediated analgesia would be a great advance in clinical pain management, together with decreasing addictive liability and overdose deaths.

Author Contributions: The manuscript was written through contributions of all authors. S.F. and M.S. designed the study and analyzed the data, and H.S. provided HS-731, for Figure 1. Experiments presented in Figure 2 were designed by M.A.-K. and K.K. and were executed and analyzed by A.M., M.B., K.K. and B.H. For Figure 3. the study was design by M.A.-K. and executed by C.C., A.M. and S.B.L. All authors have read and agreed to the published version of the manuscript.

Funding: The work was supported by The Higher Education Institutional Excellence Programme of the Ministry of Human Capacities in Hungary, within the framework of the Neurology Thematic Programme of Semmelweis University (FIKP, 2018) the National Research, Development and Innovation Office of Hungary (NKFI FK

124878), by the Economic Development and Innovation Operational Programme (GINOP 2.3.2-15-2016-00034), the European Community (EPILA, QLK6-1999-02334) and the Austrian Science Fund (FWF: I2463-B21).

Conflicts of Interest: The authors declare no conflict of interest.

References

1. Holzer, P. Opioid receptors in the gastrointestinal tract. *Regul. Pept.* **2009**, *155*, 11–17. [CrossRef] [PubMed]
2. Janson, W.; Stein, C. Peripheral opioid analgesia. *Curr. Pharm. Biotechnol.* **2003**, *4*, 270–274. [CrossRef] [PubMed]
3. Mansour, A.; Fox, C.; Akil, H.; Watson, S. Opioid-receptor mRNA expression in the rat CNS: Anatomical and functional implications. *Trends Neurosci.* **1995**, *18*, 22–29. [CrossRef]
4. Kieffer, B.L.; Befort, K.; Gaveriaux-Ruff, C.; Hirth, C.G. The delta-opioid receptor: Isolation of a cDNA by expression cloning and pharmacological characterization. *Proc. Natl. Acad. Sci. USA* **1992**, *89*, 12048–12052. [CrossRef]
5. Chen, Y.; Mestek, A.; Liu, J.; Hurley, J.A.; Yu, L. Molecular cloning and functional expression of a mu-opioid receptor from rat brain. *Mol. Pharmacol.* **1993**, *44*, 8–12. [CrossRef]
6. Minami, M.; Toya, T.; Katao, Y.; Maekawa, K.; Nakamura, S.; Onogi, T.; Kaneko, S.; Satoh, M. Cloning and expression of a cDNA for the rat kappa-opioid receptor. *FEBS Lett.* **1993**, *329*, 291–295. [CrossRef]
7. Pert, C.B.; Snyder, S.H. Opiate receptor: Demonstration in nervous tissue. *Science* **1973**, *179*, 1011–1014. [CrossRef] [PubMed]
8. Simon, E.J.; Hiller, J.M.; Edelman, I. Stereospecific binding of the potent narcotic analgesic (3H) Etorphine to rat-brain homogenate. *Proc. Natl. Acad. Sci. USA* **1973**, *70*, 1947–1949. [CrossRef] [PubMed]
9. Terenius, L. Characteristics of the "receptor" for narcotic analgesics in synaptic plasma membrane fraction from rat brain. *Acta. Pharmacol. Toxicol.* **1973**, *33*, 377–384. [CrossRef]
10. Law, P.Y.; Wong, Y.H.; Loh, H.H. Molecular mechanisms and regulation of opioid receptor signaling. *Annu. Rev. Pharmacol. Toxicol.* **2000**, *40*, 389–430. [CrossRef]
11. Lord, J.A.; Waterfield, A.A.; Hughes, J.; Kosterlitz, H.W. Endogenous opioid peptides: Multiple agonists and receptors. *Nature* **1977**, *267*, 495–499. [CrossRef]
12. Mollereau, C.; Parmentier, M.; Mailleux, P.; Butour, J.-L.; Moisand, C.; Chalon, P.; Caput, D.; Vassart, G.; Meunier, J.-C. ORL1, a novel member of the opioid receptor family. *FEBS Lett.* **1994**, *341*, 33–38. [CrossRef]
13. Wang, J.B.; Johnson, P.S.; Imai, Y.; Persico, A.M.; Ozenberger, B.A.; Eppler, C.M.; Uhl, G.R. cDNA Cloning of an orphan opiate receptor gene family member and its splice variant. *FEBS Lett.* **1994**, *348*, 75–79. [CrossRef]
14. Reinscheid, R.K.; Nothacker, H.P.; Bourson, A.; Ardati, A.; Henningsen, R.A.; Bunzow, J.R.; Grandy, D.K.; Langen, H.; Monsma, F.J.; Civelli, O. Orphanin FQ: A neuropeptide that activates an opioidlike G protein-coupled receptor. *Science* **1995**, *270*, 792–794. [CrossRef] [PubMed]
15. Burford, N.T.; Wang, D.; Sadée, W. G-protein coupling of mu-opioid receptors (OP3): Elevated basal signalling activity. *Biochem. J.* **2000**, *348*, 531–537. [CrossRef] [PubMed]
16. Dhawan, B.N.; Cesselin, F.; Raghubir, R.; Reisine, T.; Bradley, P.B.; Portoghese, P.S.; Hamon, M. International Union of Pharmacology. XII. Classification of opioid receptors. *Pharmacol. Rev.* **1996**, *48*, 567–592.
17. Bian, J.-M.; Wu, N.; Su, R.-B.; Li, J. Opioid receptor trafficking and signaling: What happens after opioid receptor activation? *Cell. Mol. Neurobiol.* **2012**, *32*, 167–184. [CrossRef]
18. Sim, L.J.; Childers, S.R. Anatomical distribution of mu, delta, and kappa opioid- and nociceptin/orphanin FQ-stimulated [35S]guanylyl-5'-O-(gamma-thio)-triphosphate binding in guinea pig brain. *J. Comp. Neurol.* **1997**, *386*, 562–572. [CrossRef]
19. Kaplovitch, E.; Gomes, T.; Camacho, X.; Dhalla, I.A.; Mamdani, M.M.; Juurlink, D.N. Sex differences in dose escalation and overdose death during chronic opioid therapy: A population-based cohort study. *PLoS ONE* **2015**, *10*, e0134550. [CrossRef]
20. Morgan, M.M.; Christie, M.J. Analysis of opioid efficacy, tolerance, addiction and dependence from cell culture to human. *Br. J. Pharmacol.* **2011**, *164*, 1322–1334. [CrossRef]
21. Hayhurst, C.J.; Durieux, M.E. Differential opioid tolerance and opioid-induced hyperalgesia. *Anesthesiology* **2016**, *124*, 483–488. [CrossRef] [PubMed]
22. Akbarali, H.I.; Inkisar, A.; Dewey, W.L. Site and mechanism of morphine tolerance in the gastrointestinal tract. *Neurogastroenterol. Motil.* **2014**, *26*, 1361–1367. [CrossRef]

23. Dumas, E.O.; Pollack, G.M. Opioid tolerance development: A pharmacokinetic/pharmacodynamic perspective. *AAPS J.* **2008**, *10*, 537–551. [CrossRef] [PubMed]
24. National Institute on Drug Abuse. Fentanyl and Other Synthetic Opioids Drug Overdose Deaths. Available online: https://www.drugabuse.gov/related-topics/trends-statistics/infographics/fentanyl-other-synthetic-opioids-drug-overdose-deaths (accessed on 22 May 2020).
25. Kanny, D.; Liu, Y.; Brewer, R.D.; Garvin, W.S.; Balluz, L. Vital signs: Binge drinking prevalence, frequency, and intensity among adults-united states, 2010. *Morb. Mortal. Wkly. Rep.* **2012**, *61*, 14–19.
26. Scholl, L.; Seth, P.; Kariisa, M.; Wilson, N.; Baldwin, G. Morbidity and mortality weekly report udrug and opioid-involved overdose deaths-nited States, 2013–2017. *MMWR Morb. Mortal. Wkly. Rep.* **2019**, *67*, 1419–1427.
27. Zoorob, M. Fentanyl shock: The changing geography of overdose in the United States. *Int. J. Drug Policy* **2019**, *70*, 40–46. [CrossRef] [PubMed]
28. Farrar, J.T.; Polomano, R.C.; Berlin, J.A.; Strom, B.L. A comparison of change in the 0-10 numeric rating scale to a pain relief scale and global medication performance scale in a short-term clinical trial of breakthrough pain intensity. *Anesthesiology* **2010**, *112*, 1464–1472. [CrossRef]
29. Buntin-Mushock, C.; Phillip, L.; Moriyama, K.; Palmer, P.P. Age-dependent opioid escalation in chronic pain patients. *Anesth. Analg.* **2005**, *100*, 1740–1745. [CrossRef]
30. Bowman, W.C.; Rand, M.J. *Textbook of Pharmacology*, 2nd ed.; Blackwell Scientific Publications: Oxford, UK, 1980; ISBN 0632099909.
31. Eisenberg, E.; McNicol, E.D.; Carr, D.B. Efficacy and safety of opioid agonists in the treatment of neuropathic pain of nonmalignant origin: Systematic review and meta-analysis of randomized controlled trials. *JAMA* **2005**, *293*, 3043–3052. [CrossRef]
32. Stein, C.; Machelska, H.; Binder, W.; Schäfer, M. Peripheral opioid analgesia. *Curr. Opin. Pharmacol.* **2001**, *1*, 62–65. [CrossRef]
33. Stein, C.; Lang, L.J. Peripheral mechanisms of opioid analgesia. *Curr. Opin. Pharmacol.* **2009**, *9*, 3–8. [CrossRef] [PubMed]
34. Fürst, S.; Riba, P.; Friedmann, T.; Tímar, J.; Al-Khrasani, M.; Obara, I.; Makuch, W.; Spetea, M.; Schütz, J.; Przewlocki, R.; et al. Peripheral versus central antinociceptive actions of 6-amino acid-substituted derivatives of 14-O-methyloxymorphone in acute and inflammatory pain in the rat. *J. Pharmacol. Exp. Ther.* **2005**, *312*, 609–618. [CrossRef] [PubMed]
35. Bileviciute-Ljungar, I.; Spetea, M.; Guo, Y.; Schutz, J.; Windisch, P.; Schmidhammer, H. Peripherally mediated antinociception of the μ-opioid receptor agonist HS-731 after subcutaneous and oral administration in rats with carrageenan-induced hindpaw inflammation. *J. Pharmacol. Exp. Ther.* **2005**, *317*, 220–227. [CrossRef] [PubMed]
36. Baillie, L.D.; Schmidhammer, H.; Mulligan, S.J. Peripheral μ-opioid receptor mediated inhibition of calcium signaling and action potential-evoked calcium fluorescent transients in primary afferent CGRP nociceptive terminals. *Neuropharmacology* **2015**, *93*, 267–273. [CrossRef]
37. Spetea, M.; Rief, S.B.; Haddou, T.B.; Fink, M.; Kristeva, E.; Mittendorfer, H.; Haas, S.; Hummer, N.; Follia, V.; Guerrieri, E.; et al. Synthesis, biological, and structural explorations of new zwitterionic derivatives of 14-O-methyloxymorphone, as potent μ/δ opioid agonists and peripherally selective antinociceptives. *J. Med. Chem.* **2019**, *62*, 641–653. [CrossRef]
38. Spahn, V.; Del Vecchio, G.; Labuz, D.; Rodriguez-Gaztelumendi, A.; Massaly, N.; Temp, J.; Durmaz, V.; Sabri, P.; Reidelbach, M.; Machelska, H.; et al. A nontoxic pain killer designed by modeling of pathological receptor conformations. *Science* **2017**, *355*, 966–969. [CrossRef]
39. Rodriguez-Gaztelumendi, A.; Spahn, V.; Labuz, D.; Machelska, H.; Stein, C. Analgesic effects of a novel pH-dependent μ-opioid receptor agonist in models of neuropathic and abdominal pain. *Pain* **2018**, *159*, 2277–2284. [CrossRef]
40. He, S.-Q.; Yang, F.; Perez, F.M.; Xu, Q.; Shechter, R.; Cheong, Y.-K.; Carteret, A.F.; Dong, X.; Sweitzer, S.M.; Raja, S.N.; et al. Tolerance develops to the antiallodynic effects of the peripherally acting opioid loperamide hydrochloride in nerve-injured rats. *Pain* **2013**, *154*, 2477–2486. [CrossRef]
41. Akbarali, H.I.; Dewey, W.L. Gastrointestinal motility, dysbiosis and opioid-induced tolerance: Is there a link? *Nat. Rev. Gastroenterol. Hepatol.* **2019**, *16*, 323–324. [CrossRef]

42. He, L.; Kim, J.A.; Whistler, J.L. Biomarkers of morphine tolerance and dependence are prevented by morphine-induced endocytosis of a mutant mu-opioid receptor. *FASEB J.* **2009**, *23*, 4327–4334. [CrossRef]
43. Lackó, E.; Riba, P.; Giricz, Z.; Váradi, A.; Cornic, L.; Balogh, M.; Király, K.; Csekő, K.; Mousa, S.A.; Hosztafi, S.; et al. New morphine analogs produce peripheral antinociception within a certain dose range of their systemic administration. *J. Pharmacol. Exp. Ther.* **2016**, *359*, 171–181. [CrossRef] [PubMed]
44. Balogh, M.; Zádori, Z.S.; Lázár, B.; Karádi, D.; László, S.; Mousa, S.A.; Hosztafi, S.; Zádor, F.; Riba, P.; Schäfer, M.; et al. The peripheral versus central antinociception of a novel opioid agonist: Acute inflammatory pain in rats. *Neurochem. Res.* **2018**, *43*, 1250–1257. [CrossRef] [PubMed]
45. Shannon, H.E.; Lutz, E.A. Comparison of the peripheral and central effects of the opioid agonists loperamide and morphine in the formalin test in rats. *Neuropharmacology* **2002**, *42*, 253–261. [CrossRef]
46. Takasuna, M.; Negus, S.S.; DeCosta, B.R.; Woods, J.H. Opioid pharmacology of the antinociceptive effects of loperamide in mice. *Behav. Pharmacol.* **1994**, *5*, 189–195. [CrossRef]
47. Brown, D.R.; Goldberg, L.I. The use of quaternary narcotic antagonists in opiate research. *Neuropharmacology* **1985**, *24*, 181–191. [CrossRef]
48. Reichert, J.A.; Daughters, R.S.; Rivard, R.; Simone, D.A. Peripheral and preemptive opioid antinociception in a mouse visceral pain model. *Pain* **2001**, *89*, 221–227. [CrossRef]
49. Martínez, V.; Abalo, R. Peripherally acting opioid analgesics and peripherally-induced analgesia. *Behav. Pharmacol.* **2020**, *31*, 136–158. [CrossRef]
50. Labuz, D.; Mousa, S.A.; Schäfer, M.; Stein, C.; Machelska, H. Relative contribution of peripheral versus central opioid receptors to antinociception. *Brain Res.* **2007**, *1160*, 30–38. [CrossRef]
51. Al-Khrasani, M.; Spetea, M.; Friedmann, T.; Riba, P.; Király, K.; Schmidhammer, H.; Furst, S. DAMGO and 6β-glycine substituted 14-O-methyloxymorphone but not morphine show peripheral, preemptive antinociception after systemic administration in a mouse visceral pain model and high intrinsic efficacy in the isolated rat vas deferens. *Brain Res. Bull.* **2007**, *74*, 369–375. [CrossRef]
52. Al-Khrasani, M.; Lackó, E.; Riba, P.; Király, K.; Sobor, M.; Timár, J.; Mousa, S.; Schäfer, M.; Fürst, S. The central versus peripheral antinociceptive effects of μ-opioid receptor agonists in the new model of rat visceral pain. *Brain Res. Bull.* **2012**, *87*, 238–243. [CrossRef]
53. Khalefa, B.I.; Shaqura, M.; Al-Khrasani, M.; Fürst, S.; Mousa, S.A.; Schäfer, M. Relative contributions of peripheral versus supraspinal or spinal opioid receptors to the antinociception of systemic opioids. *Eur. J. Pain* **2012**, *16*, 690–705. [CrossRef] [PubMed]
54. Obara, I.; Przewlocki, R.; Przewlocka, B. Local peripheral effects of μ-opioid receptor agonists in neuropathic pain in rats. *Neurosci. Lett.* **2004**, *360*, 85–89. [CrossRef] [PubMed]
55. Obara, I.; Makuch, W.; Spetea, M.; Schütz, J.; Schmidhammer, H.; Przewlocki, R.; Przewlocka, B. Local peripheral antinociceptive effects of 14-O-methyloxymorphone derivatives in inflammatory and neuropathic pain in the rat. *Eur. J. Pharmacol.* **2007**, *558*, 60–67. [CrossRef]
56. Balogh, M.; Zádor, F.; Zádori, Z.S.; Shaqura, M.; Király, K.; Mohammadzadeh, A.; Varga, B.; Lázár, B.; Mousa, S.A.; Hosztafi, S.; et al. Efficacy-based perspective to overcome reduced opioid analgesia of advanced painful diabetic neuropathy in rats. *Front. Pharmacol.* **2019**, *10*, 347. [CrossRef] [PubMed]
57. Truong, W.; Cheng, C.; Xu, Q.-G.; Li, X.-Q.; Zochodne, D.W. Mu Opioid receptors and analgesia at the site of a peripheral nerve injury. *Ann. Neurol.* **2003**, *53*, 366–375. [CrossRef] [PubMed]
58. Guan, Y.; Johanek, L.M.; Hartke, T.V.; Shim, B.; Tao, Y.-X.; Ringkamp, M.; Meyer, R.A.; Raja, S.N. Peripherally acting mu-opioid receptor agonist attenuates neuropathic pain in rats after L5 spinal nerve injury. *Pain* **2008**, *138*, 318–329. [CrossRef]
59. Shinoda, K.; Hruby, V.J.; Porreca, F. Antihyperalgesic effects of loperamide in a model of rat neuropathic pain are mediated by peripheral δ-opioid receptors. *Neurosci. Lett.* **2007**, *411*, 143–146. [CrossRef]
60. Zuckerman, A.; Bolan, E.; de Paulis, T.; Schmidt, D.; Spector, S.; Pasternak, G.W. Pharmacological characterization of morphine-6-sulfate and codeine-6-sulfate. *Brain Res.* **1999**, *842*, 1–5. [CrossRef]
61. Botros, S.; Lipkowski, A.W.; Larson, D.L.; Stark, P.A.; Takemori, A.E.; Portoghese, P.S. Opioid agonist and antagonist activities of peripherally selective derivatives of naltrexamine and oxymorphamine. *J. Med. Chem.* **1989**, *32*, 2068–2071. [CrossRef] [PubMed]
62. Lacko, E.; Varadi, A.; Rapavi, R.; Zador, F.; Riba, P.; Benyhe, S.; Borsodi, A.; Hosztafi, S.; Timar, J.; Noszal, B.; et al. A novel μ-opioid receptor ligand with high in vitro and in vivo agonist efficacy. *Curr. Med. Chem.* **2012**, *19*, 4699–4707. [CrossRef]

63. Smith, T.W.; Buchan, P.; Parsons, D.N.; Wilkinson, S. Peripheral antinociceptive effects of N-methyl morphine. *Life Sci.* **1982**, *31*, 1205–1208. [CrossRef]
64. Spetea, M.; Schmidhammer, H. Recent advances in the development of 14-alkoxy substituted morphinans as potent and safer opioid analgesics. *Curr. Med. Chem.* **2012**, *19*, 2442–2457. [CrossRef]
65. Zádor, F.; Mohammadzadeh, A.; Balogh, M.; Zádori, Z.S.; Király, K.; Barsi, S.; Galambos, A.R.; László, S.B.; Hutka, B.; Váradi, A.; et al. Comparisons of In Vivo and In Vitro Opioid Effects of Newly Synthesized 14-Methoxycodeine-6-O-sulfate and Codeine-6-O-sulfate. *Molecules* **2020**, *25*, 1370. [CrossRef] [PubMed]
66. Vadivelu, N.; Mitra, S.; Hines, R.L. Peripheral opioid receptor agonists for analgesia: A comprehensive review. *J. Opioid Manag.* **2011**, *7*, 55–68. [CrossRef] [PubMed]
67. Sehgal, N.; Smith, H.S.; Manchikanti, L. Peripherally acting opioids and clinical implications for pain control. *Pain Physician* **2011**, *14*, 249–258. [PubMed]
68. Zöllner, C.; Mousa, S.A.; Fischer, O.; Rittner, H.L.; Shaqura, M.; Brack, A.; Shakibaei, M.; Binder, W.; Urban, F.; Stein, C.; et al. Chronic morphine use does not induce peripheral tolerance in a rat model of inflammatory pain. *J. Clin. Invest.* **2008**, *118*, 1065–1073. [CrossRef] [PubMed]
69. Stein, C.; Pflüger, M.; Yassouridis, A.; Hoelzl, J.; Lehrberger, K.; Welte, C.; Hassan, A.H. No tolerance to peripheral morphine analgesia in presence of opioid expression in inflamed synovia. *J. Clin. Invest.* **1996**, *98*, 793–799. [CrossRef]
70. Allouche, S.; Noble, F.; Marie, N. Opioid receptor desensitization: Mechanisms and its link to tolerance. *Front. Pharmacol.* **2014**, *5*, 280. [CrossRef]
71. Al-Hasani, R.; Bruchas, M.R. Molecular mechanisms of opioid receptor-dependent signaling and behavior. *Anesthesiology* **2011**, *115*, 1363–1381. [CrossRef]
72. Uniyal, A.; Gadepalli, A.; Akhilesh; Tiwari, V. Underpinning the neurobiological intricacies associated with opioid tolerance. *ACS Chem. Neurosci.* **2020**, *11*, 830–839. [CrossRef]
73. Mori, M.; Oguri, K.; Yoshimura, H.; Shimomura, K.; Kamata, O.; Ueki, S. Chemical synthesis and analgesic effect of morphine ethereal sulfates. *Life Sci. I.* **1972**, *11*, 525–533. [CrossRef]
74. Kolesnikov, Y.A.; Jain, S.; Wilson, R.; Pasternak, G.W. Peripheral morphine analgesia: Synergy with central sites and a target of morphine tolerance. *J. Pharmacol. Exp. Ther.* **1996**, *279*, 502–506. [PubMed]
75. Kolesnikov, Y.; Pasternak, G.W. Topical opioids in mice: Analgesia and reversal of tolerance by a topical N-methyl-D-aspartate antagonist. *J. Pharmacol. Exp. Ther.* **1999**, *290*, 247–252. [PubMed]
76. Aley, K.O.; Levine, J.D. Dissociation of tolerance and dependence for opioid peripheral antinociception in rats. *J. Neurosci.* **1997**, *17*, 3907–3912. [CrossRef]
77. Danysz, W.; Kozela, E.; Parsons, C.G.; Sladek, M.; Bauer, T.; Popik, P. Peripherally acting NMDA receptor/glycineB site receptor antagonists inhibit morphine tolerance. *Neuropharmacology* **2005**, *48*, 360–371. [CrossRef]
78. Ben-Eliyahu, S.; Marek, P.; Vaccarino, A.L.; Mogil, J.S.; Sternberg, W.F.; Liebeskind, J.C. The NMDA receptor antagonist MK-801 prevents long-lasting non-associative morphine tolerance in the rat. *Brain Res.* **1992**, *575*, 304–308. [CrossRef]
79. Trujillo, K.A. Are NMDA receptors involved in opiate-induced neural and behavioral plasticity? *Psychopharmacology (Berl.)* **2000**, *151*, 121–141. [CrossRef]
80. Carlton, S.M.; Hargett, G.L.; Coggeshall, R.E. Localization and activation of glutamate receptors in unmyelinated axons of rat glabrous skin. *Neurosci. Lett.* **1995**, *197*, 25–28. [CrossRef]
81. Zhou, S.; Bonasera, L.; Carlton, S.M. Peripheral administration of NMDA, AMPA or KA results in pain behaviors in rats. *Neuroreport* **1996**, *7*, 895–900. [CrossRef]
82. Davidson, E.M.; Coggeshall, R.E.; Carlton, S.M. Peripheral NMDA and non-NMDA glutamate receptors contribute to nociceptive behaviors in the rat formalin test. *Neuroreport* **1997**, *8*, 941–946. [CrossRef]
83. Meuser, T.; Giesecke, T.; Gabriel, A.; Horsch, M.; Sabatowski, R.; Hescheler, J.; Grond, S.; Palmer, P.P. Mu-opioid receptor mRNA regulation during morphine tolerance in the rat peripheral nervous system. *Anesth. Analg.* **2003**, *97*, 1458–1463. [CrossRef] [PubMed]
84. Sun, J.; Chen, S.; Chen, H.; Pan, H. μ-Opioid receptors in primary sensory neurons are essential for opioid analgesic effect on acute and inflammatory pain and opioid-induced hyperalgesia. *J. Physiol.* **2019**, *597*, 1661–1675. [CrossRef]

85. Kiraly, K.; Caputi, F.F.; Hanuska, A.; Kató, E.; Balogh, M.; Köles, L.; Palmisano, M.; Riba, P.; Hosztafi, S.; Romualdi, P.; et al. A new potent analgesic agent with reduced liability to produce morphine tolerance. *Brain Res. Bull.* **2015**, *117*, 32–38. [CrossRef] [PubMed]
86. Aley, K.O.; Green, P.G.; Levine, J.D. Opioid and adenosine peripheral antinociception are subject to tolerance and withdrawal. *J. Neurosci.* **1995**, *15*, 8031–8038. [CrossRef] [PubMed]
87. Honoré, P.; Catheline, G.; Le Guen, S.; Besson, J.M. Chronic treatment with systemic morphine induced tolerance to the systemic and peripheral antinociceptive effects of morphine on both carrageenin induced mechanical hyperalgesia and spinal c-Fos expression in awake rats. *Pain* **1997**, *71*, 99–108. [CrossRef]
88. Pethő, G.; Reeh, P.W. Sensory and signaling mechanisms of bradykinin, eicosanoids, platelet-activating factor, and nitric oxide in peripheral nociceptors. *Physiol. Rev.* **2012**, *92*, 1699–1775. [CrossRef]
89. Tokuyama, S.; Inoue, M.; Fuchigami, T.; Ueda, H. Lack of tolerance in peripheral opioid analgesia in mice. *Life Sci.* **1998**, *62*, 1677–1681. [CrossRef]
90. Inoue, M.; Shimohira, I.; Yoshida, A.; Zimmer, A.; Takeshima, H.; Sakurada, T.; Ueda, H. Dose-related opposite modulation by nociceptin/orphanin FQ of substance P nociception in the nociceptors and spinal cord. *J. Pharmacol. Exp. Ther.* **1999**, *291*, 308–313.
91. Inoue, M.; Ueda, H. Protein kinase C-mediated acute tolerance to peripheral mu-opioid analgesia in the bradykinin-nociception test in mice. *J. Pharmacol. Exp. Ther.* **2000**, *293*, 662–669.
92. Shaqura, M.A.; Zöllner, C.; Mousa, S.A.; Stein, C.; Schäfer, M. Characterization of μ opioid receptor binding and g protein coupling in rat hypothalamus, spinal cord, and primary afferent neurons during inflammatory pain. *J. Pharmacol. Exp. Ther.* **2004**, *308*, 712–718. [CrossRef]
93. Stein, C. Opioid Receptors. *Annu. Rev. Med.* **2016**, *67*, 433–451. [CrossRef] [PubMed]
94. Stein, C.; Schäfer, M.; Machelska, H. Attacking pain at its source: New perspectives on opioids. *Nat. Med.* **2003**, *9*, 1003–1008. [CrossRef] [PubMed]
95. Mousa, S.A.; Straub, R.H.; Schäfer, M.; Stein, C. Beta-endorphin, Met-enkephalin and corresponding opioid receptors within synovium of patients with joint trauma, osteoarthritis and rheumatoid arthritis. *Ann. Rheum. Dis.* **2007**, *66*, 871–879. [CrossRef] [PubMed]
96. Stein, C.; Zöllner, C. Opioids and Sensory Nerves. In *Sensory Nerves*; Canning, B., Ed.; Springer: Berlin, Germany, 2009; pp. 495–518. ISBN 978-3-540-79089-1.
97. Del Vecchio, G.; Spahn, V.; Stein, C. Novel opioid analgesics and side effects. *ACS Chem. Neurosci.* **2017**, *8*, 1638–1640. [CrossRef] [PubMed]
98. Ninković, J.; Roy, S. Role of the mu-opioid receptor in opioid modulation of immune function. *Amino Acids* **2013**, *45*, 9–24. [CrossRef]
99. Fernández-Dueñas, V.; Pol, O.; García-Nogales, P.; Hernández, L.; Planas, E.; Puig, M.M. Tolerance to the antinociceptive and antiexudative effects of morphine in a murine model of peripheral inflammation. *J. Pharmacol. Exp. Ther.* **2007**, *322*, 360–368. [CrossRef]
100. Hernández, L.; Romero, A.; Almela, P.; García-Nogales, P.; Laorden, M.L.; Puig, M.M. Tolerance to the antinociceptive effects of peripherally administered opioids: Expression of β-arrestins. *Brain Res.* **2009**, *1248*, 31–39. [CrossRef]
101. Eidson, L.N.; Murphy, A.Z. Persistent peripheral inflammation attenuates morphine-induced periaqueductal gray glial cell activation and analgesic tolerance in the male rat. *J. Pain* **2013**, *14*, 393–404. [CrossRef]
102. Bruce, D.J.; Peterson, C.D.; Kitto, K.F.; Akgün, E.; Lazzaroni, S.; Portoghese, P.S.; Fairbanks, C.A.; Wilcox, G.L. Combination of a δ-opioid receptor agonist and loperamide produces peripherally-mediated analgesic synergy in mice. *Anesthesiology* **2019**, *131*, 649–663. [CrossRef]
103. Hoffman, E.M.; Watson, J.C.; St Sauver, J.; Staff, N.P.; Klein, C.J. Association of long-term opioid therapy with functional status, adverse outcomes, and mortality among patients with polyneuropathy. *JAMA Neurol.* **2017**, *74*, 773–779. [CrossRef]
104. Furlan, A.D.; Sandoval, J.A.; Mailis-Gagnon, A.; Tunks, E. Opioids for chronic noncancer pain: A meta-analysis of effectiveness and side effects. *CMAJ* **2006**, *174*, 1589–1594. [CrossRef] [PubMed]
105. Al-Khrasani, M.; Mohammadzadeh, A.; Balogh, M.; Király, K.; Barsi, S.; Hajnal, B.; Köles, L.; Zádori, Z.S.; Harsing, L.G. Glycine transporter inhibitors: A new avenue for managing neuropathic pain. *Brain Res. Bull.* **2019**, *152*, 143–158. [CrossRef] [PubMed]
106. Porreca, F.; Tang, Q.B.; Bian, D.; Riedl, M.; Elde, R.; Lai, J. Spinal opioid mu receptor expression in lumbar spinal cord of rats following nerve injury. *Brain Res.* **1998**, *795*, 197–203. [CrossRef]

107. Kohno, T.; Ji, R.-R.; Ito, N.; Allchorne, A.J.; Befort, K.; Karchewski, L.A.; Woolf, C.J. Peripheral axonal injury results in reduced mu opioid receptor pre- and post-synaptic action in the spinal cord. *Pain* **2005**, *117*, 77–87. [CrossRef] [PubMed]
108. Mansikka, H.; Zhao, C.; Sheth, R.N.; Sora, I.; Uhl, G.; Raja, S.N. Nerve injury induces a tonic bilateral mu-opioid receptor-mediated inhibitory effect on mechanical allodynia in mice. *Anesthesiology* **2004**, *100*, 912–921. [CrossRef] [PubMed]
109. Klein, A.H.; Mohammad, H.K.; Ali, R.; Peper, B.; Wilson, S.P.; Raja, S.N.; Ringkamp, M.; Sweitzer, S. Overexpression of μ-opioid receptors in peripheral afferents, but not in combination with enkephalin, decreases neuropathic pain behavior and enhances opioid analgesia in mouse. *Anesthesiology* **2018**, *128*, 967–983. [CrossRef]
110. Kayser, V.; Lee, S.H.; Guilbaud, G. Evidence for a peripheral component in the enhanced antinociceptive effect of a low dose of systemic morphine in rats with peripheral mononeuropathy. *Neuroscience* **1995**, *64*, 537–545. [CrossRef]
111. Idänpään-Heikkilä, J.J.; Guilbaud, G.; Kayser, V. Prevention of tolerance to the antinociceptive effects of systemic morphine by a selective cholecystokinin-B receptor antagonist in a rat model of peripheral neuropathy. *J. Pharmacol. Exp. Ther.* **1997**, *282*, 1366–1372.
112. Chu, L.F.; Angst, M.S.; Clark, D. Opioid-induced hyperalgesia in humans. *Clin. J. Pain* **2008**, *24*, 479–496. [CrossRef]
113. Busserolles, J.; Lolignier, S.; Kerckhove, N.; Bertin, C.; Authier, N.; Eschalier, A. Replacement of current opioid drugs focusing on MOR-related strategies. *Pharmacol. Ther.* **2020**, *210*, 107519. [CrossRef]
114. Corder, G.; Tawfik, V.L.; Wang, D.; Sypek, E.I.; Low, S.A.; Dickinson, J.R.; Sotoudeh, C.; Clark, J.D.; Barres, B.A.; Bohlen, C.J.; et al. Loss of μ opioid receptor signaling in nociceptors, but not microglia, abrogates morphine tolerance without disrupting analgesia. *Nat. Med.* **2017**, *23*, 164–173. [CrossRef] [PubMed]
115. Walker, J.; Catheline, G.; Guilbaud, G.; Kayser, V. Lack of cross-tolerance between the antinociceptive effects of systemic morphine and asimadoline, a peripherally-selective κ-opioid agonist, in CCI- neuropathic rats. *Pain* **1999**, *83*, 509–516. [CrossRef]
116. Albert-Vartanian, A.; Boyd, M.R.; Hall, A.L.; Morgado, S.J.; Nguyen, E.; Nguyen, V.P.H.; Patel, S.P.; Russo, L.J.; Shao, A.J.; Raffa, R.B. Will peripherally restricted kappa-opioid receptor agonists (pKORAs) relieve pain with less opioid adverse effects and abuse potential? *J. Clin. Pharm. Ther.* **2016**, *41*, 371–382. [CrossRef] [PubMed]
117. Trujillo, K.A.; Akil, H. Inhibition of opiate tolerance by non-competitive N-methyl-D-aspartate receptor antagonists. *Brain Res.* **1994**, *633*, 178–188. [CrossRef]
118. Tortorici, V.; Nogueira, L.; Aponte, Y.; Vanegas, H. Involvement of cholecystokinin in the opioid tolerance induced by dipyrone (metamizol) microinjections into the periaqueductal gray matter of rats. *Pain* **2004**, *112*, 113–120. [CrossRef] [PubMed]
119. Schäfer, M.; Zhou, L.; Stein, C. Cholecystokinin inhibits peripheral opioid analgesia in inflamed tissue. *Neuroscience* **1997**, *82*, 603–611. [CrossRef]
120. Ebert, B.; Thorkildsen, C.; Andersen, S.; Christrup, L.L.; Hjeds, H. Opioid analgesics as noncompetitive N-methyl-D-aspartate (NMDA) antagonists. *Biochem. Pharmacol.* **1998**, *56*, 553–559. [CrossRef]
121. Zhang, X.; de Araujo Lucas, G.; Elde, R.; Wiesenfeld-Hallin, Z.; Hökfelt, T. Effect of morphine on cholecystokinin and μ-opioid receptor-like immunoreactivities in rat spinal dorsal horn neurons after peripheral axotomy and inflammation. *Neuroscience* **1999**, *95*, 197–207. [CrossRef]
122. Kohno, T.; Kumamoto, E.; Higashi, H.; Shimoji, K.; Yoshimura, M. Actions of opioids on excitatory and inhibitory transmission in substantia gelatinosa of adult rat spinal cord. *J. Physiol.* **1999**, *518*, 803–813. [CrossRef]
123. Shaqura, M.; Khalefa, B.I.; Shakibaei, M.; Winkler, J.; Al-Khrasani, M.; Fürst, S.; Mousa, S.A.; Schäfer, M. Reduced number, G protein coupling, and antinociceptive efficacy of spinal mu-opioid receptors in diabetic rats are reversed by nerve growth factor. *J. Pain* **2013**, *14*, 720–730. [CrossRef]
124. Fisher, C.; Johnson, K.; Okerman, T.; Jurgenson, T.; Nickell, A.; Salo, E.; Moore, M.; Doucette, A.; Bjork, J.; Klein, A.H. Morphine efficacy, tolerance, and hypersensitivity are altered after modulation of SUR1 subtype KATP channel activity in mice. *Front. Neurosci.* **2019**, *13*, 1122. [CrossRef]
125. DuPont, A.W.; DuPont, H.L. The intestinal microbiota and chronic disorders of the gut. *Nat. Rev. Gastroenterol. Hepatol.* **2011**, *8*, 523–531. [CrossRef] [PubMed]

126. Sharon, G.; Sampson, T.R.; Geschwind, D.H.; Mazmanian, S.K. The central nervous system and the gut microbiome. *Cell* **2016**, *167*, 915–932. [CrossRef] [PubMed]
127. Tremaroli, V.; Bäckhed, F. Functional interactions between the gut microbiota and host metabolism. *Nature* **2012**, *489*, 242–249. [CrossRef] [PubMed]
128. Zhang, L.; Meng, J.; Ban, Y.; Jalodia, R.; Chupikova, I.; Fernandez, I.; Brito, N.; Sharma, U.; Abreu, M.T.; Ramakrishnan, S.; et al. Morphine tolerance is attenuated in germfree mice and reversed by probiotics, implicating the role of gut microbiome. *Proc. Natl. Acad. Sci. USA* **2019**, *116*, 13523–13532. [CrossRef] [PubMed]
129. Wang, F.; Meng, J.; Zhang, L.; Johnson, T.; Chen, C.; Roy, S. Morphine induces changes in the gut microbiome and metabolome in a morphine dependence model. *Sci. Rep.* **2018**, *8*, 3596. [CrossRef]
130. Mischel, R.A.; Dewey, W.L.; Akbarali, H.I. Tolerance to morphine-induced inhibition of TTX-R sodium channels in dorsal root ganglia neurons is modulated by gut-derived mediators. *iScience* **2018**, *2*, 193–209. [CrossRef]
131. Kang, M.; Mischel, R.A.; Bhave, S.; Komla, E.; Cho, A.; Huang, C.; Dewey, W.L.; Akbarali, H.I. The effect of gut microbiome on tolerance to morphine mediated antinociception in mice. *Sci. Rep.* **2017**, *7*, 42658. [CrossRef]
132. Mischel, R.A.; Muchhala, K.H.; Dewey, W.L.; Akbarali, H.I. The "culture" of pain control: A review of opioid-induced dysbiosis (OID) in antinociceptive tolerance. *J. Pain* **2019**. [CrossRef] [PubMed]
133. Meng, J.; Banerjee, S.; Li, D.; Sindberg, G.M.; Wang, F.; Ma, J.; Roy, S. Opioid exacerbation of Gram-positive sepsis, induced by gut microbial modulation, is rescued by IL-17A neutralization. *Sci. Rep.* **2015**, *5*, 10918. [CrossRef] [PubMed]
134. Banerjee, S.; Sindberg, G.; Wang, F.; Meng, J.; Sharma, U.; Zhang, L.; Dauer, P.; Chen, C.; Dalluge, J.; Johnson, T.; et al. Opioid-induced gut microbial disruption and bile dysregulation leads to gut barrier compromise and sustained systemic inflammation. *Mucosal Immunol.* **2016**, *9*, 1418–1428. [CrossRef] [PubMed]
135. Lee, K.; Vuong, H.E.; Nusbaum, D.J.; Hsiao, E.Y.; Evans, C.J.; Taylor, A.M.W. The gut microbiota mediates reward and sensory responses associated with regimen-selective morphine dependence. *Neuropsychopharmacology* **2018**, *43*, 2606–2614. [CrossRef] [PubMed]
136. Kashyap, P.C.; Marcobal, A.; Ursell, L.K.; Larauche, M.; Duboc, H.; Earle, K.A.; Sonnenburg, E.D.; Ferreyra, J.A.; Higginbottom, S.K.; Million, M.; et al. Complex interactions among diet, gastrointestinal transit, and gut microbiota in humanized mice. *Gastroenterology* **2013**, *144*, 967–977. [CrossRef] [PubMed]
137. Touw, K.; Ringus, D.L.; Hubert, N.; Wang, Y.; Leone, V.A.; Nadimpalli, A.; Theriault, B.R.; Huang, Y.E.; Tune, J.D.; Herring, P.B.; et al. Mutual reinforcement of pathophysiological host-microbe interactions in intestinal stasis models. *Physiol. Rep.* **2017**, *5*, e13182. [CrossRef] [PubMed]
138. Sharma, U.; Olson, R.K.; Erhart, F.N.; Zhang, L.; Meng, J.; Segura, B.; Banerjee, S.; Sharma, M.; Saluja, A.K.; Ramakrishnan, S.; et al. Prescription opioid induce gut dysbiosis and exacerbate colitis in a murine model of Inflammatory Bowel Disease. *J. Crohns. Colitis* **2019**. [CrossRef] [PubMed]
139. Sindberg, G.M.; Callen, S.E.; Banerjee, S.; Meng, J.; Hale, V.L.; Hegde, R.; Cheney, P.D.; Villinger, F.; Roy, S.; Buch, S. Morphine potentiates dysbiotic microbial and metabolic shifts in acute SIV infection. *J. Neuroimmune Pharmacol.* **2019**, *14*, 200–214. [CrossRef]
140. Acharya, C.; Betrapally, N.S.; Gillevet, P.M.; Sterling, R.K.; Akbarali, H.; White, M.B.; Ganapathy, D.; Fagan, A.; Sikaroodi, M.; Bajaj, J.S. Chronic opioid use is associated with altered gut microbiota and predicts readmissions in patients with cirrhosis. *Aliment. Pharmacol. Ther.* **2017**, *45*, 319–331. [CrossRef]
141. Xu, Y.; Xie, Z.; Wang, H.; Shen, Z.; Guo, Y.; Gao, Y.; Chen, X.; Wu, Q.; Li, X.; Wang, K. Bacterial diversity of intestinal microbiota in patients with substance use disorders revealed by 16S rRNA gene deep sequencing. *Sci. Rep.* **2017**, *7*, 3628. [CrossRef]
142. Kim, S.C.; Tonkonogy, S.L.; Albright, C.A.; Tsang, J.; Balish, E.J.; Braun, J.; Huycke, M.M.; Sartor, R.B. Variable phenotypes of enterocolitis in interleukin 10-deficient mice monoassociated with two different commensal bacteria. *Gastroenterology* **2005**, *128*, 891–906. [CrossRef]
143. Moon, C.; Baldridge, M.T.; Wallace, M.A.; Burnham, C.-A.D.; Virgin, H.W.; Stappenbeck, T.S. Vertically transmitted faecal IgA levels determine extra-chromosomal phenotypic variation. *Nature* **2015**, *521*, 90–93. [CrossRef]
144. Lane, E.R.; Zisman, T.L.; Suskind, D.L. The microbiota in inflammatory bowel disease: Current and therapeutic insights. *J. Inflamm. Res.* **2017**, *10*, 63–73. [CrossRef] [PubMed]

145. Geirnaert, A.; Calatayud, M.; Grootaert, C.; Laukens, D.; Devriese, S.; Smagghe, G.; De Vos, M.; Boon, N.; Van de Wiele, T. Butyrate-producing bacteria supplemented in vitro to Crohn's disease patient microbiota increased butyrate production and enhanced intestinal epithelial barrier integrity. *Sci. Rep.* **2017**, *7*, 11450. [CrossRef] [PubMed]
146. Ng, S.C.; Hart, A.L.; Kamm, M.A.; Stagg, A.J.; Knight, S.C. Mechanisms of action of probiotics: Recent advances. *Inflamm. Bowel Dis.* **2009**, *15*, 300–310. [CrossRef] [PubMed]
147. Moore, B.A.; Stewart, T.M.R.; Hill, C.; Vanner, S.J. TNBS ileitis evokes hyperexcitability and changes in ionic membrane properties of nociceptive DRG neurons. *Am. J. Physiol. Gastrointest. Liver Physiol.* **2002**, *282*, 1045-1051. [CrossRef]
148. Komla, E.; Stevens, D.L.; Zheng, Y.; Zhang, Y.; Dewey, W.L.; Akbarali, H.I. Experimental colitis enhances the rate of antinociceptive tolerance to morphine via peripheral opioid receptors. *J. Pharmacol. Exp. Ther.* **2019**, *370*, 504–513. [CrossRef]
149. Hutchinson, M.R.; Shavit, Y.; Grace, P.M.; Rice, K.C.; Maier, S.F.; Watkins, L.R. Exploring the neuroimmunopharmacology of opioids: An integrative review of mechanisms of central immune signaling and their implications for opioid analgesia. *Pharmacol. Rev.* **2011**, *63*, 772–810. [CrossRef]
150. Mahajan, S.D.; Aalinkeel, R.; Sykes, D.E.; Reynolds, J.L.; Bindukumar, B.; Fernandez, S.F.; Chawda, R.; Shanahan, T.C.; Schwartz, S.A. Tight junction regulation by morphine and HIV-1 tat modulates blood-brain barrier permeability. *J. Clin. Immunol.* **2008**, *28*, 528–541. [CrossRef]
151. Plein, L.M.; Rittner, H.L. Opioids and the immune system - friend or foe. *Br. J. Pharmacol.* **2018**, *175*, 2717–2725. [CrossRef]
152. Levy, M.; Kolodziejczyk, A.A.; Thaiss, C.A.; Elinav, E. Dysbiosis and the immune system. *Nat. Rev. Immunol.* **2017**, *17*, 219–232. [CrossRef]
153. Barbara, G.; Stanghellini, V.; Brandi, G.; Cremon, C.; Di Nardo, G.; De Giorgio, R.; Corinaldesi, R. Interactions between commensal bacteria and gut sensorimotor function in health and disease. *Am. J. Gastroenterol.* **2005**, *100*, 2560–2568. [CrossRef]

Sample Availability: Samples of the compounds are available from the authors.

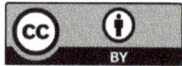

© 2020 by the authors. Licensee MDPI, Basel, Switzerland. This article is an open access article distributed under the terms and conditions of the Creative Commons Attribution (CC BY) license (http://creativecommons.org/licenses/by/4.0/).

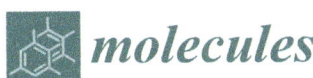

Review

Development of Diphenethylamines as Selective Kappa Opioid Receptor Ligands and Their Pharmacological Activities

Helmut Schmidhammer *, Filippo Erli, Elena Guerrieri and Mariana Spetea *

Department of Pharmaceutical Chemistry, Institute of Pharmacy and Center for Molecular Biosciences Innsbruck (CMBI), University of Innsbruck, Innrain 80-82, 6020 Innsbruck, Austria; filippo.erli@student.uibk.ac.at (F.E.); eleguerrieri@hotmail.com (E.G.)
* Correspondence: helmut.schmidhammer@uibk.ac.at (H.S.); mariana.spetea@uibk.ac.at (M.S.)

Received: 15 October 2020; Accepted: 30 October 2020; Published: 2 November 2020

Abstract: Among the opioid receptors, the kappa opioid receptor (KOR) has been gaining substantial attention as a promising molecular target for the treatment of numerous human disorders, including pain, pruritus, affective disorders (i.e., depression and anxiety), drug addiction, and neurological diseases (i.e., epilepsy). Particularly, the knowledge that activation of the KOR, opposite to the mu opioid receptor (MOR), does not produce euphoria or leads to respiratory depression or overdose, has stimulated the interest in discovering ligands targeting the KOR as novel pharmacotherapeutics. However, the KOR mediates the negative side effects of dysphoria/aversion, sedation, and psychotomimesis, with the therapeutic promise of biased agonism (i.e., selective activation of beneficial over deleterious signaling pathways) for designing safer KOR therapeutics without the liabilities of conventional KOR agonists. In this review, the development of new KOR ligands from the class of diphenethylamines is presented. Specifically, we describe the design strategies, synthesis, and pharmacological activities of differently substituted diphenethylamines, where structure–activity relationships have been extensively studied. Ligands with distinct profiles as potent and selective agonists, G protein-biased agonists, and selective antagonists, and their potential use as therapeutic agents (i.e., pain treatment) and research tools are described.

Keywords: kappa opioid receptor; diphenethylamines; design and synthesis; structure–activity relationships; agonist; partial agonist; biased agonist; antagonist; binding affinity; selectivity

---

1. Introduction

Throughout human history, opioids have been used for medicinal and recreational practices to relieve pain, cough, and diarrhea, and to induce euphoria. The mood changes produced by opioids have been the basis for their abuse [1,2]. However, it was in the 20th century when major advances were made in understanding how opioids act to produce their beneficial and harmful effects. At the same time, the efficacy of opioids to treat human diseases was significantly improved by major developments in medicinal chemistry, bioinformatics, and neurosciences. Specifically, the existence of specific receptors for opioid drugs was first demonstrated on the basis of binding assays in brain preparations [3–5]. The multiplicity of opioid receptors was reported with different classes of opioid drugs having distinct pharmacological activities [6]. Since their first characterization, four opioid receptor types, referred to as mu (μ, MOR), delta (δ, DOR), kappa (κ, KOR), and nociceptin (NOP) receptor have been defined, and their crystal structures were obtained [7–9]. Opioid receptors belong to the family of seven transmembrane G protein-coupled receptors (GPCRs) and share about 60% homology in the amino acid composition [7–9]. Parallel to the multiple opioid receptors, endogenous opioid peptides (i.e., β-endorphins, enkephalins, dynorphins, and nociceptin/orphanin FQ) were identified in mammals [7,8]. When multiple types of opioid receptors were first proposed [6], it was clear that most of the therapeutic and side effects of opioids, clinically used as analgesics, were mediated by the MOR. These drugs included morphine and other analgesics, such as oxycodone, oxymorphone, and fentanyl [10–13]. Particularly, the misuse and overdosing with MOR agonists are an ongoing public health crisis worldwide, owing to the dramatic growth, especially in the United States of America (USA), of overdose deaths and diagnoses of opioid-use disorder associated with prescription opioids [14,15]. The challenge of researchers has always been to find innovative drugs that retain analgesic efficacy without the debilitating side effects of conventional MOR agonists, especially respiratory depression, as the primary cause of opioid-related overdose mortality.

During the past decades, the KOR has emerged as an alternative pharmacotherapeutic target; opposite to the MOR activation, the KOR does not mediate the rewarding effects or the respiratory depression, and it induces fewer gastrointestinal-related complications [7,16,17]. The endogenous kappa opioid system comprises the KOR and endogenous peptide ligands, the dynorphins, named after the Greek word dynamis (power) [18]. The KOR protein contains 380 amino acids, with seven transmembrane α-helices characteristic of the GPCRs. In comparison to other species, the human protein sequence of the KOR is 91% identical to the guinea pig and 94% identical to the mouse and rat [9,16]. The KOR/dynorphin system has a widespread distribution in the central and peripheral nervous systems (CNS and PNS) and various non-neuronal tissues of different species, including humans [19–26], consistent with its functional diversity. The endogenous kappa opioid system has key functions in numerous physiological and behavioral responses, including pain inhibition, diuresis, response to stress, reward processing, regulation of mood states, cognitive function, epileptic seizures, and sensation of itch [2,16,27–31].

Differential modulation of the KOR using selective ligands targeting the receptor is regarded a viable strategy for developing therapies for human disorders where the endogenous kappa opioid system plays a central role. Activation of central and peripheral KORs by agonist ligands was demonstrated to produce therapeutic effects of analgesia [32–34], antipruritic effects [25,35], and anticonvulsant/antiseizure effects [31,36]. Recent evidence has uncovered potential therapeutic areas for KOR antagonists, such as affective disorders and addiction-related behaviors [37–44].

Although targeting the KOR for the development of new drugs is promising, the KOR is not devoid of undesirable side effects, with receptor activation causing dysphoria, sedation, diuresis, and psychotomimetic effects in humans [33,45–47], and aversion, anhedonia-like, and anxiety-like effects in animals [48,49]. The contemporary concept of "functional selectivity" or "biased agonism" at the GPCR was introduced to describe the condition wherein ligands stabilize different conformations of the GPCR and can signal through parallel or independent signaling pathways mediated by G proteins and other effectors, principle among them being β-arrestin2 [50–53]. Activation of G protein-mediated pathways upon KOR activation is recognized to be responsible for the beneficial effects of analgesia and anti-itching, while β-arrestin2 recruitment and subsequent p38 phosphorylation KOR are considered to be involved in the negative side effects of dysphoria/aversion and sedation [54,55]. These findings that independent signaling mechanisms can be linked to distinct physiological effects of the KOR and can be pharmacologically separated by biased KOR ligands offer nowadays new perspectives in the discovery of KOR-targeted therapeutics with less liability for undesirable side effects. Accumulated literature on the development of KOR biased agonists was presented in recent reviews [56–60].

The first selective KOR ligand was ketocyclazocine (after which the kappa receptor type is named [6]), which produces analgesia in animals, as well as sedation and ataxia [33]. Over the years, a diversity of KOR ligands, as natural, naturally derived, and synthetic compounds with different scaffolds, as small molecules or peptides, with short- or long-acting pharmacokinetics, and central or peripheral site of action, were made available through chemical synthesis and evaluated as potential therapeutic agents or research tools. Several KOR agonists were evaluated in human clinical trials for the treatment of pain and pruritus, whereas KOR antagonists are under clinical development for the treatment of major depressive disorders and substance use disorders. Currently, nalfurafine is the only

KOR agonist approved for clinical use as an antipruritic drug in Japan [35]. A synopsis of the literature on such developments is beyond the scope of this review; however, we recommend extended and recent reviews in the field [25,33,34,43,44,56,61–66]. Furthermore, the available crystal structures of the KOR in inactive (Protein Data Bank, PDB code 4DJH) [67] and in active conformations (PDB code 6B73) [68] and the accessibility of modern computational methods (e.g., molecular dynamics (MD) simulation) offer a unique prospect for computational drug discovery [69–71].

In this review, we present recent chemical developments and structure–activity relationships (SAR) for a new class of KOR ligands with a diphenethylamine scaffold. We also outline the in vitro and in vivo pharmacological activities of diphenethylamines with diverse profiles ranging from potent and selective agonists to G protein-biased agonists and selective antagonists; their potential use as therapeutics is also discussed.

2. Design and Synthesis of Diphenethylamines

The synthesis of diphenethylamines, **1** (RU 24213) and **2** (RU 24294) (Figure 1), was described about 40 years ago [72]. These compounds were originally developed as potential anti-Parkinson's drugs [72]. Both **1** and **2** were selective dopamine D_2 receptor agonists at doses close to apomorphine, while exhibiting a longer duration of action [73]. Compounds **1** and **2** were also reported to display moderate affinity at the KOR acting as antagonists in in vitro binding assays [74]. The N-n-C_5H_{11} analogue **3** (Figure 1) was tested in vivo and showed an antagonistic action against the KOR agonist U50,488 on diuresis and analgesic activity in rats [75].

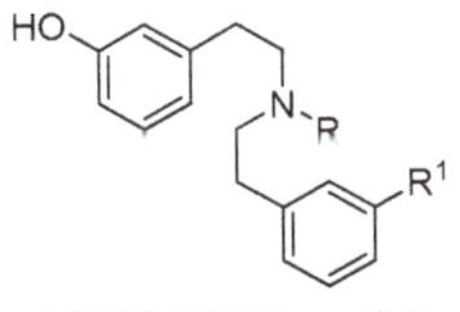

1 (RU 24213) R = n-C_3H_7, R_1 = H
2 (RU 24926) R = n-$_3H_7$, R_1 = OH
3 R = n-C_5H_{11}, R_1 = H

Figure 1. Structures of diphenethylamines 1–3.

On the basis of these earlier findings, new diphenethylamine analogues with different substituents at the nitrogen and on the phenolic moieties were designed, synthesized, and biologically evaluated [76–81]. SAR studies were reported on these new structures with several diphenethylamines emerging as highly potent and selective ligands with full/partial agonist, biased agonist, and antagonist activities at the KOR (Figure 2).

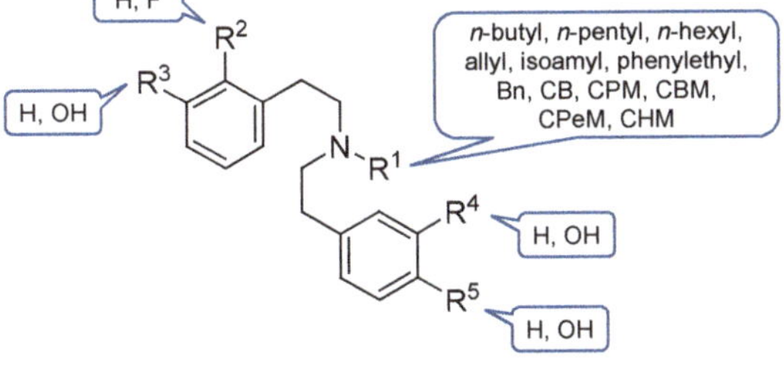

Figure 2. Design strategy of new KOR ligands with a diphenethylamine scaffold. Bn: benzyl, CB: cyclobutyl, CPM: cycloproplymethyl, CBM: cyclobutylmethyl, CPeM: cyclopentylmethyl, CHM: cyclohexylmethyl.

2.1. Synthesis of 3-Monohydroxy-Substituted Diphenethylamines

The initial design strategy of new diphenethylamines as KOR ligands targeted modifications at the nitrogen with the extension of the *n*-alkyl (*n*-C_4H_9 and *n*-C_6H_{13}) and introduction of cycloalkylmethyl (CPM and CBM) substituents in 3-monohydroxy-substituted diphenethylamines [76]. 2-(3-Methoxyphenyl)-*N*-phenethylethaneamine (**5**) was readily available from 2-(3-methoxyphenyl) ethaneamine (**4**) by alkylation with phenethyl bromide [74]. *N*-Alkylation of **5** using the respective alkyl bromides occurred, leading to compounds **6–9**, which were in turn transformed by ether cleavage with sodium ethanethiolate in *N*,*N*-dimethylformalide (DMF) at elevated temperature into the respective phenols **10–13** (Scheme 1).

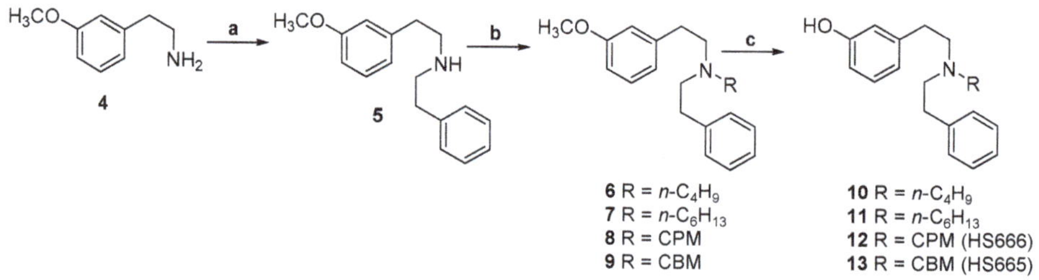

Scheme 1. Synthetic route to diphenethylamines **10–13**. (a) Compound **4** was alkylated with phenethylamine in DMF using K_2CO_3 as base to give **5**; (b) further alkylation of **5** with the respective alkyl bromides in DMF afforded **6–9**; (c) compounds **6–9** were in turn transformed by ether cleavage with sodium ethanethiolate in DMF at elevated temperature into the respective phenols **10–13**.

The synthesis of HS665 (**13**) was optimized employing an alternative route (Scheme 2). 3-Hydroxyphenylacetic acid (**14**) was reacted with 2-phenethylamine (**15**) to afford amide **16**. Boron hydrate (BH_3) reduction yielded amine **17**, which was *N*-alkylated with cyclobutylmethyl bromide to give **13** (HS665) with a higher yield (21%) than in the original procedure (17%) [76].

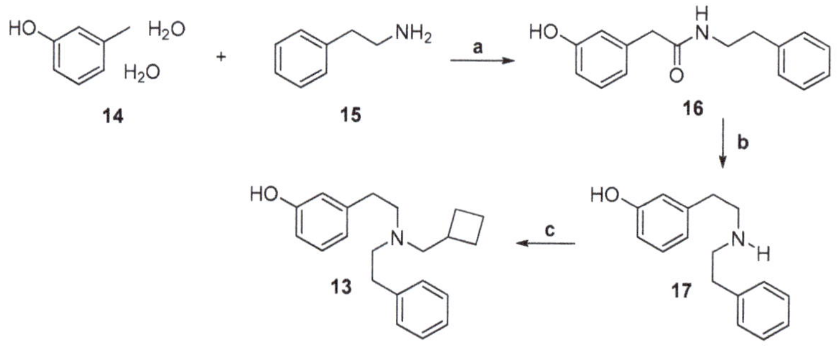

Scheme 2. Alternative synthesis of HS665 (**13**) via acetamide **16**. (a) EDCl, HOAt, CH_2Cl_2, room temperature (r.t.); (b) 1 M BH_3·tetrahydrofurane (THF), THF, reflux; (c) cyclobutylmethyl bromide, $NaHCO_3$, CH_3CN, reflux to afford HS665 (**13**).

The design of further 3-monohydroxy-substituted diphenethylamines as KOR ligands was based on HS666 (**12**) and HS665 (**13**) as lead molecules. The *N*-CPM and *N*-CBM groups in HS666 (**12**) and HS665 (**13**), respectively, were substituted by aliphatic and arylakyl groups of different sizes and lengths [77,78]. The synthesis of 3-monohydroxy-substituted diphenethylamines **18–22** started from the amine **17**, which was *N*-alkylated with cyclopentylmethyl bromide, cyclohexylmethyl bromide, benzyl bromide, isoamyl bromide, and cyclobutyl tosylate to yield the respective compounds (Scheme 3). Using this synthetical route, ether cleavage with sodium ethanethiolate was avoided.

The N-phenylethyl-substituted diphenethylamine, 24, was also prepared, where 5 was N-alkylated with phenethyl bromide to afford compound 23, which was demethylated by ether cleavage with sodium ethanethiolate in DMF to yield phenol 24 (Scheme 4).

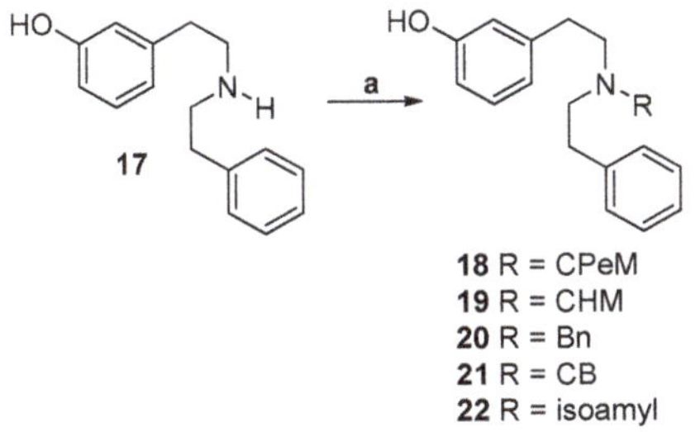

Scheme 3. Synthetic route to diphenethylamines 18–22. (a) Compounds 18–22 were prepared from 17 by N-alkylation with the respective alkyl bromide or cyclobutyl tosylate in the presence of NaHCO$_3$ in CH$_3$CN.

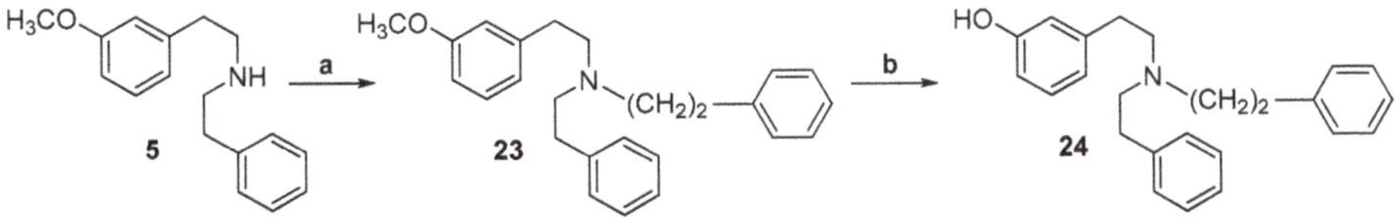

Scheme 4. Synthetic route to diphenethylamine 24. (a) Phenethyl bromide, K$_2$CO$_3$, DMF; (b) sodium ethanethiolate, DMF at elevated temperature.

2.2. Synthesis of 4-Monohydroxy-Substituted Diphenethylamines

The next design strategy evaluated the consequence of switching the hydroxyl group from position 3 to 4 in HS666 (12) and HS665 (13) on the KOR activity [77]. The 4-monohydroxy diphenethylamines 28 and 32 were synthesized (Schemes 5 and 6). Amide 26 was prepared from 4-hydroxyphenylacetic acid (25), which was treated with phenethylamine (15) in CH$_2$Cl$_2$ in the presence of EDCl and HOAt. BH$_3$ reduction yielded amine 27 that was N-alkylated with cyclobutylmethyl bromide to give 28 (Scheme 5). Alkylation of 2-(4-methoxyphenyl)ethaneamine (29) with phenethyl bromide afforded 2-(4-methoxyphenyl)-N-phenethylethaneamine (30), which was N-alkylated with cyclopropylmethyl bromide leading to 31. Compound 31 was treated at elevated temperature with ethanethiolate in DMF to yield 32 (Scheme 6).

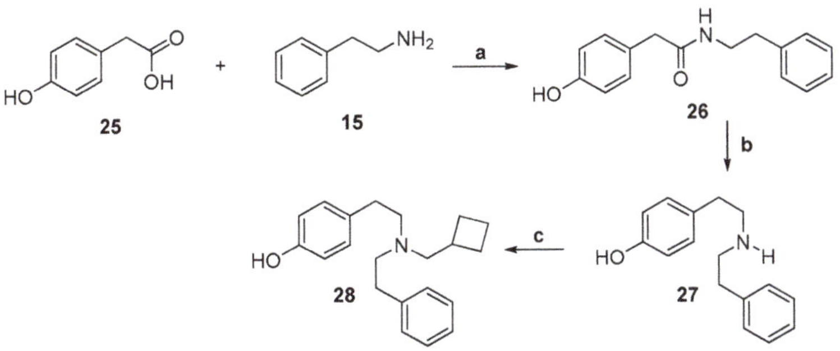

Scheme 5. Synthetic route to diphenethylamine 28. (a) EDCl, HOAt, CH$_2$Cl$_2$, r.t.; (b) 1 M BH$_3$·THF, THF, reflux; (c) cyclobutylmethyl bromide, NaHCO$_3$, CH$_3$CN, reflux to afford compound 28.

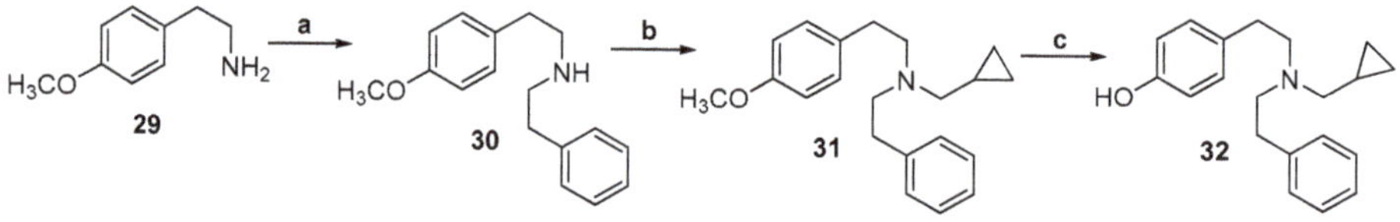

Scheme 6. Synthetic route to diphenethylamine **32**. (**a**) Compound **29** was alkylated with phenethylamine in DMF to give **30**; (**b**) alkylation of **30** with cyclopropylmethyl bromide in DMF afforded **31**; (**c**) compound **31** was in turn transformed by ether cleavage with sodium ethanethiolate in DMF into **32**.

2.3. Synthesis of 3,3′-Dihydroxy-Substituted Diphenethylamines

RU 24294 (**2**) is the analogue of RU 24213 (**1**) having two hydroxyl groups at positions 3 and 3′ of the two phenyl rings (Figure 1). This compound was also found to be a selective KOR antagonist in in vitro binding assays [74]. The subsequent design strategy targeted the effect of an introduction of an additional hydroxyl group in position 3′ on the KOR activity [78]. Several 3,3′-dihydroxy diphenethylamines substituted at the nitrogen with CPM (**37**), CBM (**38**), allyl (**39**), cyclopentylmethyl (CPeM) (**46**), cyclohexylmethyl (CHM) (**47**), and isoamyl (**48**) were synthesized (Schemes 7 and 8). The synthesis of the 3,3′-dihydroxy derivatives **37–39** started from N-(3-methoxyphenethyl)-2-(3-methoxyphenyl)ethaneamine (**33**) [72], which was alkylated with the respective alkyl bromides or allyl bromide to afford **34–36**. Ether cleavage with sodium ethanethiolate in DMF resulted in 3,3′-dihydroxy-substituted diphenethylamines **37–39** (Scheme 7). 3-Hydroxyphenylacetic acid (**14**) was reacted with 3-methoxyphenylethylamine (**40**) to provide amide **41**. BH$_3$ reduction in THF gave amine **42**, which was N-alkylated with the respective cyclopentylmethyl, cyclohexylmethyl, and isoamyl bromide to give **43–45**. Ether cleavage afforded **46–48** (Scheme 8).

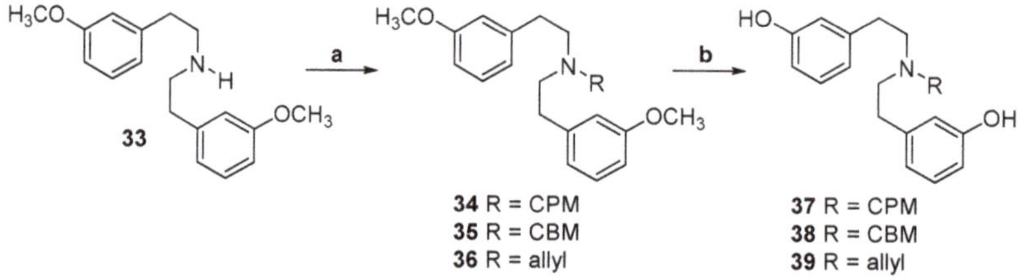

Scheme 7. Synthetic route to diphenethylamines **37–39**. (**a**) Compound **33** [72] was alkylated with the respective alkyl or allyl bromide, K$_2$CO$_3$, DMF, N$_2$, 80 °C; (**b**) sodium ethanethiolate, DMF, N$_2$, 130 °C.

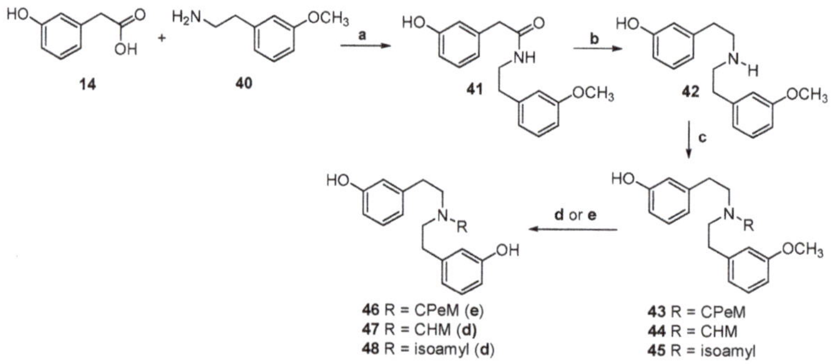

Scheme 8. Synthetic route to diphenethylamines **46–48**. (**a**) EDCl and HOAt in CH$_2$Cl$_2$, N$_2$, r.t.; (**b**) BH$_3$·THF 1 M in THF, N$_2$, reflux; (**c**) respective alkyl bromide, NaHCO$_3$, CH$_3$CN, N$_2$, reflux; (**d**) sodium ethanethiolate, DMF, N$_2$, 130 °C; (**e**) BBr$_3$ 1 M CH$_2$Cl$_2$ solution in CH$_2$Cl$_2$, −15 °C [82].

2.4. Synthesis of 3,4′-Dihydroxy-Substituted Diphenethylamines

Diphenethylamines with 3,4′-dihydroxy groups were designed to explore the influence of the orientation of the additional hydroxyl group on the KOR activity [78]. 3,4′-Dihydroxy diphenethylamines substituted with N-allyl (**55**), N-CPM (**56**), N-CBM (**57**), and N-CHM (**58**) were synthesized (Scheme 9). Treatment of 4-hydroxyphenylacetic acid (**25**) with 3-methoxyphenylethylamine (**40**) in the presence of EDCl and HOAt provided **49**. BH_3 reduction of **49** in THF gave amine **50**, which was alkylated with the respective allyl or alkyl bromides **51–54**. Ether cleavage afforded diphenetylamines **55–58** (Scheme 9).

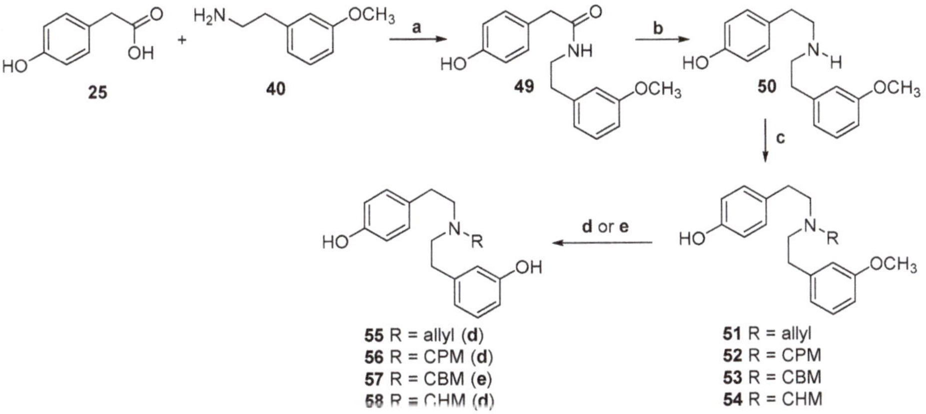

Scheme 9. Synthetic route to diphenethylamines **55–58**. (**a**) EDCl and HOAt in CH_2Cl_2, N_2, r.t.; (**b**) BH_3·THF 1 M in THF, N_2, reflux; (**c**) respective alkyl or allyl bromide, $NaHCO_3$, CH_3CN, N_2, reflux; (**d**) sodium ethanethiolate, DMF, N_2, 130 °C; (**e**) BBr_3 1 M CH_2Cl_2 solution in CH_2Cl_2, −15 °C.

2.5. Synthesis of 2-Fluoro-Substituted Diphenethylamines

The high strength and large dipole moment of the C–F bond, along with the strong electronegativity, small size, and modest lipophilicity of fluorine, all subtend versatility in the drug design [83]. Different 2-fluoro-substituted derivatives were designed in order to assess the effect of the presence of fluorine in position 2 in diphenethylamines on the KOR activity and physicochemical properties [78]. The inclusion of a 2-fluoro substitution initially targeted the 3-monohydroxy N-CBM-substituted HS665 (**13**) resulting in derivative **64** (Scheme 10). Other 2-fluoro-substituted diphenethylamines were prepared including the 3-monohydroxy N-CHM-substituted **65** (Scheme 10), the 3,3′-dihydroxy N-CBM-substituted **69** (Scheme 11), and the 3,4′-dihydroxy N-CBM-substituted **74** (Scheme 12). It was also expected that the blood–brain barrier (BBB) penetration may be slightly restricted due to the fluoro substituent in the proximity to the 3-hydroxyl group, which results in a lower calculated pKa value of the 3-OH group of **64** in comparison to the calculated pKa value of the 3-OH group of **13** (cpKa = 9.77 for **13** vs. 8.35 for **64**, MarvinSketch 17.10, ChemAxon) [78]. According to the calculated partition coefficients (clogP) and distribution coefficients at pH 7.4 ($clogD_{7.4}$) (MarvinSketch 17.10, Chem Axon), fluorinated compounds **64**, **65**, **69**, and **74** had similar values to analogues HS665 (**13**), **19**, **38**, and **57**, respectively, and a good capability to pass the BBB [78]. 2-Fluoro-3-methoxyphenylacetic acid (**59**) was treated with phenethylamine (**15**) in CH_2Cl_2 in the presence EDCl and HOAt to afford amide **60**. BH_3 reduction yielded amine **61**, which was N-alkylated with the respective cyclobutylmethyl and cyclohexylmethyl bromide to give **62** and **63**. Ether cleavage with BBr_3 afforded **64** and **65** (Scheme 10).

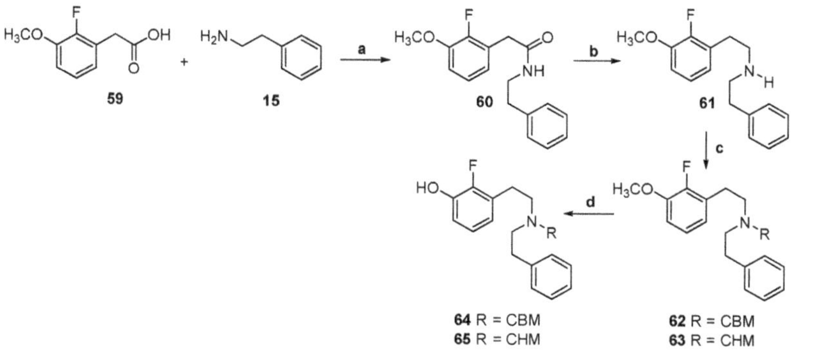

Scheme 10. Synthetic route to diphenethylamines **64** and **65**. (**a**) EDCl and HOAt in CH_2Cl_2, N_2, r.t.; (**b**) $BH_3 \cdot THF$ 1 M in THF, N_2, reflux; (**c**) respective alkyl bromide, $NaHCO_3$, CH_3CN, N_2, reflux; (**d**) BBr_3 1 M CH_2Cl_2 solution in CH_2Cl_2, −15 °C.

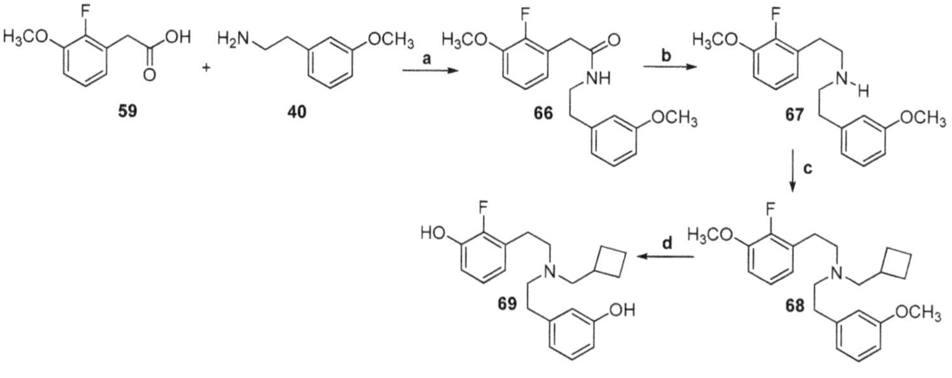

Scheme 11. Synthetic route to diphenethylamine **69**. (**a**) EDCl and HOAt in CH_2Cl_2, N_2, rt; (**b**) $BH_3 \cdot THF$ 1 M in THF, N_2, reflux; (**c**) cyclobutylmethyl bromide, $NaHCO_3$, CH_3CN, N_2, reflux; (**d**) BBr_3 1 M CH_2Cl_2 solution in CH_2Cl_2, −15 °C.

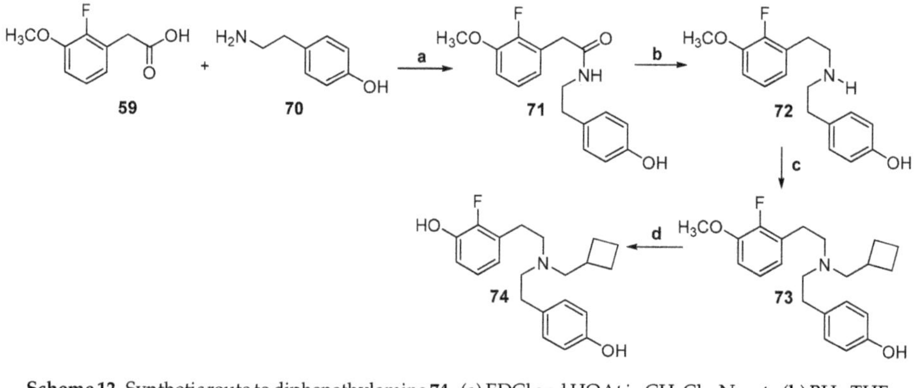

Scheme 12. Synthetic route to diphenethylamine **74**. (**a**) EDCl and HOAt in CH_2Cl_2, N_2, r.t.; (**b**) $BH_3 \cdot THF$ 1 M in THF, N_2, reflux; (**c**) cyclobutylmethyl bromide, $NaHCO_3$, CH_3CN, N_2, reflux; (**d**) BBr_3 1 M CH_2Cl_2 solution in CH_2Cl_2, −15 °C.

2-Fluoro-3-methoxyphenylacetic acid (**59**) was reacted with 3-methoxyphenethylamine (**40**) to provide amide **66**. BH$_3$ reduction in THF gave amine **67**, which was *N*-alkylated with cyclobutylmethyl bromide to provide **68**. Ether cleavage with BBr$_3$ afforded **69** (Scheme 11). Amide **71** was prepared from 2-fluoro-3-methoxyphenylacetic acid (**59**), which was treated with 3-methoxyphenethylamine (**70**) in CH$_2$Cl$_2$ in the presence of EDCl and HOAt. BH$_3$ reduction yielded amine **72**, which was *N*-alkylated with cyclobutylmethyl bromide to give **73**. Ether cleavage with BBr$_3$ afforded **74** (Scheme 12).

2.6. Synthesis of an Aromatic Unsubstituted Diphenethylamine

To extend the understanding of the role of phenolic functions on the KOR activity, the aromatic unsubstituted diphenethylamine **78** was synthesized [78]. Amide **76** was prepared from phenylacetic acid (**75**), which was treated with 2-diphenethylamine (**15**) in CH$_2$Cl$_2$ in the presence EDCl and HOAt. BH$_3$ reduction yielded amine **77**, which was *N*-alkylated with cyclobutylmethyl bromide to give **78** (Scheme 13).

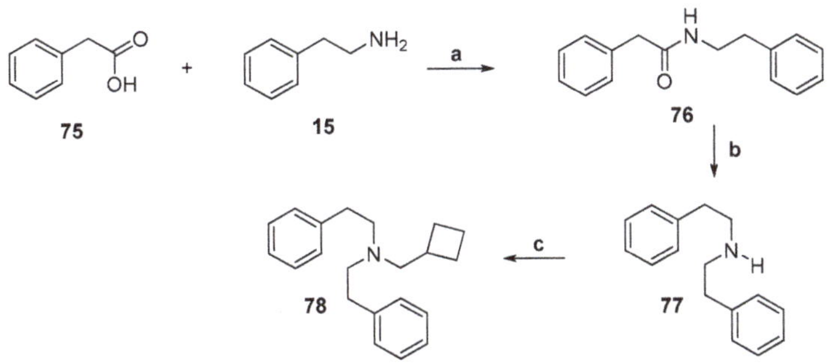

Scheme 13. Synthetic route to diphenethylamine **78**. (**a**) EDCl and HOAt in CH$_2$Cl$_2$, N$_2$, r.t.; (**b**) BH$_3$·THF 1 M in THF, N$_2$, reflux; (**c**) cyclobutylmethyl bromide, NaHCO$_3$, CH$_3$CN, N$_2$, reflux.

2.7. Synthesis of [^{3}H]HS665

In addition to their potential as therapeutics for the treatment of human disorders where the KOR has a key function, KOR ligands with a diphenethylamine scaffold may be of significant value as research tools in investigating KOR pharmacology in vitro and in vivo. Radioligands are essential tools in the GPCR research, and the field of opioid drug discovery has benefited significantly from the structural and functional insights afforded by radiolabeled ligands [84,85]. Typically, tritium labeling of small molecules and opioid peptides has a long tradition and is a well-established method to obtain labeled compounds [84,85]. Precursors for tritiation can be prepared by a number of chemical modifications, resulting in derivatives that can be reduced by tritium to obtain tritium-labeled molecules. One of the most common chemical modifications is bromination. Tritium-labeled HS665 (**13**), [^{3}H]HS665, was prepared using this strategy [86]. The 2,4-dibrominated compound (**79**) was prepared from HS665 (**13**) using *N*-bromosuccinimide (NBS) and diisoproplyamine (DIPA) in CH$_2$Cl$_2$, and dehalotritiation of **79** was performed (Scheme 14) to yield [^{3}H]HS665 with a specific activity of 30.65 Ci/mmol. [^{3}H]HS665 specifically labeled the recombinant and neuronal KOR [86], and was employed as research probe for assessing in vitro KOR activity of new ligands [87–92].

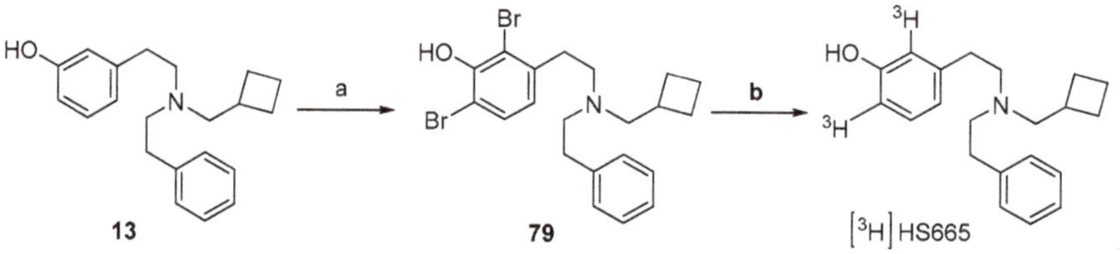

Scheme 14. Synthetic route to [³H]HS665. (**a**) DIPA, NBS, CH$_2$Cl$_2$, r.t.; (**b**) Triethylamine (TEA), PdO/BaSO$_4$ catalyst, tritium gas, r.t. HS665 (**13**) was first brominated using NBA and DIPA in CH$_2$Cl$_2$ to afford the dibrominated analogue **79**. A mixture of **79**, DMF, TEA, and PdO/BaSO$_4$ catalyst was reacted with tritium gas at r.t. The crude product was obtained with 216 mCi in ethanol. This product was purified by RP-HPLC to afford [³H]HS665 with a radioactive purity of ≥95% and with a specific activity of 30.65 Ci/mmol.

2.8. Synthesis of Structurally Related Diphenethylamines

Two structurally related diphenethylamines included the 2-pyridyl analogues 3G1 (**80**) and 3G2 (**81**) (Figure 3) [80], as derivatives of the reported 3-monohydroxy, N-CPeM-substituted **18** and 3-monohydroxy, N-CHM-substituted **19** (Scheme 3) [78]. The synthesis of **80** and **81** was performed by a contract research organization (WuXi Apptech, Shanghai, China) using methods reported by the Schmidhammer and Spetea group [78], and they were described as ligands with KOR agonist activity [80].

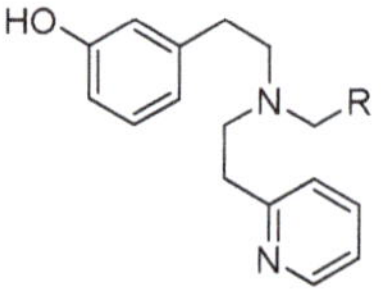

80 (3G1) R = CPeM
81 (3G2) R = CHM

Figure 3. Structures of 2-pyridyl analogues **80** and **81**.

3. Pharmacological Activities of Diphenethylamines at the KOR

3.1. Agonists and Partial Agonists

The first strategy used for designing KOR ligands with a diphenethylamine scaffold targeted the extension of the *n*-alkyl substituent at the nitrogen in the 3-monohydroxy-substituted RU 24213 (**1**) and **3** (Figure 1), specifically, substitution of the *n*-C$_3$H$_7$ group in **1** with an *n*-C$_4$H$_9$ group (**10**) and *n*-C$_5$H$_{11}$ group in **3** with an *n*-C$_6$H$_{13}$ group (**11**) (Table 1) [76]. In vitro binding studies demonstrated that replacing the N-*n*-C$_3$H$_7$ group with an N-*n*-C$_4$H$_9$ substituent (**1** vs. **10**) resulted in comparable affinity and potency at the KOR, albeit with a lower selectivity of **10** for the human KOR expressed in Chinese hamster ovary (CHO-hKOR) cells ((Table 1). Lengthening of the N-substituent in the *n*-C$_5$H$_{11}$ analogue **3** by one methylene group resulting in the *n*-C$_6$H$_{13}$ analogue **11** produced an additional reduction in both affinity and selectivity for the KOR. 3-Monohydroxy-substituted **1** and **3** were reported to display moderate affinity and selectivity at the KOR in the rat brain [74,75], whereas a higher KOR affinity was measured to the recombinant human receptor (Table 1) [76]. In vitro assays using rat brain membranes established diphenethylamines **1** and **3** as KOR antagonists on the basis of the decreased ligand affinity in the presence of NaCl/guanosine triphosphate [74,75]. In the guanosine-5′-O(3-[³⁵S]thio)-triphosphate ([³⁵S]GTPγS) binding studies using CHO-hKOR cell membranes, **1** and **3** had moderate KOR potencies and low efficacies, with a KOR partial agonist profile [76]. Extension of the N-*n*-alkyl substituent in 3-monohydroxy-substituted **1** and **3** conserved the KOR partial agonism character with a moderate potency for **10** and **11**, respectively (Table 1).

Table 1. In vitro activities of differently substituted diphenethylamines as full and partial agonists at the KOR.

Ligand	R¹, R², R³, R⁴, R⁵	KOR Binding [a]		KOR Activity [b]	
		K_i (nM)	K_i ratio KOR/MOR/DOR	EC_{50} (nM)	%Stim.
3-Monohydroxy-substituted					
1 (RU 24213)	n-C₃H₇, H, OH, H, H	8.13	1/73/457	49.1	21.1
3	n-C₅H₁₁, H, OH, H, H	12.6	1/26/104	86.4	36.2
10	n-C₄H₉, H, OH, H, H	10.9	1/38/223	46.2	45.5
11	n-C₆H₁₃, H, OH, H, H	141	1/5.6/25	647	24.0
12 (HS666)	CPM, H, OH, H, H	5.90	1/140/>1700	35.0	53.4
13 (HS665)	CBM, H, OH, H, H	0.49	1/1106/>20000	3.62	90.0
18	CPeM, H, OH, H, H	0.017	1/16118/133471	3.87	82.8
19	CHM, H, OH, H, H	0.061	1/8803/35066	0.23	61.9
20	Bn, H, OH, H, H	0.71	1/652/2623	4.65	79.5
21	CB, H, OH, H, H	10.3	1/65/344	46.1	50.7
22	isoamyl, H, OH, H, H	2.69	1/96/1020	22.1	74.7
4-Monohydroxy-substituted					
28	CBM, H, OH, H, H	36.3	1/20/59	109	43.8
3,3′-Dihydroxy-substituted					
37	CPM, H, OH, OH, H	4.62	1/137/617	20.6	51.3
38	CBM, H, OH, OH, H	0.38	1/605/8789	4.44	71.1
39	allyl, H, OH, OH, H	19.1	1/19/39	154	37.5
46	CPeM, H, OH, OH, H	0.31	1/1884/8952	13.7	80.4
47	CHM, H, OH, OH, H	0.14	1/1193/10229	17.6	91.1
48	isoamyl, H, OH, OH, H	2.10	1/100/699	16.6	65.6
3,4′-Dihydroxy-substituted					
55	allyl, H, OH, H, OH	43.5	1/4/25	248	29.8
57	CBM, H, OH, H, OH	3.43	1/5/125	22.2	76.4
58	CHM, H, OH, H, OH	1.85	1/126/885	22.2	84.3
2-Fluoro-substituted					
64	CBM, F, OH, H, H	0.072	1/5529/>138000	6.90	66.1
65	CHM, F, OH, H, H	0.040	1/21275/>250000	2.77	88.9
69	CBM, F, OH, OH, H	0.12	1/4642/>83000	1.49	57.5
74	CBM, F, OH, H, OH	3.37	1/155/389	36.7	69.1
Unsubstituted					
78	CBM, H, H, H, H	79.1	1/13/28	359	91.9

[a] Determined in competition binding assays using membranes from CHO cells stably expressing human opioid receptors. [b] Determined in the [³⁵S]GTPγS binding assay using CHO-hKOR cell membranes. Data from [76–78]. K_i, inhibition constant; EC_{50}, 50% effective concentration; %Stim, percentage stimulation relative to U69,593 (reference KOR full agonist).

The subsequent design strategy evaluated the character of the *N*-substituent in 3-monohydroxy-substituted diphenethylamines (alkyl vs. cycloalkylmethyl vs. arylakyl) on KOR activities (Table 1) [76,78,81]. The *N*-CPM substituent in derivative **12** (HS666) and an *N*-CBM group in analogue **13** (HS665) were found to be more favorable for ligand binding at the KOR than the *N*-*n*-alkyl groups in **1**, **3**, **10**, and **11**, by increasing affinity and selectivity at the KOR, as well as showing better

KOR agonist potency and efficacy (Table 1). HS665 (**13**) was the first 3-monohydroxy-substituted diphenethylamine reported with a KOR full agonist activity [76].

The available structures of the human KOR [67,68], together with efficient computational methods (i.e., molecular docking and molecular dynamics (MD) simulations), currently enable investigating ligand–receptor interactions, revealing structural features that promote binding and selectivity, and developing structure–affinity and structure–function relationships [69,70]. Molecular docking studies using the crystal structure of the human KOR (PDB code 4DJH) [67] and an active-like structure of the KOR attained by MD simulations explored binding modes of the 3-monohydroxy-substituted diphenethylamines, **1**, **3**, and **10–13** at the KOR [77]. In silico studies established that the size of the N-substituent hosted by the hydrophobic pocket formed by the residues Val108, Ile316, and Tyr320 influenced ligand binding and selectivity to the receptor, with the N-CPM group in **12** (HS666) and N-CBM substituent in **13** (HS665) having the optimal size. The hydrogen bond formed by the phenolic 3-hydroxyl group of N-CBM-substituted HS665 (**13**) with His291 was crucial for binding affinity and agonist activity at the KOR [77]. Using mutant KOR models, where Val108 was virtually mutated into Ala, the corresponding residue in MOR and DOR, confirmed the experimentally demonstrated KOR selectivity of HS665 (**13**). Docking of HS665 (**13**) to the mutant receptor showed the loss of the crucial hydrogen bond of the phenolic group with His291 [77]. Molecular modeling studies also established that the n-alkyl size limit of the N-substituent is five carbon atoms, as KOR affinities of the N-substituted n-C$_3$H$_7$, n-C$_4$H$_9$, and n-C$_5$H$_{11}$ analogues were in the same range, whereas the presence of an n-C$_6$H$_{13}$ chain at the nitrogen caused a larger reduction in the binding affinity (Table 1) [77].

The design of new 3-monohydroxy-substituted diphenethylamines was based on HS666 (**12**) and HS665 (**13**) as leads, where the N-CPM substituent in HS666 (**12**) and N-CBM substituent in HS665 (**13**) were exchanged by aliphatic and arylakyl groups of different sizes and lengths [77,78]. Interesting SAR observations were reported in this series (compounds **18–22**) with regard to the KOR binding affinity, selectivity, and functional activity (Table 1). The presence of bulkier N-substituents, such as N-CPeM (**18**) and N-CHM (**19**) groups, resulted in the largest increase in the KOR affinity, in the picomolar range, and excellent KOR selectivity (Table 1) [78]. Introduction of an N-benzyl group resulted in very high affinity and selectivity at the KOR of analogue **20**, albeit less prominent than derivatives with N-CBM (**13**), N-CPeM (**18**), and N-CHM (**19**) substitutions. In the [^{35}S]GTPγS binding assay using CHO-hKOR cell membranes, the 3-monohydroxy-substituted diphenethylamines **18** and **20** were potent and full agonist at the KOR, while derivative **19** had a profile of a potent KOR partial agonist (Table 1) [78]. Introduction of N-cyclobutyl (**21**) and N-isoamyl (**22**) substitutions was reported to produce a further decrease in the KOR affinity and selectivity and to behave as KOR partial agonists. It was established that N-CPeM and N-CHM substitutions are highly favorable in terms of interaction with the KOR [78].

Shifting the position of the phenolic hydroxyl group from position 3 to 4 in HS665 (**13**) significantly decreased affinity and selectivity at the KOR of **28** (Table 1) [77]. Differential functional activity at the KOR regarding the G protein activation was also observed after switching the hydroxyl group, with **13** as a highly potent and full KOR agonist and the 4-hydroxy modification in **28** resulting in a low potency and efficacy KOR partial agonist.

Within the 3,3′-dihydroxy diphenethylamine series (compounds **37–39** and **46–48**, Table 1), N-CBM (**38**), N-CPeM (**46**), and N-CHM (**47**) groups resulted in derivatives with very high KOR affinity and selectivity [78]. An additional hydroxyl group at position 3′ in N-CPM-substituted HS666 (**12**) and N-CBM-substituted HS665 (**13**) did not change the affinity and selectivity at the KOR of the resulting analogues **37** and **38**, respectively, but changed the full agonist profile of **13** into a potent KOR partial agonist **38**, with no change in the KOR partial agonism of **37** vs. **12**. Similar observation of the lack of alterations in the KOR activity was reported for the 3,3′-dihydroxy N-isoamyl-substituted **48** and its counterpart **22** (Table 1). The 3,3′-dihydroxy, N-CHM-substituted **47** had decreased KOR affinity, selectivity, and potency compared to its analogue **19**, with a shift from a partial agonist of **19** to a full agonist profile for **47**. A more significant reduction in affinity, selectivity, and potency at the KOR was found for the 3,3′-dihydroxy, N-CPeM derivative **46** compared to its analogue **18**, with both compounds being full agonists at the KOR. It was reported that an *N*-allyl substitution (**39**) was least favorable for the interaction with the KOR within the series of 3,3′-dihydroxy diphenethylamines (Table 1) [78].

Further SAR studies described the consequence of shifting the 3′-hydroxy group to position 4′ with a decrease in both KOR binding affinity and selectivity for *N*-allyl-substituted **55**, *N*-CBM-substituted **57**, and *N*-CHM-substituted **58** when compared to their 3,3′-dihydroxy analogues **39**, **38**, and **47**, respectively (Table 1) [78]. In vitro functional activity studies indicated that the 3′-OH to 4′-OH shift did not change the KOR partial agonist (**39** vs. **55** and **38** vs. **57**) or full agonist activity (**47** vs. **58**).

Within the series of 2-fluorinated diphenethylamines, the *N*-CBM-substituted **64** and *N*-CHM-substituted **65** with a single 3-hydroxyl group were reported having very high affinities at the KOR, in the picomolar range, and an extraordinary KOR selectivity (Table 1) [78]. Compound **65** was the most selective KOR ligand in the series and a very potent full agonist. An *N*-CBM substitution together with a 2-fluoro substituent (**64**) significantly improved both KOR affinity and selectivity in comparison to HS665 (**13**), while it converted a full agonist (**13**) into a potent KOR partial agonist (**64**). A substantial increase in the KOR selectivity was reported for the 2-fluorinated *N*-CHM-substituted **65** compared to analogue **19**, with both compounds showing very good KOR affinity (K_i values of 0.061 nM for **19** and 0.040 nM for **65**), whereas **65** was also a potent full agonist. Furthermore addition of a 2-fluoro substituent into the 3,3′-dihydroxy, *N*-CBM derivative **38** increased binding affinity and potency at the KOR to **69**, together with an increase in the KOR selectivity for **69**, without changing the KOR partial agonism (Table 1). Whereas the 3,4′-dihydroxy, *N*-CBM-substituted **74** had comparable affinity to **14** at the KOR, the presence of a 2-fluoro substituent in **74** improved KOR selectivity and left the KOR partial agonist profile unaffected. According to these SAR observations, a fluorine substitution at position 2 in this class of diphenethylamines appears as highly advantageous with regard to the KOR activity profile [78].

The role of phenolic functions in diphenethylamines related to the KOR activity was also demonstrated, where the aromatic unsubstituted analogue **76** was synthesized and reported as having the lowest binding affinity and selectivity at the KOR within the series, showing that the presence of a 3-hydroxyl group is required for the interaction with the KOR in vitro (Table 1) [78].

Two structurally related diphenethylamines to the series presented in Table 1, the *N*-CPeM-substituted **80** and *N*-CHM-substituted **81** were reported (Figure 3, Table 2) [80]. Both compounds **80** and **81** were described as KOR full agonists in the [^{35}S]GTPγS binding assay using membranes for U2OS cell stably expressing the human KOR (U2OS-hKOR) [80]. However, they had reduced agonist potencies than *N*-CPeM and *N*-CHM analogues **18** and **19**, respectively, indicating that a pyridine ring in **80** and **81** is less favorable than a phenyl ring in **18** and **19** (Tables 1 and 2). Binding affinities and selectivities at the KOR of **80** and **81** are yet to be reported.

3.2. Biased Agonists

As outlined in the introduction, in addition to the G protein-mediated signaling, another important signaling event following agonist stimulation of the KOR activation is β-arrestin2 recruitment, with increasing evidence that this signaling pathway mediates the negative side effects (i.e., dysphoria/aversion, sedation, motor incoordination) associated with receptor activation. Therefore, the concept of biased agonism at the KOR has gained significance to drug discovery, with diverse chemical approaches being evaluated toward the design of G protein-biased KOR agonists as effective and safer therapeutics (for reviews, see [56–60]).

In vitro functional studies described diphenethylamines **10**, **12**, **13**, and **18**, as well as structurally related **80** and **81**, as G protein-biased KOR agonists with different degrees of bias (Table 2) [79,80,93]. Studies compared ligand potency and efficacy through two functional assays measuring G protein activation (the [^{35}S]GTPγS binding assay) and β-arrestin2 recruitment (PathHunter β-arrestin2 assay) at the human KOR (Table 2). The *N*-*n*-C_4H_9 substituted **10** was found to be a KOR agonist in the [^{35}S]GTPγS binding assay, without inducing any stimulation of β-arrestin2 recruitment [79]. The *N*-CPM-substituted HS666 (**12**) was reported as a KOR partial agonist in the G protein coupling assay with minor (E_{max} of 24% of the reference KOR agonist U69,593) [93] to no measurable β-arrestin2 recruitment [80]. The N-CBM- and the N-CPeM-substituted HS665 (**13**) and **18**, respectively, showed weak partial agonism for the KOR-induced β-arrestin2 recruitment, while they were very potent and fully efficacious in promoting KOR-dependent G protein activation [79,93]. A similar profile was reported for the two structurally related diphenethylamines **80** and **81** (Table 2).

Table 2. Comparison of in vitro potencies and efficacies of KOR agonists from the class of diphenethylamines to induce G protein activation and β-arrestin2 recruitment.

Ligand	G Protein Activation [a]		β-Arrestin2 Recruitment [b]		References
	EC_{50} (nM)	E_{max} (%) [c]	EC_{50} (nM)	E_{max} (%) [c]	
10	14 (GTPγS, U2OS-hKOR)	94	–[d] (PathHunter, U2OS-hKOR-β-arrestin2)	–[d]	[79]
12 (HS666)	35.7 (GTPγS, CHO-hKOR)	50	449 (PathHunter, U2OS-hKOR-β-arrestin2)	24	[93]
13 (HS665)	4.987 (GTPγS, CHO-hKOR)	88	463 (PathHunter, U2OS-hKOR-β-arrestin2)	55	[93]
18	0.64 (GTPγS, U2OS-hKOR)	100	720 (PathHunter, U2OS-hKOR-β-arrestin2)	55	[79]
80	8.2 (GTPγS, U2OS-hKOR)	86.7	3956 (PathHunter, U2OShKOR-β-arrestin2)	61.2	[80]
81	11.8 (GTPγS, U2OS-hKOR)	81.6	2082 (PathHunter, U2OShKOR-β-arrestin2)	57.7	[80]

[a] Determined in the [^{35}S]GTPγS binding assay at the human KOR. [b] Determined in the PathHunter β-arrestin2 recruitment assay at the human KOR. [c] Percentage relative to the maximal effect of U69,593. –[d] denotes no stimulation. For structures of compounds **10**, **12**, **13**, and **18**, refer to Table 1; for structures of compounds **80** and **81**, refer to Figure 3.

3.3. Antinociceptive and Behavioral Effects of Agonists from the Class of Diphenethylamines

Pharmacological in vivo studies on KOR agonists from the class of diphenethylamines reported on their antinociceptive activities in mouse models of acute thermal nociception (warm-water tail-withdrawal assay) [93] and visceral pain (acetic acid-induced writhing test) [76,78]. Evaluation of the antinociceptive effects showed that the N-CPM-substituted HS666 (**12**) and N-CBM-substituted HS665 (**13**) produced dose-dependent effects in the warm-water tail-withdrawal assay mice after central, intracerebroventricular (i.c.v.) administration (50% Effective dose, ED_{50} = 6.02 nmol for **12**, and 3.74 nmol for **13**, vs. ED_{50} = 7.21 nmol for U50,488) [93]. In the same study [93], no antinociception was detected in KOR-knockout (KO) mice, indicating that the effects of compounds **12** and **13** were KOR-specific. The first diphenethylamine reported as a potent antinociception agent following subcutaneous (s.c.) administration was the KOR full agonist HS665 (**13**) [76]. In the writing test, HS665 (**13**) was equipotent to U50,488 (Table 3). In the mouse model of visceral pain, the KOR partial agonist HS666 (**13**) was also described as having antinociceptive efficacy after s.c. administration, with a potency twofold lower than that of U50,488 (Table 3) [78]. The antiwrithing effects of HS666 (**12**) and HS665 (**13**) were blocked by pretreatment with the KOR antagonist, nor-binaltorphimine (nor-BNI), which confirmed the KOR-specific effect [76,78].

Additional diphenethylamines with a KOR agonism profile were reported as effective antinociceptive agents with a KOR-mediated effect in the acetic acid-induced writhing test in mice after s.c. administration (Table 3) [78]. Interesting SAR observations were drawn from these studies regarding in vitro and in vivo agonist activities. In the series of 3-monohydoxy substituted diphenethylamines, the N-CPeM-substituted **18**, which was the most potent KOR agonist in vitro (Table 1), was described as the most effective in producing an antinociceptive effect (Table 3). The N-CHM-substituted **19**, a KOR partial agonist in vitro, was highly effective and only twofold less potent than its analogue **18**, while it was equipotent to the N-Bn-substituted **20** [78]. Introduction of an N-isoamyl group (**22**) caused a reduction in the antinociceptive potency, albeit comparable to the potencies of the leads HS666 (**12**) and HS665 (**13**) (Table 3).

In the series of 3,3′-dihydroxy-substituted diphenethylamines, increasing the size of the cycloalkylmethyl substituent at the nitrogen did not significantly alter the in vivo agonist potencies, with the *N*-CBM- (**38**), *N*-CPeM- (**46**)**,** and *N*-CHM-substituted (**47**) derivatives showing similar potencies in inhibiting the writhing response in mice after s.c. administration (Table 3) [78]. However, a reduction in the in vivo potency (twofold) was presented by the 3,3′-dihydroxy *N*-CPeM-substituted **46** compared to its 3-monohydroxy analogue **18**, an SAR observation that likely relates to the decreased in vitro KOR agonist potency of **46** (Table 1). This reduction in the antinociceptive potency was not observed for the *N*-CBM (**38**), *N*-CHM (**47**), and *N*-isoamyl (**48**) derivatives when compared to their 3-monohydroxy analogues HS665 (**13**), **19**, and **22**, respectively. It was also reported that switching the 3′-hydroxyl group to position 4′ resulted in a lower antinociceptive potency for the *N*-CHM-substituted **58** than its analogue **47** (ED_{50} = 0.95 mg/kg for **47** vs. ED_{50} = 1.90 mg/kg for **58**), whereas no difference was observed between the *N*-CBM derivatives **38** and **57** (ED_{50} = 1.71 mg/kg for **38** vs. ED_{50} = 1.73 mg/kg for **57**) (Table 3) [78].

Table 3. Antinociceptive potencies of differently substituted diphenethylamines in mice.

Ligand	R^1, R^2, R^3, R^4, R^5	Antinociception [a] ED_{50} (mg/kg, s.c.) [a]
U50,488	-	1.54
12 (HS666)	CPM, H, OH, H, H	3.23
13 (HS665)	CBM, H, OH, H, H	1.91
18	CPeM, H, OH, H, H	0.49
19	CHM, H, OH, H, H	1.01
20	Bn, H, OH, H, H	1.21
22	isoamyl, H, OH, H, H	2.78
37	CPM, H, OH, OH, H	4.73
38	CBM, H, OH, OH, H	1.71
46	CPeM, H, OH, OH, H	1.19
47	CHM, H, OH, OH, H	0.95
48	isoamyl, H, OH, OH, H	2.63
57	CBM, H, OH, H, OH	1.73
58	CHM, H, OH, H, OH	1.90
64	CBM, F, OH, H, H	2.64
65	CHM, F, OH, H, H	1.33
69	CBM, F, OH, OH, H	2.25
74	CBM, F, OH, H, OH	2.14

[a] Determined in the acetic acid-induced writhing assay in mice after s.c. administration. Data from [76,78].

Several diphenethylamines with a 2-fluoro substitution were reported to be highly efficacious in the writhing test in mice after s.c. administration (Table 3) [78]. Replacement of the *N*-CBM substituent in 2-fluorinated analogue **64** by the *N*-CHM group in **65** changed the in vitro agonist activity by converting a KOR partial agonist **64** into a full agonist **65** (Table 1), but also improved the antinociceptive activity of **65**. In mice, the 2-fluorinated, *N*-CHM-substituted **65** was more potent in the acetic acid-induced writhing test than its analogue **64** (Table 3). The 2-fluorinated analogues with a CBM substituent at the nitrogen, **69** and **74**, had comparable antinociceptive potencies to their *N*-CBM derivatives **38** and **57**, respectively, with all compounds reported as KOR partial agonists in vitro [78]. The 2-fluorinated, N-CBM-substituted **64** was slightly less potent than its analogue HS665 (**13**), associated with the reduced in vitro KOR agonist potency and efficacy of **64** (Tables 1 and 3) [78].

In addition to antinociceptive activities of KOR agonists from the class of diphenethylamines, other behavioral responses in mice were reported (Table 4) [78–80,93]. Particularly, diphenethylamine derivatives with a G protein-biased agonists profile (Table 2) were evaluated for KOR-mediated side effects of sedation/motor dysfunction and aversive-like behavior. It is well recognized that agonists at the KOR cause sedation in humans, while, in animals, a decrease in locomotor activity can be measured (for reviews, see [16,33]). First in vivo studies on the N-CPM-substituted HS666 (**12**) and the N-CPM-substituted HS665 (**13**), given i.c.v. to mice at antinociceptive ED_{90} doses effective in the warm-water tail-withdrawal assay, reported on the absence of a significant effect on the motor performance in the rotarod test [93]. It was also reported that HS666 (**12**), HS665 (**13**), and two other 3-monohydroxy-substituted analogues, the N-CPeM- (**18**) and N-CHM-substituted (**19**), did not cause locomotor impairment at systemic s.c. doses up to fivefold of the antinociceptive ED_{50} doses in the writing assay (Table 4) [78]. Intraperitoneal (i.p.) administration of HS665 (**13**) and **18** in a higher dose of 30 mg/kg to mice produced a significant decrease in the rotarod performance, but less than U50,488 [79,80]. These compounds have varying biased signaling toward G protein activation in vitro, with HS666 (**12**) as a -G protein-biased KOR partial agonist with an efficacy in β-arrestin2 recruitment ranging from 0–24% [80,93], and HS665 (**13**) and **18** as G protein-biased KOR full agonists with a partial agonist activity for β-arrestin2 signaling (efficacy between 30–55% for **13** and between 55–73% for **18**) [79,80,93].

Table 4. Behavioral effects in mice of KOR agonists from the class of diphenethylamines.

Ligand	Antinociception (Test, ED_{50}, Route, Strain)	Locomotor Activity (rotarod test) (Dose, Route, Strain)	Aversion (CPA) (Dose, Route, Strain)	References
10	n.d.	30 mg/kg, i.p., C57/BL6	n.d.	[79,80]
12 (HS666)	tail-withdrawal, 6.02 nmol, i.c.v., C57/BL6J writhing, 3.23 mg/kg, s.c., CD1	30 nmol, i.c.v., C57/BL6J 10 and 20 mg/kg, s.c., CD1	CPA, 150 nmol, i.c.v., C57/BL6J n.d.	[93] [78]
13 (HS665)	tail-withdrawal, 3.74 nmol, i.c.v., C57/BL6J writhing, 1.91 mg/kg, s.c., CD1	10 nmol, i.c.v., C57/BL6J 5 and 10 mg/kg, s.c., CD1 30 mg/kg, i.p., C57/BL6	CPA, 30 nmol, i.c.v. C57/BL6J n.d.	[93] [76,78] [79,80]
18	writhing, 0.49 mg/kg, s.c., CD1	2.5 mg/kg, s.c., CD1 30 mg/kg, i.p., C57/BL6	n.d.	[78] [79,80]
19	writhing, 1.01 mg/kg, s.c., CD1	5 mg/kg, s.c., CD1	n.d.	[78]
64	writhing, 2.64 mg/kg, s.c., CD1	15 mg/kg, s.c., CD1	n.d.	[78]
65	writhing, 1.33 mg/kg, s.c., CD1	7.5 mg/kg, s.c., CD1	n.d.	[78]
80	n.d.	30 mg/kg, i.p., C57/BL6	n.d.	[80]
81	n.d.	30 mg/kg, i.p., C57/BL6	n.d.	[80]

For structures of compounds **10**, **12**, **13**, **18**, **19**, **64**, and **65**, refer to Table 1; for structures of compounds **80** and **81**, refer to Figure 3. CPA, conditioned place aversion; i.c.v., intracerebroventricular; s.c., subcutaneous; i.p., intraperitoneal; n.d., not determined.

In the rotarod test, the N-n-C_4H_9-substituted **10**, which does not measurably recruit β-arrestin2, did not cause locomotor incoordination following i.p. administration to mice at a dose of 30 mg/kg [79,80]. Diphenethylamines with a 2-fluoro substitution and an N-CBM group (**64**) or an N-CHM group (**65**) also produced no significant changes in the motor function of mice at doses equivalent to fivefold the effective antinociceptive ED_{50} dose in the writhing assay (Table 4) [78]. Structurally related diphenethylamines **80** and **81**, as partial agonists for β-arrestin2 signaling, caused a modest motor impairment at doses of 30 mg/kg, i.p., without reaching the level of deficiency produced by U50,488 in the rotarod test [80]. Until now, there are no data available on the antinociceptive potencies of diphenethylamines derivatives **10**, **80**, and **81**; therefore, it is difficult to evaluate the safety profile of these compounds. The in vivo findings related to the impact on the motor function of diphenethylamines **10**, HS666 (**12**),

HS665 (**13**), **18**, **80**, and **81** shows a possible correlation between the level of biased agonism and KOR agonism-induced motor incoordination.

A major side effect related to the KOR activation is dysphoria, reported already in early human studies [45,46]. Because dysphoria cannot be directly measured in animals, the aversive response of a drug can be assessed using the conditioned place aversion (CPA) paradigm [48,49]. Conventional, unbiased KOR agonists (i.e., U50,488, U69,593, and salvinorin A) produce marked aversive effects in rodents in the CPA test [36,93–96]. The KOR-specific aversive effects were described to be linked with the recruitment of β-arrestin2 to the receptor, with G protein-biased KOR agonists expected to achieve the beneficial effect of analgesia and to be devoid of dysphoric/aversive effects.

First studies on the potential to induce KOR-specific aversive behavior in the CPA test were reported for the N-CPM-substituted HS666 (**12**) and the N-CPM-substituted HS665 (**13**) following central i.c.v. administration in mice [93]. Neither preference nor aversion was measured in mice after treatment with HS666 (**13**) up to 25-fold the antinociceptive ED_{50} doses effective in the warm-water tail-withdrawal assay. In the same study, HS665 (**13**) was found to induce aversive-like effects in mice in a dose eightfold higher than the effective antinociceptive ED_{50} dose in the tail-withdrawal assay [93]. The in vivo pharmacological profile of HS665 (**13**) appeared to be alike to that of the G protein biased-KOR agonist RB-64 [94], including antinociception effects with no motor incoordination, but with aversive-like actions in mice [93,94]. Furthermore, this is a notable profile, as HS665 (**13**) appears to activate favorably KOR-mediated G proteinactivation over β-arrestin2 signaling, albeit with higher efficacy for β-arrestin2 recruitment than HS666 (**12**) (Table 2) [93].

A recent study using high-throughput phosphoproteomics compared the phosphoproteomes of the mouse striatum after central, intracisternal (i.c.) injection of HS666 (**12**) and HS665 (**13**) and other KOR agonists, U50,488 [97], 6′-guanidinonaltrindole (6′-GNTI) [98], and RB-64 [99], given at doses effective in behavioral studies [95]. It was found that, compared to the aversive, β-arrestin2recruiting KOR agonists U50,488 [36,93,96], RB-64 [94,100], and HS665 (**12**) [93], the nonaversive, G protein-biased HS666 (**12**) [93] and 6′-GNTI [36,101,102] had a differential dynamic phosphorylation pattern of synaptic proteins and did not activate mTOR signaling [95]. This study proposed that the mammalian target of rapamycin (mTOR) signaling pathway may be involved in mediating aversion caused by KOR agonists. The KOR-specific mechanism was demonstrated by the lack of significant phosphorylation changes in the KOR-KO mouse striatum [95].

3.4. Antagonists

Diphenethylamines displaying antagonist activity at the KOR were reported [77,78]. The first diphenethylamine was the N-phenylethyl-substituted **24**, which showed no substantial agonist activity at the KOR in vitro, and antagonized U69,593-induced [^{35}S]GTPγS binding with relatively low potency (Table 5) [77]. In vitro binding studies with CHO-hKOR cell membranes established that an N-phenylethyl group (**24**) also resulted in a decreased binding affinity at the KOR compared to other diphenethylamine derivatives and a complete loss of binding at the MOR and DOR (Table 5).

Switching the 3-hydroxyl group to position 4 in N-CPM-substituted **12** converted the KOR partial agonist HS666 (**12**) into a KOR antagonist (**32**) (Table 5) [77]. The 4-hydroxy, N-CBM-substituted **32** had higher KOR antagonist potency than the N-phenylethyl-substituted **24** in the [^{35}S]GTPγS binding assay. The in vitro profiles of diphenethylamines **24** and **32** were supported by molecular docking studies [77] using the inactive structure of the human KOR (PDB code 4DJH) [67]. The N-phenylethyl group in **24** is relatively bulky to be hosted by the hydrophobic pocket formed by the residues Val108, Ile316, and Tyr320, which resulted in a different orientation of the phenolic moiety compared to the full agonist HS665 (**13**), making this compound a weak KOR antagonist. Diphenethylamine **32** with a phenolic 4-hydroxy group did not form the hydrogen bond with His291, an important residue for affinity and agonist activity at the KOR [77].

It was also reported that introduction of an additional hydroxyl group at position 4′ in HS666 (**13**) also changed the in vitro functional activity of **13**, from a KOR partial agonist to an antagonist

56 (Table 5) [78]. An interesting observation was that an additional hydroxyl group in position 3′ into N-CPM-substituted 32 retained the high antagonist potency at the KOR in vitro, while it also increased affinity and selectivity of analogue 56 at the KOR (Table 5). The in vivo KOR antagonist activity of 3,4′-dihydroxy, N-CPM derivative 56 was also demonstrated [78]. Pretreatment of mice with 56 (10 mg/kg, s.c.), 15 min before the KOR agonist U50,488, produced a complete reversal of U50,488-induced antinociception in the acetic acid-induced writhing assay. The absence of an agonist activity was further demonstrated for 56, as it did not affect writhing pain behavior after s.c. administration to mice [78].

Table 5. In vitro activities of differently substituted diphenethylamines as antagonists at the KOR.

Ligand	R^1, R^2, R^3, R^4, R^5	KOR Binding [a]		KOR Activity [b]
		K_i (nM)	K_i Ratio KOR/MOR/DOR	K_e (nM)
24	(CH$_2$)$_2$Ph, H, OH, H, H	211	1/>47/>47	1311
32	CPM, H, H, H, OH	218	1/8/10	32.1
56	CPM, H, OH, H, OH	3.56	1/129/>2800	24.3

[a] Determined in competition binding assays using membranes of CHO cells stably expressing human opioid receptors. [b] Determined in the [^{35}S]GTPγS binding assay using CHO hKOR cell membranes. Data from [77,78].

4. Summary and Conclusions

Potent and selective KOR ligands have been targeted since the discovery of multiple opioid receptor types, with increased attention in the 21st century paid to the discovery of novel ligands targeting the receptor and their potential to treat human disorders involving the kappa opioid system. This field has significantly advanced with an understanding of the function of the endogenous kappa opioid system in physiological and neuropsychiatric behaviors. Furthermore, future drug development in the KOR field is expected to significantly benefit from the available active and inactive KOR crystal structures and access to powerful computational systems and technologies.

In this review, we focused on a new class of KOR ligands with a diphenethylamine scaffold. We highlighted chemical advances in the functionalization and modification of the diphenethylamines toward the development of KOR ligands with distinct profiles, ranging from potent and selective agonists to G protein-biased agonists and selective antagonists. The first leads were HS666 (12) and HS665 (13), a selective KOR partial agonist and a full agonist, respectively [76]. The emerged SAR studies showed that KOR selectivity can be affected by simple structural modifications. The 3-hydroxyl function is required for the interaction with the KOR in vitro, and the character of the N-substituent plays an important role on the binding and activation of the KOR. The SAR established that an N-CPM substitution in HS666 (12) and an N-CBM substitution in HS665 (13) are more favorable for the interaction with KOR than n-alkyl groups causing an increase in KOR affinity and selectivity, as well as in KOR agonist potency and efficacy. Bulkier substituents at the nitrogen, such as CPeM and CHM (compounds 18 and 19, respectively, Table 1), resulted in the largest increase (in the picomolar range) in binding affinity and excellent selectivity for the KOR. Furthermore, modification with a 2-fluoro substitution in N-CBM- and N-CHM-substituted diphenethylamines (64 and 65, respectively, Table 1) led to compounds with very high affinities (in the picomolar range) at the KOR and an additional increase in the KOR selectivity. These properties make such compounds valuable research tools in investigating KOR pharmacology. The 3-OH→4-OH switch resulted in reduced KOR binding.

Additional hydroxyl groups at positions 3' or 4' had different consequences on the KOR activity, with the 3,4'-dihydroxy, *N*-CBM-substituted **58** (Table 4) as a high affinity and selective KOR ligand with in vitro and in vivo antagonism. Among the diphenethylamine derivatives, G protein-biased KOR agonists with different degrees of bias were identified.

Pain represents a primary clinical indication for KOR agonists, with the evidence that agonists at the KOR have analgesic properties with lower abuse potential than MOR agonists. Diphenethylamines with a KOR agonist profile (full, partial, or G protein-biased) were demonstrated as highly efficacious antinociceptive agents with a KOR-specific mechanism of action in mouse models of acute thermal nociception and visceral pain. Furthermore, behavioral studies established these ligands as potential antinociceptives with reduced liability for KOR-mediated adverse effects in mice (aversion, sedation/locomotor impairment) [78,93].

Whereas KOR antagonists are important research tools for studying the in vitro and in vivo KOR pharmacology, evidence on their antidepressant, anxiolytic, and antiaddictive effects support the potential therapeutic applications of KOR antagonists in the treatment of human disease states (i.e., depression, anxiety, and addiction). Selective KOR ligands from the class of diphenethylamines were reported with in vitro and in vivo antagonism, with future studies remaining to establish their therapeutic value.

In summary, a combination of target drug design, synthetical efforts, and pharmacological assessments of diphenethylamines as a class of structurally distinct, selective KOR ligands, enabled the identification of structural elements that determine the distinct activity profiles, with the prospective as candidates for future drug development for the treatment of pain and other neuropsychiatric illnesses.

Author Contributions: The manuscript was written through contributions of all the authors. All authors read and agreed to the published version of the manuscript.

Funding: The authors thank the Austrian Science Fund (FWF: P30433, P30592, and 14697) and the University of Innsbruck for support.

Acknowledgments: Open Access Funding by the Austrian Science Fund (FWF).

Conflicts of Interest: The authors declare no competing interests.

References

1. Evans, C.J. Secrets of opium poppy revealed. *Neuropharmacology* **2004**, *47*, 293–299. [CrossRef]
2. Darcq, E.; Kieffer, B.L. Opioid receptors: Drivers to addiction. *Nature* **2018**, *19*, 499–514. [CrossRef] [PubMed]
3. Pert, C.B.; Snyder, S.H. Properties of opiate-receptor binding in rat brain. *Science* **1973**, *70*, 2243–2247. [CrossRef] [PubMed]
4. Simon, E.J.; Hiller, J.M.; Edelman, I. Stereospecific binding of the potent narcotic analgesic [^{3}H]etorphine to rat-brain homogenate. *Proc. Natl. Acad. Sci. USA* **1973**, *70*, 1947–1949. [CrossRef]
5. Terenius, L. Stereospecific interaction between narcotic analgesics and a synaptic plasma membrane fraction of rat cerebral cortex. *Acta Pharmacol. Toxicol.* **1973**, *32*, 317–320. [CrossRef] [PubMed]
6. Martin, W.R.; Eades, C.G.; Thompson, J.A.; Huppler, R.E.; Gilbert, P.E. The effects of morphine- and nalorphine-like drugs in the nondependent and morphine-dependent chronic spinal dog. *J. Pharmacol. Exp. Ther.* **1976**, *197*, 517–532. [PubMed]
7. Stein, C. Opioid receptors. *Annu. Rev. Med.* **2016**, *67*, 433–451. [CrossRef] [PubMed]
8. Corder, G.; Castro, D.C.; Bruchas, M.R.; Scherrer, G. Endogenous and exogenous opioids in pain. *Annu. Rev. Neurosci.* **2018**, *41*, 453–473. [CrossRef]
9. Waldoher, M.; Bartlett, S.E.; Whistler, J.L. Opioid receptors. *Annu. Rev. Biochem.* **2004**, *73*, 953–990. [CrossRef] [PubMed]
10. Casy, A.F.; Parfitt, R.T. *Opioid Analgesics: Chemistry and Receptors*; Plenum Press: New York, NY, USA, 1986.
11. Fürst, S.; Hosztafi, S. The chemical and pharmacological importance of morphine analogues. *Acta Physiol. Hung.* **2008**, *95*, 3–44. [CrossRef]

12. Spetea, M.; Asim, M.F.; Wolber, G.; Schmidhammer, H. The μ opioid receptor and ligands acting at the μ opioid receptor, as therapeutics and potential therapeutics. *Curr. Pharm. Des.* **2013**, *19*, 7415–7434. [CrossRef] [PubMed]
13. Pasternak, G.W. Mu opioid pharmacology: 40 years to the promised land. *Adv. Pharmacol.* **2018**, *82*, 261–291.
14. Volkow, N.D.; Jones, E.B.; Einstein, E.B.; Wargo, E.M. Prevention and treatment of opioid misuse and addiction: A review. *JAMA Psychiatry* **2019**, *76*, 208–216. [CrossRef]
15. Stevens, G.W. Receptor-centric solutions for the opioid epidemic: Making the opioid user impervious to overdose death. *J. Neurosci. Res.* **2020**. [CrossRef] [PubMed]
16. Lemos, C.J.; Chavkin, C. Kappa opioid receptor function. In *The Opiate Receptors*, 2nd ed.; Pasternak, C.W., Ed.; Humana Press: Totowa, NJ, USA, 2011; pp. 265–305.
17. Imam, M.Z.; Kuo, A.; Ghassabian, S.; Smith, M.T. Progress in understanding mechanisms of opioid-induced gastrointestinal adverse effects and respiratory depression. *Neuropharmacology* **2018**, *131*, 238–255. [CrossRef]
18. Goldstein, A.; Tachibana, S.; Lowney, L.I.; Hunkapiller, M.; Hood, L. Dynorphin-(1-13), an extraordinarily potent opioid peptide. *Proc. Natl. Acad. Sci. USA* **1979**, *76*, 6666–6670. [CrossRef]
19. Stein, C.; Millan, M.J.; Shippenberg, T.S.; Peter, K.; Herz, A. Peripheral opioid receptors mediating antinociception in inflammation. Evidence for involvement of mu, delta and kappa receptors. *J. Pharmacol. Exp. Ther.* **1989**, *248*, 1269–1275.
20. Ji, R.R.; Zhang, Q.; Law, P.Y.; Low, H.H.; Elde, R.; Hökfelt, T. Expression of μ-, δ-, and κ-opioid receptor-like immunoreactivities in rat dorsal root ganglia after carrageenan-induced inflammation. *J. Neurosci.* **1995**, *15*, 8156–8166. [CrossRef]
21. Mansour, A.; Fox, C.A.; Akil, H.; Watson, S.J. Opioid-receptor mRNA expression in the rat CNS: Anatomical and functional implications. *Trends Neurosci.* **1995**, *18*, 22–29. [CrossRef]
22. McCarthy, L.; Wetzel, M.; Sliker, J.K.; Eisenstein, T.K.; Rogers, T.J. Opioids, opioid receptors, and the immune response. *Drug Alcohol Depend.* **2001**, *62*, 111–123. [CrossRef]
23. Holzer, P. Opioid receptors in the gastrointestinal tract. *Regul. Pept.* **2009**, *155*, 11–17. [CrossRef]
24. Peng, J.; Sarkar, S.; Chang, S. Opioid receptor expression in human brain and peripheral tissues using absolute quantitative real-time RT-PCR. *Drug Alcohol Depend.* **2012**, *124*, 223–228. [CrossRef]
25. Cowan, A.; Kehner, G.B.; Inan, S. Targeting itch with ligands selective for κ opioid receptors. *Handb. Exp. Pharmacol.* **2015**, *226*, 291–314.
26. Snyder, L.M.; Chiang, M.C.; Loeza-Alcocer, E.; Omori, Y.; Hachisuka, J.; Sheahan, T.D.; Gale, J.R.; Adelman, P.C.; Sypek, E.I.; Fulton, S.A.; et al. Kappa opioid receptor distribution and function in primary afferents. *Neuron* **2018**, *99*, 1274–1288. [CrossRef]
27. Van't Veer, A.; Carlezon, W.A. Role of kappa-opioid receptors in stress and anxiety-related behavior. *Psychopharmacology* **2013**, *229*, 435–452. [CrossRef] [PubMed]
28. Cahill, C.M.; Taylor, A.M.W.; Cook, C.; Ong, E.; Morón, J.A.; Evans, C.J. Does the kappa opioid receptor system contribute to pain aversion? *Front. Pharmacol.* **2014**, *253*, 1–15. [CrossRef] [PubMed]
29. Lalanne, L.; Ayranci, G.; Kieffer, B.L.; Lutz, P.E. The kappa opioid receptor: From addiction to depression, and back. *Front. Psychiatry* **2014**, *170*, 1–17. [CrossRef]
30. Crowley, N.A.; Kash, T.L. Kappa opioid receptor signaling in the brain: Circuitry and implications for treatment. *Prog. Neuropsychopharmacol. Biol. Psychiatry* **2015**, *62*, 51–60. [CrossRef]
31. Burtscher, J.; Schwarzer, C. The opioid system in temporal lobe epilepsy: Functional role and therapeutic potential. *Front. Mol. Neurosci.* **2017**, *10*, 245. [CrossRef]
32. Kivell, B.; Prisinzano, T.E. Kappa opioids and the modulation of pain. *Psychopharmacology* **2010**, *210*, 109–119. [CrossRef]
33. Albert-Vartanian, A.; Boyd, M.R.; Hall, A.L.; Morgado, S.J.; Nguyen, E.; Nguyen, V.P.; Patel, S.P.; Russo, L.J.; Shao, A.J.; Raffa, R.B. Will peripherally restricted κ opioid receptor agonists (pKORAs) relieve pain with less opioid adverse effects and abuse potential? *J. Clin. Pharm. Ther.* **2016**, *41*, 371–382. [CrossRef]
34. Beck, T.C.; Dix, T.A. Targeting peripheral κ-opioid receptors for the non-addictive treatment of pain. *Future Drug Discov.* **2019**, *1*, FDD17. [CrossRef] [PubMed]
35. Shigeki, I. Nalfurafine hydrochloride to treat pruritus: A review. *Clin. Cosmet. Investig. Dermatol.* **2015**, *8*, 249–255.

36. Zangrandi, L.; Burtscher, J.; MacKay, J.P.; Colmers, W.F.; Schwarzer, C. The G-protein biased partial κ opioid receptor agonist 6′GNTI blocks hippocampal paroxysmal discharges without inducing aversion. *Br. J. Pharmacol.* **2016**, *173*, 1756–1767. [CrossRef]
37. Spetea, M.; Asim, M.F.; Noha, S.; Wolber, G.; Schmidhammer, H. Current k-opioid receptor ligands and discovery of a new molecular scaffold as a k-opioid receptor antagonist using pharmacophore-based virtual screening. *Curr. Pharm. Des.* **2013**, *19*, 7362–7372. [CrossRef]
38. Carroll, F.I.; Carlezon, W.A., Jr. Development of κ opioid receptor antagonists. *J. Med. Chem.* **2013**, *56*, 2178–2195. [CrossRef]
39. Rorick-Kehn, L.M.; Witkin, J.M.; Statnick, M.A.; Eberle, E.L.; McKinzie, J.H.; Kahl, S.D.; Forster, B.M.; Wong, C.J.; Li, X.; Crile, R.S.; et al. LY2456302 is a novel, potent, orally-bioavailable small molecule kappa-selective antagonist with activity in animal models predictive of efficacy in mood and addictive disorders. *Neuropharmacology* **2014**, *77*, 131–144. [CrossRef]
40. Urbano, M.; Guerrero, M.; Rosen, H.; Roberts, E. Antagonists of the kappa opioid receptor. *Bioorg. Med. Chem. Lett.* **2014**, *24*, 2021–2032. [CrossRef] [PubMed]
41. Simonson, B.; Morani, A.S.; Ewald, A.W.; Walker, L.; Kumar, N.; Simpson, D.; Miller, J.H.; Prisinzano, T.E.; Kivell, B.M. Pharmacology and anti-addiction effects of the novel κ opioid receptor agonist Mesyl Sal B, a potent and long-acting analogue of salvinorin A. *Br. J. Pharmacol.* **2015**, *172*, 515–531. [CrossRef] [PubMed]
42. Carlezon, W.A., Jr.; Krystal, A.D. Kappa-opioid antagonists for psychiatric disorders: From bench to clinical trials. *Depress. Anxiety* **2016**, *33*, 895–906. [CrossRef]
43. Browne, C.A.; Lucki, I. Targeting opioid dysregulation in depression for the development of novel therapeutics. *Pharmacol. Ther.* **2019**, *201*, 51–76. [CrossRef] [PubMed]
44. Jacobson, M.L.; Browne, C.A.; Lucki, I. Kappa opioid receptor antagonists as potential therapeutics for stress-related disorders. *Annu. Rev. Pharmacol. Toxicol.* **2020**, *60*, 615–636. [CrossRef] [PubMed]
45. Pande, A.C.; Pyke, R.E.; Greiner, M.; Wideman, G.L.; Benjamin, R.; Pierce, M.W. Analgesic efficacy of enadoline versus placebo or morphine in postsurgical pain. *Clin. Neuropharmacol.* **1996**, *19*, 451–456. [CrossRef]
46. Pfeiffer, A.; Brantl, V.; Herz, A.; Emrich, H.M. Psychotomimesis mediated by kappa opiate receptors. *Science* **1986**, *233*, 774–776. [CrossRef]
47. Ranganathan, M.; Schnakenberg, A.; Skosnik, P.D.; Cohen, B.M.; Pittman, B.; Sewell, R.A.; D'Souza, D.C. Dose-related behavioral, subjective, endocrine, and psychophysiological effects of the κ opioid agonist Salvinorin A in humans. *Biol. Psychiatry* **2012**, *72*, 871–879. [CrossRef]
48. Land, B.B.; Bruchas, M.R.; Lemos, J.C.; Xu, M.; Melief, E.J.; Chavkin, C. The dysphoric component of stress is encoded by activation of the dynorphin kappa-opioid system. *J. Neurosci.* **2008**, *28*, 407–414. [CrossRef] [PubMed]
49. Tejeda, H.A.; Counotte, D.S.; Oh, E.; Ramamoorthy, S.; Schultz-Kuszak, K.N.; Bäckman, C.M.; Chefer, V.; O'Donnell, P.; Shippenberg, T.S. Prefrontal cortical kappa-opioid receptor modulation of local neurotransmission and conditioned place aversion. *Neuropsychopharmacology* **2013**, *38*, 1770–1779. [CrossRef] [PubMed]
50. Rankovic, Z.; Brust, T.F.; Bohn, L.M. Biased agonism: An emerging paradigm in GPCR drug discovery. *Bioorg. Med. Chem. Lett.* **2016**, *26*, 241–250. [CrossRef]
51. Wootten, D.; Christopoulos, A.; Marti-Solano, M.; Babu, M.M.; Sexton, P.M. Mechanisms of signalling and biased agonism in G protein-coupled receptors. *Nat. Rev. Mol. Cell Biol.* **2018**, *19*, 638–653. [CrossRef]
52. Mores, K.L.; Cassell, R.J.; van Rijn, R.M. Arrestin recruitment and signaling by G protein-coupled receptor heteromers. *Neuropharmacology* **2019**, *152*, 15–21. [CrossRef]
53. Seyedabadi, M.; Ghahremani, M.H.; Albert, P.R. Biased signaling of G protein coupled receptors (GPCRs): Molecular determinants of GPCR/transducer selectivity and therapeutic potential. *Pharmacol. Ther.* **2019**, *200*, 148–178. [CrossRef] [PubMed]
54. Bruchas, M.R.; Schindler, A.G.; Shankar, H.; Messinger, D.I.; Miyatake, M.; Land, B.B.; Lemos, J.C.; Hagan, C.E.; Neumaier, J.F.; Quintana, A.; et al. Selective p38alpha MAPK deletion in serotonergic neurons produces stress resilience in models of depression and addiction. *Neuron* **2011**, *71*, 498–511. [CrossRef]
55. Ehrich, J.M.; Messinger, D.I.; Knakal, C.R.; Kuhar, J.R.; Schattauer, S.S.; Bruchas, M.R.; Zweifel, L.S.; Kieffer, B.L.; Phillips, P.E.; Chavkin, C. Kappa opioid receptor-induced aversion requires p38 MAPK activation in VTA dopamine neurons. *J. Neurosci.* **2015**, *35*, 1291–12931. [CrossRef] [PubMed]

56. Bruchas, M.R.; Roth, B.L. New technologies for elucidating opioid receptor function. *Trends Pharmacol. Sci.* **2016**, *37*, 279–289. [CrossRef] [PubMed]
57. Bohn, L.M.; Aubé, J. Seeking (and finding) biased ligands of the kappa opioid receptor. *ACS Med. Chem. Lett.* **2017**, *8*, 694–700. [CrossRef]
58. Mores, K.L.; Cummins, B.R.; Cassell, R.J.; van Rijn, R.M. A review of the therapeutic potential of recently developed G protein-biased kappa agonists. *Front. Pharmacol.* **2019**, *10*, 407. [CrossRef]
59. Turnaturi, R.; Chiechio, S.; Salerno, L.; Rescifina, A.; Pittalà, V.; Cantarella, G.; Tomarchio, E.; Parenti, C.; Pasquinucci, L. Progress in the development of more effective and safer analgesics for pain management. *Eur. J. Med. Chem.* **2019**, *183*, 111701. [CrossRef]
60. Faouzi, A.; Varga, B.R.; Majumdar, S. Biased opioid ligands. *Molecules* **2020**, *25*, 4257. [CrossRef]
61. Aldrich, J.V.; McLaughlin, J.P. Opioid peptides: Potential for drug development. *Drug Discov. Today Technol.* **2012**, *9*, e23–e31. [CrossRef]
62. Chavkin, C.; Martinez, D. Kappa antagonist JDTic in phase 1 clinical trial. *Neuropsychopharmacology* **2015**, *40*, 2057–2058. [CrossRef]
63. Helal, M.A.; Habib, E.S.; Chittiboyina, A.G. Selective kappa opioid antagonists for treatment of addiction, are we there yet? *Eur. J. Med. Chem.* **2017**, *141*, 632–647. [CrossRef] [PubMed]
64. Roach, J.J.; Shenvi, R.A. A review of salvinorin analogs and their kappa-opioid receptor activity. *Bioorg. Med. Chem. Lett.* **2018**, *28*, 1436–1445. [CrossRef]
65. Turnaturi, R.; Marrazzo, A.; Parenti, C.; Pasquinucci, L. Benzomorphan scaffold for opioid analgesics and pharmacological tools development: A comprehensive review. *Eur. J. Med. Chem.* **2018**, *148*, 410–422. [CrossRef]
66. Coffeen, U.; Pellicer, F. *Salvia divinorum*: From recreational hallucinogenic use to analgesic and anti-inflammatory action. *J. Pain Res.* **2019**, *12*, 1069–1076. [CrossRef]
67. Wu, H.; Wacker, D.; Mileni, M.; Katritch, V.; Won Han, G.; Vardy, E.; Liu, W.; Thompson, A.A.; Huang, X.P.; Carroll, F.I.; et al. Structure of the human κ-opioid receptor in complex with JDTic. *Nature* **2012**, *485*, 327–332. [CrossRef] [PubMed]
68. Che, T.; Majumdar, S.; Zaidi, S.A.; Ondachi, P.; McCorvy, J.D.; Wang, S.; Mosier, P.D.; Uprety, R.; Vardy, E.; Krumm, B.E.; et al. Structure of the nanobody-stabilized active state of the κ opioid receptor. *Cell* **2018**, *172*, 55–67. [CrossRef]
69. Ferré, G.; Czaplicki, G.; Demange, P.; Milon, A. Structure and dynamics of dynorphin peptide and its receptor. *Vitam. Horm.* **2019**, *111*, 17–47.
70. Filizola, M. Insights from molecular dynamics simulations to exploit new trends for the development of improved opioid drugs. *Neurosci. Lett.* **2019**, *700*, 50–55. [CrossRef]
71. Manglik, A. Molecular basis of opioid action: From structures to new leads. *Biol. Psychiatry* **2020**, *87*, 6–14. [CrossRef]
72. Nedelec, L.; Dumont, C.; Oberlander, C.; Frechet, D.; Laurent, J.; Boissier, J.R. Synthèse et étude de l'activité dopaminergique de dérivés de la di(phénéthyl)amine. *Eur. J. Med. Chem. Chim. Ther.* **1978**, *13*, 553–563.
73. Euvrard, C.; Ferland, L.; Di Paolo, T.; Beaulieu, M.; Labrie, F.; Oberlander, C.; Raynaud, J.P.; Boissier, J.R. Activity of two new dopaminergic agonists at the striatal and anterio pituitary levels. *Neuropharmacology* **1980**, *19*, 379–386. [CrossRef]
74. Fortin, M.; Degryse, M.; Petit, F.; Hunt, P.F. The dopamine D_2 agonist RU 241213 and RU 24926 are also kappa-opioid receptor antagonists. *Neuropharmacology* **1991**, *30*, 409–412. [CrossRef]
75. Cosquer, P.; Delevallee, F.; Droux, S.; Fortin, M.; Petit, F. Amine Compounds. US Patent 5,141,962, 25 August 1992.
76. Spetea, M.; Berzetei-Gurske, I.P.; Guerrieri, E.; Schmidhammer, H. Discovery and pharmacological evaluation of a diphenethylamine derivative (HS665), a highly potent and selective κ opioid receptor agonist. *J. Med. Chem.* **2012**, *55*, 10302–10306. [CrossRef]
77. Guerrieri, E.; Bermudez, M.; Wolber, G.; Berzetei-Gurske, I.P.; Schmidhammer, H.; Spetea, M. Structural determinants of diphenethylamines for interaction with the κ opioid receptor: Synthesis, pharmacology and molecular modeling studies. *Bioorg. Med. Chem. Lett.* **2016**, *26*, 4769–4774. [CrossRef]
78. Erli, F.; Guerrieri, E.; Ben Haddou, T.; Lantero, A.; Mairegger, M.; Schmidhammer, H.; Spetea, M. Highly potent and selective new diphenethylamines interacting with the κ-opioid receptor: Synthesis, pharmacology, and structure-activity relationships. *J. Med. Chem.* **2017**, *60*, 7579–7590. [CrossRef] [PubMed]

79. Dunn, A.D.; Reed, B.; Guariglia, C.; Dunn, A.M.; Hillman, J.M.; Kreek, M.J. Structurally related kappa opioid receptor agonists with substantial differential signaling bias: Neuroendocrine and behavioral effects in C57BL6 mice. *Int. J. Neuropsychopharmacol.* **2018**, *21*, 847–857. [CrossRef]
80. Dunn, A.D.; Reed, B.; Erazo, J.; Ben-Ezra, A.; Kreek, M.J. Signaling properties of structurally diverse kappa opioid receptor ligands: Toward in vitro models of in vivo responses. *ACS Chem. Neurosci.* **2019**, *10*, 3590–3600. [CrossRef]
81. Schmidhammer, H.; Spetea, M.; Guerrieri, E. Diphenethylamine Derivatives which are Inter Alia Useful as Analgesics and Methods for their Production. US Patent 10,377,698, 13 August 2019.
82. Rice, K.C. A rapid, high-yield conversion of codeine to morphine. *J. Med. Chem.* **1977**, *20*, 164–165. [CrossRef] [PubMed]
83. Johnson, B.M.; Shu, Y.-Z.; Zhuo, X.; Meanwell, N.A. Metabolic and pharmaceutical aspects of fluorinated compounds. *J. Med. Chem.* **2020**, *63*, 6315–6386. [CrossRef]
84. Tóth, G.; Mallareddy, J.R.; Tóth, F.; Lipkowski, A.W.; Tourwe, D. Radiotracers, tritium labeling of neuropeptides. *ARKIVOC* **2012**, 163–174. [CrossRef]
85. Tóth, G.; Mallareddy, J.R. Tritiated opioid receptor ligands as radiotracers. *Curr. Pharm. Des.* **2013**, *19*, 7461–7472. [CrossRef]
86. Guerrieri, E.; Mallareddy, J.R.; Tóth, G.; Schmidhammer, H.; Spetea, M. Synthesis and pharmacological evaluation of [^{3}H]HS665, a novel, highly selective radioligand for the kappa opioid receptor. *ACS Chem. Neurosci.* **2015**, *6*, 456–463. [CrossRef]
87. Dumitrascuta, M.; Ben Haddou, T.; Guerrieri, E.; Noha, S.M.; Schläfer, L.; Schmidhammer, H.; Spetea, M. Synthesis, pharmacology, and molecular docking studies on 6-desoxo-N-methylmorphinans as potent µ-opioid receptor agonists. *J. Med. Chem.* **2017**, *60*, 9407–9412. [CrossRef] [PubMed]
88. Erdei, A.I.; Borbély, A.; Magyar, A.; Taricska, N.; Perczel, A.; Zsíros, O.; Garab, G.; Szűcs, E.; Ötvös, F.; Zádor, F.; et al. Biochemical and pharmacological characterization of three opioid-nociceptin hybrid peptide ligands reveals substantially differing modes of their actions. *Peptides* **2018**, *99*, 205–216. [CrossRef]
89. Martin, C.; Dumitrascuta, M.; Mannes, M.; Lantero, A.; Bucher, D.; Walker, K.; Van Wanseele, Y.; Oyen, E.; Hernot, S.; Van Eeckhaut, A.; et al. Biodegradable amphipathic peptide hydrogels as extended-release system for opioid peptides. *Med. Chem.* **2018**, *61*, 9784–9789. [CrossRef]
90. Dumitrascuta, M.; Bermudez, M.; Ben Haddou, T.; Guerrieri, E.; Schläfer, L.; Ritsch, A.; Hosztafi, S.; Lantero, A.; Kreutz, C.; Massotte, D.; et al. N-Phenethyl substitution in 14-methoxy-N-methylmorphinan-6-ones turns selective µ opioid receptor ligands into dual µ/δ opioid receptor agonists. *Sci. Rep.* **2020**, *10*, 5653. [CrossRef]
91. Szűcs, E.; Marton, J.; Szabó, Z.; Hosztafi, S.; Kékesi, G.; Tuboly, G.; Bánki, L.; Horváth, G.; Szabó, P.T.; Tömböly, C.; et al. Synthesis, biochemical, pharmacological characterization and in silico profile modelling of highly potent opioid orvinol and thevinol derivatives. *Eur. J. Med. Chem.* **2020**, *191*, 112–145. [CrossRef]
92. Szűcs, E.; Stefanucci, A.; Dimmito, M.P.; Zádor, F.; Pieretti, S.; Zengin, G.; Vécsei, L.; Benyhe, S.; Nalli, M.; Mollica, A. Discovery of kynurenines containing oligopeptides as potent opioid receptor agonists. *Biomolecules* **2020**, *10*, 284. [CrossRef]
93. Spetea, M.; Eans, S.O.; Ganno, M.L.; Lantero, A.; Mairegger, M.; Toll, L.; Schmidhammer, H.; McLaughlin, J.P. Selective κ receptor partial agonist HS666 produces potent antinociception without inducing aversion after i.c.v. administration in mice. *Br. J. Pharmacol.* **2017**, *174*, 2444–2456. [CrossRef] [PubMed]
94. White, K.L.; Robinson, J.E.; Zhu, H.; DiBerto, J.F.; Polepally, P.R.; Zjawiony, J.K.; Nichols, D.E.; Malanga, C.J.; Roth, B.L. The G protein-biased kappa-opioid receptor agonist RB-64 is analgesic with a unique spectrum of activities in vivo. *J. Pharmacol. Exp. Ther.* **2015**, *352*, 98–109. [CrossRef] [PubMed]
95. Liu, J.J.; Sharma, K.; Zangrandi, L.; Chen, C.; Humphrey, S.J.; Chiu, Y.-T.; Spetea, M.; Liu-Chen, L.Y.; Schwarzer, C.; Mann, M. In vivo brain GPCR signaling elucidated by phosphoproteomics. *Science* **2018**, *360*, eaao4927. [CrossRef]
96. Liu, J.J.; Chiu, Y.T.; DiMattio, K.M.; Chen, C.; Huang, P.; Gentile, T.A.; Muschamp, J.W.; Cowan, A.; Mann, M.; Liu-Chen, L.Y. Phosphoproteomic approach for agonist-specific signaling in mouse brains: mTOR pathway is involved in κ opioid aversion. *Neuropsychopharmacology* **2019**, *44*, 939–949. [CrossRef] [PubMed]
97. Von, P.F.V.; Lewis, R.A. U-50,488, a selective kappa opioid agonist: Comparison to other reputed kappa agonists. *Prog. Neuropsychopharmacol. Biol. Psychiatry* **1982**, *6*, 467–470.

98. Sharma, S.K.; Jones, R.M.; Metzger, T.G.; Ferguson, D.M.; Portoghese, P.S. Transformation of a kappa-opioid receptor antagonist to a kappa agonist by transfer of a guanidinium group from the 5'- to 6'-position of naltrindole. *J. Med. Chem.* **2001**, *44*, 2073–2079. [CrossRef]
99. Yan, F.; Bikbulatov, R.V.; Mocanu, V.; Dicheva, N.; Parker, C.E.; Wetsel, W.C.; Mosier, P.D.; Westkaemper, R.B.; Allen, J.A.; Zjawiony, J.K.; et al. Structure-based design, synthesis, and biochemical and pharmacological characterization of novel salvinorin A analogues as active state probes of the kappa-opioid receptor. *Biochemistry* **2009**, *48*, 6898–6908. [CrossRef]
100. White, K.L.; Scopton, A.P.; Rives, M.L.; Bikbulatov, R.V.; Polepally, P.R.; Brown, P.J.; Kenakin, T.; Javitch, J.A.; Zjawiony, J.K.; Roth, B.L. Identification of novel functionally selective κ-opioid receptor scaffolds. *Mol. Pharmacol.* **2014**, *85*, 83–90. [CrossRef] [PubMed]
101. Rives, M.L.; Rossillo, M.; Liu-Chen, L.Y.; Javitch, J.A. 6'-Guanidinonaltrindole (6'-GNTI) is a G protein-biased κ-opioid receptor agonist that inhibits arrestin recruitment. *J. Biol. Chem.* **2012**, *287*, 27050–27054. [CrossRef] [PubMed]
102. Schmid, C.L.; Streicher, J.M.; Groer, C.E.; Munro, T.A.; Zhou, L.; Bohn, L.M. Functional selectivity of 6'-guanidinonaltrindole (6'-GNTI) at κ-opioid receptors in striatal neurons. *J. Biol. Chem.* **2013**, *288*, 22387–22398. [CrossRef]

Publisher's Note: MDPI stays neutral with regard to jurisdictional claims in published maps and institutional affiliations.

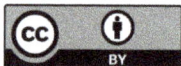

© 2020 by the authors. Licensee MDPI, Basel, Switzerland. This article is an open access article distributed under the terms and conditions of the Creative Commons Attribution (CC BY) license (http://creativecommons.org/licenses/by/4.0/).

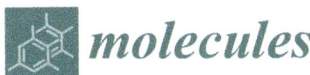

Article

Heteromerization of Endogenous Mu and Delta Opioid Receptors Induces Ligand-Selective Co-Targeting to Lysosomes

Lyes Derouiche [1], Florian Pierre [1], Stéphane Doridot [2], Stéphane Ory [1] and Dominique Massotte [1,*]

[1] French National Centre for Scientific Research, Institut des Neurosciences Cellulaires et Intégratives, University of Strasbourg, 67000 Strasbourg, France; lyes.derouiche@gmail.com (L.D.); florianb.pierre@gmail.com (F.P.); ory@inci-cnrs.unistra.fr (S.O.)
[2] French National Centre for Scientific Research, Chronobiotron, 67200 Strasbourg, France; doridot@inci-cnrs.unistra.fr
* Correspondence: d.massotte@unistra.fr

Academic Editor: Mariana Spetea
Received: 30 July 2020; Accepted: 29 September 2020; Published: 30 September 2020

Abstract: Increasing evidence indicates that native mu and delta opioid receptors can associate to form heteromers in discrete brain neuronal circuits. However, little is known about their signaling and trafficking. Using double-fluorescent knock-in mice, we investigated the impact of neuronal co-expression on the internalization profile of mu and delta opioid receptors in primary hippocampal cultures. We established ligand selective mu–delta co-internalization upon activation by 1-[[4-(acetylamino)phenyl]methyl]-4-(2-phenylethyl)-4-piperidinecarboxylic acid, ethyl ester (CYM51010), [D-Ala2, NMe-Phe4, Gly-ol5]enkephalin (DAMGO), and deltorphin II, but not (+)-4-[(αR)-α-((2S,5R)-4-Allyl-2,5-dimethyl-1-piperazinyl)-3-methoxybenzyl]-N,N-diethylbenzamide (SNC80), morphine, or methadone. Co-internalization was driven by the delta opioid receptor, required an active conformation of both receptors, and led to sorting to the lysosomal compartment. Altogether, our data indicate that mu–delta co-expression, likely through heteromerization, alters the intracellular fate of the mu opioid receptor, which provides a way to fine-tune mu opioid receptor signaling. It also represents an interesting emerging concept for the development of novel therapeutic drugs and strategies.

Keywords: mu opioid receptor; delta opioid receptor; heteromer; internalization; primary hippocampal culture; lysosomes

1. Introduction

The opioid system modulates a large number of functions including nociception, emotional responses, reward and motivation, and cognition, as well as neuroendocrine physiology and autonomic functions [1,2]. It is composed of three G-protein-coupled receptors, mu, delta, and kappa, and three families of opioid peptides, the enkephalins, dynorphins, and endorphins [3]. Several decades of pharmacology have uncovered the complexity of the opioid pharmacology and evidenced functional interactions between receptors that can take place at different levels, including within the cell [4,5]. This led to postulate the formation of functional association between different opioid receptor types to generate a novel entity with specific pharmacological, signaling, and trafficking properties called heteromers [6]. Heteromers within the opioid family were postulated for the first time about 20 years ago involving the delta and the kappa opioid receptors [7]. Heteromerization of mu and delta opioid receptors was then proposed shortly after [8] and extensively studied in co-transfected cells [9]. Mu and delta opioid receptors have different intracellular fate when internalized, with mu opioid receptors being recycled quickly to the plasma membrane [10,11] and delta opioid receptors being degraded in the lysosomal compartment [12–14]. In co-transfected HEK293 cells, co-internalization of mu and delta opioid receptors was reported following activation by the mu agonists [D-Ala^2, NMe-Phe^4, Gly-ol^5]enkephalin (DAMGO) [15–18] or methadone [19] or following activation by the delta agonists SNC80 [17,18], [H-Dmt-Tic-NH-CH(CH2-COOH)-Bid] (UFP512) [17], deltorphin I [18], deltorphin II [16–18], or D-Pen2, D-Pen5 -enkephalin (DPDPE) [17]. Co-targeting to the lysosomal compartment was observed following activation by deltorphin I [18] or methadone [19]. However, differences in the cellular content are known to exist between cell types that may impact receptor functioning [20,21] and underline the need for studies on endogenous receptors. Although a previous report indicated that the mu agonist DAMGO induced co-internalization and co-recycling of mu and delta opioid receptors in Dorsal root ganglia (DRG) cultures pretreated with morphine, suggesting that mu–delta heteromerization may affect the trafficking of the delta opioid receptor in these conditions [22], little is known so far regarding the consequences the trafficking of mu–delta heteromers in neurons.

Using double-fluorescent knock-in mice co-expressing functional mu and delta opioid receptors respectively fused to the red fluorescent protein mCherry or the green fluorescent protein eGFP, we previously mapped neurons co-expressing mu and delta opioid receptors [11]. In the hippocampus, they corresponded to γ-aminobutyric acid (GABA) interneurons with 70% being parvalbumin-positive [23]. We also established close physical proximity of the two receptors in the hippocampus, a prerequisite to mu–delta heteromerization [11]. Here, we took advantage of the double-fluorescent knock-in mice to examine whether mu–delta physical proximity was also associated with functional changes by monitoring mu and delta receptor internalization in primary hippocampal cultures. We showed ligand-specific mu–delta receptor co-internalization induced by the mu–delta-biased agonist CYM51010 [24,25], the mu agonist DAMGO, and the delta agonist deltorphin II, but not the mu agonists morphine and methadone or the delta agonist SNC80. We also established the sorting of mu–delta heteromers to the lysosomal compartment indicating that mu–delta heteromerization affects the intracellular fate of the mu opioid receptor in its native environment. These data point to mu–delta heteromerization as a means to fine-tune mu opioid receptor signaling and neuronal activity.

2. Results

2.1. Endogenous Mu–Delta Heteromers Are Present at the Neuronal Surface under Basal Conditions

In agreement with our previous reports using the fluorescent knock-in mice expressing delta-eGFP and/or mu-mCherry [11,13,26,27], both mu and delta opioid receptors were detected at the plasma membrane in primary hippocampal neurons under basal conditions (Figure 1A). Quantification of the receptor density using the ICY bioimaging software [28] indicated that the fluorescence density at the cell surface was 2.5-fold higher compared to the cytoplasm for either receptor (Figure 1B). Merged images highlighted an overlay of the green and red fluorescence at the surface of the neuron, and quantification of the density of receptor co-localization indicated higher co-localization at the plasma membrane compared to the cytoplasm (Figure 1C), with only 10% of the receptors co-localized in the cytoplasm (Figure 1D).

Our data, thus, indicate close physical proximity of endogenous mu and delta opioid receptors at the plasma membrane of hippocampal neurons and suggest constitutive mu–delta heteromerization at the surface of neurons.

2.2. CYM51010 Induces Mu–Delta Receptor Co-Internalization and Co-Localization in the Late Endosomal Compartment in Primary Hippocampal Cultures

CYM51010 was reported as a mu–delta-biased agonist because its antinociceptive effect was blocked by an antibody selective for mu–delta heteromers and its activity was reduced in mice deficient for the mu or delta opioid receptor [24,25]. We, therefore, tested whether activation by this ligand (concentration range 10 nM to 10 µM) triggered mu and delta receptor internalization in primary hippocampal cultures from double-fluorescent knock-in mice. CYM51010 concentrations equivalent to, or higher than, 400 nM induced mu-mCherry and delta-eGFP internalization as seen from the decrease in fluorescence density associated with the plasma membrane and the appearance of fluorescent intracellular vesicles (Figure 1A,B). Quantification of the extent of co-localization 15, 30, and 60 min after agonist administration showed that the fraction of mu and delta opioid receptors that co-localized at the plasma membrane significantly decreased (Figure 1C), whereas mu–delta receptor co-localization increased in the cytoplasm at the three time points (Figure 1D), establishing co-internalization of the receptors. Triple immunofluorescence labeling with Lysosomal-associated membrane protein 1 (LAMP1) as a marker of the late endosomal–lysosomal compartment showed increased co-localization with mu-mCherry and delta-eGFP 60 min after activation by CYM51010 (Figure 2), suggesting that mu and delta opioid receptors are targeted together to the degradation pathway.

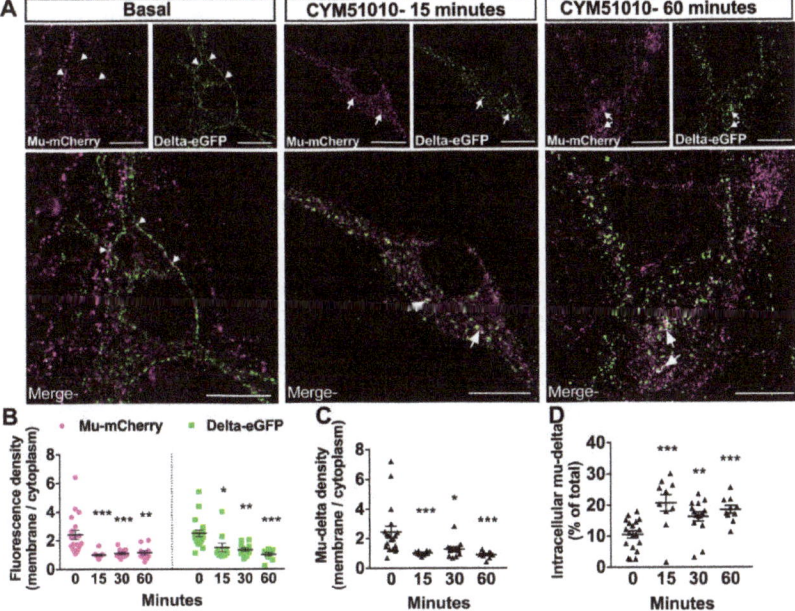

Figure 1. Mu and delta opioid receptors co-internalize upon CYM51010 activation in primary hippocampal cultures. (**A**) Representative confocal images showing mu-mCherry and delta-eGFP fluorescence localized at the plasma membrane (arrowheads) under basal condition or internalized in vesicle-like structures 15 or 60 min after CYM51010 (400 nM) application (arrows). Scale bar = 10 µm. (**B**) Receptor internalization induced by CYM51010 application (400 nM) expressed as a ratio of membrane-associated versus intracellular fluorescence densities for each receptor. Two-way ANOVA $F_{treatment}$ (3, 94) = 17.98; $p < 0.0001$. $F_{receptor}$ (1, 94) = 1.06; $F_{interaction}$ (3, 94) = 0.54. Tukey's post hoc test for mu-mCherry, *** $p < 0.001$, ** $p = 0.01$. Tukey's post hoc test for delta-eGFP, * $p = 0.02$, ** $p = 0.002$, *** $p < 0.001$; n = 10 to 20 neurons per group from at least three independent cultures. (**C**) Subcellular redistribution of mu–delta heteromers expressed as a ratio of membrane-associated versus intracellular fluorescence densities for co-localized mu-mCherry and delta-eGFP receptors. One-way ANOVA (F (3, 48) = 13.64; $p < 0.0001$) followed by multiple-comparison Dunn's post hoc test. * $p = 0.03$, *** $p < 0.001$; n = 10–20 neurons per group from at least three independent cultures. (**D**) Fraction of cytoplasmic mu-delta heteromers expressed as the percentage of mu-mCherry and delta-eGFP overlapping objects detected in vesicle-like structures at the different times. Kruskal Wallis test ($p < 0.0001$) followed with multiple comparisons Dunn's test. ** $p < 0.01$, 30 min vs basal, *** $p < 0.001$ 15 min and 60 min vs basal. N = 10 to 20 neurons per group from at least 3 independent cultures.

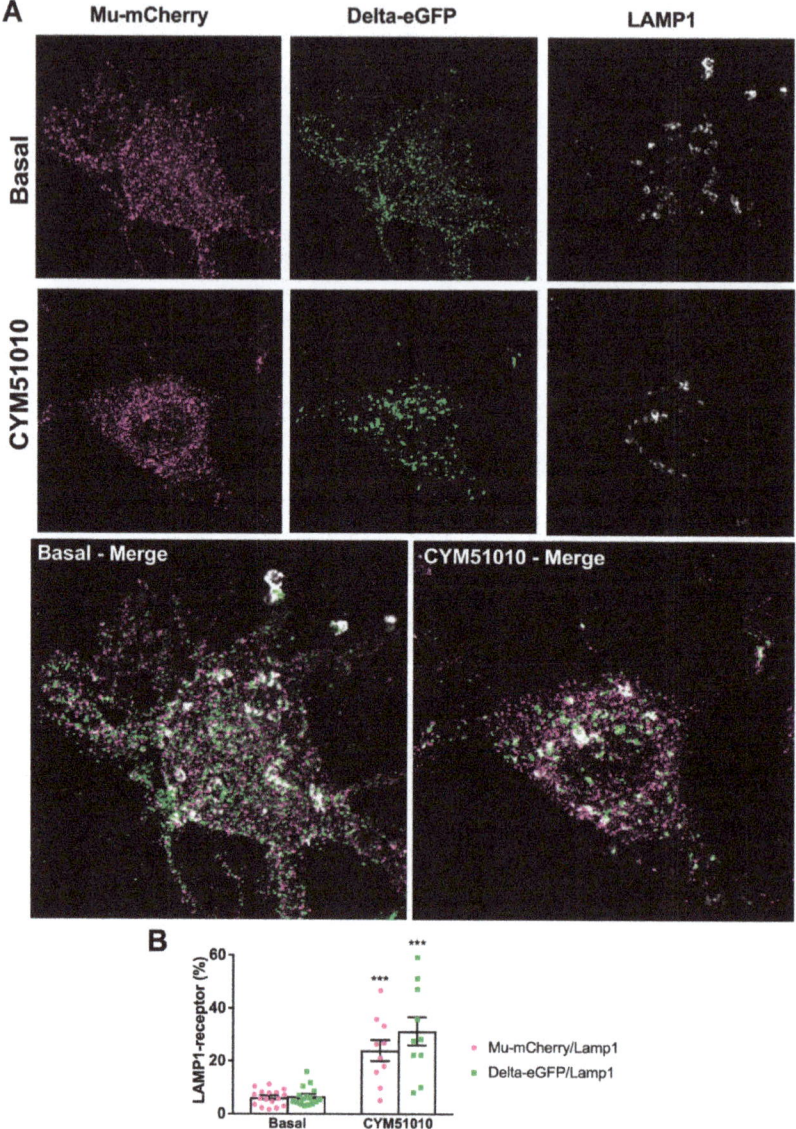

Figure 2. Mu and delta opioid receptors co-localize in the lysosomal compartment upon CYM51010 activation in primary hippocampal cultures. (**A**) Representative confocal images showing mu-mCherry–delta-eGFP colocalization with LAMP1 immunoreactive compartment under basal conditions or 60 min after CYM51010 application (400 nM). Scale bar = 10 μm (inset scale bar = 2.5 μm). (**B**) Drug treatment induces statistically significant increase in the amount of colocalization of mu-mCherry/delta-eGFP colocalization with LAMP1 labeling. Two-way ANOVA $F_{drug\ treatment}$ (1, 49) = 62.70; $p < 0.0001$. $F_{receptor}$ (1, 49) = 2.12, $p = 0.15$; $F_{interaction}$ (1, 49) = 3.65, $p = 0.2$. Tukey's post hoc test: *** $p < 0.001$ for both mu-mCherry and delta-eGFP; n = 10–20 neurons per group from at least three independent cultures.

We then sought to investigate whether internalization of the mu opioid receptor by CYM51010 was promoted by its association with the delta opioid receptor. In primary hippocampal cultures from single fluorescent knock-in animals expressing mu-mCherry and deficient for the delta opioid receptor, CYM51010 concentrations up to 1 µM failed to induce mu-mCherry internalization (Figure 3A,B) with only limited mu opioid receptor clustering and subcellular redistribution at 10 µM (Figure 3B).

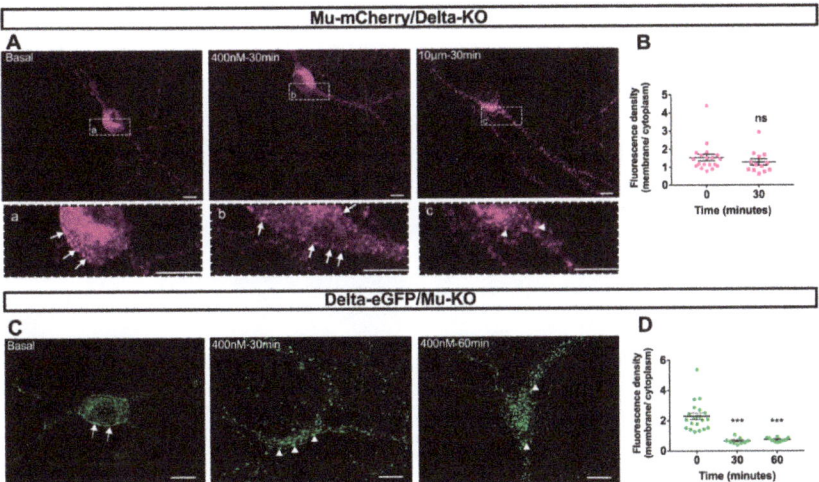

Figure 3. CYM51010 internalization of mu or delta opioid receptors in primary hippocampal cultures from mice deficient for one of the receptors. (**A**) Representative confocal images showing that mu-mCherry is associated with the plasma membrane (arrows) in basal conditions and 30 min after CYM51010 (400 nM) addition in delta-knockout (KO) mice. Scale bar = 10 µm. (**B**) Mu-mCherry internalization induced by CYM51010 application expressed as a ratio of membrane-associated versus intracellular fluorescence densities. Mann–Whitney test, $p = 0.20$; $n = 13$ to 20 neurons per group from at least three independent cultures. (**C**) Representative confocal images showing that delta-eGFP is predominantly associated with the plasma membrane in basal conditions (arrows) in mu-KO mice, whereas the association is mostly intracellular at 30 and 60 min after CYM51010 (400 nM) addition (arrowheads). Scale bar = 10 µm. (**D**) Delta-eGFP internalization induced by CYM51010 application expressed as a ratio of membrane-associated versus intracellular fluorescence densities. Kruskal–Wallis test ($p < 0.0001$) followed by Dunn's multiple comparison test. Significant differences after multiple-comparison tests are expressed as $p < 0.001$ (***) compared to basal group; $n = 9$–20 neurons per group from at least three independent cultures.

We also examined whether internalization of the delta opioid receptor upon activation by CYM51010 required mu opioid receptor co-expression. In primary hippocampal cultures from single fluorescent knock-in animals expressing delta-eGFP and deficient for the mu opioid receptor, CYM51010 (400 nM) induced internalization of the delta opioid receptor (Figure 3C). In addition, predominant intracellular localization was observed 30 and 60 min after agonist application (Figure 3D) in agreement with kinetics described for the delta selective agonist SNC80 [12,13,26], indicating that CYM51010 was able to promote delta opioid receptor internalization despite the lack of mu opioid receptor expression.

Together, these data establish that mu opioid receptor internalization by CYM51010 is dependent on mu–delta receptor co-expression and directs the mu opioid receptor to the late endocytic compartment.

2.3. CYM51010-Induced Mu–Delta Receptor Co-Internalization Is Blocked by Pretreatment with Mu- or Delta-Selective Antagonists

In neurons expressing one receptor only, CYM51010 activation led to the internalization of delta but not mu opioid receptors (Figure 3). We, therefore, sought to determine whether co-internalization by CYM51010 required the two receptors to be in an active conformation. To this aim, we examined the impact of pretreatment for 15 min with the mu-selective antagonists beta-funaltrexamine (β-FNA) (20 nM) orCTAP (200 nM). Both antagonists prevented mu opioid receptor cellular redistribution but did not block delta opioid receptor internalization (Figure 4A,C,D). These results suggest that an active conformation of the mu opioid receptor is required for mu–delta co-internalization.

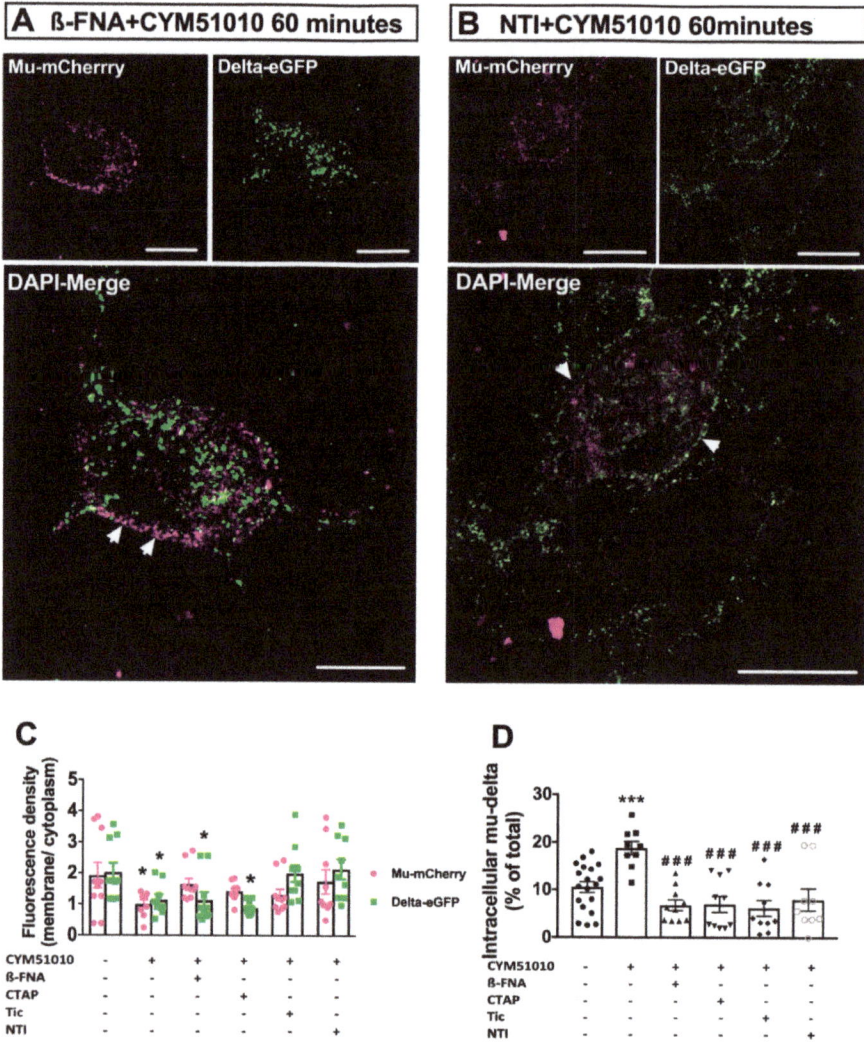

Figure 4. Antagonist pretreatment abolishes mu–delta opioid receptor co-internalization by CYM51010 in primary hippocampal cultures. (**A**) Representative confocal images showing mu-mCherry predominant localization at the plasma membrane and delta-eGFP extensive internalization after pretreatment with the mu antagonist β-FNA (200 nM) for 15 min, followed by incubation for 60 min with CYM51010 (400 nM).

Scale bar = 10 µm. (**B**) Representative confocal images showing mu-mCherry and delta-eGFP predominant localization at the plasma membrane after pretreatment with delta antagonist naltrindole (200 nM) (NTI) for 15 min, followed by incubation for 60 min with CYM51010 (400 nM). Scale bar = 10 µm. (**C**) Pretreatment with the mu antagonists β-FNA or CTAP (200 nM) blocks mu-mCherry but not delta-eGFP internalization, whereas pretreatment with the delta antagonists naltrindole (NTI) and tic-deltorphin (tic) (200 nM) prevent internalization of both mu-mCherry and delta-eGFP. Receptor internalization is expressed as a ratio of membrane-associated versus intracellular fluorescence densities for each receptor. Two-way ANOVA $F_{treatment}$ (5, 104) = 4.73, p = 0.0001. $F_{receptor}$ (1, 104) = 0.1, p = 0.84; $F_{interaction}$ (5, 100) = 1.96; p = 0.0006. Multiple comparisons with Tukey's post hoc test, * p = 0.04 basal vs. CYM51010 for mu-mCherry, * p = 0.04 basal vs. CYM51010, * p = 0.04 basal vs. β-FNA, * p = 0.04 basal vs. CTAP; n = 9–20 neurons per group from at least three independent cultures. (**D**) Mu-mCherry/delta-eGFP co-internalization is prevented by treatment with either mu or delta antagonists. Percentage of colocalized receptors in the cytoplasm after drug treatment. The fraction of cytoplasmic mu–delta heteromers is expressed as the percentage of mu-mCherry and delta-eGFP overlapping objects detected in vesicle-like structures 60 min after CYM51010 application. One-way ANOVA (p < 0.0001) followed by multiple-comparison Dunnett's test. Significant differences after multiple comparisons tests are expressed as *** p < 0.001 when compared to basal group and ### p < 0.001 when compared to CYM51010 without antagonists; n = 9–20 neurons per group from at least three independent cultures.

We evaluated the need for delta opioid receptor activation in the co-internalization process. Whereas pretreatment with mu antagonists blocked mu but not delta opioid receptor internalization, pretreatment with the selective delta antagonists naltrindole or tic-deltorphin 200 nM blocked the internalization of both delta and mu opioid receptors (Figure 4B–D). This indicates that mu–delta cellular redistribution is driven by delta opioid receptor expression and activation.

Together, this result indicates that mu–delta receptor co-internalization upon CYM51010 activation is driven by delta opioid receptors and requires both mu and delta opioid receptors to be in an active conformation.

2.4. Mu–Delta Receptor Co-Internalization Is Ligand-Specific

We examined whether other synthetic opioid agonists were able to promote mu–delta receptor co-internalization in primary hippocampal cultures. Mu–delta receptor co-localization in the cytoplasm was increased 30 min after stimulation with the mu agonist DAMGO (1 µM) or the delta agonist deltorphin II (100 nM), but not upon stimulation with the delta agonist SNC 80 (100 nM) or the mu agonists morphine (10 µM) or methadone (1 µM) (Figure 5). These data establish ligand-specific internalization of endogenous mu–delta heteromers by exogenous opioids.

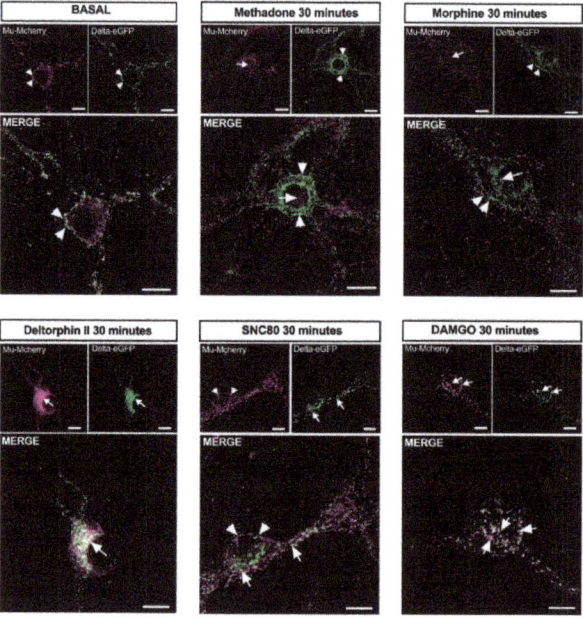

Figure 5. Mu–delta opioid receptor co-internalization is ligand-selective in primary hippocampal cultures. Representative confocal images showing mu-mCherry and delta-eGFP fluorescence at the plasma membrane (arrowheads) under basal conditions or co-internalized in vesicle-like structures (arrows) 30 min after DAMGO (1 µM) or deltorphin II (100 nM), but not SNC80 (100 nM), morphine (10 µM), or methadone (1 µM). Scale bar = 10 µm.

3. Discussion

In this study, we used primary hippocampal cultures of double-fluorescent knock-in mice to investigate the impact of neuronal co-expression on the internalization of native mu and delta opioid receptors.

3.1. Mu–Delta Co-Internalization Is Induced by Different Ligands in Native or Co-Transfected Cells

We showed here that co-internalization of endogenous mu and delta opioid receptors was ligand-dependent and took place following activation by the mu–delta-biased agonist CYM51010, the mu agonist DAMGO, or the delta agonist deltorphin II, but not following activation by the mu agonist morphine. This is consistent with previous reports in co-transfected HEK293 cells in which co-internalization of the receptors was promoted by DAMGO [15–18] or deltorphin II [16–18], but not morphine [19]. No co-internalization of mu and delta opioid receptors was observed following activation by the delta agonist SNC80, in agreement with the absence of receptor co-internalization in the spinal cord of delta-eGFP knock-in mice following SNC80 (10 mg/kg intraperitoneal (i.p.)) administration [29]. These results obtained in native environment are, however, in marked contrast to the reported mu–delta co-internalization in co-transfected cells [17,18]. Furthermore, we did not evidence mu–delta co-internalization by the mu agonist methadone although this ligand induced mu–delta co-trafficking in in co-transfected cells [19]. Collectively, these observations highlight the difficulty to draw definite conclusions from data collected in heterologous systems. Differences between native and heterologous environments may reflect distinct cellular contents [20]. Internalization of the delta opioid receptor was dependent on G protein coupled receptor kinase 2 (GRK2) in cortical neurons but not in transfected HEK293 cells, although the latter expressed GRK2 and supported

GRK2-mediated internalization of other GPCRs [30]. Similarly, the ability of ligands to differentially activate signaling pathways in AtT20 neuroblastoma and CHO cell lines uncovered clear influence of the cellular background on mu opioid receptor signaling [31]. Expression of high levels of receptors in a non-native environment can also artificially elicit interactions that would not occur in vivo and could subsequently affect functional responses. Accordingly, low levels of mu (10–15 fmol/mg protein) [32,33] and delta opioid receptors (30–50 fmol/mg protein) [32–35] are present in the mouse hippocampus, whereas heterologous receptors are most often expressed in the picomolar range.

A potential influence resulting from the C-terminal fusion to a fluorescent protein is also to be considered. Addition of the fluorescent tag did not modify the expression level of the mu opioid receptor [11] but induced a twofold increase in delta opioid receptor expression [12]. In particular, strong surface expression of the delta-eGFP construct in the hippocampus could alter receptor trafficking and signaling. However, no overt change in the neuroanatomical distribution, pharmacological, and signaling properties or behavioral response has been evidenced so far in the knock-in mice expressing the delta-eGFP and/or mu-mcherry fluorescent fusions (reviewed in [36]). Importantly, delta-eGFP surface expression varies across the nervous system and is increased upon chronic morphine administration [27] or in neuropathic pain conditions [37], as previously reported for wild-type receptors (reviewed in [5,36]). Moreover, the use of the delta-eGFP fusion enabled detecting in vivo partial receptor internalization in response to a physiological stimulation [26] or upregulation following Pavlovian training [38]. The fluorescent knock-in mice, therefore, appear to be well-suited reporters for native opioid receptor studies.

3.2. CYM51010 Activation Induces Co-Targeting of Mu and Delta Receptors to the Lysosomal Compartment

Native mu opioid receptors rapidly recycle back to the plasma membrane [10,11], whereas native delta opioid receptors are slow-recycling receptors that are degraded in the lysosomal compartments [13]. Here, we observed that native mu–delta heteromers were targeted to the lysosomal compartment in primary neurons triggering a change in the mu opioid receptor intracellular fate following activation by CYM51010. Although CYM51010 was reported as a mu–delta heteromer biased agonist [24], it also binds to mu or delta opioid receptors expressed alone. Previous reports suggested that CYM51010 would not activate delta opioid receptors because [^{35}S]GTPγS activation by CYM51010 was not prevented by antibodies specific for the delta opioid receptor [24], and CYM51010 administration did not modify mechanical or thermal allodynia in neuropathic mu knockout animals [25]. However, our data revealed that CYM51010 promoted delta opioid receptor internalization in mu knockout mice indicating that it could activate this receptor in the absence of the mu opioid receptor. CYM51010 could also activate mu opioid receptors because antibodies specific for the mu opioid receptor reduced [^{35}S]GTPγS activation by CYM51010, although to a lesser extent than mu–delta-specific antibodies [24]. Moreover, CYM51010 had analgesic properties in delta knockout mice [25]. As shown here, activation of the mu opioid receptor by CYM51010 was not associated with internalization when the receptor was expressed alone. On the other hand, CYM51010 induced internalization of the mu opioid receptor when associated with the delta opioid receptor, suggesting that its binding triggered a different conformation of the mu opioid receptor that allowed beta-arrestin recruitment. Mu-selective (CTAP, cyprodime, β-FNA) or delta-selective (naltrindole, tic-deltorphin) antagonists prevented endogenous mu–delta co-internalization in agreement with previously reported inhibition of the mu or delta receptor, respectively, by a delta or a mu selective antagonist in co-transfected HEK293 cells [17]. These observations strongly suggest that co-trafficking requires both receptors in an active conformation and that mu–delta co-internalization did not result from random nonfunctional contacts elicited by receptor close proximity in the membrane.

Interestingly, delta antagonists blocked mu–delta receptor co-internalization, whereas mu antagonists only blocked mu opioid receptor internalization without affecting delta opioid receptor internalization and degradation. These data indicate that co-internalization was driven by the delta opioid receptor, possibly through constitutive β-arrestin recruitment [39,40]. Delta antagonists could, therefore, inhibit co-sequestration of the receptors by disrupting contacts between delta opioid receptors and β-arrestins, which would in turn destabilize the interface between the mu and delta opioid receptors.

3.3. Mu and Delta Opioid Receptors Form Functional Heteromers in the Hippocampus

Physical proximity of the receptors was established by co-immunoprecipitation in the hippocampus, where neuronal co-expression of mu and delta opioid receptors was mostly detected in parvalbumin-positive neurons [11]. Here, we confirmed co-expression of the two receptors at the plasma membrane in basal conditions. We also established that CYM51010, an agonist that preferentially binds mu–delta heteromers [24], induced co-internalization of the two receptors. In addition, co-internalization changed the intracellular fate of the mu opioid receptor compared to neurons where the receptor was expressed alone. Indeed, the mu opioid receptor was targeted to the lysosomal compartment instead of being recycled to the plasma membrane. Altogether, these observations satisfy the criteria for receptor heteromerization as defined by the International Union of Basic and Clinical Pharmacology (IUPHAR) [41] and establish the presence of functional mu–delta heteromers in hippocampal neurons.

4. Materials and Methods

4.1. Animals

Double knock-in mice co-expressing fluorescent mu and delta opioid receptors (mu-mCherry/delta-eGFP) were obtained by crossing previously generated single fluorescent knock-in mice expressing delta-eGFP or mu-mCherry, as described previously [11]. Single-fluorescent knock-in mice deficient for the other receptor were generated by crossing delta-eGFP with mu-knockout mice or mu-mCherry with delta knockout mice. The genetic background of all animals was 50:50 C57BL6/J:129svPas. Male and female adult mice (8–12 weeks old) were used for in vivo experiments.

Mice were housed in an animal facility under controlled temperature (21 ± 2 °C) and humidity (45% ± 5%) under a 12 h/12 h dark–light cycle with food and water ad libitum. All experiments were performed in agreement with the European legislation (directive 2010/63/EU acting on protection of laboratory animals) and received agreement from the French ministry (APAFIS 20 1503041113547 (APAFIS#300).02).

4.2. Drugs

$$\overline{\text{D-Phe–Cys–Tyr–D-Trp–Pen–Thr–NH}_2}$$

(CTAP) (C-6352), beta-funaltrexamine (β-FNA) (O-003), fentanyl citrate (F3886), naltrindole (N-2893), [D-Ala^2, NMe-Phe^4, Gly-ol^5]enkephalin (DAMGO) (E-7384), and deltorphin II (T-0658) were purchased from Sigma. (+)-4-[(αR)-α-((2S,5R)-4-Allyl-2,5-dimethyl-1-piperazinyl)-3-methoxybenzyl]-N,N-diethylbenzamide (SNC80) (cat n° 0764) was obtained from Tocris bioscience, 1-[[4-(acetylamino)phenyl]methyl]-4-(2-phenylethyl)-4-piperidinecarboxylic acid, ethyl ester (CYM51010) (ML-335) was obtained from Cayman chemical, and tic-deltorphin was synthesized as reported in [42]. Morphine hydrochloride was from Francopia, and methadone (M-0267) was from Sigma.

4.3. Primary Neuronal Culture

Primary neuronal cultures were performed as previously described [28]. Briefly, P0–P3 mice pups were decapitated, and their hippocampi were dissected and digested with papain (20 U/mL, Worthington cat. no. LS003126). Cells were plated (8–10 × 10^4 cells/well) on polylysine (PLL, Sigma)-coated coverslips in 24-well plates. Cultures were maintained for 15 days in vitro (DIV) with half of the medium (Neurobasal A medium supplemented with 2% B27 (GIBCO, cat. no. 17504044), 2 mM glutamax (GIBCO, cat. no. 35050061), 0.5 mM glutamine and penicillin/streptomycin) changed every 5–7 days. Fully matured primary neurons (DIV 10 to 14) were used for all studies.

4.4. Drug Administration and Sample Preparation

DAMGO, naltrindole, CTAP, deltorphin II, morphine, methadone, and tic-deltorphin were dissolved in sterile milliQ water, CYM51010 was dissolved in saline solution with Dimethyl sulfoxide (DMSO) (0.2% final volume) and Tween-80 (1% final volume), and SNC 80 was dissolved in DMSO at 10 mg/mL. Drugs were added to the culture medium of mature neurons (as 1% of the total culture volume) (12–15 days in vitro) and incubated at 37 °C as indicated. Antagonists were added to the culture medium 15 min before agonist treatment.

For immunofluorescence studies, cultures were washed in cold 0.1 M phosphate-buffered saline pH 7.4 (PBS) and fixed with 4% paraformaldehyde in PBS. Cells were washed three times with cold PBS and kept at 4 °C until processing.

4.5. Fluorescent Detection with Antibodies

Primary neuronal cultures or brain sections were incubated in the blocking solution PBST (PBS with 0.2% Tween-20 (Sigma)) and 5% normal goat serum (Sigma)) for 1 h at room temperature (20–22 °C) and then overnight at 4 °C in the blocking solution with chicken anti-GFP (1/1000, Aves GFP-1020), rabbit anti ds-red (1/1000, Clontech 632496), and rat anti-LAMP1 (1/500, BD Biosciences 553792) when applicable. Cells were washed three times in PBST and incubated for 2 h in PBST with goat anti-chicken antibodies coupled to AlexaFluor 488 (1/2000, Molecular Probes A11039), goat anti-rabbit coupled to AlexaFluor 594 (1/2000, Molecular Probes A11012), and goat anti-rat coupled to DyLight 650 (1/500, Invitrogen SA5-100021). After three washes in PBST, nuclei were stained with 4,6′-diamidino-2-phenylindole (DAPI) (1 µg/mL in PBS) for 5 min. Samples were mounted with ProLong™ Gold Antifade mounting medium (Molecular Probes) and kept at −20°, protected from light, until confocal imaging.

4.6. Image Acquisition and Analysis

Confocal images were acquired (Leica SP5) using a 63× (Numerical aperture (NA) 1.4) oil immersion objective and analyzed with ICY software (http://icy.bioimageanalysis.org/) as previously described [28]. Briefly, quantification was performed on a single-plane image from a z-stack within two sequential steps. First, the plasma membrane and cytoplasmic compartment were defined for each neuron. Each neuron was carefully delineated using the "free-hand area" tool. This initial Region of interest (ROI) was filled with the "fill holes in ROI" plugin to define the total cell area (ROI $_{total}$). ROIs were then processed to generate two ROIs corresponding to the cell periphery and the cytoplasm. On the basis of staining in basal conditions, we estimated that most of the plasma membrane staining was found over an 8 pixel thickness. Therefore, we automatically eroded, with the "Erode ROI" plugin, the ROI $_{total}$ by 8 pixels and subtracted this new ROI (ROI $_{cyto}$) from ROI $_{total}$ to obtain a ROI corresponding to the cell periphery (ROI $_{peri}$).

The spots were then detected in each channel and the amount of co-localization determined in each region of interest. To detect the specific signal in each ROI, we used the "spot detector" plugin which relies on the wavelet transform algorithm [43]. By carefully setting the sensitivity threshold and the scale of objects to detect, it allows the detection of spots even in images with low signal-to-noise ratio. In our conditions, the sensitivity threshold was fixed between 50 and 60, and the scale of objects was set at 2 (pixel size 3) for mu and delta receptors. Once parameters were defined, images were processed with the tool "protocol" in ICY, which is a graphical interface for automated image processing. Data including the number of spots detected in each channel and ROI, the number of co-localized objects, and the ROI area were automatically collected in excel files. Objects were considered co-localized if the distance of their centroid was equal to or less than 3 pixels. The protocol used in these analyses is available online (http://icy.bioimageanalysis.org/protocol/newcolocalizer-with-binary-and-excel-output-v1_batch/). To obtain histograms, we calculated object densities for each receptor reported to the surface of each ROI. Membrane-to-cytoplasm density ratios were calculated to illustrate the subcellular distribution of each receptor. The extent of co-localization was calculated according to the following formula for each ROI: % colocalization $= 100 \times \left(\frac{\text{colocalized mu and delta objects}}{\sum (\text{detected mu and delta objects})} \right)$. The extent of internalization is expressed as the ratio of membrane/cytoplasm immunoreactivity densities for each receptor or co-localized mu–delta. Co-localization of the two receptors is expressed as the percentage of co-localized mu-mCherry and delta-eGFP signals reported to the total immunoreactivity.

4.7. Statistical Analysis

Statistical analyses were performed with Graphpad Prism V7 software (GraphPad, San Diego, CA, USA). Normality of the distributions and homogeneity of the variances were checked before statistical comparison to determine appropriate tests. One-way nonparametric (Kruskal–Wallis followed by Dunn's multiple-comparison test) or parametric one-way ANOVA test (followed by Dunnett's multiple-comparison test) were used to compare different experimental groups. A two-way ANOVA followed by post hoc Tukey's test for multiple comparisons was used for multiple factor comparisons. Results in graphs and histograms are illustrated as means ± standard error of the mean (SEM).

5. Conclusions

Our data demonstrate for the first time that co-expression of native mu and delta opioid receptors in hippocampal neurons alters the intracellular fate of the mu opioid receptor in a ligand-selective manner. This observation supports functional heteromerization of the two receptors that would contribute to the fine-tuning of mu opioid receptor signaling. It, therefore, highlights an interesting emerging concept for the development of novel therapeutic drugs and strategies. Importantly, our study also emphasizes the need to perform pharmacological studies on native receptors due to the limited translational value of data collected in co-transfected cells.

Author Contributions: Conceptualization, D.M. and L.D.; methodology, D.M., L.D., and S.O.; software, S.O.; validation, D.M., L.D., and S.O.; formal analysis, D.M., F.P., L.D., and S.O.; investigation, D.M., F.P., and L.D.; resources, S.D.; writing—original draft preparation, D.M.; writing—review and editing, D.M., L.D., and S.O.; visualization, D.M. and L.D.; supervision, D.M.; funding acquisition, D.M. All authors have read and agreed to the published version of the manuscript.

Funding: This research was funded by the Fondation pour la Recherche Médicale (DPA20140129364), the CNRS, and the University of Strasbourg. L. Derouiche was the recipient of an IDEX postdoctoral fellowship from the University of Strasbourg.

Acknowledgments: The authors would like to thank the Chronobiotron animal facility (UMS 3415 CNRS) and the in vitro imaging platform of the Institut des Neurosciences Cellulaires et Intégratives (UPS 3156 CNRS) for their assistance.

Conflicts of Interest: The authors declare no conflict of interest.

References

1. Gaveriaux-Ruff, C.; Kieffer, B.L. Opioid receptor genes inactivated in mice: The highlights. *Neuropeptides* **2002**, *36*, 62–71. [CrossRef] [PubMed]
2. Feng, Y.; He, X.; Yang, Y.; Chao, D.; H Lazarus, L.; Xia, Y. Current research on opioid receptor function. *Curr. Drug Targets* **2012**, *13*, 230–246. [CrossRef] [PubMed]
3. Charbogne, P.; Kieffer, B.L.; Befort, K. 15 years of genetic approaches in vivo for addiction research: Opioid receptor and peptide gene knockout in mouse models of drug abuse. *Neuropharmacology* **2014**, *76 Pt B*, 204–217. [CrossRef]
4. Zhang, Z.; Pan, Z.Z. Synaptic mechanism for functional synergism between delta- and mu-opioid receptors. *J. Neurosci.* **2010**, *30*, 4735–4745. [CrossRef] [PubMed]
5. Gendron, L.; Mittal, N.; Beaudry, H.; Walwyn, W. Recent advances on the delta opioid receptor: From trafficking to function. *Br. J. Pharmacol.* **2015**, *172*, 403–419. [CrossRef] [PubMed]
6. Fujita, W.; Gomes, I.; Devi, L.A. Revolution in GPCR Signaling: Opioid receptor heteromers as novel therapeutic targets. *Br. J. Pharmacol.* **2014**, *171*, 4155–4176. [CrossRef]

7. Jordan, B.A.; Devi, L.A. G-protein-coupled receptor heterodimerization modulates receptor function. *Nature* **1999**, *399*, 697–700. [CrossRef]
8. Gomes, I.; Jordan, B.A.; Gupta, A.; Trapaidze, N.; Nagy, V.; Devi, L.A. Heterodimerization of mu and delta opioid receptors: A role in opiate synergy. *J. Neurosci.* **2000**, *20*, 1–5. [CrossRef]
9. Fujita, W.; Gomes, I.; Devi, L.A. Mu-Delta opioid receptor heteromers: New pharmacology and novel therapeutic possibilities. *Br. J. Pharmacol.* **2015**, *172*, 375–387. [CrossRef]
10. Trafton, J.A.; Abbadie, C.; Marek, K.; Basbaum, A.I. Postsynaptic signaling via the [mu]-opioid receptor: Responses of dorsal horn neurons to exogenous opioids and noxious stimulation. *J. Neurosci.* **2000**, *20*, 8578–8584. [CrossRef]
11. Erbs, E.; Faget, L.; Scherrer, G.; Matifas, A.; Filliol, D.; Vonesch, J.L.; Koch, M.; Kessler, P.; Hentsch, D.; Birling, M.C.; et al. A mu-delta opioid receptor brain atlas reveals neuronal co-occurrence in subcortical networks. *Brain Struct. Funct.* **2015**, *220*, 677–702. [CrossRef] [PubMed]
12. Scherrer, G.; Tryoen-Tóth, P.; Filliol, D.; Matifas, A.; Laustriat, D.; Cao, Y.Q.; Basbaum, A.I.; Dierich, A.; Vonesh, J.L.; Gavériaux-Ruff, C.; et al. Knockin mice expressing fluorescent delta-opioid receptors uncover G protein-coupled receptor dynamics in vivo. *Proc. Natl. Acad. Sci. USA* **2006**, *103*, 9691–9696. [CrossRef] [PubMed]
13. Pradhan, A.A.; Becker, J.A.; Scherrer, G.; Tryoen-Toth, P.; Filliol, D.; Matifas, A.; Massotte, D.; Gavériaux-Ruff, C.; Kieffer, B.L. In vivo delta opioid receptor internalization controls behavioral effects of agonists. *PLoS ONE* **2009**, *4*, e5425. [CrossRef] [PubMed]
14. Whistler, J.L.; Enquist, J.; Marley, A.; Fong, J.; Gladher, F.; Tsuruda, P.; Murray, S.R.; Von Zastrow, M. Modulation of postendocytic sorting of G protein-coupled receptors. *Science* **2002**, *297*, 615–620. [CrossRef]
15. Rozenfeld, R.; Devi, L.A. Receptor heterodimerization leads to a switch in signaling: Beta-arrestin2-mediated ERK activation by mu-delta opioid receptor heterodimers. *FASEB J.* **2007**, *21*, 2455–2465. [CrossRef]
16. Hasbi, A.; Nguyen, T.; Fan, T.; Cheng, R.; Rashid, A.; Alijaniaram, M.; Rasenick, M.M.; O'Dowd, B.F.; George, S.R. Trafficking of preassembled opioid mu-delta heterooligomer-Gz signaling complexes to the plasma membrane: Coregulation by agonists. *Biochemistry* **2007**, *46*, 12997–13009. [CrossRef]
17. Kabli, N.; Martin, N.; Fan, T.; Nguyen, T.; Hasbi, A.; Balboni, G.; O'Dowd, B.F.; George, S.R. Agonists at the delta-opioid receptor modify the binding of micro-receptor agonists to the micro-delta receptor hetero-oligomer. *Br. J. Pharmacol.* **2010**, *161*, 1122–1136. [CrossRef]
18. He, S.Q.; Zhang, Z.N.; Guan, J.S.; Liu, H.R.; Zhao, B.; Wang, H.B.; Li, Q.; Yang, H.; Luo, J.; Li, Z.Y.; et al. Facilitation of mu-opioid receptor activity by preventing delta-opioid receptor-mediated codegradation. *Neuron* **2011**, *69*, 120–131. [CrossRef]
19. Milan-Lobo, L.; Whistler, J.L. Heteromerization of the mu- and delta-opioid receptors produces ligand-biased antagonism and alters mu-receptor trafficking. *J. Pharmacol. Exp. Ther.* **2011**, *337*, 868–875. [CrossRef]
20. Benredjem, B.; Dallaire, P.; Pineyro, G. Analyzing biased responses of GPCR ligands. *Curr. Opin. Pharmacol.* **2017**, *32*, 71–76. [CrossRef]
21. Broad, J.; Maurel, D.; Kung, V.W.; Hicks, G.A.; Schemann, M.; Barnes, M.R.; Kenakin, T.P.; Granier, S.; Sanger, G.J. Human native kappa opioid receptor functions not predicted by recombinant receptors: Implications for drug design. *Sci. Rep.* **2016**, *6*, 30797. [CrossRef] [PubMed]
22. Ong, E.W.; Xue, L.; Olmstead, M.C.; Cahill, C.M. Prolonged morphine treatment alters delta opioid receptor post-internalization trafficking. *Br. J. Pharmacol.* **2015**, *172*, 615–629. [CrossRef] [PubMed]
23. Pierre, F.; Ugur, M.; Faivre, F.; Doridot, S.; Veinante, P.; Massotte, D. Morphine-dependent and abstinent mice are characterized by a broader distribution of the neurons co-expressing mu and delta opioid receptors. *Neuropharmacology* **2019**, *152*, 30–41. [CrossRef] [PubMed]
24. Gomes, I.; Fujita, W.; Gupta, A.; Saldanha, S.A.; Negri, A.; Pinello, C.E.; Eberhart, C.; Roberts, E.; Filizola, M.; Hodder, P.; et al. Identification of a mu-delta opioid receptor heteromer-biased agonist with antinociceptive activity. *Proc. Natl. Acad. Sci. USA* **2013**, *110*, 12072–12077. [CrossRef]
25. Tiwari, V.; He, S.Q.; Huang, Q.; Liang, L.; Yang, F.; Chen, Z.; Tiwari, V.; Fujita, W.; Devi, L.A.; Dong, X.; et al. Activation of micro-delta opioid receptor heteromers inhibits neuropathic pain behavior in rodents. *Pain* **2020**, *161*, 842–855. [CrossRef]
26. Faget, L.; Erbs, E.; Le Merrer, J.; Scherrer, G.; Matifas, A.; Benturquia, N.; Noble, F.; Decossas, M.; Koch, M.; Kessler, P.; et al. In vivo visualization of delta opioid receptors upon physiological activation uncovers a distinct internalization profile. *J. Neurosci.* **2012**, *32*, 7301–7310. [CrossRef]

27. Erbs, E.; Faget, L.; Ceredig, R.A.; Matifas, A.; Vonesch, J.L.; Kieffer, B.L.; Massotte, D. Impact of chronic morphine on delta opioid receptor-expressing neurons in the mouse hippocampus. *Neuroscience* **2016**, *313*, 46–56. [CrossRef]
28. Derouiche, L.; Ory, S.; Massotte, D. Double fluorescent knock-in mice to investigate endogenous mu-delta opioid heteromer subcellular distribution. In *Receptor-Receptor Interactions in the Central Nervous System*; Fuxe, K., Borroto Escuela, D., Eds.; Springer: New York, NY, USA, 2018; pp. 149–162.
29. Wang, D.; Tawfik, V.L.; Corder, G.; Low, S.A.; François, A.; Basbaum, A.I.; Scherrer, G. Functional Divergence of Delta and Mu Opioid Receptor Organization in CNS Pain Circuits. *Neuron* **2018**, *98*, 90–108.e5. [CrossRef]
30. Charfi, I.; Nagi, K.; Mnie-Filali, O.; Thibault, D.; Balboni, G.; Schiller, P.W.; Trudeau, L.E.; Pineyro, G. Ligand- and cell-dependent determinants of internalization and cAMP modulation by delta opioid receptor (DOR) agonists. *Cell Mol. Life Sci.* **2014**, *71*, 1529–1546. [CrossRef]
31. Thompson, G.L.; Lane, J.R.; Coudrat, T.; Sexton, P.M.; Christopoulos, A.; Canals, M. Systematic analysis of factors influencing observations of biased agonism at the mu-opioid receptor. *Biochem. Pharmacol.* **2016**, *113*, 70–87. [CrossRef]
32. Kitchen, I.; Slowe, S.J.; Matthes, H.W.; Kieffer, B. Quantitative autoradiographic mapping of mu-, delta- and kappa-opioid receptors in knockout mice lacking the mu-opioid receptor gene. *Brain Res.* **1997**, *778*, 73–88. [CrossRef]
33. Lesscher, H.M.; Bailey, A.; Burbach, J.P.H.; Van Ree, J.M.; Kitchen, I.; Gerrits, M.A. Receptor-selective changes in mu-, delta- and kappa-opioid receptors after chronic naltrexone treatment in mice. *Eur. J. Neurosci.* **2003**, *17*, 1006–1012. [CrossRef]
34. Goody, R.J.; Oakley, S.M.; Filliol, D.; Kieffer, B.L.; Kitchen, I. Quantitative autoradiographic mapping of opioid receptors in the brain of delta-opioid receptor gene knockout mice. *Brain Res.* **2002**, *945*, 9–19. [CrossRef]
35. Chung, P.C.S.; Keyworth, H.L.; Martin-Garcia, E.; Charbogne, P.; Darcq, E.; Bailey, A.; Filliol, D.; Matifas, A.; Scherrer, G.; Ouagazzal, A.M.; et al. A novel anxiogenic role for the delta opioid receptor expressed in GABAergic forebrain neurons. *Biol. Psychiatry* **2015**, *77*, 404–415. [CrossRef] [PubMed]
36. Ceredig, R.A.; Massotte, D. Fluorescent knock-in mice to decipher the physiopathological role of G protein-coupled receptors. *Front. Pharmacol.* **2014**, *5*, 289. [CrossRef]
37. Ceredig, R.A.; Pierre, F.; Doridot, S.; Alduntzin, U.; Salvat, E.; Yalcin, I.; Gaveriaux-Ruff, C.; Barrot, M.; Massotte, D. Peripheral delta opioid receptors mediate duloxetine antiallodynic effect in a mouse model of neuropathic pain. *Eur. J. Neurosci.* **2018**, *48*, 2231–2246. [CrossRef]
38. Bertran-Gonzalez, J.; Laurent, V.; Chieng, B.C.; Christie, M.J.; Balleine, B.W. Learning-related translocation of delta-opioid receptors on ventral striatal cholinergic interneurons mediates choice between goal-directed actions. *J. Neurosci.* **2013**, *33*, 16060–16071. [CrossRef]
39. Bradbury, F.A.; Zelnik, J.C.; Traynor, J.R. G protein independent phosphorylation and internalization of the delta-opioid receptor. *J. Neurochem.* **2009**, *109*, 1526–1535. [CrossRef]
40. Law, P.Y.; Maestri-El Kouhen, O.; Solberg, J.; Wang, W.; Erickson, L.J.; Loh, H.H. Deltorphin II-induced rapid desensitization of delta-opioid receptor requires both phosphorylation and internalization of the receptor. *J. Biol. Chem.* **2000**, *275*, 32057–32065. [CrossRef]
41. Pin, J.P.; Neubig, R.; Bouvier, M.; Devi, L.; Filizola, M.; Javitch, J.A.; Lohse, M.J.; Milligan, G.; Palczewski, K.; Parmentier, M.; et al. International Union of Basic and Clinical Pharmacology. LXVII. Recommendations for the recognition and nomenclature of G protein-coupled receptor heteromultimers. *Pharmacol. Rev.* **2007**, *59*, 5–13. [CrossRef]
42. Salvadori, S.; Guerrini, R.; Balboni, G.; Bianchi, C.; Bryant, S.D.; Cooper, P.S.; Lazarus, L.H. Further studies on the Dmt-Tic pharmacophore: Hydrophobic substituents at the C-terminus endow delta antagonists to manifest mu agonism or mu antagonism. *J. Med. Chem.* **1999**, *42*, 5010–5019. [CrossRef] [PubMed]
43. Olivo-Marin, J.C. Extraction of spots in biological images using multiscale products. *Pattern Recogn.* **2002**, *35*, 1989–1996. [CrossRef]

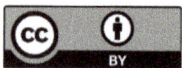

© 2020 by the authors. Licensee MDPI, Basel, Switzerland. This article is an open access article distributed under the terms and conditions of the Creative Commons Attribution (CC BY) license (http://creativecommons.org/licenses/by/4.0/).

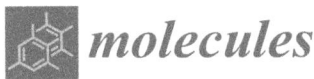

Article

Synthesis and Pharmacological Evaluation of Hybrids Targeting Opioid and Neurokinin Receptors

Karol Wtorek [1], Anna Adamska-Bartłomiejczyk [1], Justyna Piekielna-Ciesielska [1], Federica Ferrari [2], Chiara Ruzza [2], Alicja Kluczyk [3], Joanna Piasecka-Zelga [4], Girolamo Calo' [2] and Anna Janecka [1,*]

[1] Department of Biomolecular Chemistry, Medical University of Lodz, Mazowiecka 6/8, 92-215 Lodz, Poland; karol.wtorek@umed.lodz.pl (K.W.); anna.adamska@umed.lodz.pl (A.A.-B.); justyna.piekielna@umed.lodz.pl (J.P.-C.)
[2] Department of Medical Sciences, Section of Pharmacology, University of Ferrara, 44121 Ferrara, Italy; frrfrc2@unife.it (F.F.); rzzchr@unife.it (C.R.); clg@unife.it (G.C.)
[3] Faculty of Chemistry, University of Wroclaw, 50-383 Wroclaw, Poland; alicja.kluczyk@chem.uni.wroc.pl
[4] Institute of Occupational Medicine, Research Laboratory for Medicine and Veterinary Products in the GMP Head of Research Laboratory for Medicine and Veterinary Products, 91-348 Lodz, Poland; Joanna.Zelga@imp.lodz.pl
* Correspondence: anna.janecka@umed.lodz.pl

Academic Editors: Mariana Spetea and Helmut Schmidhammer
Received: 28 October 2019; Accepted: 2 December 2019; Published: 5 December 2019

Abstract: Morphine, which acts through opioid receptors, is one of the most efficient analgesics for the alleviation of severe pain. However, its usefulness is limited by serious side effects, including analgesic tolerance, constipation, and dependence liability. The growing awareness that multifunctional ligands which simultaneously activate two or more targets may produce a more desirable drug profile than selectively targeted compounds has created an opportunity for a new approach to developing more effective medications. Here, in order to better understand the role of the neurokinin system in opioid-induced antinociception, we report the synthesis, structure–activity relationship, and pharmacological characterization of a series of hybrids combining opioid pharmacophores with either substance P (SP) fragments or neurokinin receptor (NK1) antagonist fragments. On the bases of the in vitro biological activities of the hybrids, two analogs, opioid agonist/NK1 antagonist Tyr-[D-Lys-Phe-Phe-Asp]-Asn-D-Trp-Phe-D-Trp-Leu-Nle-NH$_2$ (**2**) and opioid agonist/NK1 agonist Tyr-[D-Lys-Phe-Phe-Asp]-Gln-Phe-Phe-Gly-Leu-Met-NH$_2$ (**4**), were selected for in vivo tests. In the writhing test, both hybrids showed significant an antinociceptive effect in mice, while neither of them triggered the development of tolerance, nor did they produce constipation. No statistically significant differences in in vivo activity profiles were observed between opioid/NK1 agonist and opioid/NK1 antagonist hybrids.

Keywords: opioid receptors; neurokinin-1 receptor; peptide synthesis; receptor binding studies; functional assay; writhing test; tolerance

1. Introduction

Due to their role in pain perception and modulation, opioid receptors (μ, δ, and κ, or MOR, DOR, and KOR, respectively) are very important targets in medicinal chemistry. The plant alkaloid morphine and its derivatives, which elicit their analgesic effect mostly through the activation of MOR [1], are often the only choice for the management of severe pain [2]. However, the long-term use of these drugs in chronic pain states causes the development of tolerance, which in turn necessitates dose escalation [3]. As a result, the development of side effects, including the inhibition of gastrointestinal transit, respiratory depression, and physical dependence, occurs [4]. Therefore, the dissociation of analgesia from the adverse side effects elicited by MOR agonists is the main goal in the search for better and safer analgesics.

In the past decade the efforts of chemists in synthesizing new opioid analogs have been concentrated on obtaining multifunctional opioid ligands, interacting simultaneously with more than one opioid receptor type [5–7]. For example, compounds with a MOR agonist/DOR antagonist profile showed fewer side effects and enhanced efficacy [8].

Since opioid peptides are not the only modulators of pain signals in the central nervous system (CNS), a new approach in the search for more efficient analgesics with limited side effects is to combine opioids with other neurotransmitters involved in pain perception (e.g., cholecystokinin, neurotensin, substance P, etc.) [9–12]. Such novel chimeras, also known as multitarget ligands, may interact independently with their respective receptors and potentially produce more effective antinociception [13].

The tachykinin undecapeptide substance P (SP: Arg-Pro-Lys-Pro-Gln-Gln-Phe-Phe-Gly-Leu-Met-NH$_2$) is a neurotransmitter/neuromodulator which is known to transmit pain signaling from the periphery to the CNS. SP acts through the activation of neurokinin 1 receptor (NK1), which is found in both the central and peripheral nervous systems and is associated with pain responses related to noxious stimuli [14]. Antagonism at the NK1 blocks the signals induced by SP and can inhibit the enhanced secretion of SP and increased expression of NK1 in prolonged pain states. That makes NK1 antagonists potential therapeutic agents for pain relief [15–17].

The pharmacological blockade of NK1 with an antagonist seems logical in the design of hybrid peptides with improved activity. The rationale for the synthesis of opioid/NK1 antagonist hybrids is also supported by the documented co-localization of opioids and NK1 in nervous structures in the transmission of nociceptive impulses [12].

Several hybrid opioid/NK1 antagonists have been reported so far. As the opioid part, fragments or analogs of [Met]enkephalin [18], biphalin [19], dermorphin [20], or other opioids [21,22] have been used and connected with NK1 antagonists. One example of such a MOR agonist/NK1 antagonist is the compound Dmt-D-Arg-Aba-Gly-*N*-methyl-*N*-3′,5′-di(trifluoromethyl)benzyl, which produced potent analgesic effects upon chronic administration but still manifested a tolerance profile similar to that of morphine [23].

In contrast to the hyperalgesic effects of SP, it was demonstrated that in low doses, SP can intensify opioid-mediated analgesia in a naloxone-reversible manner, probably by triggering endogenous opioid peptide release [24]. Linking the *C*-terminal SP fragments with morphine or opioid peptides gave hybrids which produced a strong analgesic effect, with low or no tendency to develop opioid tolerance following central administration to rats [25–28].

Foran et al. [25] described the endomorphin-2 (EM-2)/SP-7-11 chimera (ESP7) with overlapping Phe-Phe residues, which produced opioid-dependent antinociception without loss of potency over a five-day period, suggesting that co-activation of MOR and NK1 is essential for maintaining opioid responsiveness.

Kream et al. [26] synthesized a hybrid of morphine covalently conjugated through a succinic acid linker to SP$_{3-11}$ (designated MSP9). This analog was shown to activate MOR and KOR, as well as NK1, and its antinociceptive effect most likely depended on the potent functional coupling of NK1 with both opioid receptors.

Small peptides are in general not suitable as drugs, since they are metabolically unstable and often degrade in a few minutes. Among other strategies, cyclization has turned out to be a useful tool for generating analogs with enhanced chemical and enzymatic stability, as well as improved pharmacodynamic properties [29]. In the last several years, we focused our research on the synthesis of cyclic analogs based on the sequence of endomorphin-2 (EM-2; Tyr-Pro-Phe-Phe-NH$_2$), with incorporated bifunctional amino acids that make ring closure possible. The cyclic peptide Tyr-c[D-Lys-Phe-Phe-Asp]NH$_2$ (1) displayed a mixed MOR/KOR affinity profile, enzymatic stability, and strong and long-lasting antinociceptive activity after either intracerebroventricular (icv) or peripheral administration, which indicated its ability to cross the blood–brain barrier (BBB) [30,31].

Here, we report the synthesis and pharmacological evaluation of hybrids combining this cyclopeptide with either the SP pharmacophore or NK1 antagonist (spantide II) fragments in order to compare the antinociceptive potential of these two types of hybrids and to enhance our knowledge on the cross-talk between opioid and neurokinin systems in pain perception and regulation.

The largest obstacle in joining two molecules is possible interference between them, which may lead to partial or even complete loss of affinity at the respective receptors. In this report, the binding and activation profiles of the hybrid analogs at the opioid and NK1 receptors were investigated, followed by in vivo studies of antinociceptive activity and tolerance development in mice.

2. Results

2.1. Chemistry

The structures of the new hybrids are presented in Figure 1. The peptides were synthesized by the solid-phase procedure using Fmoc/tBu chemistry with the hyper-acid labile Mtt/O-2 PhiPr groups for selective protection of amine/carboxyl side-chain groups engaged in the formation of the cyclic fragment. TBTU (2-(1H-benzotriazole-1-yl)-1,1,3,3-tetramethylaminium tetrafluoroborate) was used for coupling reactions. All compounds were purified by semipreparative RP HPLC (reverse phase high-performance liquid chromatography), and their identity was confirmed by high-resolution mass spectrometry (ESI-HRMS). The purity of the compounds characterized by analytical RP HPLC was determined to be ≥95%. The detailed analytical data of the synthesized peptides are provided in the Supplementary Materials (Table S1, Figures S1–S6).

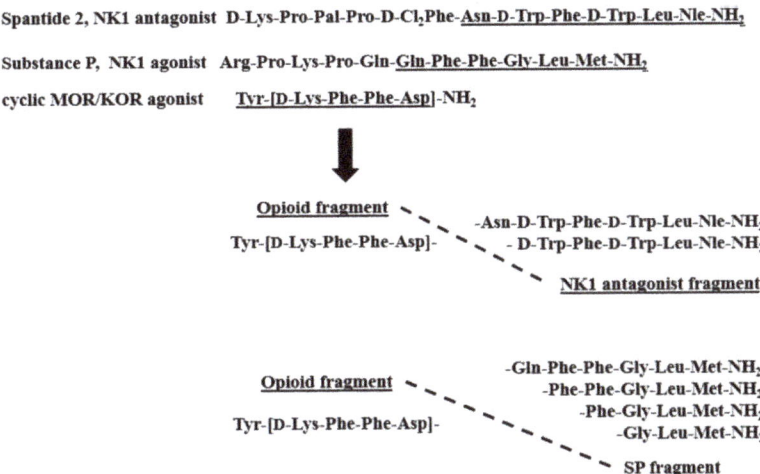

Figure 1. Sequences of hybrid analogs.

2.2. Receptor Binding Affinity

A radioligand binding assay was performed to determine the opioid receptor (OR) binding affinities of the novel analogs using commercially available membranes of Chinese hamster ovary cells (CHO) transfected with human recombinant ORs. [^{3}H]DAMGO, [^{3}H]deltorphin-2, and [^{3}H]U-69593 were used as the radioligands for MOR, DOR, and KOR, respectively. The results are summarized in Table 1. Tyr-[D-Lys-Phe-Phe-Asp]NH$_2$ (**1**) was used as a reference opioid compound. The novel hybrids, with the exception of **3,** showed MOR affinity in the nanomolar range. None of them acquired significant DOR affinity. At the KOR, analog 7, containing the shortest SP fragment, exhibited the strongest binding.

Table 1. Receptor affinities of hybrid opioid/NK1 antagonist/agonist analogs at MOR, DOR, KOR, and NK1.

No.	Sequence	K_i [nM]			
		MOR [a]	DOR [a]	KOR [a]	NK1 [b]
1	Tyr-[D-Lys-Phe-Phe-Asp]-NH$_2$	0.35 ± 0.02	170.8 ± 3.50	1.12 ± 0.20	Inactive
2	Tyr-[D-Lys-Phe-Phe-Asp]-Asn-D-Trp-Phe-D-Trp-Leu-Nle-NH$_2$	5.99 ± 0.70	201.6 ± 2.50	7.46 ± 0.60	10.48 ± 0.60
3	Tyr-[D-Lys-Phe-Phe-Asp]-D-Trp-Phe-D-Trp-Leu-Nle-NH$_2$	28.24 ± 1.45	212.6 ± 6.31	2.85 ± 0.44	12.82 ± 0.92
4	Tyr-[D-Lys-Phe-Phe-Asp]-Gln-Phe-Phe-Gly-Leu-Met-NH$_2$	7.98 ± 0.97	224.8 ± 14.0	10.76 ± 0.85	15.6 ± 1.23
5	Tyr-[D-Lys-Phe-Phe-Asp]-Phe-Phe-Gly-Leu-Met-NH$_2$	4.90 ± 0.34	96.6 ± 3.8	28.34 ± 1.71	51.6 ± 4.2
6	Tyr-[D-Lys-Phe-Phe-Asp]-Phe-Gly-Leu-Met-NH$_2$	2.98 ± 0.14	28.7 ± 1.01	2.7 ± 0.12	2332 ± 189
7	Tyr-[D-Lys-Phe-Phe-Asp]-Gly-Leu-Met-NH$_2$	1.14 ± 0.21	113.2 ± 4.6	0.89 ± 0.04	8128 ± 724
8	SP	ND	ND	ND	3.24 ± 0.43

[a] Displacement of [^{3}H]DAMGO, [^{3}H]deltorphin-2, and [^{3}H]U-69593 from membranes of CHO cells transfected with the human opioid receptors MOR, DOR, and KOR. [b] Displacement of [^{3}H][Sar^9, Met(O$_2$)^{11}]SP from membranes of CHO cells transfected with the human NK1 receptor. All values are expressed as mean ± SEM, $n \geq 3$. ND-not determined.

The binding assay was also used to examine the affinity of the synthesized hybrids for NK1 in commercial membranes of CHO cells stably expressing human NK1. [^{3}H][Sar^9, Met(O$_2$)^{11}]SP was used as a competing radioligand. SP was included as a parent agonist (Table 1).

2.3. Calcium Mobilization Functional Assay

The functional activity of the hybrids was evaluated at all three ORs in calcium mobilization assay in which CHO cells co-expressing human recombinant opioid receptors and chimeric G proteins were used to monitor changes in intracellular calcium levels [32,33]. These changes reflect activation of the G-protein-coupled receptors (GPCR) and can be used for the pharmacological characterization of novel agonist and antagonist ligands [34,35].

The concentration–response curves were obtained for all hybrids (Figure S7, Supplementary Materials). The agonist potencies (pEC$_{50}$) and efficacies (α) of the tested ligands are summarized in Table 2.

Table 2. Agonist potencies (pEC$_{50}$) and efficacies (α) of analogs **1–7** determined on MOR, DOR, and KOR coupled with calcium signaling.

Peptide	MOR		DOR		KOR	
	pEC$_{50}$ (CL$_{95\%}$)	α ± SEM	pEC$_{50}$ (CL$_{95\%}$)	α ± SEM	pEC$_{50}$ (CL$_{95\%}$)	α ± SEM
EM-2	8.22 (7.87–8.56)	1.00	Inactive		Inactive	
DPDPE	Inactive		7.29 (7.16–7.43)	1.00	Inactive	
Dynorphin A	6.67 (6.17–7.17)	0.83 ± 0.10	7.73 (7.46–8.00)	0.99 ± 0.04	8.86 (8.59–9.12)	1.0
1	8.98 (8.50–9.45)	0.98 ± 0.01	Crc incomplete		8.66 (8.56–8.76)	0.96 ± 0.02
2	7.50 (7.28–7.71)	0.66 ± 0.04	Crc incomplete		8.01 (7.56–8.46)	0.99 ± 0.05
3	6.76 (6.46–7.06)	0.72 ± 0.04	Crc incomplete		8.45 (7.56–9.34)	1.05 ± 0.05
4	7.46 (7.26–8.00)	0.90 ± 0.04	Crc incomplete		7.85 (7.60–8.11)	0.92 ± 0.05
5	7.63 (7.12–7.80)	0.86 ± 0.03	6.41 (5.82–7.01)	0.50 ± 0.01	7.17 (7.02–7.31)	0.64 ± 0.04
6	8.04 (7.89–8.20)	0.81 ± 0.05	6.82 (5.97–7.66)	0.65 ± 0.05	8.33 (7.96–8.69)	0.92 ± 0.02
7	8.69 (8.23–9.16)	0.85 ± 0.05	6.44 (5.80–7.08)	0.38 ± 0.04	8.80 (8.46–9.14)	1.06 ± 0.06

"Crc incomplete" means that the maximal effect could not be determined due to the low potency of a compound; endomorphin-2 (EM-2), DPDPE, and dynorphin A were used as reference agonists for calculating intrinsic activity at MOR, DOR, and KOR, respectively. Data are expressed as mean ± SEM, $n = 5$.

At the MOR, the parent analog **1** showed full efficacy and potency (pEC$_{50}$ = 8.98, α = 0.98), even higher than EM-2 (pEC$_{50}$ = 8.22, α = 1.00). Analogs **2** and **3** containing NK1 antagonist fragments showed lower efficacy (α = 0.66 and 0.72, respectively) and much lower potency (30- and 100-fold, respectively) as compared with **1**. For hybrids **4–7**, containing hexa-, penta-, tetra-, and tri-peptide

C-terminal fragments of SP, activation of MOR depended on the length of the SP fragment, with the highest pEC$_{50}$ value observed for analog **7**, containing the shortest SP sequence (Gly-Leu-Met-NH$_2$).

Consistent with the binding results, analogs **1–4** were able to increase intracellular calcium levels at DOR only at the highest concentration tested, and peptides **5–7** showed potency an order of magnitude lower than that of [D-Pen^{2,5}]enkephalin (DPDPE), used as a reference DOR ligand. At the KOR, the cyclic opioid **1**, hybrids **2** and **3** containing NK1 antagonist fragments, and **6** and **7** with SP fragments all stimulated calcium release with high potency and efficacy. Especially, analog **7** mimicked the stimulatory effect of dynorphin A, showing maximal effect and a similar value of potency (pEC$_{50}$ = 8.80).

The calcium mobilization assay results were well correlated with the results of the binding assays.

Calcium mobilization studies were also performed for all new hybrids using CHO cells expressing the human NK1 (CHO$_{NK1}$). In these cells, SP, used as a standard, stimulated intracellular calcium mobilization in a concentration-dependent manner with high maximal effect and potency (pEC$_{50}$ = 9.08). Analog **4** mimicked the stimulatory effects of SP with a fourfold lower potency value (pEC$_{50}$ = 8.45), while all other hybrids were much less active, with potency decreasing in the same order as SP fragment length. These data are summarized in Table 3.

Table 3. Agonist potencies (pEC$_{50}$) and efficacies (α) of SP and analogs **2–7** determined on NK1 coupled with calcium signaling.

No.	NK1	
	pEC$_{50}$ (CL$_{95\%}$)	$\alpha \pm$ SEM
SP	9.08 (8.83–9.34)	1.00
2	Inactive	
3	Inactive	
4	8.45 (8.00–8.91)	0.96 $\pm$ 0.05
5	7.80 (7.45–8.15)	1.11 $\pm$ 0.05
6	6.11 (5.73–6.49)	1.03 $\pm$ 0.05
7	5.68 (5.35–6.01)	0.99 $\pm$ 0.08

SP was used as a reference agonist for calculating intrinsic activity at NK1. $N = 5$.

Compounds 2 and 3, which were inactive as agonists, were then tested as antagonists in inhibition response experiments against SP, and the effects were compared with an NK1 antagonist, aprepitant. Aprepitant tested as an agonist up to 10 µM did not modify per se the intracellular calcium levels in the CHONK1 cells. In inhibition response experiments, increasing concentrations of aprepitant and analogs 2 and 3 (0.01 nM to 10 µM) were tested against 10 nM SP. All three compounds inhibited the effect of SP in a concentration-dependent manner (Figure 2). The pKB values of these compounds are summarized in Table 4.

Table 4. Antagonist potencies (pK$_B$) of aprepitant and analogs **2** and **3**.

No.	pK$_B$ (CL$_{95\%}$)
aprepitant	10.11 (9.48–10.74)
2	7.33 (7.03–7.63)
3	7.63 (7.25–8.00)

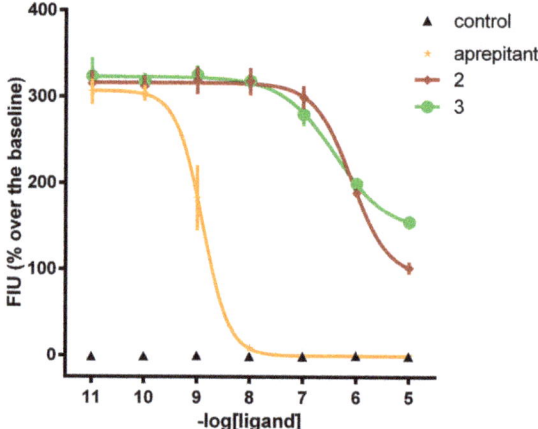

Figure 2. Calcium mobilization assay. Inhibition response curves to aprepitant and analogs **2** and **3** against SP (10 nM). Aprepitant alone was used as a control; $n \geq 3$.

2.4. Antinociceptive Activity

For the assessment of antinociceptive activity, two hybrid analogs were chosen, one with an opioid agonist/NK1 antagonist profile (**2**) and one with an opioid agonist/NK1 agonist domain (**4**). For comparison, cyclic opioid analog **1** was included in the study as a positive control. This analog was shown in our previous paper [30] to exert a very strong antinociceptive effect in the hot-plate test, much stronger than EM-2. The writhing test was used as an acute pain model. This test involves intraperitoneal (i.p.) injection of acetic acid which results in abdominal constriction, causing the mice to writhe. Peptides or saline (control) were administered i.p. over a concentration range of 0.3 to 5 mg/kg at 15 min before the injection of acetic acid (0.5%, 10 mL/kg). The baseline number of writhes in the saline-treated animals was about 35. The i.p. administration of peptides to mice not treated with acetic acid did not evoke any writhes (data not shown). All three tested analogs (**1**, **2**, and **4**) significantly decreased the number of writhes (down to averages of 6.4, 12.4, and 4.5, respectively) at the dose of 5 mg/kg, and the effect was dose-dependent (Figure 3).

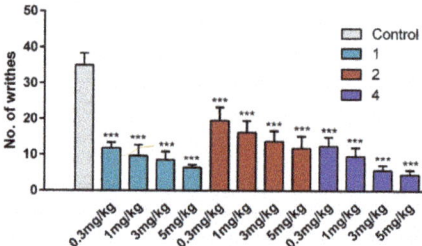

Figure 3. The effect of opioid analog **1** and hybrids **2** and **4** at the doses of 5, 3, 1, and 0.3 mg/kg, administered intraperitoneally (i.p.), on the number of pain-induced behaviors in mice. Peptides or vehicle were administered 15 min before the i.p. injection of acetic acid (0.5%, 10 mL/kg). The number of writhes was determined 5 min after acetic acid injection over a period of 15 min. The data represent mean ± SEM, $n = 10$. Statistical significance was assessed using one-way ANOVA and a post hoc multiple comparison by the Student–Newman–Keuls test. *** $p < 0.001$, as compared to control.

2.5. Tolerance

To examine whether mice developed tolerance to hybrids **2** and **4**, these analogs and analog **1** for comparison were injected once daily (5 mg/kg) for seven consecutive days. After repeated administration, the antinociceptive effect was determined on Day 7, performing the writhing test as above. The analgesic activity of opioid analog **1** was drastically reduced (number of writhes increased from 6 to 17). In contrast, on the seventh day of administration, hybrids **2** and **4** still produced as strong an antinociceptive effect as on Day 1, indicating that they did not cause tolerance development (Figure 4).

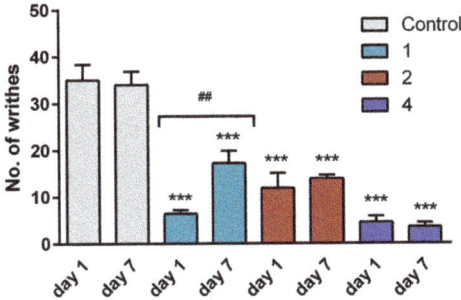

Figure 4. A comparison of the antinociceptive effect of single (Day 1) and repeated (Day 7) i.p. injections of opioid analog **1** and hybrids **2** and **4** at the dose of 5 mg/kg in the writhing test in mice. The data represent mean ± SEM, $n = 10$. Statistical significance was assessed using one-way ANOVA and a post hoc multiple comparison by the Student–Newman–Keuls test. *** $p < 0.001$, as compared to control.

2.6. Stool Mass and Consumption of Food and Water

In order to determine the influence of prolonged administration of the tested compounds on gastrointestinal passage, stool was collected for six days from mice used in the tolerance development test. Opioid analog **1**, used as a positive control, was shown to cause serious constipation in mice compared to the control group. For both hybrids **2** and **4**, no statistically significant differences in stool mass were observed.

Animals injected daily with saline or the tested compounds were also used to determine the influence of analogs on food and water consumption. Stool water content and food and water consumption were unchanged in all tested groups compared with the control (Figure 5).

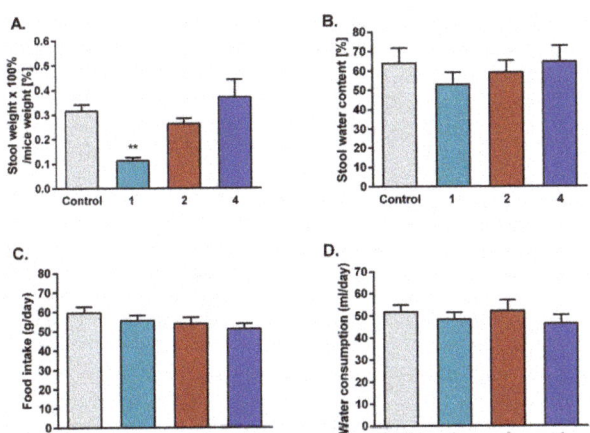

Figure 5. Effect of repeated i.p. injections of saline and the tested peptides on stool mass (**A**), stool water content (**B**), food intake (**C**), and water consumption (**D**). The data represent mean ± SEM, $n = 10$. Statistical significance was assessed using one-way ANOVA and a post hoc multiple comparison by the Student–Newman–Keuls test. *** $p < 0.001$, as compared to control.

3. Discussion

Opioid and NK1 receptors are highly expressed in the CNS [36], and both play important roles in the direct and indirect control of pain signal transmission and modulation [37].

Here, we report on the synthesis and the initial pharmacological testing of several hybrid peptides with opioid agonist/NK1 antagonist and opioid agonist/NK1 agonist profiles. We performed structure affinity/activity relationship studies, seeking hybrids that could simultaneously and potently bind opioid and NK1 receptors. Both types of hybrids were designed with the same opioid fragment to make the comparison of their activity easier. It was already documented in the literature that simultaneous activation of both MOR and KOR intensifies the analgesic effect of pure MOR agonists [38]. Therefore, for the construction of the hybrids, opioid peptide **1**, displaying mixed MOR/KOR affinity, very good enzymatic stability, and antinociceptive activity even stronger than that of MOR-selective EM-2, was chosen [30]. This cyclic opioid was linked with either NK1 antagonist or agonist fragments of various length. As NK1 antagonists, C-terminal hexa- or pentapeptide portions of spantide II were used. NK1 agonists were represented by hexa-, penta-, tetra-, or tripeptide C-terminal fragments of SP. All new hybrids displayed reduced but still high binding affinity and agonist activity at the MOR which could be attributed to the opioid portion and which was crucial in order to achieve in vivo analgesia. The affinity for MOR of the hybrids linking opioid and SP fragments increased inversely to the length of the SP fragment. All new hybrids also retained quite high affinity for KOR, only slightly decreased in comparison to parent peptide **1**. Significant affinity for NK1 was acquired for only hybrids with penta- and hexapeptide fragments of spantide II and a hexapeptide fragment of SP. Spantide-II-containing chimeras **2** and **3** were shown to bind with quite good affinity to NK1 but were inactive in the functional test, suggesting that they could be NK1 antagonists. This assumption was confirmed in the inhibition response experiments against SP. Taken together, the obtained results showed that opioid/NK1 antagonist hybrids stimulated opioid receptors and simultaneously behaved as antagonists at NK1.

On the basis of these data, we can conclude that the attachment of SP or spantide II fragments to the opioid peptide did not prevent binding of the hybrids to MOR and KOR, and the K_i values were, with one exception (hybrid **3**), only 3- to 23-fold higher when compared to the parent opioid. Activation of the NK1 receptor required a hexapeptide fragment of SP.

Hybrids **2** and **4**, which could interact with both opioid and NK1 receptors, were selected for the in vivo assay, which was conducted in an acute pain model (writhing test) in mice. Despite the lower affinity of the hybrids for opioid and NK1 receptors, the analgesic effect they evoked was comparable with that of parent opioid **1**. No statistically significant differences in the in vivo activity profile were observed between opioid/NK1 agonist and opioid/NK1 antagonist hybrids bearing the same opioid fragment. None of the hybrids caused tolerance or constipation development, unlike **1**.

We can assume that hybrid **2** blocked the pronociceptive signals induced by the endogenous SP, which in turn enhanced the effect produced by the opioid part. Hybrid **4** could intensify the antinociception by triggering the release of endogenous opioids, as reported for the co-administration of morphine with small doses of SP [24]. Signaling cross-talk between opioid receptors mediating analgesia [39,40] and the NK1 receptor which is responsible for pain perception is well documented [41,42]. The co-administration of NK1 antagonists together with opioids was considered an option in chronic pain management, since NK1 blockade might be able to reduce the development of opioid tolerance, physical dependence, and withdrawal [43,44]. In preclinical animal studies, NK1 antagonists showed a promising profile, attenuating the nociceptive responses caused by inflammation or nerve damage [15–17,45]. However, they failed to exhibit efficacy in clinical trials [46]. On the other hand, NK1 agonists were reported to counteract the development of opioid tolerance which is linked to desensitization of the opioid receptors. The desensitization is caused by the administration of opioids, especially when it is prolonged, and results in the progressive reduction of signal transduction [47]. Interestingly, in some cases an NK1 agonist, SP, can increase the recycling and enhance the resensitization of MOR [48,49]. Moreover, it was shown that either morphine or DAMGO promoted rapid endocytosis of MOR in striatal neurons, whereas the simultaneous activation of NK1 with SP inhibited this regulatory process. Therefore, bivalent hybrids which bind simultaneously with opioid and NK1 receptors seem to be the reasonable choice for studying complicated interactions between these two systems.

Further experiments including conformational analyses and molecular docking studies will be performed to disclose the structural determinants responsible for the binding of both types of hybrids to opioid receptors.

4. Materials and Methods

4.1. General Methods

Most of the chemicals and solvents were obtained from Sigma Aldrich (Poznan, Poland). Protected amino acids were provided by Trimen Co (Lodz, Poland), and MBHA Rink-Amide peptide resin (100–200 mesh, 0.8 mmol/g) was provided by NovaBiochem. Opioid radioligands, [^{3}H]DAMGO, [^{3}H]deltorphin-2, and [^{3}H]U-69593, and human recombinant ORs and NK1 receptor came from PerkinElmer (Krakow, Poland). GF/B glass fiber strips were purchased from Whatman (Brentford, UK). Analytical and semi-preparative RP HPLC was performed using a Waters Breeze instrument (Milford, MA, USA) with a dual absorbance detector (Waters 2487). The ESI-MS experiments were performed on a Bruker FTICR (Fourier transform ion cyclotron resonance) Apex-Qe Ultra 7 T mass spectrometer equipped with a standard ESI source. The instrument was operated in the positive ion mode and calibrated with the Tunemix™ mixture (Agilent Technologies, CA, USA). The structures of peptides were confirmed using a Shimadzu LCMS-IT-TOF (ion trap–time-of-flight) hybrid mass spectrometer with auto-tuning in the positive ion mode.

4.2. Peptide Synthesis

All peptide hybrids were synthesized by the standard solid-phase procedure on MBHA Rink-Amide peptide resin using the N^α-Fmoc strategy and TBTU as a coupling reagent, according to the method described elsewhere [50]. Final products were purified by RP-HPLC on a Vydac C_{18} column (10 µm, 22 × 250 mm) at a flow rate of 2 mL/min, using as an eluent a linear gradient of 0.1% TFA in water (A) and 80% acetonitrile in water containing 0.1% TFA (B) ranging from 0% to 100% B over 25 min. The purity of the analogs was at least 95%, as determined on the basis of analytical RP HPLC (Vydac C_{18}, 5 µm, 4.6 × 250 mm column, 1 mL/min over 50 min) and ESI-HRMS for exact mass determination (see also Supplementary Materials).

4.3. Radioligand Binding Assays

To determine the affinity of peptide analogs to respective receptors, competition binding experiments were performed, as described in detail elsewhere [51].

Commercial membranes of CHO cells stably expressing either human ORs or NK1 receptor were used. [^{3}H]DAMGO, [^{3}H]deltorphin-2, and [^{3}H]U-69593 were employed as the competing radioligands for MOR, DOR, and KOR, respectively, while [^{3}H][Sar^9, Met(O$_2$)^{11}]SP was utilized for the NK1 receptor. Membranes were incubated in a 0.5 mL volume of 50 mM Tris/HCl (pH = 7.4), 0.5% bovine serum albumin (BSA), with a number of peptidase inhibitors (bacitracin, bestatin, captopril) and various concentrations of radioligands for 2 h at 25 °C. Nonspecific binding was assessed in the presence of 10 mM naloxone for ORs or SP for NK1 receptor.

4.4. Cell Culture

All transfected cell lines (obtained in the Department of Medical Sciences, University of Ferrara) were maintained in culture medium consisting of Dulbecco's MEM/HAM'S F-12 (50/50) supplemented with 10% fetal bovine serum (FBS) and streptomycin (100 µg/mL), penicillin (100 IU/mL), L-glutamine (2 mmol/L), geneticin (G418; 200 µg/mL), fungizone (1 µg/mL), and hygromycin B (100 µg/mL). Cell cultures were kept at 37 °C in 5% CO_2 humidified air. When confluence was reached (3–4 days), cells were subcultured as required using trypsin/EDTA and used for testing.

4.5. Calcium Mobilization Functional Assay

Calcium mobilization assay was performed as reported in detail elsewhere [51]. For the experiments, CHO cells stably co-expressing the human MOR or KOR and the C-terminally modified $G\alpha_{qi5}$, CHO cells co-expressing DOR and the $G\alpha_{qG66Di5}$ protein, and CHO cells expressing NK1 receptor were used. Cells co-expressing ORs and the chimeric G proteins were generated as described [34]. Cells expressing NK_1 receptor were a generous gift from the laboratory of Prof. T. Costa (ISS, Rome, It). Briefly, cells incubated for 24 h in 96-well black, clear-bottom plates were loaded with medium supplemented with probenecid (2.5 mmol/L), calcium-sensitive fluorescent dye Fluo-4 AM (3 μmol/L), and pluronic acid (0.01%) and kept for 30 min at 37 °C. Following aspiration of the loading solution and a washing step, serial dilutions of peptide stock solutions were added. Fluorescence changes were measured using the FlexStation II (Molecular Device, Union City, CA, USA). The maximal change in fluorescence, expressed as the percentage over the baseline fluorescence, was used to determine the agonist response. In antagonism-type experiments, tested hybrids were injected into the wells 24 min before adding an agonist (SP).

4.6. Animals

All animal care and experimental procedures were performed in accordance with the Medical University of Lodz recommendations, described in the Guide for the Care and Use of Laboratory Animals, and complied with the Animal Research: Reporting of In Vivo Experiments (ARRIVE) guidelines [52]. Local Bioethical Committee approval number 61/ŁB708/2017.

Male Balb/c mice (Animal Facility of Nofer Institute of Occupational Medicine, Lodz, Poland) weighing 22–25 g were used in the study. The animals were housed under standard conditions (22 ± 1 °C, 12 h light/dark cycle) with food and water ad libitum for five days before the experiments.

4.7. Assessment of Antinociception by Writhing Test

Antinociceptive activity was assessed by the writhing test. Mice were divided into groups of 10 animals each. A single i.p. injection of saline or a tested compound (at doses 0.3, 1, 3, or 5 mg/kg) was followed (after 15 min) by the i.p. administration of acetic acid (0.65% in 0.9% NaCl, 10 mL/kg) [53]. After 5 min recovery, specific spontaneous behaviors characterized by elongation of the body ("writhes") were counted for 15 min.

4.8. Assessment of Tolerance Development

Peptides were administered at the highest dose (5 mg/kg) used before in the writhing test. In the experiment, four new groups of animals (10 mice per group, housed in one cage) underwent repeated injections (i.p.) of saline or the tested compounds (Days 1–7). On Day 7, following saline or peptide administration, the writhing test was performed, as described above. The antinociceptive activity of a compound was compared to the activity obtained after a single injection of this compound in the corresponding dose (5 mg/kg).

Immediately after the sessions with acetic acid, mice were anesthetized via 3% isoflurane (AErrane) inhalation and euthanized by cervical dislocation.

4.9. Stool Collection

After the i.p. injections of saline or peptides (Days 1–6), mice were placed in a separate clean cages and stool was collected for a period of 90 min. Fecal pellets were collected immediately after expulsion to avoid evaporation and placed in closed 1.5 mL tubes. Tubes were weighed to obtain the wet weight of the stool. Then, the tubes were opened and stool was dried overnight at 65 °C and reweighed to obtain the dry weight. The stool water content was calculated from the difference between the wet and dry stool weights.

4.10. Food and Water Consumption

Every day at the same hour (8:00 a.m.) from Day 1 to 6, the mass of consumed food (g) and water (mL) was calculated from the difference in weights of the food and water supply at the beginning and the end of the 24 h observation period.

4.11. Statistical Analysis and Terminology

The pharmacological terminology adopted in this paper is consistent with International Union of Basic and Clinical Pharmacology (IUPHAR) recommendations [54]. All data are expressed as mean ± SEM from *n*-many experiments, as shown in the table and figure legends. Concentration–response curves were analyzed by nonlinear regression using Graph Pad Prism 6.0 (La Jolla, CA, USA). In displacement binding assays, the values of the inhibitory constants (K_i) were obtained from displacement curves and calculated using the Cheng and Prusoff equation [55] {$\log[EC_{50}/(1 + [L]/K_d)]$} where EC_{50} is the concentration of the ligand that displaces 50% of the radioligand, [L] is the radioligand concentration, and K_d is the dissociation constant of the radioligand. In functional experiments, agonist potency was expressed as pEC_{50}, which is the negative logarithm to base 10 of the agonist molar concentration that produces 50% of the maximal possible effect of that agonist. Concentration–response curves were fitted with the four-parameter logistic nonlinear regression model

$$\text{Effect} = \text{baseline} + \frac{E_{max} - \text{baseline}}{1 + 10^{(\log EC_{50} - X) \cdot n}} \quad (1)$$

where X is the agonist concentration and n is the Hill coefficient. Ligand efficacy was expressed as intrinsic activity (α) calculated as a ratio of the peptide E_{max} to the E_{max} of the standard agonist (Supplementary Materials, Figure S7). The antagonist potency for ligands in inhibition response experiments was expressed as pK_B, which was calculated as the negative logarithm to base 10 of the K_B from the following Equation:

$$K_B = \left[\frac{IC_{50}}{\left(\left[2 + \left(\frac{[A]}{EC_{50}} \right)^n \right]^{1/n} - 1 \right)} \right] \quad (2)$$

where IC_{50} is the concentration of antagonist that produces 50% inhibition of the agonist response, [A] is the concentration of agonist, EC_{50} is the concentration of agonist producing a 50% maximal response, and *n* is the slope coefficient of the concentration–response curve to the agonist [56]. All statistical analyses were performed using Graph Pad Prism 6.0 (La Jolla, CA, USA). Differences between groups were analyzed with one-way ANOVA and a post hoc multiple comparison by the Student–Newman–Keuls test. A probability level of 0.05 or smaller was used to indicate statistical significance.

Supplementary Materials: The following are available online, Table S1: Physicochemical characterization of analogs 2–7, Figure S1–S6: High resolution MS spectra, Figure S7: Concentration-response curves of hybrid analogs 2–7 in the functional assay.

Author Contributions: Conceptualization, K.W., J.P.-C., G.C., and A.J.; Investigation, K.W., A.A.-B., J.P.-C., F.F., C.R., A.K., and J.P.-Z.; Methodology, K.W., A.A.-B. and J.P.-C.; Supervision, G.C. and A.J.; Writing—original draft, A.J., J.P.-C. and K.W.; Writing—review and editing, G.C. and A.J.

Funding: This work was supported by a grant from the National Science Center (No. 2015/17/B/ST5/00153) and a grant from the Medical University of Lodz (No. 503/1-156-02/503-11-002). The authors would like to thank Andrzej Reszka (Shim-Pol, Poland) for providing access to the Shimadzu IT-TOF instrument.

Conflicts of Interest: The authors have no conflict of interest to declare.

References

1. Spetea, M.; Asim, M.F.; Wolber, G.; Schmidhammer, H. The μ opioid receptor and ligands acting at the μ opioid receptor, as therapeutics and potential therapeutics. *Curr. Pharm. Des.* **2013**, *19*, 7415–7434. [CrossRef]
2. Smith, H.S.; Peppin, J.F. Toward a systematic approach to opioid rotation. *J. Pain Res.* **2014**, *7*, 589–608. [PubMed]
3. Ueda, H.; Ueda, M. Mechanisms underlying morphine analgesic tolerance and dependence. *Front. Biosci.* **2009**, *14*, 5260–5272. [CrossRef] [PubMed]
4. Morgan, M.M.; Christie, M.J. Analysis of opioid efficacy, tolerance, addiction and dependence from cell culture to human. *Br. J. Pharmacol.* **2011**, *164*, 1322–1334. [CrossRef] [PubMed]
5. Turnaturi, R.; Aricò, G.; Ronsisvalle, G.; Parenti, C.; Pasquinucci, L. Multitarget opioid ligands in pain relief: New players in an old game. *Eur. J. Med. Chem.* **2016**, *108*, 211–228. [CrossRef]
6. Giri, A.K.; Hruby, V.J. Investigational peptide and peptidomimetic μ and δ opioid receptor agonists in the relief of pain. *Expert Opin. Investig. Drugs* **2014**, *23*, 227–241. [CrossRef]
7. Mollica, A.; Pinnen, F.; Costante, R.; Locatelli, M.; Stefanucci, A.; Pieretti, S.; Davis, P.; Lai, J.; Rankin, D.; Porreca, F.; et al. Biological active analogues of the opioid peptide biphalin: Mixed α/β(3)-peptides. *J. Med. Chem.* **2013**, *56*, 3419–3423. [CrossRef]
8. Morphy, R.; Rankovic, Z. Designing multiple ligands-medicinal chemistry strategies and challenges. *Curr. Pharm. Des.* **2009**, *15*, 587–600. [CrossRef]
9. Ballet, S.; Pietsch, M.; Abell, A.D. Multiple ligands in opioid research. *Protein Pept. Lett.* **2008**, *15*, 668–682. [CrossRef]
10. Fujii, H. Twin and triplet drugs in opioid research. *Top. Curr. Chem.* **2011**, *299*, 239–275.
11. Kleczkowska, P.; Lipkowski, A.W.; Tourwé, D.; Ballet, S. Hybrid opioid/non-opioid ligands in pain research. *Curr. Pharm. Des.* **2013**, *19*, 7435–7450. [CrossRef] [PubMed]
12. Kleczkowska, P.; Nowicka, K.; Bujalska-Zadrozny, M.; Hermans, E. Neurokinin-1 receptor-based bivalent drugs in pain management: The journey to nowhere? *Pharmacol. Ther.* **2019**, *196*, 44–58. [CrossRef] [PubMed]
13. Dvoracsko, S.; Stefanucci, A.; Novellino, E.; Mollica, A. The design of multitarget ligands for chronic and neuropathic pain. *Future Med. Chem.* **2015**, *7*, 2469–2483. [CrossRef] [PubMed]
14. Garcia-Recio, S.; Gascón, P. Biological and pharmacological aspects of the NK1-receptor. *Biomed. Res. Int.* **2015**, *2015*, 495704. [CrossRef]
15. Corrêa, J.M.X.; Soares, P.C.L.R.; Niella, R.V.; Costa, B.A.; Ferreira, M.S.; Junior, A.C.S.; Sena, A.S.; Sampaio, K.M.O.R.; Silva, E.B.; Silva, F.L.; et al. Evaluation of the antinociceptive effect of maropitant, a neurokinin-1 receptor antagonist, in cats undergoing ovariohysterectomy. *Vet. Med. Int.* **2019**, *2019*, 9352528. [CrossRef]
16. Liu, X.; Zhu, Y.; Zheng, W.; Qian, T.; Wang, H.; Hou, X. Antagonism of NK-1R using aprepitant suppresses inflammatory response in rheumatoid arthritis fibroblast-like synoviocytes. *Artif. Cells Nanomed. Biotechnol.* **2019**, *47*, 1628–1634. [CrossRef]
17. Prasoon, P.; Gupta, S.; Kumar, R.; Gautam, M.; Kaler, S.; Ray, S.B. Role of fosaprepitant, a neurokinin Type 1 receptor antagonist, in morphine-induced antinociception in rats. *Indian J. Pharmacol.* **2016**, *48*, 394–398.
18. Yamamoto, T.; Nair, P.; Largent-Milnes, T.M.; Jacobsen, N.E.; Davis, P.; Ma, S.W.; Yamamura, H.I.; Vanderah, T.W.; Porreca, F.; Lai, J.; et al. Discovery of a potent and efficacious peptide derivative for δ/μ opioid agonist/neurokinin 1 antagonist activity with a 2′,6′-dimethyl-L-tyrosine: In vitro, in vivo, and NMR-based structural studies. *J. Med. Chem.* **2011**, *54*, 2029–2038. [CrossRef]
19. Bonney, I.M.; Foran, S.E.; Marchand, J.E.; Lipkowski, A.W.; Carr, D.B. Spinal antinociceptive effects of AA501, a novel chimeric peptide with opioid receptor agonist and tachykinin receptor antagonist moieties. *Eur. J. Pharmacol.* **2004**, *488*, 91–99. [CrossRef]
20. Guillemyn, K.; Kleczkowska, P.; Novoa, A.; Vandormael, B.; Van den Eynde, I.; Kosson, P.; Asim, M.F.; Schiller, P.W.; Spetea, M.; Lipkowski, A.W.; et al. In vivo antinociception of potent mu opioid agonist tetrapeptide analogues and comparison with a compact opioid agonist-neurokinin 1 receptor antagonist chimera. *Mol. Brain* **2012**, *5*, 4. [CrossRef]

21. Giri, A.K.; Apostol, C.R.; Wang, Y.; Forte, B.L.; Largent-Milnes, T.M.; Davis, P.; Rankin, D.; Molnar, G.; Olson, K.M.; Porreca, F.; et al. Discovery of novel multifunctional ligands with μ/δ opioid agonist/neurokinin-1 (NK1) antagonist activities for the treatment of pain. *J. Med. Chem.* **2015**, *58*, 8573–8583. [CrossRef] [PubMed]
22. Nair, P.; Yamamoto, T.; Cowell, S.; Kulkarni, V.; Moye, S.; Navratilova, E.; Davis, P.; Ma, S.W.; Vanderah, T.W.; Lai, J.; et al. Discovery of tripeptide-derived multifunctional ligands possessing delta/mu opioid receptor agonist and neurokinin 1 receptor antagonist activities. *Bioorg. Med. Chem. Lett.* **2015**, *25*, 3716–3720. [CrossRef] [PubMed]
23. Guillemyn, K.; Kleczkowska, P.; Lesniak, A.; Dyniewicz, J.; Van der Poorten, O.; Van den Eynde, I.; Keresztes, A.; Varga, E.; Lai, J.; Porreca, F.; et al. Synthesis and biological evaluation of compact, conformationally constrained bifunctional opioid agonist-neurokinin-1 antagonist peptidomimetics. *Eur. J. Med. Chem.* **2015**, *92*, 64–77. [CrossRef] [PubMed]
24. Kream, R.M.; Kato, T.; Shimonaka, H.; Marchand, J.E.; Wurm, W.H. Substance P markedly potentiates the antinociceptive effects of morphine sulfate administered at the spinal level. *Proc. Natl. Acad. Sci. USA* **1993**, *90*, 3564–3568. [CrossRef] [PubMed]
25. Foran, S.E.; Carr, D.B.; Lipkowski, A.W.; Maszczynska, I.; Marchand, J.E.; Misicka, A.; Beinborn, M.; Kopin, A.S.; Kream, R.M. A substance P-opioid chimeric peptide as a unique nontolerance-forming analgesic. *Proc. Natl. Acad. Sci. USA* **2000**, *97*, 7621–7626. [CrossRef] [PubMed]
26. Kream, R.M.; Liu, N.L.; Zhuang, M.; Esposito, P.L.; Esposito, T.R.; Stefano, G.B.; Witmeyer, J.J., 3rd. Synthesis and pharmacological analysis of a morphine/substance P chimeric molecule with full analgesic potency in morphine-tolerant rats. *Med. Sci. Monit.* **2007**, *13*, 25–31.
27. Varamini, P.; Hussein, W.M.; Mansfeld, F.M.; Toth, I. Synthesis, biological activity and structure-activity relationship of endomorphin-1/substance P derivatives. *Bioorg. Med. Chem.* **2012**, *20*, 6335–6343. [CrossRef]
28. Kowalczyk, A.; Kleczkowska, P.; Rękawek, M.; Kulik, K.; Lesniak, A.; Erdei, A.; Borics, A.; Martin, C.; Pawlik, K.; Lipkowski, A.W.; et al. Biological evaluation and molecular docking studies of AA3052, a compound containing a μ selective opioid peptide agonist DALDA and d-Phe-Phe-d-Phe-Leu-Leu-NH2, a substance P analogue. *Eur. J. Pharm. Sci.* **2016**, *93*, 11–20. [CrossRef]
29. Piekielna, J.; Perlikowska, R.; Gach, K.; Janecka, A. Cyclization in opioid peptides. *Curr. Drug Targets* **2013**, *14*, 798–816. [CrossRef]
30. Perlikowska, R.; do-Rego, J.C.; Cravezic, A.; Fichna, J.; Wyrebska, A.; Toth, G.; Janecka, A. Synthesis and biological evaluation of cyclic endomorphin-2 analogs. *Peptides* **2010**, *31*, 339–345. [CrossRef]
31. Perlikowska, R.; Malfacini, D.; Cerlesi, M.C.; Calo', G.; Piekielna, J.; Floriot, L.; Henry, T.; do-Rego, J.C.; Tömböly, C.; Kluczyk, A. Pharmacological characterization of endomorphin-2-based cyclic pentapeptides with methylated phenylalanine residues. *Peptides* **2014**, *55*, 145–150. [CrossRef] [PubMed]
32. Ma, Q.; Ye, L.; Liu, H.; Shi, Y.; Zhou, N. An overview of Ca2+ mobilization assays in GPCR drug discovery. *Expert Opin. Drug Discov.* **2017**, *12*, 511–523. [CrossRef] [PubMed]
33. Caers, J.; Peymen, K.; Suetens, N.; Temmerman, L.; Janssen, T.; Schoofs, L.; Beets, I. Characterization of G protein-coupled receptors by a fluorescence-based calcium mobilization assay. *J. Vis. Exp.* **2014**, *89*, e51516. [CrossRef] [PubMed]
34. Camarda, V.; Calo', G. Chimeric G proteins in fluorimetric calcium assays: Experience with opioid receptors. *Methods Mol. Biol.* **2013**, *937*, 293–306.
35. Camarda, V.; Fischetti, C.; Anzellotti, N.; Molinari, P.; Ambrosio, C.; Kostenis, E.; Regoli, D.; Trapella, C.; Guerrini, R.; Severo, S.; et al. Pharmacological profile of NOP receptors coupled with calcium signaling via the chimeric protein G alpha qi5. *Naunyn-Schmiedebergs Arch. Pharmacol.* **2009**, *379*, 599–607. [CrossRef]
36. Millan, M.J. Descending control of pain. *Prog. Neurobiol.* **2002**, *66*, 355–474. [CrossRef]
37. Pinto, M.; Sousa, M.; Lima, D.; Tavares, I. Participation of mu-opioid, GABA(B), and NK1 receptors of major pain control medullary areas in pathways targeting the rat spinal cord: Implications for descending modulation of nociceptive transmission. *J. Comp. Neurol.* **2008**, *510*, 175–187. [CrossRef]
38. Greedy, B.M.; Bradbury, F.; Thomas, M.P.; Grivas, K.; Cami-Kobeci, G.; Archambeau, A.; Bosse, K.; Clark, M.J.; Aceto, M.; Lewis, J.W.; et al. Orvinols with mixed kappa/mu opioid receptor agonist activity. *J. Med. Chem.* **2013**, *56*, 3207–3216. [CrossRef]
39. Lao, L.; Song, B.; Chen, W.; Marvizón, J.C. Noxious mechanical stimulation evokes the segmental release of opioid peptides that induce mopioid receptor internalization in the presence of peptidase inhibitors. *Brain Res.* **2008**, *1197*, 85–93. [CrossRef]

40. Chen, W.; Marvizón, J.C.G. Acute inflammation induces segmental, bilateral, supraspinally mediated opioid release in the rat spinal cord, as measured by mu-opioid receptor internalization. *Neuroscience* **2009**, *161*, 157–172. [CrossRef]
41. De Felipe, C.; Herrero, J.F.; O'Brien, J.A.; Palmer, J.A.; Doyle, C.A.; Smith, A.J.; Laird, J.M.; Belmonte, C.; Cervero, F.; Hunt, S.P. Altered nociception, analgesia and aggression in mice lacking the receptor for substance P. *Nature* **1998**, *392*, 394–397. [CrossRef] [PubMed]
42. Perl, E.R. Ideas about pain, a historical view. *Nat. Rev. Neurosci.* **2007**, *8*, 71–80. [CrossRef] [PubMed]
43. George, D.T.; Gilman, J.; Hersh, J.; Thorsell, A.; Herion, D.; Geyer, C.; Peng, X.; Kielbasa, W.; Rawlings, R.; Brandt, J.E.; et al. Neurokinin 1 receptor antagonism as a possible therapy for alcoholism. *Science* **2008**, *319*, 1536–1539. [CrossRef] [PubMed]
44. Huang, S.C.; Korlipara, V.L. Neurokinin-1 receptor antagonists: A comprehensive patent survey. *Expert Opin. Ther. Pat.* **2010**, *20*, 1019–1045. [CrossRef]
45. Gallantine, E.L.; Meert, T.F. Attenuation of the gerbil writhing response by mu-, kappa-and deltaopioids, and NK-1, -2 and -3 receptor antagonists. *Pharmacol. Biochem. Behav.* **2004**, *79*, 125–135. [CrossRef]
46. Hill, R. NK1 (substance P) receptor antagonists—Why are they not analgesic in humans? *Trends Pharmacol. Sci.* **2000**, *21*, 244–246. [CrossRef]
47. Allouche, S.; Noble, F.; Marie, N. Opioid receptor desensitization: Mechanisms and its link to tolerance. *Front. Pharmacol.* **2014**, *5*, 280. [CrossRef]
48. Bowman, S.L.; Soohoo, A.L.; Shiwarski, D.J.; Schulz, S.; Pradhan, A.A.; Puthenveedu, M.A. Cellautonomous regulation of Mu-opioid receptor recycling by substance P. *Cell Rep.* **2015**, *10*, 1925–1936. [CrossRef]
49. Xiao, J.; Zeng, S.; Wang, X.; Babazada, H.; Li, Z.; Liu, R.; Yu, W. Neurokinin 1 and opioid receptors: Relationships and interactions in nervous system. *Transl. Perioper. Pain Med.* **2016**, *1*, 11–21.
50. Perlikowska, R.; Fichna, J.; Wyrebska, A.; Poels, J.; Vanden Broeck, J.; Toth, G.; Storr, M.; do Rego, J.C.; Janecka, A. Design, synthesis and pharmacological characterization of endomorphin analogues with non-cyclic amino acid residues in position 2. *Basic Clin. Pharmacol. Toxicol.* **2010**, *106*, 106–113. [CrossRef]
51. Wtorek, K.; Artali, R.; Piekielna-Ciesielska, J.; Koszuk, J.; Kluczyk, A.; Gentilucci, L.; Janecka, A. Endomorphin-2 analogs containing modified tyrosines: Biological and theoretical investigation of the influence on conformation and pharmacological profile. *Eur. J. Med. Chem.* **2019**, *179*, 527–536. [CrossRef] [PubMed]
52. Kilkenny, C.; Browne, W.; Cuthill, I.C.; Emerson, M.; Altman, D.G. NC3Rs Reporting Guidelines Working Group. Animal research: Reporting in vivo experiments: The ARRIVE guidelines. *Br. J. Pharmacol.* **2010**, *160*, 1577–1579. [CrossRef] [PubMed]
53. Fichna, J.; Sibaev, A.; Sałaga, M.; Sobczak, M.; Storr, M. The cannabinoid-1 receptor inverse agonist taranabant reduces abdominal pain and increases intestinal transit in mice. *Neurogastroenterol. Motil.* **2013**, *25*, e550–e559. [CrossRef] [PubMed]
54. Neubig, R.; Spedding, M.; Kenakin, T.; Christopoulos, A. International Union of Pharmacology Committee on Receptor Nomenclature and Drug Classification. XXXVIII. Update on terms and symbols in quantitative pharmacology. *Pharmacol. Rev.* **2003**, *55*, 597–606. [CrossRef]
55. Cheng, Y.-C.; Prusoff, W.H. Relationship between the inhibition constant (K_I) and the concentration of inhibitor which causes 50% inhibition (IC_{50}) of an enzymatic reaction. *Biochem. Pharmacol.* **1973**, *22*, 3099–3108.
56. Kenakin, T.; Williams, M. Defining and characterizing drug/compound function. *Biochem. Pharmacol.* **2014**, *87*, 40–63. [CrossRef]

Sample Availability: Samples of the compounds 1–7 are available from the authors.

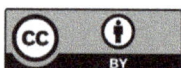

© 2019 by the authors. Licensee MDPI, Basel, Switzerland. This article is an open access article distributed under the terms and conditions of the Creative Commons Attribution (CC BY) license (http://creativecommons.org/licenses/by/4.0/).

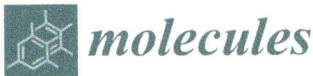

Review
Biased Opioid Ligands

Abdelfattah Faouzi, Balazs R. Varga and Susruta Majumdar *

Center for Clinical Pharmacology, St. Louis College of Pharmacy and Washington University School of Medicine, St. Louis, MO 63131, USA; abdelfattah.faouzi@stlcop.edu (A.F.); balazs.varga@stlcop.edu (B.R.V.)
* Correspondence: susrutam@email.wustl.edu; Tel.: +1-314-446-8162

Academic Editors: Mariana Spetea and Helmut Schmidhammer
Received: 7 August 2020; Accepted: 12 September 2020; Published: 16 September 2020

Abstract: Achieving effective pain management is one of the major challenges associated with modern day medicine. Opioids, such as morphine, have been the reference treatment for moderate to severe acute pain not excluding chronic pain modalities. Opioids act through the opioid receptors, the family of G-protein coupled receptors (GPCRs) that mediate pain relief through both the central and peripheral nervous systems. Four types of opioid receptors have been described, including the µ-opioid receptor (MOR), κ-opioid receptor (KOR), δ-opioid receptor (DOR), and the nociceptin opioid peptide receptor (NOP receptor). Despite the proven success of opioids in treating pain, there are still some inherent limitations. All clinically approved MOR analgesics are associated with adverse effects, which include tolerance, dependence, addiction, constipation, and respiratory depression. On the other hand, KOR selective analgesics have found limited clinical utility because they cause sedation, anxiety, dysphoria, and hallucinations. DOR agonists have also been investigated but they have a tendency to cause convulsions. Ligands targeting NOP receptor have been reported in the preclinical literature to be useful as spinal analgesics and as entities against substance abuse disorders while mixed MOR/NOP receptor agonists are useful as analgesics. Ultimately, the goal of opioid-related drug development has always been to design and synthesize derivatives that are equally or more potent than morphine but most importantly are devoid of the dangerous residual side effects and abuse potential. One proposed strategy is to take advantage of biased agonism, in which distinct downstream pathways can be activated by different molecules working through the exact same receptor. It has been proposed that ligands not recruiting β-arrestin 2 or showing a preference for activating a specific G-protein mediated signal transduction pathway will function as safer analgesic across all opioid subtypes. This review will focus on the design and the pharmacological outcomes of biased ligands at the opioid receptors, aiming at achieving functional selectivity.

Keywords: G-protein bias; arrestin recruitment; opioid receptors; respiration; mitragynine; analgesia

1. Introduction

G-protein coupled receptors (GPCRs) are a 7 transmembrane-spanning evolutionary conserved superfamily that has been well described in the literature and the subject of extensive studies for the last couple of decades [1,2]. They can bind to a very large variety of signaling molecules and consequently play an incredible array of function in the human body [2]. It has been estimated that more than one-third of the drugs currently marketed interact with GPCRs [3].

Among this class of molecules, the opioid receptors represent one of the biggest targets in modern medicine [4]. Indeed, the current "opioid crisis" is one the biggest challenges in therapeutics, especially in the United States [5]. To this day, several questions about these receptors remain unanswered, which is the main reason behind the inability to treat addiction efficiently and/or synthesize pain-relieving agents devoid of side effects. This prompts further research to specifically understand the entire physiology and mechanisms of action linked to the opioid receptors and GPCRs in general. This distinct class of molecules encompasses the MOR (μ-opioid receptor), KOR (κ-opioid receptor), DOR (δ-opioid receptor), the NOP (nociceptin opioid receptor) and can be activated by both endogenous or exogenous opioids ligands, with morphine being the prototypic agent [2,6]. Upon activation, GPCRs are known to experience conformational changes, subsequently leading to different corresponding signaling pathways [2,6]. GPCRs transduction signaling is dependent on the receptor-mediated activation of heterotrimeric G proteins, which are composed of three subunits, Gα, Gβ, and Gγ respectively [1]. When bound to GDP, Gα associates with the Gβγ dimer in order to form the inactive heterotrimer. Receptor activation promotes the engagement of the GDP-bound heterotrimer that accelerates GDP dissociation from Gα. Subsequently, the Gα subunit undergoes conformational changes resulting in the dissociation of the Gα and Gβγ subunits. Both subunits have been shown to modulate the activity of different downstream effector proteins with Gα targeting effectors including adenylyl cyclases or cGMP phosphodiesterase while Gβγ recruits GRKs to the membrane and regulates G-protein-coupled phosphoinosite 3 kinase (PI3K) or mitogen-activated protein kinases (MAPK). The final step of this cycle consists of a GTP to GDP hydrolyzation process promoted by the Gα subunit GTPase intrinsic activity, which then re-associates with Gβγ to complete the G-protein activation circle [1].

The ability to elicit a preferential signaling pathway depending on the spatial molecular rearrangement towards an orthosteric ligand is called "biased agonism" or "functional selectivity" [7–10]. This concept remains unclear and is very disputed within the scientific community in terms of reaching general consensus about its exact definition. Nonetheless, the discovery of such phenomenon has been of tremendous interest in the fields of drug discovery, academia, and the drug industry [11]. Most importantly, it offers a therapeutic alternative to conventional opioid analgesics (in particular to the ones targeting the MOR such as morphine) which are well known for inducing several adverse reactions such as tolerance, dependence, constipation in addition to respiratory depression and addiction.

It is now well established that the activation of opioid receptors triggers two main transducing pathways with more or less preference: the β-arrestin 2 or/and the G-protein pathway [12,13]. The β-arrestin 2 (ubiquitously expressed) regulates opioid receptors signaling through desensitization and internalization, while the G-protein pathway is the "classical" signaling route and will promote different effects depending on the opioid receptor subtype, including analgesia [7,14]. Additionally, it has now been reported that biased opioid receptors ligands induce conformational changes of the receptor, activating a specific signaling pathway. In fact, several structural studies showed that G protein-biased ligands stabilize a certain opioid receptor conformation distinct from the conformation stabilized by β-arrestin biased ligands, which correlates with an equilibrium between the active and inactive states of the receptor and dictates the selective engagement between G-protein and β-arrestin [1,15,16]. These studies provide invaluable insights into the binding mode of these proteins and shed light on which specific residues are involved in these processes. However, further investigations are required in order to truly comprehend this phenomenon which is drawing even more growing interest to this field [17]. The concept of functional selectivity in its simplest form is represented in Figure 1.

The primary aim of this article will be to provide a non-exhaustive list of biased agonists of all the opioid receptors with an understanding of the limitations and advantages both in vitro and in vivo that they can provide. Also, we will focus on the significance and potential future avenues for the development of biased ligands and their analogs targeting the opioid receptors.

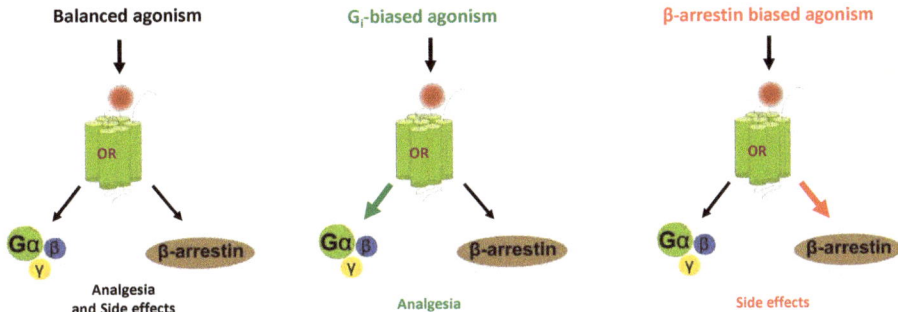

Figure 1. Functional selectivity correlation of opioid agonists. Ligands not recruiting β-arrestin 2 at all opioid subtypes are proposed to dissociate subtype selective adverse effects from its pain-relieving properties. In the case of the μ-opioid receptor (MOR), biased ligands will have less tolerance. For KOR, ligands should have less sedation and anhedonia. Biased DOR agonists should separate convulsions from analgesia while role of biased NOP receptor ligands is less well characterized, although it is possible that memory impairment, sedation, and hypothermia may be dissociated.

2. MOR Biased Agonism

For more than 20 years now, the synthesis of biased agonists targeting the MOR has been considered as a credible strategy in order to mitigate analgesia from the classical opioids side effects. It started in 1999, when Bohn et al. demonstrated an improved antinociceptive effect of morphine in β-arrestin 2 (or arrestin-3) KO mice [18]. Determining the extent of β-arrestin 2 involvement in the development of side effects was the focus of follow-up studies, which demonstrated reduced gastrointestinal, respiratory depressant effects, and tolerance of morphine in β-arrestin 2 KO mice [19,20]. These results were recapitulated in mice by knocking down β-arrestin 2 with antigene RNA and siRNA. While antinociception was found to be prolonged, tolerance was diminished [21,22].

These results were significant in the opioid field and created a whole new approach in the design of G protein-biased agonists, thought to be "better opioids" with an improved safety profile targeting the MOR (Figure 2 shows a list of these ligands targeting MOR). In all cases, DAMGO ((D-Ala(2)-mephe(4)-gly-ol(5))enkephalin) is considered as the standard balanced agonist as the comparator, unless otherwise stated. A non-exhaustive list of MOR biased ligands with potency and efficacy at the G-protein and the β-arrestin2 pathways is shown in Table 1.

Table 1. Ligands targeting the MOR.

Ligand	Functional Selectivity	G-Protein EC_{50} (nM)	E_{max}	β-Arrestin2 EC_{50} (nM)	E_{max}	PubChem ID	Ref
TRV130	G-protein	8.1 (cAMP)	84	7.3 (PathHunter)	15	66553195	[23]
Morphine	Balanced agonist	7.4 (cAMP)	100	6.3 (PathHunter)	100	5288826	[23]
TRV130	G-protein	7.97 (Glosensor)	75	8.02 (BRET)	26	66553195	[24]
DAMGO	Balanced agonist	8.58 (Glosensor)	100	8.3 (BRET)	100	5462471	[24]
TRV130	G-protein	7.9 (cAMP)	86	Inactive (PathHunter)	NQ	66553195	[25]
DAMGO	Balanced	8.4 (cAMP)	100	6.7 (PathHunter)	100	5462471	[25]

Table 1. Cont.

Ligand	Functional	G-Protein	E_{max}	β-Arrestin2	E_{max}	PubChem	Ref
TRV130	agonist G-protein partial agonist	8.66 (cAMP)	86	7.71 (BRET)	58	66553195	[26]
DAMGO	Balanced agonist	8.48 (cAMP)	100	7.55 (BRET)	100	5462471	[26]
PZM21	G-protein	7.73 (Glosensor)	83	7.68 (BRET)	32	121596705	[24]
DAMGO	Balanced agonist	8.58 (Glosensor)	100	8.3 (BRET)	100	5462471	[24]
PZM21	G-protein	110 (BRET)	39	450 (BRET)	18	121596705	[27]
DAMGO	Balanced agonist	390 (BRET)	100	1200 (BRET)	100	5462471	[27]
PZM21	G-protein partial agonist	8.64 (cAMP)	84	7.56 (BRET)	59	121596705	[26]
DAMGO	Balanced agonist	8.48 (cAMP)	100	1200 (BRET)	100	5462471	[26]
7-OH	G-protein	34.5 (BRET)	47	Inactive (BRET)	NQ	44301524	[28]
DAMGO	Balanced agonist	1 (BRET)	100	NA (BRET)	100	5462471	[28]
7-OH	G-protein	53 (GTPγS)	77	Inactive (PathHunter)	NQ	44301524	[29]
DAMGO	Balanced agonist	19 (GTPγS)	100	106 (PathHunter)	100	5462471	[29]
7OH	G-protein	7.8 (cAMP)	84	Inactive (PathHunter)	NQ	44301524	[25]
DAMGO	Balanced agonist	8.4 (cAMP)	100	6.7 (PathHunter)	100	5462471	[25]
	Selectivity	EC_{50} (nM)		EC_{50} (nM)		ID	
Mitragynine pseudoindoxyl	G-protein	1.7 (CHO)	82	Inactive PathHunter	NQ	44301701	[29]
DAMGO	Balanced agonist	19 (GTPγS)	100	106 (PathHunter)	100	5462471	[29]
Herkinorin	G-protein	500 (CHO)	130	No internalization of βarr2-GFP	NQ	11431898	[30]
Herkamide	Balanced agonist	360 (CHO)	134	Internalization of βarr2-GFP seen	NQ	NA	[30]
DAMGO	Balanced agonist	40 (CHO)	100	Internalization of βarr2-GFP seen	NQ	5462471	[30]
Herkinorin	Balanced agonist	7.08 (Glosensor)	104	7.15 (BRET)	104	11431898	[24]
DAMGO	Balanced agonist	8.58 (Glosensor)	100	8.3 (BRET)	100	5462471	[24]
Kurkinorin	G-protein	1.2 (cAMP)	100	140 (PathHunter)	96	132079904	[31]
DAMGO	Balanced agonist	0.6 (cAMP)	100	42 (PathHunter)	100	5462471	[31]
1	G-protein	0.03 (cAMP)	100	14 (PathHunter)	81	NA	[32]
DAMGO	Balanced agonist	0.6 (cAMP)	100	42 (PathHunter)	100	5462471	[32]
SR-11501	β-arrestin2	7.9 (cAMP)	98	374 (PathHunter)	59	146025598	[33]
SR-17018	G-protein	76 (cAMP)	105	>10,000 (PathHunter)	10	130431397	[33]
DAMGO	Balanced agonist	5.2 (cAMP)	100	229 (PathHunter)	100	5462471	[33]
SR-11501	β-arrestin2	133 (GTPγS)	98	374 (PathHunter)	59	146025598	[33]

Table 1. *Cont.*

Ligand	Functional	G-Protein	E_{max}	β-Arrestin2	E_{max}	PubChem	Ref
SR-17018	G-protein	193 (GTPγS)	72	>10,000 (PathHunter)	10	130431397	[33]
DAMGO	Balanced agonist	34 (GTPγS)	100	229 (PathHunter)	100	5462471	[33]
SR-17018	G-protein partial agonist	7.67 (cAMP)	62	6.48 (BRET)	49	130431397	[26]
DAMGO	Balanced agonist	8.48 (cAMP)	100	1200 (BRET)	100	5462471	[26]
2	G-protein	91 (GTPγS)	74	>10,000 (PathHunter)	66	NA	[34]
3	G-protein	153 (GTPγS)	91	>10,000 (PathHunter)	12	NA	[34]
DAMGO	Balanced agonist	34 (GTPγS)	100	229 (PathHunter)	100	5462471	[34]
DAMGO	Balanced agonist	8.4 (cAMP)	100	6.7 (PathHunter)	100	5462471	[25]
MP102	G-protein	5.4 (cAMP)	88	5.2 (PathHunter)	16	NA	[25]
MP103	Balanced agonist	6.5 (cAMP)	90	6.3 (PathHunter)	63	146025824	[25]
MP105	Balanced agonist	6.7 (cAMP)	87	6.6 (PathHunter)	54	146025825	[25]

Assessment of G-protein and βarrestin-2 recruitment of ligands targeting MOR. G-protein biased ligands shown in bold along with control balanced agonist. G-protein biased ligands shown in bold along with control balanced agonist. NQ-not quantified; NA-not available.

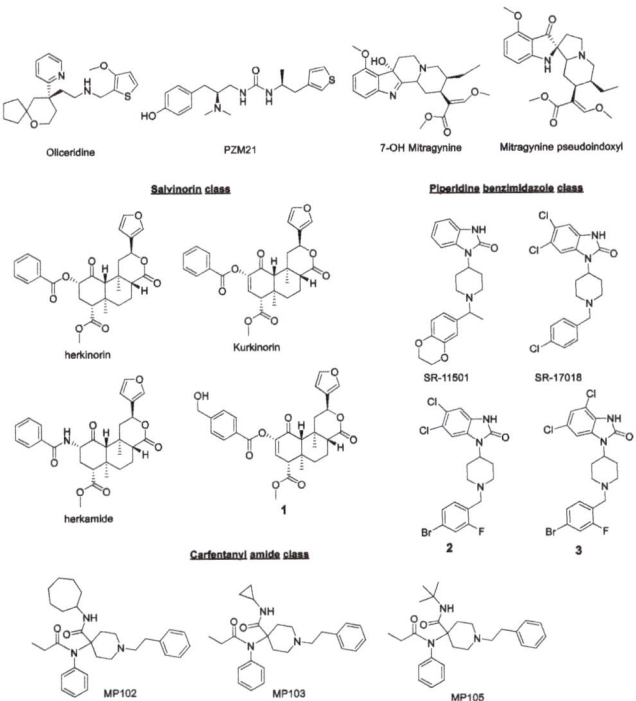

Figure 2. Structures of MOR biased ligands reported having different levels of β-arrestin 2 recruitment.

Oliceridine/TRV130

[(3-methoxythiophen-2-yl)methyl]({2-[(9R)-9-(pyridin-2-yl)-6-oxaspiro[4.5]decan-9-yl]ethyl)amine), also known as TRV130 or Oliceridine was the first G-protein biased ligand developed by the pharmaceutical company Trevena in 2013 [23]. The discovery of this agent was the result of a high-throughput screening (HTS) of their chemical library followed by further optimization for potency, ligand bias, and selectivity toward the MOR. In their initial study, the authors found that TRV130 was a G-protein partial agonist of the MOR which exhibited a 3-fold preference for the G-pathway over the β-arrestin 2, relative to morphine and fentanyl [23]. In HEK cells, Oliceridine was uncovered to be more potent for G-protein stimulation (EC_{50} = 8 nM vs. 50 nM for morphine) but less active on β-arrestin 2 recruitment compared to morphine (14% of morphine efficacy). TRV130 signaling has been studied by other groups too (See Table 1 for details). Perhaps due to its ability to act as a G-protein weak partial agonist, Oliceridine also displayed a very safe side effects profile in vivo with reduced constipation and respiratory depression in these initial findings. Additionally, the measurements of antinociception proved that this agent was a powerful analgesic in rodents in the hot plate assay for mice (ED_{50} = 0.9 mg/kg vs. ED_{50} = 4.9 mg/kg for morphine) and in several assays for rats such as the tail-flick or the rat hindpaw incisional pain model.

Consequently, Oliceridine advanced through several phases of clinical trials, was outvoted in 2018 initially, and was finally approved by the U.S. Food and Drug Administration (FDA) in 2020 [35].

In earlier clinical trials, it produced opioid-like subjective effects in humans, suggesting abuse liability [36] consistent with recent reports in the literature on TRV130 in rodents shows mixed results with the drug showing constipation, addictive properties, and tolerance similar to classical MOR agonists in rodents while also showing less signs of somatic withdrawal, raising doubts about the drug's safety profile [37,38]. However, with the recent FDA approval, the potential of G-biased agonism can now finally be tested in humans and findings may help the field to either call it a day on MOR biased agonsim or push for the development of additional biased agonists.

PZM21

1-[(2S)-2-(dimethylamino)-3-(4-hydroxyphenyl)propyl]-3-[(2S)-1-(thiophen-3-yl)propan-2-yl]urea, also known as PZM21 was the first in class structure-based discovered G-protein biased agonist of the MOR by a group of scientists from the University of Stanford, UCSF, UNC-Chapel Hill and, Friedrich-Alexander-Universität Erlangen-Nürnberg in 2016 [24]. Over 3 million molecules were computationally docked against the inactive structure of MOR which led to the identification of PZM21 as a non-prototypical potent G_i activator at MOR with minimal β-arrestin 2 recruitment (see Table 1 for PZM21 signaling studies by other groups). PZM21 also showed great selectivity for MOR over other 330 other off-targets [24]. The investigations on PZM21 as a potential analgesic also showed long-lasting potent antinociception in the hot plate and formalin injection assays, but, curiously, no effect was detected in the tail-flick assay. It is well-described in the literature that the (mice or rat) tail-flick test is a measure of spinal reflexes response which would mean that PZM21 only triggers a supraspinal effect in vivo [39]. Moreover, PZM21 analgesia was completely abolished in MOR KO mice which proved that the effect was MOR-mediated. Finally, the authors showed that PZM21 did induce constipation but to a lower extent compared to morphine and, impressively, did not cause respiratory depression, conditioned place preference (CPP), nor significantly increased locomotion.

In contrast, a follow-up study from another group in 2018 proved that although PZM21 was indeed a potent analgesic, it caused significant, rapid, and persistent respiratory depression in C57/BL and CD-1 mice when injected intraperitoneally or subcutaneously [27]. This effect was comparable to that of a 10 mg/kg equianalgesic dose of morphine.

Another recent study confirmed that PZM21 caused long-lasting dose-dependent antinociception and did not induce reward- and reinforcement-related behavior [40]. However, the authors showed that PZM21 led to the development of antinociceptive tolerance and naloxone-precipitated withdrawal symptoms after multiple administrations. They also showed that pretreatment with PZM21 could increase morphine-induced antinociception and attenuate the expression of morphine reward. In contrast to the initial investigations of this agent, they expressed concerns about PZM21 clinical applications.

Intrathecal opiate use with drugs like morphine is usually impacted by the risk of producing space-occupying intrathecal masses through Mas-related G-protein coupled receptor (MRGPR) signaling. A recent study by the Yaksh group shows that PZM21 does not produce mast cell degranulation or activation of fibroblasts because it doesn't activate MRGs, unlike morphine, suggesting that MOR biased ligands could be useful for intrathecal therapies [41].

7-OH mitragynine/Mitragynine pseudoindoxyl

The psychoactive plant *Mitragyna speciosa* (also known as "kratom") has been used in Southeast Asian traditional medicine as a tea or directly chewed for centuries in order to treat a large range of pathologies due to its opioid properties and stimulant-like effects [42]. Numerous alkaloids have been isolated from this plant, including the primary constituent indole-scaffold based mitragynine and the oxidized derivative 7-hydroxymitragynine (7-OH). This latter compound has been well documented in the literature and a series of papers from a group of Chiba University researchers reported its activity as a MOR selective agonist which produced a full antinociceptive effect in the mouse-tail flick at a 5 mg/kg or 10 mg/kg concentration when administered subcutaneously or orally, respectively [43]; an effect antagonized by naloxone injection. Classical opioid-like side effects were reported in the same study, such as withdrawal, constipation (albeit less than morphine), and tolerance [44,45]. Another study from 2016 looked more closely at the pharmacology of mitragynine and 7-OH [28]. The authors proved that both agents were G_i-biased partial agonist of the MOR which did not recruit β-arrestin 2. Moreover, the authors claimed that the very weak signal obtained in β-arrestin 2 recruitment assays did not allow for bias quantification. The G-protein bias of 7-OH has been replicated independently by two groups (See Table 1) [25,29]. Another collaborative effort between the Memorial Sloan Kettering Cancer Center and the University of Florida in the same year also proved that 7-OH was 5 times more potent than morphine when administered subcutaneously [29]. Furthermore, this study drew attention to another oxidized derivative from mitragynine, namely mitragynine pseudoindoxyl (MP) [29]. The authors showed that MP is a high affinity agonist at MOR in [^{35}S]GTPγS assays while it shows no β-arrestin 2 recuitment. In vivo in mice, MP was at least 1.5 and 3-5 times more potent than morphine after intracerebroventricular and subcutaneous administration, respectively, in different strains of mice (CD1, C57BL/6, and 129Sv6). Side effect analyses additionally emphasized the development of analgesic tolerance but showed that it was far slower compared to morphine (29 days vs. 5) and the same observation could be made with constipation and dependence. Finally, this agent failed to show either aversive or rewarding effect when tested in the conditioned place preference paradigm. Finally, a follow-up study from 2019 proved that mitragynine is converted to 7-OH by cytochrome P450 through an hepatic metabolism-dependent mechanism and that high concentration of this agent could be retrieved in the plasma/brains of mice, which explains its analgesic properties [46]. The study also conclusively showed 7-OH analgesic actions being MOR-dependent and KOR- and DOR-independent using opioid subtype KO mice. Recent studies showed that 7-OH is self-administered in rats like other MOR modulators suggestive that bias at MOR may not dissociate addiction from analgesia [47].

Herkinorin/Kurkinorin

Methyl(2S,4aR,6aR,7R,9S,10aS,10bR)-9-(benzoyloxy)-2-(furan-3-yl)-6a,10b-dimethyl-4,10-dioxododecahydro-2H-benzo[f]isochromene-7-carboxylate and methyl (2S,4aR,6aR,9S,10aR,10bR)-9-(benzoyloxy)-2-(furan-3-yl)-6a,10b-dimethyl-4,10-dioxo 1,4,4a,5,6,6a,9,10,10a,10b-decahydro-2H-benzo[f]isochromene-7-carboxylate, more commonly known as Herkinorin and Kurkinorin, respectively, are analogs of the natural product Salvinorin A described as an agonist of the KOR [48]. The SAR of Sal A was vastly studied and subsequent chemical modification allowed for the synthesis of other opioid receptors ligands, including herkinorin and kurkinorin [49]. Interestingly, these agents were described as the first non-nitrogenous MOR agonists, and displayed strong affinity toward the MOR (K_i = 1.2 nM and 40 nM for Kurkinorin and

Herkinorin, respectively) [50]; both compounds did not recruit β-arrestin 2 while Herkenorin in addition did not promote receptor internalization [30,48]. The arrestin recruitment of Herkenorin at MOR has been recently been challenged (Table 1) [24]. Follow up studies from the Prisinzano group yielded several analogs on the Sal A template which were then biologically tested in vitro and in vivo [32]. One particular analog of interest was herkamide, where the phenyl ester was replaced by a phenyl amide substituent. Herkamide in contrast to herkenorin robustly recruited β-arrestin 2 and internalized MOR. Similar studies on Kurkinorin proved that it was a G_i-protein biased agonist of the MOR, which demonstrated potent centrally-mediated antinociception in the hot water tail-flick test in male B6-SJL mice equal to morphine while Herkinorin acted as a peripherally restricted analgesic (active in the rodent formalin test but no activity detected in the tail flick-assays) [31]. Pre-treatment with naloxone blocked the antinociceptive effect of Kurkinorin, proving that the effect was indeed MOR specific. Of note, the authors raised questions about the CNS penetrating potential of Kurkinorin compared to Herkinorin given the strong similarities in the chemical scaffolds, cLogP, and PSA of both entities. Side effects profiling showed that Kurkinorin induced tolerance but significantly less compared to morphine. Similarly, using the rotarod behavioral assay, it was shown that Kurkinorin impaired motor coordination but considerably less compared to morphine, while Herkinorin had no effect, which was in accordance with the non-CNS penetrating ability of this agent. Finally, the addition of a lesser rewarding effect of Kurkinorin compared to morphine (assessed through condition place preference paradigm) highlights these agents as very promising alternatives to the classical opioid therapies, but further studies need to be undertaken in order to shed light on the exact mechanism of action and mitigate centrally-induced side effects. A recent report from the same group showed an analog of Kurkinorin with a p-CH_2OH substitutent (Methyl (2S,4aR,6aR,7R,10aR,10bR)-2-(furan-3-yl)-9-((4-(hydroxymethyl)benzoyl)oxy)-6a,10b-dimethyl-4,10-dioxo-1,4,4a,5,6,6a,7,10,10a,10bdecahydro-2H-benzo[f]isochromene-7-carboxylate, **1**, Figure 2 and Table 1) retaining the G-protein bias at MOR and low analgesic tolerance potential of the parent template. This compound was 100-fold more potent over morphine both in vitro and in vivo [32].

Piperidine benzimidazoles

In 2017, a collaboration from two groups of the Scripps Research Institute led to the development of a series of substituted piperidine benzimidazole with high agonistic affinity for the MOR [33]. This very thorough study explored the SARs of these agents which resulted in the identification of several analogs with high G-protein bias and showed that halogen substituents (grafted on different parts of the scaffold) favored MOR conformations that promote robust [^{35}S]GTPγS binding while disfavoring β-arrestin 2 signaling. Most notably, SR-17018, SR-15098, and SR-15099 were completely inactive in the β-arrestin 2 recruitment assay, which was an issue in order to quantify bias factors as fairly stated by the authors. As such, and in order to make sure none of the synthesized analogs were merely potent partial agonist, the quantification model was modified accordingly and the authors looked at the ability of these agents to block a stimulatory 10 µM dose of DAMGO. In addition, G-protein activation was measured through two different assays: forskolin-stimulated cAMP accumulation in CHO-hMOR cells and stimulation of [^{35}S]GTPγS binding in membranes. As a result, G-protein bias was preserved for all these derivatives with the exception of SR-11501 which appeared to be a balanced agonist of the MOR. In vivo studies in mouse brainstem confirmed the activity of the piperidine benzimidazoles as G-protein agonists of the MOR with SR-11501 being the least potent (which was in agreement with previous in vitro assays) while no activity was detected in MOR KO mice, proving the high selectivity of the whole series. Noteworthy, the authors emphasized that bias quantification can differ significantly when the inhibition of cAMP stimulation is used as a measure of G-protein signaling. The SR MOR agonists were also uncovered to be long-lasting, brain penetrant (after intraperitoneal administration), and to promote potent antinociception in both the hot plate and warm water tail withdrawal assays equal to morphine and fentanyl. Interestingly, when these agents were tested for respiratory depression, the derivatives with the highest G-protein bias displayed the lowest respiratory depression, below to that of morphine at a same equi-antinociceptive dose. Finally, this work showed that bias factors can correlate with therapeutic window, and a strong linear correlation was established between these two features. A recent report, however, challenges the bias hypothesis as a mechanism for the lower respiratory depression potential of SR-17018 compared to morphine (also see Table 1). In 2018, a follow-up study from the same groups looked at iteratively optimizing and expanding the SARs of this series (with modification of the substituents and the central ring size) while analyzing bias factors, which the authors referred to as "bias-focused SAR study" [34]. This work also shed light on other DMPK parameters such as cytochrome P450 inhibition, suitable half-life, and even microsomal stability. As a result, they managed to identify structural features such as the presence of halogens and a central piperidine which positively impacts bias and safety profiles. As in the initial Cell paper study, a pair of interesting compounds were identified. Compound **2** with di-Cl groups ortho to each other (5,6-Dichloro-1-(1-(4-bromo-2-fluorobenzyl)piperidin-4-yl)-1*H*-benzo[*d*]imidazol-2(3*H*)-one) showed high G-protein bias (β-arrestin 2 E_{max} = 12%) compared to compound **3** where di-Cl groups (4,6-Dichloro-1-(1-(4-bromo-2-fluorobenzyl)piperidin-4-yl)-1*H*-benzo[*d*]imidazol-2(3*H*)-one) were meta (β-arrestin 2 E_{max} = 66%) to each other (Figure 2, Table 1b). Both compounds had similar G-protein potency and efficacy. Taking together comparative bias studies with biased/balanced agonist pairs, namely SR 17018 and SR11501 [51] and compounds **2** and **3** on this template, shows how small changes of chemical structure can lead to the engagement and disengagement of β-arrestin 2 while retaining G-protein potency. Additional studies are still ongoing, which the authors hope will guide the design of safer analgesics in the near future.

Carfentanyl amides

Compounds in the fentanyl class are believed to recruit β-arrestin 2 and are arrestin biased [33]. The introduction of a cycloheptyl amide substituent (*N*-cycloheptyl-1-phenethyl-4-(*N*-phenylpropionamido) piperidine-4-carboxamide, **MP102**) into the fentanyl moiety leads to MOR agonists which retain G protein signaling but lose arrestin signaling. Interestingly, two analogs in the same series with a t-butyl amide group (*N*-(*tert*-butyl)-1-phenethyl-4-(*N*-phenylpropionamido)piperidine-4-carboxamide, **MP105**) and cyclopropyl amide group (*N*-cyclopropyl-1-phenethyl-4-(*N*-phenylpropionamido)piperidine-4-carboxamide, **MP103**) instead of cycloheptyl amide moiety showed higher efficacy in the β-arrestin 2 assay compared to **MP102**, again suggesting that small changes in structure of the analog lead to differential signaling (Table 1). A lead compound in this series **MP102** [25,52] exhibited moderately potent analgesia with significantly reduced respiratory depression, constipation, and physical dependence while showing analgesic tolerance and reward behavior. The role of DOR agonism in the actions of **MP102** may play a key role in vivo and needs to be investigated with future analog design.

Controversy on biased agonists of the MOR

The whole concept which states that G-protein biased agonists of the MOR that do not recruit β-arrestin could significantly improve the therapeutic window and are less prone to the development of classical opioids side effects still remains under very sensitive scrutiny. Indeed, several recent studies ask for very careful consideration of the in vitro/in vivo data, given that β-arrestin 2 signaling might not be directly or indirectly involved in opioid-induced respiratory depression, constipation, or withdrawal [27,53,54]. Among the most important findings, the respiration of morphine was found to be β-arrestin 2-independent. In addition, mice with mutations in the C-tail with a series of serine- and threonine-to-alanine mutations that is likely to lead to less recruitment of β-arrestin 2 still retained respiratory depression, constipation, and withdrawal of opioids. The results contrast with KO mice data from β-arrestin 2 in the S129/C57BL/6 mixed strain mice. Consistent with past results, tolerance was attenuated, and the analgesic duration of action was prolonged in these mutant mice. These controversial results mainly emphasize the critical need for novel pharmacological tools, which could help in probing the opioid-signaling system.

3. KOR Biased Agonism

The ubiquitous distribution of κ-opioid receptors (KORs) across the peripheral and central nervous system and their involvement in a wide array of functions such as motor control, nociception, and consciousness have made KOR a promising target in the pain management field [55]. Interestingly, KOR agonists do not produce the common side effects associated with classical opioids such as respiratory depression and overdose, and do not activate the reward pathway [55]. However, the therapeutic utility of full KOR agonists is decreased by other effects including dysphoria, sedation, anxiety, and depression which have restricted the clinical development of such drugs. Nevertheless, recent studies proved that β-arrestin 2 recruitment and subsequent p38 phosphorylation is required in order to trigger aversion [56,57], whereas this is not the case for the analgesic effect. In addition, targeting KOR have been associated with reducing itch/pruritis as potential therapeutic action [58]. These findings suggest that functionally selective KOR agonists that are able to selectively activate G-protein signaling without activating p38α MAPK and thus causing side effects may have therapeutic potential as non-dysphoric antipruritic analgesics or could be used as adjuvants to potentiate MOR-targeting analgesics such as morphine. A list of ligands not recruiting β-arrestin 2 at KOR is shown in Figure 3. In this case U50,488H and Sal A are considered balanced agonist comparator drugs. A non-exhaustive list of KOR biased ligands with potency and efficacy at the G-protein and the β-arrestin2 pathways is shown in Table 2.

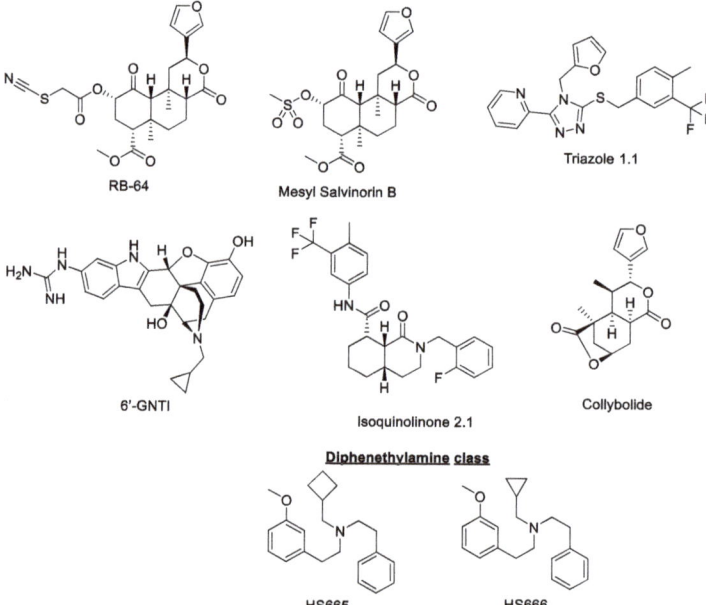

Figure 3. Structures of KOR biased ligands reported having different levels of β-arrestin 2 recruitment.

Table 2. Ligands targeting the KOR.

Ligand	Functional Selectivity	G-Protein EC$_{50}$ (nM)	E$_{max}$	β-Arrestin2 EC$_{50}$ (nM)	E$_{max}$	PubChem ID	Ref
RB64	G-protein	5.2 (cAMP)	99	1130 (Tango)	126	73347341	[59]
Salvinorin A	Balanced agonist	4.73 (cAMP)	100	10.5 (Tango)	100	128563	[59]
Mesyl Salvinorin B	G-protein	0.12 (cAMP)	101	236 (PathHunter)	90	11271318	[60]
U50,488H	Balanced agonist	0.23 (cAMP)	100	162 (PathHunter)	100	3036289	[60]
Triazole 1.1	G-protein	77 (GTPγS)	101	4995 (PathHunter)	98	46245518	[61]
U50,488H	Balanced agonist	24 (GTPγS)	100	52.7 (PathHunter)	100	3036289	[61]
HS665	G-protein	4.98 (GTPγS)	88	463 (PathHunter)	55	71452041	[62]
HS666	G-protein	35.7 (GTPγS)	50	449 (PathHunter)	24	71452040	[62]
U69,693	Balanced agonist	18.2 (GTPγS)	100	67.7 (PathHunter)	100	105104	[62]
6'GNTI	G-protein	1.6 (BRET)	64	Inactive (BRET)	NQ	146673012	[63]
U50,488H	Balanced agonist	43 (BRET)	100	2000 (BRET)	100	3036289	[63]
6'GNTI	G-protein	2.1 (GTPγS)	37	5.9 (PathHunter)	12	146673012	[64]
U50,488H	Balanced agonist	69 (GTPγS)	100	59 (PathHunter)	100	3036289	[64]
Isoquinolinone 2.1	G-protein	84.7 (GTPγS)	89	Inactive (PathHunter)	NQ	121231409	[65]
U69,693	Balanced agonist	51 (GTPγS)	100	131 (PathHunter)	100	105104	[65]
Collybolide	G-protein	2 (GTPγS)	124 *	NA	NA	21669398	[66]
Salvinorin A	Balanced agonist	0.2 (GTPγS)	136 *	NA	NA	128563	[66]

Assesment of G-protein and βarrestin-2 recruitment of ligands targeting KOR. G-protein biased ligands shown in bold along with control balanced agonist. * %Basal, NQ-notquantified, NA-not available.

RB64

22-thiocyanatosalvinorin A, or RB-64, was first synthesized in the laboratory of Dr. Jordan Zjawiony as a semi synthetic structural derivative of the centrally active salvinorin A (extracted from the plant *Salvia divinorum*) compound [59]. This agent was described as a G-protein biased full agonist of the KOR with a bias towards G-protein signaling relative to salvinorin A by the Bryan Roth laboratory. In vitro studies showed indeed that RB-64 recruits β-arrestin 2 but acts primarily as a very potent agonist of the G-protein pathway. In the same study, the antinociceptive effect of RB-64 was tested in the hot plate assay along with U69593 and salvinorin A in wild-type, β-arrestin 2 KO, and KOR KO mice. RB-64 showed a significant and long-lasting analgesic effect in wild-type and β-arrestin 2 KO mice while no antinociception was detected in KOR KO mice, suggesting that this effect was essentially KOR-mediated.

Surprisingly, and in contrast to expectations, this agent (along with salvinorin A and U69593) produced significant aversion when it was tested in the CPP/CPA paradigm in both wild-type and β-arrestin 2 KO mice. Thus, these findings would suggest that G-protein pathway mediates KOR-induced dysphoria. Another feature of this study was that RB-64, even at a very high dose, did not impair motor coordination and the rotarod performances in wild-type and β-arrestin 2 KO mice contrarily to the two other unbiased standards. Given that salvinorin A and U69593 do recruit β-arrestin 2, this would mean an important role for β-arrestin 2 in the locomotor circuitry.

Mesyl salvinorin B

Similar to RB-64, ((2S,4aR,6aR,7R,9S,10aS,10bR)-9-(methanesulfonyloxy)-2-(3- furanyl)dodecahydro-6a-10b-dimethyl-4,10-dioxy-2H-napto-[2,1-c]pyran-7-carboxylic acid methyl ester), or Mesyl salvinorin B, is a semi-synthetic structural derivative of Salvinorin A which was synthesized in the laboratory of Dr. Thomas E. Prinsinzano in order to improve Salvinorin A's poor pharmacological profile [60]. Mesyl salvinorin B has a mesylate substitution at the C-2 position on its scaffold and has similar binding affinity for KOR compared to Salvinorin A (Mesyl Sal B K_i = 2.3 ± 0.1 nM and Sal A K_i = 1.9 ± 0.2 nM in CHO KOR) [60]. It has been shown to act as a G-biased full agonist of the KOR and induce both β-arrestin 2 recruitment and G-protein stimulation in vitro, the latter with a stronger potency. This agent has also been found to display a wide array of therapeutic effects such as the antinociception or attenuation of drug seeking behavior in rodents. Indeed, in the tail-withdrawal assay, Mesyl salvinorin B displayed antinociception but appeared to be a weaker analgesic with reduced potency (EC_{50} = 3.0 mg/kg, Sal A EC_{50} = 2.1 mg/kg) and efficacy (E_{Max} = 38%, Sal A E_{Max} = 87%) compared to its parent derivative Sal A. The same study also revealed a significant effect of this agent on cocaine-induced hyperactivity and seeking behavior. Mesyl salvinorin B did not negatively affect sucrose self-administration, which is a preclinical measure of anhedonia in male Sprague Dawley rats. Interestingly, this agent did also not induce aversion when tested for CPA and did not impair locomotor activity on the rotarod. Additionally, another study showed that Mesyl salvinorin B significantly reduced excessive alcohol drinking [67].

Triazole 1.1

[2-(4-(furan-2-ylmethyl)-5-((4-methyl-3-(trifluoromethyl)benzyl)thio)-4H-1,2,4-triazol-3-yl)pyridine], or triazole 1.1, is a compound that was first discovered in 2013 as the result of a collaboration between 5 different research institutes [65,68]. It was selected after high-throughput screening (HTS) of a huge library of KOR agonists because of its high degree of bias within the collection, its efficacy in the warm water tail immersion assay, and its ability to cross the blood–brain barrier efficiently when administered systemically. Triazole 1.1 is a full agonist of the KOR, which, compared to both U50,488H and U69,593, displayed remarkable G-biased agonism. This agent exhibited a potent antinociceptive effect in the warm water tail withdrawal assay that was comparable to that achieved with U50,488H in mice. In the same study, Norbinaltorphimine (NorBNI) was found to fully reverse the analgesia produced by triazole 1.1 and no effect was observed in KOR KO mice, which demonstrated that this effect was KOR mediated. KOR agonists are known for their potential antipruritic activity, which is why this compound was also tested in the mouse non-histamine pruritis model [58,69]. Triazole 1.1 was uncovered to significantly suppress chloroquine phosphate–induced scratching with an effect comparable to that of U50,488H. The antipruritic effects of triazole 1.1 were also blocked by a 24h pretreatment with NorBNI, which confirmed that the effect was KOR-specific. However, a very recent study on the effects of typical and atypical KOR agonists underlined that triazole 1.1 had no effect on its own, albeit reducing overall levels of scratching during time course determination [70]. In addition, an analysis of the locomotor activity showed that treatment with Triazole 1.1 did not affect locomotion at any of the doses tested, which was in contrast to what was observed with U50,488H. The same study also analyzed dopamine concentrations in the nucleus accumbens ((NAcc) which can be linked to both sedation and dysphoria in animals [61]. Contrary to the balanced agonist U50,488H, triazole 1.1 did not alter dopamine release in the brain nor affected significantly ICCS in rats at doses which induced in vivo analgesia.

Diphenethylamines HS665 and HS666

The first series of diphenethylamine derivatives was reported in 2012 by Drs. Helmut Schmidhammer and Mariana Spetea research groups as novel selective KOR ligands on the basis of previous work on the Dopamine D_2 receptor agonist RU 24213 [71,72]. This agent displayed moderate activity on KOR and acted as an antagonist of the KOR. Further chemical derivatizations led to the identification of two leads, namely HS665 and HS666 (with an N-cyclobutylmethyl (N-CBM) and a N-cyclopropylmethyl (N-CPM) moiety, respectively), which exhibited great affinity and potency toward the KOR. More specifically, HS665 acted as a highly selective and full KOR agonist, while HS666 was a selective KOR partial agonist. Both these agents exhibited very weak partial agonism for β-arrestin 2 recruitment in contrast to U69,593 which robustly recruited β-arrestin 2 (using the DiscoveRx PathHunter β-arrestin 2 assay). In the warm water tail withdrawal assay, both compounds elicited dose-dependent potent analgesic effect characterized by a short onset in wild-type and MOR-KO C57BL/6J mice (WT ED_{50} = 3.74 (2.90–4.78) nmol and 6.02 (4.51–8.08) nmoL for HS665 and HS666, respectively). The same experiments were conducted in KOR-KO mice with no antinociception detected, which proved that the effects was KOR-specific. Noteworthy, these agents and the standard U69,593 were all administered intracerebroventricularly. The same study investigated the behavioral effects of HS665 and HS666 in vivo. Interestingly, neither of these agents significantly impacted motor performance at any time point and HS666 did not induce CPP/CPA (Conditioned Place Preference/Conditioned Place Aversion) while HS665 produced significant place aversion when administered 5 times their analgesic ED_{90} [62]. It is not clear if HS666 did not show CPA because it was a partial agonist or if this was because of its G-protein bias. The pharmacological profile of HS665 matched RB64. Another study from the same group focused on the development of novel derivatives based on the same structural scaffold and expanded the structure-activity relationships (SARs) of the original series [73]. In this study, HS665 and HS666 pharmacology was studied subcutaneously in CD1 mice. Both drugs showed analgesic action in acetic acid writhing assay while demonstrating no sedation or motor impairment. In addition, the introduction of bulkier N-substituents and additional hydroxyl groups resulted in the identification of novel, very potent (picomolar activity), and selective KOR ligands which displayed analgesia with a reduced liability profile, reflected by the lack of sedation and motor impairment. β-Arrestin 2 was not measured with any analogs in this series and CPA with lead compounds was also not evaluated. Similarly, the Kreek group evaluated additional N-substituents (N-cyclopentyl and N-cyclohexyl) and substituted the phenyl ring with a pyridine ring [74]. All analogs still retained the G-biased signaling seen with the parent HS666 on which these analogs were based upon. Detailed evaluations on these compounds are awaited.

6′-GNTI

Originally synthesized by Dr. Philip S. Portoghese and his research group in 2001, 6′-guanidinyl-17-(cyclopropylmethyl)-6,7-dehydro-4,5α-epoxy-3,14-dihydroxy-6,7-2′,3′-indolomorphinan dihydrochloride, more commonly known as 6′GNTI [75], is a derivative of the highly potent DOR-selective antagonist Naltrindole (NTI). It was initially proposed to act as a potent DOR-KOR heteromer selective ligand and was found to interact differently with the KOR and DOR owing to its guanidinium side chain in the 6′ position.

Interestingly, a close derivative known as 5′-GNTI was found to be a selective antagonist of the KOR. Recent studies suggest 6′-GNTI is a KOR biased agonist with preferential activation of the G-protein over the β-arrestin 2 pathway [76]. More specifically, 6′-GNTI acts as a G-protein partial agonist of the KOR at low µM concentrations and does not stimulate β-arrestin 2 recruitment in the sub-mM range, acting as a β-arrestin 2 antagonist. These results were confirmed by another group that looked at drug-induced receptor internalization levels as an indirect measure of β-arrestin 2 recruitment [63]. While U50,488 and EKC led to robust receptor internalization, 6′-GNTI did not have a significant impact and potently inhibited EKC KOR-induced internalization. Additionally, 6′-GNTI was proven to be a potent analgesic in several assays and strains of rodents. It was found to produce potent analgesia in the radiant heat tail-flick assay in 129S6 and CD-1 mice and was also effective in completely blocking PGE_2-induced thermal allodynia when administered to BK-pretreated hind paws in rats. Perhaps due to its lack of selectivity for the KOR, the analgesic effects were completely reversed when prior pretreatments with either NorBNI or Naltrindole (NTI) were administered in vivo.

Additional biological studies on the striatal neurons showed that the stimulation of the KOR by 6′-GNTI triggers the activation of the Akt pathway but not the phosphorylation of the ERK1/2 proteins, which is unusual when compared to a non-biased agonist such as bremacozine or U69,593. The same study also showed that in striatal neurons from β-arrestin 2 knockout mice, there was residual ERK stimulation by 6′-GNTI and that this phenomenon was β-arrestin 2-dependent [64]. In contrast, Akt phosphorylation was symptomatic of the G-protein pathway activation.

At last, a study from 2016 investigated the potential of 6′-GNTI as an anticonvulsant/antiseizure agent, which is another area of interest for the development of KOR agonists. The authors showed that (10–30 nmol) 6′-GNTI significantly reduced paroxysmal activity in the mouse model of intra-hippocampal injection of kainic acid (acute seizures), with an effect almost comparable to that of U50,488H. The effects were also completely reversed after administration of the selective KOR antagonist 5′-GNTI. They finally also confirmed that 6′-GNTI does not induce CPA nor influence motor activity, in contrast to U50,488H which displayed strong place avoidance [77].

Isoquinolinone 2.1

2-(2-Fluorobenzyl)-*N*-(4-methyl-3-(trifluoromethyl)phenyl)-1-oxo-octahydroisoquinoline-8- carboxamide, or Isoquinolinone 2.1, is an agent that was first published in 2013 as the result of a study led by two teams from the Scripps Research Institute and the University of Kansas [65]. Initially, the isoquinolinone scaffold emerged from a 72-member library prepared by a tandem Ugi reaction and Diels–Alder addition reaction and screening for binding at potential GPCR targets by the NIMH Psychoactive Drug Screening Program [78]. Further SARs and chemical optimizations through domino acylation/Diels–Alder addition led to the identification of Isoquinolinone 2.1 as a potential lead [79]. Like Salvinorin A, this agent lacks the basic nitrogen center common in small molecule KOR ligands scaffolds. Isoquinolinone 2.1 was reported to act as a potent and highly selective KOR agonist, biased toward the G-protein signaling pathway with minimal β-arrestin 2 recruitment. In their study, the authors assessed G-protein signaling and β-arrestin 2 recruitment in different cell lines (CHO-hKOR and U2OS-hKOR-β-arrestin 2-EFC or U2OS-hKOR- β-arrestin 2-GFP) and found this agent to be G-protein biased [65]. Downstream ERK1/2 phosphorylation was also investigated as an additional measure of β-arrestin 2 recruitment, with no visible recruitment detected. Of importance, ERK1/2 activation can be misleading in quantifying β-arrestin 2 recruitment given its involvement in various signaling pathways, which was judiciously pointed out by the authors.

Finally, the intraperitoneal administration of 30 mg/kg of this drug produced potent antinociceptive effect in the warm water tail-flick assay similar to that seen with the selective KOR agonist U50,488H, with the effects peaking at 20 min post drug treatment in C57BL/6J mice.

The study, however, did not include any side effects or behavior profiling, thus it is difficult to evaluate the safety profile of this compound compared to other KOR modulators.

Collybolide

Initially extracted from the mushroom *Collybia maculata* (*Basidomycota*) in 1974 by the group of Dr. Pierre Potier, Collybolide (Colly) is a natural product pertaining to the class of sesquiterpenes [80]. It was only later in 2016 that a study demonstrated the potential of Colly and its diastereoisomers (9-epi-Colly) in pain attenuation [66]. Due to its structural similarities with Salvinorin A (a common furyl-δ-lactone motif), this agent was tested on human hMOR, hDOR, and hKOR and was found to be very selective of KOR. When the authors looked at functional selectivity, they showed that Colly was a very potent agonist in [^{35}S]GTPγS assays ($EC_{50} \approx 1$ nM) and dose-dependently inhibited adenylyl cyclase activity, but was also potent for ERK1/2 phosphorylation suggesting that it acts as a biased agonist of the hKOR though β-arrestin 2 recruitment with this natural product remains unknown [66]. The effects were reversed upon treatment with NorBNI showing a KOR-mediated effect. Interestingly, the epimerization of Colly at C9 reduced the agonistic activity and signaling which would indicate that the C9 position is critical to the full binding and signaling of Colly on hKOR. More importantly, Colly was found to exhibit potent antinociceptive effect in the tail-flick assay but was also aversive in mice (when tested in the CPA paradigm), which is similar to what was observed with Salvinorin A. However, at the same doses of both Colly and Salvinorin A (2 mg/kg), only Colly was uncovered to significantly attenuate chloroquine-mediated scratching behavior, with the effects here again reversed upon the administration of NorBNI. Finally, the authors noticed that this agent could exhibit antidepressant and anxiogenic activity in the forced swim test and open field test instead of prodepressant and anxiolytic phenotype expected of classical KOR agonists [66].

4. Biased Agonism on DOR

The first unambiguous evidence for DOR action in antinociception came with the isolation of the classical DOR ligand deltorphin II (Tyr-D-Ala-Phe-Glu-Val-Val-Gly-NH2, naturally occurring and stable DOR peptide) with 0.8 nM potency in mouse vas deferens, first isolated from the skin of a Phyllomedusa species in 1989 by Erspamer and coworkers [81]. It proved to be 13 times more potent than the other selective DOR ligand DPDPE ([D-Pen2, D-Pen5] enkephalin) in a mouse tail-flick test upon intracerebroventricular administration with peak effect close to 10 min and antinociceptive duration of 40 to 60 min. It also displayed 15 times improved selectivity to DOR over MOR [81], making it an extremely useful tool in untangling DOR function.

Later investigations revealed that DOR agonists are poor analgesics in acute pain but they are effective in animal models of chronic inflammatory and neuropathic pain, and specifically alleviate persistent pain [82]. DOR agonists also show anti-allodynic and anti-hyperalgesic properties. There is also an inhibitory DOR tone, which reduces nociceptive responses under the conditions of persistent pain [83]. The lack of DOR receptors results in anxiogenic and depressive-like behavior [84], while DOR opioid receptor agonists produce anxiolytic and anti-depressant effects [85], demonstrating the importance of DOR in regulating emotional responses.

Under basal conditions, DOR is located predominantly intracellularly, but inflammation produces a dramatic change in DOR density leading to up-regulation and membrane targeting of the receptor [86]. Unlike MOR, DOR are predominantly targeted for degradation upon internalization [87].

Agonist activity on DOR does not lead to adverse effects associated with MOR agonists like respiratory depression, addiction, or constipation [88], but agonists were thought to display proconvulsive activity [89]. However, more recent research indicates that this adverse effect is ligand-specific and only SNC80 and AZD2327 evoke convulsions, hyperlocomotion, and receptor sequestration [90,91].

DOR activation reverses the decrease in TrkB protein expression after ischemia and reduces brain ischemic infarction while DOR inhibition aggravates the ischemic damage [92].

Unlike MOR and KOR, which have been heavily investigated for biased signaling, there is a paucity of ligands at DOR which exhibit G-protein bias. Also, in addition to β-arrestin 2, β-arrestin 1 also plays a key role in DOR mediated behaviors. This section will attempt to provide a mechanistic view of bias and evaluate the ligands which are known to display bias in vitro.

DOR and biased signaling: mechanistic overview

The high-resolution (1.8 Å) crystal structure of the human DOR in the inactive state was presented by Fenalti and coworkers in 2014 [93]. Similar to the NOP receptor structure, the ICL3 adopts a closed inactive state conformation stabilized with an H-bond network, unlike in many GPCR structures where the inactive state is stabilized by an "ionic lock". The DOR sodium ion cavity is formed by 16 residues, 15 of which are conserved over class A GPCRs. A polar interaction network in the seven-transmembrane bundle core around the sodium ion stabilizes a reduced agonist affinity state modulating signal transduction. Disrupting this interaction network through mutagenesis transform classical DOR antagonists such as naltrindole into potent β-arrestin2 -biased agonists, possibly opening up new routes towards biased signaling [93]. Active-like state DOR structures in complex with a peptide (2.8 Å resolution) and a small-molecule agonist (3.3 Å resolution) obtained in 2019 revealed polar networks around the conserved $D128^{3.32}$ residue with rearrangements in the agonist-bound binding pocket upon DOR activation [94]. This residue is crucial for receptor activation as opioid agonists that contain a basic nitrogen interacting with $D^{3.32}$ extend deeper into the binding pocket compared to structurally similar antagonists. They also found changes in the nonconserved ECL3 during activation, which makes $R291^{ECL3}$ available for binding pocket interactions, notably upon the binding of endogenous peptides. Unlike peptides, DOP-selective small molecules address the nonconserved extracellular ends of helices VI and VII with their N,N-diethylbenzamide moiety, which leads to their selectivity over MOP and KOP due to steric clashes in the same region of the latter receptors [94].

In the 1990s, there was growing evidence that DOR receptors are differentially desensitized by different agonists. Notably, in 1999, Allouche and co-workers noted that in SK-N-BE cells pre-challenged either with alkaloid or peptide agonist, cross-desensitization occurred that was less marked when cells were pretreated with peptide agonists and then challenged with etorphine than the other way around. Later developments showed that the DOR receptor arrestin-mediated internalization seems to be linked to the development of analgesic tolerance and low-internalizing agonists might have a decreased tendency to induce convulsions [85].

Bradbury and co-workers showed in HEK cells expressing high number of DOR that the degree of DOR Ser^{363} phosphorylation stimulated by different agonists and the ability of the agonist to induce internalization are related, while there was no correlation between G-protein activation and receptor phosphorylation/internalization [95].

Another study revealed that Ser^{363} in the δ-opioid receptor (DOR) determines the different abilities of the DOR agonists DPDPE and TIPP to activate ERK by G-protein- or β-arrestin-dependent pathways [96]. DPDPE employed G protein as the primary mediator to activate the ERK cascade in a Src-dependent manner, whereas TIPP mediated through the β-arrestin 1/2- mediated pathway. When Ser^{363} was mutated, DPDPE gained the ability to utilize β-arrestin 1/2 as scaffolds to assemble a complex with kinases of the ERK cascade accompanied by a decrease in the desensitization of ERK signaling, indicating that β-arrestin-dependent ERK activation might play a role in preventing DOR desensitization [96].

Qiu and co-workers showed on an all Ala mutant of DOR phosphorylation sites that DOR can undergo phosphorylation-independent receptor desensitization and internalization as well. Without phosphorylation, agonist-activated DOR interacted with β-arrestin 1 and β-arrestin 2 similarly, whereas phosphorylation promoted the receptor selectivity for β-arrestin 2 over β-arrestin 1, presumably through the phosphorylated Thr/Ser residues of the carboxyl tail of DOR. The all Ala mutant displayed no interaction between β-arrestins and the carboxyl tail [97].

Aguila demonstrated that the human DOR is differentially regulated via β-arrestin 1-biased mechanisms depending on the ligand [98]. Namely, the reduction of the endogenous level of β-arrestin 1 in SK-N-BE cells only diminished peptide-induced (DPDPE and deltorphin I) hDOR desensitization, while etorphine induced desensitization remained at the same level. However, when examining endocytosis, β-arrestin 1 depletion led exactly to the opposite effect, diminishing only etorphine induced endocytosis. Given that DOR binds β-arrestin via two distinct domains [99], it is possible that the two regions would be differentially unmasked upon binding of peptidic or alkaloid ligands at the receptor, either leading to receptor uncoupling (in case of peptides) or to receptor endocytosis (in case of etorphine) [98].

Pradhan and coworkers showed DOR receptors are in a pre-engaged complex with β-arrestin 2 at the cell membrane [100]. High-internalizing agonists like SNC80 seem to induce receptor phosphorylation, preferentially recruit β-arrestin 1, and result in receptor internalization and degradation. Low-internalizing agonists like ARM390 and JNJ20788560 rather strengthen the engagement between DOR and β-arrestin 2, protecting against acute behavioral tolerance.

They also reported that the anti-allodynic effects of the high-internalizing agonist SNC80 were modulated by β-arrestin 1 and not β-arrestin 2. KO of β-arrestin 1 resulted in increased drug potency, duration of action, and decreased acute tolerance. No change in the antihyperalgesic effect of SNC80 was observed in β-arrestin 2 KOs. In contrast, β-arrestin 2 KO resulted in a gain of acute tolerance to low-internalizing agonists, suggesting that β-arrestin 2 enhances delta opioid receptor resensitization.

In the same study, live-cell imaging revealed that there is a basal engagement between DOR and β-arrestin 2 at the cell membrane, an interaction not observed with β-arrestin 1. The β-arrestin 2 interaction was strengthened with ARM390, while binding of a high-internalizing agonist produces preferential interaction between the receptor and β-arrestin 1 [100].

Similarly, Vicente-Sanchez found that β-arrestin 1 mediates the development of tolerance to the antihyperalgesic and convulsive effects of SNC80, but not tolerance to the antihyperalgesic effects of ARM390 and that DOR remained functionally coupled to G-proteins in β-arrestin 1 KO mice chronically treated with SNC80 [101].

In 2018, Dripps and coworkers showed [102] that DOR-induced convulsions are mediated with different signaling mechanisms than antihyperalgesia and antidepressant-like effects, notably that $G_{\alpha o}$, but not arrestins play a role in regulating the acute antihyperalgesic and antidepressant-like effects while β-arrestin 1 negatively regulates DOR-mediated convulsions, $G_{\alpha o}$ not playing a function in this respect. Similarly, the loss of RGS4 potentiated the antinociceptive, antihyperalgesic, and antidepressant effects of SNC 80 likely due to prolongation of DOR-mediated G protein signaling, while it did not affect convulsions. SNC80-induced convulsions were unaffected in β-arrestin 2 knockout mice but potentiated in β-arrestin 1 knockout mice [102].

Altogether, it seems there are two distinct types of DOR agonists, one, like SNC80 leading to convulsions, hyperlocomotion, and receptor sequestration, ultimately leading to tolerance to the analgesic as well as to locomotor effects. The other type of agonists, which constitute the majority, does not lead to sequestration and only leads to tolerance to the analgesic effects upon chronic treatment [90]. A part of these effects but not all could be linked to variable efficacy for arrestin-receptor interactions [103]. Ultimately, while receptor sequestration shuts down signaling at the plasma membrane, it might open up new therapeutic opportunities. A recent article by Jimenez-Vargas showed that SNC80 and DADLE ([D-Ala^2, D-Leu^5]-Enkephalin), both of which strongly internalize DOR, activate $G_{\alpha i/o}$ in endosomes and recruit β-arrestin 1/2 both to the plasma membrane and endosomes [104]. Furthermore, nanoparticle-encapsulated agonists (DADLE) target endosomal DOR and provide long-lasting antinociception through the long-lasting inhibition of mechanically evoked activation of colonic nociceptors, providing evidence that DOR in endosomes might be a superior therapeutic target for inflammatory pain [104]. The structures of DOR ligands are shown in Figure 4, while data available in the literature is summarized in Table 3.

Table 3. Ligands targeting the DOR.

Ligand	Functional Selectivity	G-Protein EC$_{50}$ (nM)	E$_{max}$	β-Arrestin2 EC$_{50}$ (nM)	E$_{max}$	PubChem ID	Ref
PN6047	G-protein	8.9 (BRET)	128	145 (BRET)	115	121430051	[105]
DADLE	Balanced agonist	2.5 (BRET)	100	69 (BRET)	100	6917707	[105]
2S-LP2	G-protein	32 (BRET)	93	1862 (BRET)	72	146025789	[106]
DADLE	Balanced agonist	59 (BRET)	100	20 (BRET)	100	6917707	[106]
TAN-67	G-protein	2.5 (cAMP)	100	12.6 (PathHunter)	41	9950038	[107]
KNT-127	G-protein	2 (cAMP)	100	3.2 (PathHunter)	71	275705784	[107]
ARM390	G-protein	126 (cAMP)	100	316 (PathHunter)	103	9841259	[107]
DPDPE	Balanced agonist	6.3 (cAMP)	100	25.1 (PathHunter)	100	104787	[107]
ARM390	G-protein	110 (BRET)	120	832 (BRET)	137	9841259	[105]
DADLE	Balanced agonist	2.5 (BRET)	100	69 (BRET)	100	6917707	[105]
JNJ20788560	G-protein	5.6 (GTPγS)	92	NA	NA	46911863	[88]
SNC80	Balanced	5.4 (GTPγS)	100	NA	NA	123924	[88]

Assestment of G-protein and βarrestin-2 recruitment of ligands targeting DOR. G-protein biased ligands shown in bold along with control balanced agonist. NA-not available.

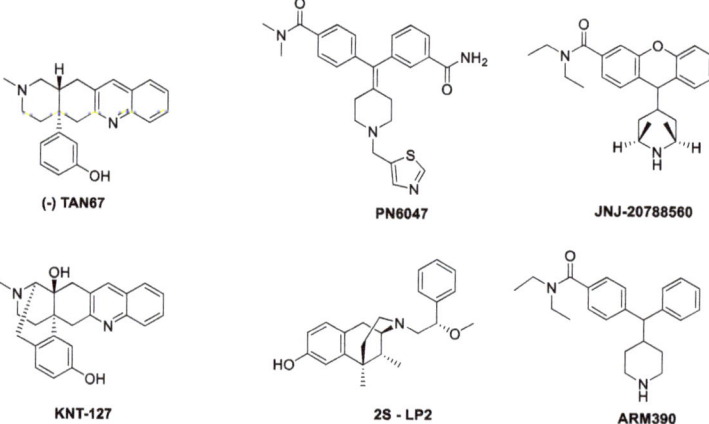

Figure 4. Structures of DOR biased ligands reported having different levels of β-arrestin 2 recruitment.

TAN67

TAN67 was designed in 1998 by Nagase and coworkers as an enantiomeric mixture based on the "message-address" concept. With a high affinity (K$_i$ = 1.12 nM) and potency (IC$_{50}$ = 6.61 nM in mouse vas deferens), it shows 2070-and 1600-fold selectivity on DOR over MOR and KOR, respectively. When administered subcutaneously, it produces an inhibition of the acetic acid induced abdominal constriction response. Later, Nagase and coworkers showed that the antinociceptive effects originate from the (-) isomer [108].

TAN67 seems to have similar potency as Leu-enkephalin both in the cAMP (around 3 nM) and β arrestin-2 recruitment assays (10–30 nM range) but has a significantly lower efficacy (41% compared to Leu-enkephalin) in the β-arrestin 2 recruitment assay [107]. As DOR agonists, both compounds alleviate alcohol withdrawal induced anxiety in mice, but only TAN67 reduced alcohol consumption [109], which might be a consequence of its diminished ability to recruit β-arrestin 2 [107].

PN6047

PN6047 is an orally bioavailable, DOR-selective G-protein biased agonist with potent antihyperalgesic efficacy in preclinical models of chronic pain. PN6047 elicited a maximal response in the BRET G-protein activation assay equivalent to that of SNC80, but with 10-fold greater potency. PN6047 is significantly biased toward G-protein activation over β-arrestin recruitment, being a particularly weak recruiter of β-arrestin 1, relative to SNC80.

In line with its G-protein efficacy, PN6047 elicited ERK1/2 activation equivalent to that of SNC80, but as a result of its limited ability to recruit arrestins, it is a partial agonist with respect to internalization.

PN6047 does not appear to have proconvulsive activity or induce analgesic tolerance. Unlike SNC80, repeated administration of PN6047 does not induce analgesic tolerance over a 16-day dosing regimen, maybe as a consequence of its limited ability to induce internalization. Like other DOR agonists, the action of PN6047 is selective for chronic pain states. In the forced swim test, PN6047 decreased immobility, consistent with the antidepressant-like effects of DOR agonists [105].

KNT127

KNT-127 displays high in vitro affinity for DOR (Ki = 0.16 nM) [110] with a potency of 2.0 nM in the cAMP assay, 3.3 nM in β-arrestin 2 recruitment assay, but with a diminished efficacy when compared to DPDPE (6.3 nM in cAMP, 12.6 nM in β-arrestin 2 recruitment assay)[107], and low affinity for MOR and KOR receptors (Ki = 21.3 and 153 nM) [110]. Its administration leads to a strong analgesia in mouse chemical pain assays [111] and significant antidepressant effects, while not causing convulsion, locomotor activation, amnesia, or coordination deficits [112].

KNT-127 (5 mg/kg) fully reversed both thermal hyperalgesia and mechanical allodynia at first administration, and this effect gradually diminished over 5 days, and tolerance to the analgesic effects of KNT-127 develops independently from pain modality and mouse strain. Chronic KNT-127 induces in vivo tolerance to DOR receptor analgesia. Altogether, the KNT-127 profile is similar to that of other agonists like AR-M1000390, ADL5747, and ADL5857 [90].

JNJ 20788560

JNJ 20788560 has an affinity of 2.0 nM for DOR (rat brain cortex binding assay) and a potency of 7.6 mg/kg p.o. In a rat zymosan radiant heat test and of 13.5 mg/kg p.o. In a rat Complete Freund's adjuvant RH test while being inactive in an uninflamed radiant heat test. Similar to ARM290, it does not recruit β-arrestin 1 but strengthens the receptor β-arrestin 2 interaction [100]. JNJ-20788560 does not produce gastrointestinal (GI) erosion, neither does it lead to the slowing of GI transit. JNJ-20788560 does not exhibit side effects like respiratory depression, withdrawal signs, self-administration behavior, muscular rigidity, or the development of tolerance [88].

2S-LP2

2S-LP2 is a biased agonist at MOR and mainly at DOR, showing a significant improvement over the *R* isomer of this compound.

During BRET studies in SH-SY5Y cell membranes DADLE promoted MOR/G-protein interaction with a potency of 6.89 and maximal effect of 81%. 2S-LP2 mimicked the maximal effect of DADLE (pEC$_{50}$ = 6.89) but was 30 times more potent (pEC$_{50}$ = 8.33, respectively). DADLE stimulated the interaction of the MOR with β-arrestin 2 with pEC$_{50}$ of 5.86 and maximal effect of 57%. 2S-LP2 mimicked the stimulatory response of DADLE with slightly lower efficacy but 9 times higher potency. 2S-LP2 displayed a modest (<10 times) bias toward G-protein.

On DOR, DADLE displayed a pEC$_{50}$ value of 7.23 and maximal effect of 42%. 2S-LP2 behaved similarly to DADLE. DADLE stimulated the interaction of the DOR with β-arrestin 2 with pEC$_{50}$ of 7.69 and maximal effect of 47%. 2S-LP2 mimicked the maximal effects of DADLE, however, being less potent. 2S-LP2 showed a statistically significant and large (200-times) bias toward G-protein.

A robust antinociceptive effect was achieved at very low doses of 2S-LP2, with an ED_{50} of 0.6 mg/kg i.p. that revealed its highest effect already at 30 min post- administration. 2S-LP2 did not significantly affect behavior responses (i.e., locomotor activity and sedation) [106].

ARM390

ARM390 is a close analogue of prototypical DOR agonist SNC80. **ARM390** in the neuroblastoma cell line SK-N-BE expressing only human DOR receptors experiments showed a weak affinity (K_i = 106 ± 34 nM) and potency (EC_{50} = 111 ± 31 nM) in cAMP assay. Like SNC80, ARM390 reduces CFA induced inflammatory pain, but unlike SNC80, it retains analgesic response for subsequent agonist injection [113] and does not cause convulsions or motor coordination deficits [90] Exposure to maximal inhibitory concentration of ARM390 leads to a rapid and strong DOR desensitization caused by uncoupling, as opposed to DPDE, Deltorphin I, and SNC-80 which desensitize through internalization [114].

ARM390 being a low-internalizing DOR opioid agonist has been suggested to be a consequence of its limited β-arrestin recruitment [100]. ARM390, while being a full agonist, exhibits lower potency than the other agonists and is significantly less potent than SNC80 in the β-arrestin recruitment assays.

5. Biased Agonism on NOP Receptor

In 1994, multiples groups reported a fourth member of the opioid receptor family that did not bind any natural or synthetic opioid ligands. Its natural ligand, N/OFQ, was first isolated the following year from hypothalamic tissue using a reverse pharmacology approach by Civelli in the CNS Department of Hoffmann-La Roche in Basel, Switzerland, and by the groups of Jean-Claude Meunier from the University of Toulouse, France, and Gilbert Vassart from the University of Brussels, Belgium.

Unlike the other natural opioid peptides that start with the canonical sequence YGGF (Tyr-Gly-Gly-Phe) at the N terminus (message domain of the peptide), N/OFQ sequence starts with FGGF (Phe-Gly-Gly-Phe).

NOP receptor is a Class A GPCR having similar intracellular coupling mechanisms to opioid receptors. N/OFQ produces anti-opioid hyperalgesic effects in supraspinal pain pathways, but analgesic effects in spinal pain pathways [115].

NOP is coupled to the inhibition of cAMP, activation of MAPK, activation of K^+ conductance, inhibition of Ca^{2+} conductance, and the inhibition of neurotransmitter release like GABA, dopamine, and acetylcholine [115].

Unlike classical opioids, NOP receptor agonists affect nociceptive transmission in a site-specific and agonist-dependent manner, but effects also depend on the species tested, and the pain state of the animal [116].

NOP receptors and N/OFQ play an active role in pain transmission, and a mixed NOP receptor/MOR agonist is now in clinical trials, and selective NOP receptor agonists are examined as possible analgesics, although they are often very sedative [117]. Notable exemptions are cebranopadol and AT-121, perhaps due to ligand bias, although we were unable to locate a bias factor for the latter in the literature [118,119]. NOP receptor agonists are more effective in blocking chronic than acute pain for unknown reasons.

The activation of the N/OFQ-NOP system leads to anxiolysis [115,120] while its blockade produces antidepressant-like effects, and this effect can be reversed by NOP receptor agonists [121]. It has been suggested that antidepressant effects of NOP receptor antagonists are linked to restoring hippocampal neurogenesis by counteracting the inhibitory effects of the endogenous N/OFQ on monoaminergic systems and increasing the expression of neuronal factors such as FGF-2 [122].

Asth and coworkers showed that NOP receptor ligands are able to promote NOP receptor /β-arrestin 2 interaction are also able to induce anxiolytic-like effects in EPM (elevated plus maze), but compounds that inhibited the NOP receptor /β-arrestin 2 interaction produced antidepressant-like effects in the FST (forced swim test) in mice [123]. This implies that the action of NOP receptor ligands on emotional states is better predicted based on their β-arrestin 2 rather than G-protein efficacy. It is possible that NOP receptor antagonists also induce antidepressant effects by blocking the recruitment of β-arrestin 2 [123].

N/OFQ blocks opioid induced supraspinal analgesia and morphine reward in the CPP paradigm [124] and reduces morphine induced Dopamine (DA) release in the nucleus accumbens of conscious rats [125].

Treatment with selective NOP receptor antagonists prevented the development of tolerance following chronic treatment with morphine. Acute treatment with N/OFQ was unable to prevent the intravenous self-infusion rate of heroin ([115] and references therein).

N/OFQ attenuates the reinforcing and motivating effects of ethanol, perhaps due to its ability to alleviate negative affective states. N/OFQ prevents the expression of somatic and affective alcohol withdrawal in ethanol dependent rats. However, 3 weeks post intoxication, N/OFQ gave rise to anxiogenic like actions in ethanol dependent rats, while continuing to exert anxiolytic like effects in non-dependent control ([115] and references therein). It should be noted that similarly to NOP receptor agonism, NOP receptor blockade reduced alcohol drinking and seeking in laboratory animals and in humans. Thus, it has been proposed that the beneficial effect of NOP receptor agonists may depend upon rapid desensitization of the N/OFQ-NOP receptor system following administration [126].

Mechanism of biased signaling on NOP receptor

NOP receptors functionally recruit both β-arrestin 1 and β-arrestin 2, the kinetics of the recruitment being ligand specific [127]. There is evidence that β-arrestin 2 is involved in NOP receptor internalization processes [128]. The endocytotic activity of NOP receptor agonists is associated with their ability to induce receptor phosphorylation at Ser^{346}, Ser^{351}, and Thr^{362}/Ser^{363}; a direct positive linear correlation was observed between the phosphorylation at Thr^{362}/Ser^{363} and receptor internalization as well as between phosphorylation at Thr^{362}/Ser^{363} and GIRK channel activation. This phosphorylation pattern in the C-terminal domain proved to be agonist selective [129].

Besides the agonist and cell type, tissue environment might have a significant impact on NOP receptor internalization and arrestin recruitment properties [130]. In most cases, NOP receptor internalization starts rapidly with robust internalization at 1h post treatment in transfected cells [128]. Following endocytosis, NOP receptor may be targeted to either recycling endosomes for return to the cell surface or lysosomes/proteosomes for proteolytic degradation and downregulation [131].

Chang and coworkers were the first to identify biased signaling at NOP receptor. While they identified G-protein bias for multiple compounds, no arrestin biased compounds could be identified, which might suggest that arrestin recruitment to the receptor is dependent of G-protein activation, and may be consequential and conformationally additive to the activated receptor/G protein complex [127].

A more systematic study on bias of NOP receptor agonists was performed by Malfacini and coworkers in 2015 using bioluminescence resonance energy transfer (BRET) technology to measure the interactions of the NOP receptor with either G-proteins or β-arrestin 2. In contrast to previous studies on the constitutive activity of MOR [132], NOP receptor did not display spontaneous coupling between the NOP receptor and G-proteins. Malfacini and coworkers showed that NOP receptor internalization requires a clathrin-dependent endocytosis mechanism that is mediated by arrestins. Most NOP receptor agonists tested show a bias for the G-protein-mediated signaling interactions, and partial agonists on the G-pathway behaved as pure competitive antagonists of receptor/arrestin interactions [130].

Due to the lack of arrestin biased signaling, the relative role of G-protein and arrestin in mediating different actions is not completely understood. The structures of biased ligands at NOP receptor are shown in Figure 5, while data available in the literature is summarized in Table 4.

Table 4. Ligands targeting the NOP.

Ligand	Functional Selectivity	G-Protein EC$_{50}$ (nM)	E$_{max}$	β-Arrestin2 EC$_{50}$ (nM)	E$_{max}$	PubChem ID	Ref
Ro 65-6570	G-protein	17 (BRET)	96	427 (BRET)	84	15512229	[130]
OFQ/N	Balanced agonist	3.6 (BRET)	100	9.6 (BRET)	100	6324645	[130]
Ro 65-6570	G-protein	6.8 (BRET)	92	102 (BRET)	64	15512229	[133]
Cebranopadol	G-protein	3.2 (BRET)	86	Inactive (BRET)	NQ	11848225	[133]
OFQ/N	Balanced agonist	6.9 (BRET)	100	6.6 (BRET)	100	6324645	[133]
MCOPPB	G-protein	0.025 (cAMP)	105	1585 (BRET)	99	24800108	[127]
SCH221,510	G-protein	4.3 (cAMP)	103	4266 (BRET)	87	9887077	[127]
NNC 63-0532	G-protein	26.3 (cAMP)	74	Inactive (BRET)	NQ	9803475	[127]
RTI-819	G-protein	72.4 (cAMP)	75	Inactive (BRET)	NQ	146034954	[127]
RTI-856	G-protein	7.24 (cAMP)	77	Inactive (BRET)	NQ	146034955	[127]
OFQ/N	Balanced agonist	0.2 (cAMP)	100	204 (BRET)	100	6324645	[127]
BPR1M97	G-protein	1.8 (cAMP)	109	5100 (PathHunter)	14	137541784	[134]
OFQ/N	Balanced agonist	0.4 (cAMP)	100	3 (PathHunter)	100	6324645	[134]

Assesment of G-protein and βarrestin-2 recruitment of ligands targeting NOP. G-protein biased ligands shown in bold along with control balanced agonist. NQ- not quantified.

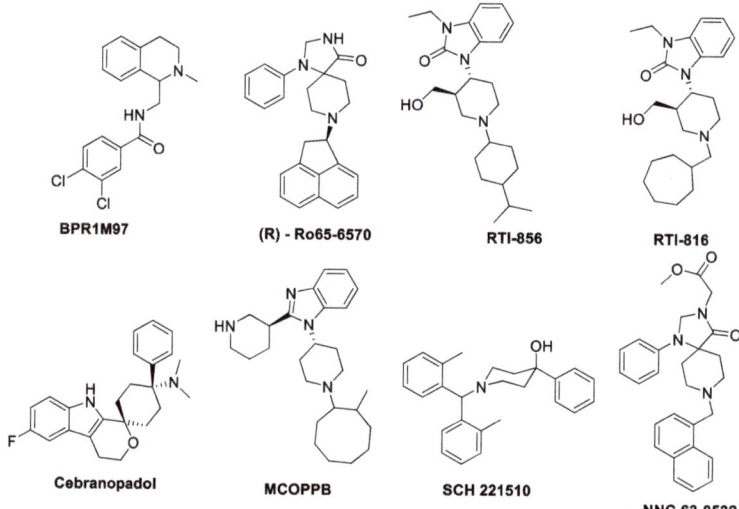

Figure 5. Structures of NOP receptor biased ligands reported having different levels of β-arrestin 2 recruitment.

BPR1M97

BPR1M97 was first identified at the National Health Research Institutes of Taiwan and proved to be a potent MOR agonist and KOR agonist with moderate activity [135]. Later, the same group showed that it behaves as a balanced full agonist in cell-based MOR assays, similar in potency and maximal efficacy to dermorphine, but as a G-protein-biased full agonist of NOP receptor having slightly lower potency at decreasing the cAMP level than that of N/OFQ, while having a similar E$_{Max}$ in HEK cells. Thus, it behaves as a dual NOP receptor/MOR agonist with 3-fold higher potency on the MOR system. BPR1M97 failed to trigger β-arrestin 2 recruitment altogether in CHO–NOP receptor.

BPR1M97 exerts faster thermal antinociceptive effects at 10 min after subcutaneous injection and shows superior antinociceptive effect of mechanical and cold allodynia (acute pain) in cancer-induced pain than morphine, while causing less respiratory, cardiovascular, and gastrointestinal dysfunction at equi-antinociceptive doses. Notably, BPR1M97-treated mice recovered respiratory frequency at 30 min post-injection as opposed to morphine, where decreasing respiratory frequency could be observed until 60 min. In addition, BPR1M97 decreased global locomotor activity as compared with morphine, and induced less withdrawal jumping precipitated by naloxone, and showed lower cross tolerance in morphine-tolerant mice than morphine in BPR1M97-tolerant mice [134]. It is difficult to assess if NOP receptor bias plays a role in the in vivo actions of this drug, but most likely the polypharmacology with actions at NOP receptor and opioid receptors mediate these effects.

Ro 65-6570

Ro 65-6570 was reported by Wichmann in 1999, and proved to have a 10- to100-fold increased affinity towards NOP receptor as opposed to the opioid receptors as expressed by the pKi values (9.6 for NOP receptor and 8.4, 7.7, and 7.0 for MOR, KOR, and DOR receptors, respectively) from competitive binding experiments with [^{3}H]-orphanin for N/OFQ in HEK293 cells, [^{3}H]-naloxone (MOR, KOR), and [^{3}H]-deltorphin (DOR) in BHK cell membranes [136]. In a BRET assay on HEK293 cell membranes, Ro 65-6570 exhibited a maximal effect not significantly different from that of N/OFQ, but was 5 fold less potent in the G-protein pathway [130]. In the NOP receptor /β-arrestin 2 assay, Ro 65-6570 showed a 50-fold loss of potency compared to N/OFQ. Comparing the ligand efficacy at G protein and β-arrestin 2 suggested that Ro 65-6570 behaves as a G-protein biased agonist.

Spontaneous locomotion in the elevation maze plus test and force motor performance were not significantly affected by Ro 65-6570 treatment [137,138]. Ro 65-6570 does not induce place preference, but co-administration (i.e., both compounds administered directly before the conditioning trial) reduced acquisition of condition place preference induced by opioids, but not by psychostimulants. Reduction of the rewarding effect of tilidine and oxycodone by Ro 65-6570 was reversed by the NOP receptor antagonist J-113397 [139].

SCH221510

SCH221510 displays at least 217-fold binding selectivity and 57-fold functional selectivity for the NOP receptor site, compared with the other opioid receptors, having a binding affinity of 0.3 nM in CHO cells which is 15-fold lower than the affinity of N/OFQ (0.02 nM), and has a functional in vitro potency (EC_{50}) of 12 nM as measured by [^{35}S] GTPγS binding to CHO cell membranes expressing NOP receptor. In the BRET assays in HEK293 cells, on the other hand, SCH-221510 displayed similar maximal effects but a 2-fold lower potency compared to N/OFQ in the G-protein assay, while it was able to promote NOP receptor/ β-arrestin 2 interactions with 10-fold less potency than N/OFQ. It displayed an almost 6-fold bias for the G-protein activation [130]. In preclinical animal models, SCH221510 produces robust and broad ranging anxiolytic-like effects in rat, gerbil, and guinea pig, that are similar to the effects produced by the benzodiazepine CDP, and do not decrease after a chronic dosing regimen. It produces anxiolytic-like activity at doses that do not produce nonspecific disruption of locomotor activity [140].

Cebranopadol

Cebranopadol behaves as a G-protein biased agonist at MOR where it recruits β-arrestin 2 with a 20-fold lower potency than for the activation of the G-protein pathway and particularly at NOP receptor, where it does not recruit β-arrestin 2. Meanwhile, its potency at MOR is 15-fold greater than at NOP receptors (0.18 nM and 3.24 nM, respectively, as compared to 6.92 nM for OFQ/N and 3.02 nM for dermorphin in the same BRET assay in HEK 293 cells). In vivo, cebranopadol exhibits highly potent and extremely long-lasting antinociceptive effects originating from both MOR and NOP receptors displaying higher analgesic potency against inflammatory than nociceptive pain, without eliciting sedation. The effects of cebranopadol in the tail withdrawal assay were sensitive to both SB-612111 and naloxone [133].

Cebranopadol, despite being a potent MOR agonist, produces only little opioid-type physical dependence in mice and rats, potentially due to its NOP receptor agonistic effects [141]. Linz and coworkers proved in 2017 that cebranopadol limits the respiratory depressant effect of its μ-opioid receptor agonist activity in rats is due to its NOP receptor agonist activity [118]. In some ways, the effects are similar to buprenorphine which shows a ceiling effect in respiratory depression with its NOP receptor actions being responsible for its particular pharmacological profile. Cebranopadol exerts potent antihyperalgesic, antiallodynic, and antinociceptive effects after local/peripheral, spinal, and supraspinal administration. After central administration of cebranopadol, antihyperalgesic efficacy is reached at doses that are not yet antinociceptive [142]. Cebranopadol was also shown to not induce either phosphorylation, or NOP receptor internalization [129].

MCOPPB

NOP receptor selective ligand MCOPPB is a G-protein biased full agonist, approximately 10-fold more potent than nociceptin and markedly less potent in arrestin recruitment displaying ~ 10^5-fold decrease in potency for arrestin coupling compared with G protein activation. MCOPPB shows a concentration-dependent or potency bias, as the ligand is a full agonist in both signaling pathways but distinguishes itself in its potency at G-protein versus arrestin signaling [127]. MCOPPB is a very potent agonist to activate the NOP receptor GIRK channels with an EC_{50} of 0.06 nM compared to N/OFQ (EC_{50} of 1.5 nM) for GIRK activation [129]. MCOPPB has an anxiolytic activity comparable to that of the benzodiazepine diazepam, but did not affect motor activity or memory function nor did it interact with alcohol at an anxiolytic dose in mice [143].

NNC 63-0532

NNC 63-0532 was reported by Thomsen in 2000 [144], and it shows moderate to high activity (70% inhibition in the cAMP assay) for MOR and KOR and for DOR and D_2, D_3 and D_4 receptors. NNC 63-0532 showed about 20-fold selectivity for NOP receptor in radioligand binding assays over MOR and KOR (respective Ki values were 7.3 nM, 140 nM and 405 nM) and 14-fold when measuring displacement of radioligand binding to D_2, D_3 and D_4 receptors (respective Ki values were 209 nM, 133 nM and 107 nM).

Besides its a NOP receptor selectivity, its arrestin recruitment could not be measured in HEK cells using BRET, which makes it a G protein-biased agonist exhibiting partial agonist activity with an efficacy of 71% and relatively low potency as indicated by a 130 fold shift in the value of EC_{50} in comparison with N/OFQ in cAMP inhibition assay in HEK cells [127]. NNC 63-0532 was not able to induce multisite phosphorylation of the NOP receptor [129].

RTI–819 and RTI–856

Both compounds show high selectivity for NOP receptor over all other opioid receptors (lowest ~30 fold on MOR for RTI–819 and ~100 fold for KOR for RTI–856)

Both RTI-819 and RTI-856 are partial agonists exhibiting similar efficacies (both around 75%) with respect to N/OFQ, but have a ~10-fold difference in potency in the G-protein pathway (72.4 nM and 7.24 nM respectively as compared to 0.20 nM for N/OFQ), while they only very weakly induced βarrestin 1 and βarrestin-2 recruitment. In the same fashion as all other G-protein partial agonists, they show bias towards G-protein signaling owing to their very weak recruitment of arrestins. This might be an indication of arrestin not being recruited at detectable levels until a threshold level of G-protein receptor activation/saturation and G-protein-coupled receptor kinase phosphorylation is reached [127].

6. Future Directions and Conclusions

Ligand bias at opioid receptors has come a long way, yet many questions remain unanswered. At MOR, the response is mixed with attenuation of respiratory depression not correlating with βarrrestin-2 recruitment. The low respiratory depression of mitragynine(s) discussed in this manuscript may be a result of other targets, like DOR antagonism. Newer reports are emerging which suggest that low intrinsic efficacy maybe responsible for the lower respiratory depression of PZM21 and SR17108 [26] compared to fentanyl. Similarly, a possible reason why ligands appear as biased maybe due to the use of highly amplified systems where a partial agonist appears like a full agonist. Going forward, a potency biased model where a ligand shows an E_{Max} > 70% in both G and arrestin is proposed instead of an efficacy biased model where a ligand with <20% E_{Max} in the arrestin pathway ligand is characterized as biased [145]. It should be noted that the attenuation of side effects in β-arrestin 2 KO mice was only seen with morphine but not with methadone, oxycodone, or fentanyl, suggesting that how the ligand stabilizes the receptor may be more important and additional signaling circuits cannot be ruled out [146].

There is a desperate need for arrestin biased ligands at all opioid subtypes (MOR, KOR, DOR, and NOP receptor) to truly understand the pharmacology of the arrestin pathway with ligands. To the best of our knowledge, only fentanyl is arrestin biased at MOR. No such ligands exist at KOR, DOR, or NOP receptor. In a mice behavioral assay an arrestin biased agonist will ideally have a phenotype opposite to that of a G-biased agonist. For example, a MOR arrestin biased ligand should show lower analgesic efficacy and higher tolerance compared to a G-biased MOR agonist. Similarly, the propensity to cause convulsions for a DOR arrestin biased ligand will be higher over a G-biased agonist and a KOR arrestin biased agonist will have more sedation. At the neuronal as well as the cellular level, these arrestin biased drugs should lead to greater internalization of the receptor.

The synthesis and pharmacology of PR6047 suggests that bias at DOR may still hold potential in investigating functional selectivity and dissociating receptor induced adverse effects from its analgesia. Newer biased ligands with high selectivity for NOP receptor over MOR are required to correlate the in vivo pharmacology with ligand bias in the NOP receptor class.

A rational drug design of biased ligands is still lacking. Some correlations of bias can be drawn out of the MP1104-KOR structure where mutation of Y312W led to transformation of balanced agonist IBNtxA into a biased agonist at KOR [147]. The stabilization of the amide carbonyl group of IBNtxA [148] through H-bonding with the phenol of 'Y' holds the iodophenyl amide arm of the ligand in the TM2-TM3 region of KOR. Mutation of 'Y' to 'W' leads to loss of this interaction and flips the amide arm towards TM5-ECL2. The investigators hypothesized that ligands binding in this TM5-ECL2 region may lead to biased agonism, while ligands orienting towards TM2-TM3 may lead to balanced agonism. The same ligand IBNtxA at MOR was a biased agonist because the aminophenyl arm was oriented towards TM5-ECL2 region. Older studies from DOR inactive state structures (D95A, N131A) as well as KOR active state structures (N141A) [147] suggest that mutations in the Na^+ binding pocket flip function of DOR antagonist as well non-selective opioid antagonists naloxone and nalterexone to β-arrestin 2 biased ligands suggesting another subpocket which may control arrestin engagement [93]. Not surprisingly, MOR variants in the C-tail of MOR also controls arrestin recruitment and control tolerance/dependence in vivo in mice as shown in elegant studies by Pan and co-workers at MSKCC [149]. The structures of biased ligands at opioids are presently missing and it is hoped that such structures of such biased ligands will greatly aid in structure-based design of biased opioids. Together, these studies are essential to identify receptor hot spots that lead to arrestin engagement and disengagement and to understand functional selectivity better.

Author Contributions: The manuscript was written through contributions of all the authors. All authors have read and agreed to the published version of the manuscript.

Funding: S.M. is supported by funds from NIH grants DA045884, DA046487, DA048379 and start-up funds from Center for Clinical Pharmacology, St. Louis College of Pharmacy and Washington University.

Conflicts of Interest: S.M. is the cofounder of Sparian Inc. and has patents related to mitragyna alkaloids and its derivatives. The other authors report no other conflict of interest.

References

1. Hilger, D.; Masureel, M.; Kobilka, B.K. Structure and dynamics of GPCR signaling complexes. *Nat. Struct. Mol. Biol.* **2018**, *25*, 4–12. [CrossRef] [PubMed]
2. Liu, X.; Xu, X.; Hilger, D.; Aschauer, P.; Tiemann, J.K.S.; Du, Y.; Liu, H.; Hirata, K.; Sun, X.; Guixà-González, R.; et al. Structural Insights into the Process of GPCR-G Protein Complex Formation. *Cell* **2019**, *177*, 1243–1251. [CrossRef] [PubMed]
3. Ma, P.; Zemmel, R. Value of novelty? *Nat. Rev. Drug Discov.* **2002**, *1*, 571–572. [CrossRef] [PubMed]
4. Bruchas, M.R.; Roth, B.L. New Technologies for Elucidating Opioid Receptor Function. *Trends Pharmacol. Sci.* **2016**, *37*, 279–289. [CrossRef] [PubMed]
5. DeWeerdt, S. Tracing the US opioid crisis to its roots. *Nature* **2019**, *573*, S10–S12. [CrossRef]
6. Deupi, X.; Kobilka, B. Activation of G Protein–Coupled Receptors. In *Advances in Protein Chemistry*; Elsevier: Amsterdam, the Netherlands, 2007; Volume 74, pp. 137–166. ISBN 978-0-12-034288-4.
7. Raehal, K.M.; Schmid, C.L.; Groer, C.E.; Bohn, L.M. Functional Selectivity at the -Opioid Receptor: Implications for Understanding Opioid Analgesia and Tolerance. *Pharmacol. Rev.* **2011**, *63*, 1001–1019. [CrossRef]
8. Franco, R.; Aguinaga, D.; Jiménez, J.; Lillo, J.; Martínez-Pinilla, E.; Navarro, G. Biased receptor functionality versus biased agonism in G-protein-coupled receptors. *Biomol. Concepts* **2018**, *9*, 143–154. [CrossRef]
9. Azzam, A.A.H.; McDonald, J.; Lambert, D.G. Hot topics in opioid pharmacology: Mixed and biased opioids. *Br. J. Anaesth.* **2019**, *122*, e136–e145. [CrossRef]
10. Wootten, D.; Christopoulos, A.; Marti-Solano, M.; Babu, M.M.; Sexton, P.M. Mechanisms of signalling and biased agonism in G protein-coupled receptors. *Nat. Rev. Mol. Cell Biol.* **2018**, *19*, 638–653. [CrossRef]
11. Stanczyk, M.A.; Kandasamy, R. Biased agonism: The quest for the analgesic holy grail. *PAIN Rep.* **2018**, *3*, e650. [CrossRef]
12. Al-Hasani, R.; Bruchas, M.R. Molecular Mechanisms of Opioid Receptor-dependent Signaling and Behavior. *Anesthesiology* **2011**, *1*. [CrossRef] [PubMed]
13. Mores, K.L.; Cassell, R.J.; van Rijn, R.M. Arrestin recruitment and signaling by G protein-coupled receptor heteromers. *Neuropharmacology* **2019**, *152*, 15–21. [CrossRef] [PubMed]
14. Fields, H.L. The Doctor's Dilemma: Opiate Analgesics and Chronic Pain. *Neuron* **2011**, *69*, 591–594. [CrossRef] [PubMed]
15. Rasmussen, S.G.F.; DeVree, B.T.; Zou, Y.; Kruse, A.C.; Chung, K.Y.; Kobilka, T.S.; Thian, F.S.; Chae, P.S.; Pardon, E.; Calinski, D.; et al. Crystal structure of the β2 adrenergic receptor–Gs protein complex. *Nature* **2011**, *477*, 549–555. [CrossRef] [PubMed]
16. Zhou, X.E.; He, Y.; de Waal, P.W.; Gao, X.; Kang, Y.; Van Eps, N.; Yin, Y.; Pal, K.; Goswami, D.; White, T.A.; et al. Identification of Phosphorylation Codes for Arrestin Recruitment by G Protein-Coupled Receptors. *Cell* **2017**, *170*, 457–469. [CrossRef] [PubMed]
17. Michel, M.C.; Charlton, S.J. Biased Agonism in Drug Discovery—Is It Too Soon to Choose a Path? *Mol. Pharmacol.* **2018**, *93*, 259–265. [CrossRef] [PubMed]
18. Bohn, L.M.; Lefkowitz, R.J.; Gainetdinov, R.R.; Peppel, K.; Caron, M.G.; Lin, F.T. Enhanced morphine analgesia in mice lacking beta-arrestin 2. *Science* **1999**, *286*, 2495–2498. [CrossRef] [PubMed]
19. Bohn, L.M.; Gainetdinov, R.R.; Lin, F.-T.; Lefkowitz, R.J.; Caron, M.G. μ-Opioid receptor desensitization by β-arrestin-2 determines morphine tolerance but not dependence. *Nature* **2000**, *408*, 720–723. [CrossRef] [PubMed]
20. Raehal, K.M. Morphine Side Effects in -Arrestin 2 Knockout Mice. *J. Pharmacol. Exp. Ther.* **2005**, *314*, 1195–1201. [CrossRef]
21. Li, Y.; Liu, X.; Liu, C.; Kang, J.; Yang, J.; Pei, G.; Wu, C. Improvement of Morphine-Mediated Analgesia by Inhibition of β-Arrestin 2 Expression in Mice Periaqueductal Gray Matter. *Int. J. Mol. Sci.* **2009**, *10*, 954–963. [CrossRef]
22. Yang, C.-H.; Huang, H.-W.; Chen, K.-H.; Chen, Y.-S.; Sheen-Chen, S.-M.; Lin, C.-R. Antinociceptive potentiation and attenuation of tolerance by intrathecal β-arrestin 2 small interfering RNA in rats. *Br. J. Anaesth.* **2011**, *107*, 774–781. [CrossRef] [PubMed]

23. Chen, X.-T.; Pitis, P.; Liu, G.; Yuan, C.; Gotchev, D.; Cowan, C.L.; Rominger, D.H.; Koblish, M.; DeWire, S.M.; Crombie, A.L.; et al. Structure–Activity Relationships and Discovery of a G Protein Biased μ Opioid Receptor Ligand, [(3-Methoxythiophen-2-yl)methyl]({2-[(9 R)-9-(pyridin-2-yl)-6-oxaspiro-[4.5]decan-9-yl]ethyl})amine (TRV130), for the Treatment of Acute Severe Pain. *J. Med. Chem.* **2013**, *56*, 8019–8031. [CrossRef] [PubMed]
24. Manglik, A.; Lin, H.; Aryal, D.K.; McCorvy, J.D.; Dengler, D.; Corder, G.; Levit, A.; Kling, R.C.; Bernat, V.; Hübner, H.; et al. Structure-based discovery of opioid analgesics with reduced side effects. *Nature* **2016**, *537*, 185–190. [CrossRef]
25. Gutridge, A.M.; Robins, M.T.; Cassell, R.J.; Uprety, R.; Mores, K.L.; Ko, M.J.; Pasternak, G.W.; Majumdar, S.; van Rijn, R.M. G protein-biased kratom-alkaloids and synthetic carfentanil-amide opioids as potential treatments for alcohol use disorder. *Br. J. Pharmacol.* **2020**, *177*, 1497–1513. [CrossRef] [PubMed]
26. Gillis, A.; Gondin, A.B.; Kliewer, A.; Sanchez, J.; Lim, H.D.; Alamein, C.; Manandhar, P.; Santiago, M.; Fritzwanker, S.; Schmiedel, F.; et al. Low intrinsic efficacy for G protein activation can explain the improved side effect profiles of new opioid agonists. *Sci. Signal.* **2020**, *13*, eaaz3140. [CrossRef]
27. Hill, R.; Disney, A.; Conibear, A.; Sutcliffe, K.; Dewey, W.; Husbands, S.; Bailey, C.; Kelly, E.; Henderson, G. The novel μ-opioid receptor agonist PZM21 depresses respiration and induces tolerance to antinociception: PZM21 depresses respiration. *Br. J. Pharmacol.* **2018**, *175*, 2653–2661. [CrossRef]
28. Kruegel, A.C.; Gassaway, M.M.; Kapoor, A.; Váradi, A.; Majumdar, S.; Filizola, M.; Javitch, J.A.; Sames, D. Synthetic and Receptor Signaling Explorations of the *Mitragyna* Alkaloids: Mitragynine as an Atypical Molecular Framework for Opioid Receptor Modulators. *J. Am. Chem. Soc.* **2016**, *138*, 6754–6764. [CrossRef]
29. Váradi, A.; Marrone, G.F.; Palmer, T.C.; Narayan, A.; Szabó, M.R.; Le Rouzic, V.; Grinnell, S.G.; Subrath, J.J.; Warner, E.; Kalra, S.; et al. Mitragynine/Corynantheidine Pseudoindoxyls As Opioid Analgesics with Mu Agonism and Delta Antagonism, which Do Not Recruit β-Arrestin-2. *J. Med. Chem.* **2016**, *59*, 8381–8397. [CrossRef]
30. Tidgewell, K.; Groer, C.E.; Harding, W.W.; Lozama, A.; Schmidt, M.; Marquam, A.; Hiemstra, J.; Partilla, J.S.; Dersch, C.M.; Rothman, R.B.; et al. Herkinorin Analogues with Differential β-Arrestin-2 Interactions. *J. Med. Chem.* **2008**, *51*, 2421–2431. [CrossRef]
31. Crowley, R.S.; Riley, A.P.; Sherwood, A.M.; Groer, C.E.; Shivaperumal, N.; Biscaia, M.; Paton, K.; Schneider, S.; Provasi, D.; Kivell, B.M.; et al. Synthetic Studies of Neoclerodane Diterpenes from *Salvia divinorum*: Identification of a Potent and Centrally Acting μ Opioid Analgesic with Reduced Abuse Liability. *J. Med. Chem.* **2016**, *59*, 11027–11038. [CrossRef]
32. Crowley, R.S.; Riley, A.P.; Alder, A.F.; Anderson, R.J.; Luo, D.; Kaska, S.; Maynez, P.; Kivell, B.M.; Prisinzano, T.E. Synthetic Studies of Neoclerodane Diterpenes from *Salvia divinorum*: Design, Synthesis, and Evaluation of Analogues with Improved Potency and G-protein Activation Bias at the μ-Opioid Receptor. *ACS Chem. Neurosci.* **2020**, *11*, 1781–1790. [CrossRef] [PubMed]
33. Schmid, C.L.; Kennedy, N.M.; Ross, N.C.; Lovell, K.M.; Yue, Z.; Morgenweck, J.; Cameron, M.D.; Bannister, T.D.; Bohn, L.M. Bias Factor and Therapeutic Window Correlate to Predict Safer Opioid Analgesics. *Cell* **2017**, *171*, 1165–1175. [CrossRef] [PubMed]
34. Kennedy, N.M.; Schmid, C.L.; Ross, N.C.; Lovell, K.M.; Yue, Z.; Chen, Y.T.; Cameron, M.D.; Bohn, L.M.; Bannister, T.D. Optimization of a Series of Mu Opioid Receptor (MOR) Agonists with High G Protein Signaling Bias. *J. Med. Chem.* **2018**, *61*, 8895–8907. [CrossRef] [PubMed]
35. Commissioner, O. FDA Approves New Opioid for Intravenous Use in Hospitals, Other Controlled Clinical Settings. Available online: https://www.fda.gov/news-events/press-announcements/fda-approves-new-opioid-intravenous-use-hospitals-other-controlled-clinical-settings (accessed on 7 September 2020).
36. Pedersen, M.F.; Wróbel, T.M.; Märcher-Rørsted, E.; Pedersen, D.S.; Møller, T.C.; Gabriele, F.; Pedersen, H.; Matosiuk, D.; Foster, S.R.; Bouvier, M.; et al. Biased agonism of clinically approved μ-opioid receptor agonists and TRV130 is not controlled by binding and signaling kinetics. *Neuropharmacology* **2020**, *166*, 107718. [CrossRef] [PubMed]
37. Liang, D.-Y.; Li, W.-W.; Nwaneshiudu, C.; Irvine, K.-A.; Clark, J.D. Pharmacological Characters of Oliceridine, a μ-Opioid Receptor G-Protein–Biased Ligand in Mice. *Anesth. Analg.* **2019**, *129*, 1414–1421. [CrossRef]
38. Altarifi, A.A.; David, B.; Muchhala, K.H.; Blough, B.E.; Akbarali, H.; Negus, S.S. Effects of acute and repeated treatment with the biased mu opioid receptor agonist TRV130 (oliceridine) on measures of antinociception, gastrointestinal function, and abuse liability in rodents. *J. Psychopharmacol.* **2017**, *31*, 730–739. [CrossRef]

39. Deuis, J.R.; Dvorakova, L.S.; Vetter, I. Methods Used to Evaluate Pain Behaviors in Rodents. *Front. Mol. Neurosci.* **2017**, *10*, 284. [CrossRef]
40. Kudla, L.; Bugno, R.; Skupio, U.; Wiktorowska, L.; Solecki, W.; Wojtas, A.; Golembiowska, K.; Zádor, F.; Benyhe, S.; Buda, S.; et al. Functional characterization of a novel opioid, PZM21, and its effects on the behavioural responses to morphine. *Br. J. Pharmacol.* **2019**, *176*, 4434–4445. [CrossRef]
41. Yaksh, T.L.; Eddinger, K.A.; Kokubu, S.; Wang, Z.; DiNardo, A.; Ramachandran, R.; Zhu, Y.; He, Y.; Weren, F.; Quang, D.; et al. Mast Cell Degranulation and Fibroblast Activation in the Morphine-induced Spinal Mass: Role of Mas-related G Protein-coupled Receptor Signaling. *Anesthesiology* **2019**, *131*, 132–147. [CrossRef]
42. Hassan, Z.; Muzaimi, M.; Navaratnam, V.; Yusoff, N.H.M.; Suhaimi, F.W.; Vadivelu, R.; Vicknasingam, B.K.; Amato, D.; von Hörsten, S.; Ismail, N.I.W.; et al. From Kratom to mitragynine and its derivatives: Physiological and behavioural effects related to use, abuse, and addiction. *Neurosci. Biobehav. Rev.* **2013**, *37*, 138–151. [CrossRef]
43. Matsumoto, K.; Horie, S.; Ishikawa, H.; Takayama, H.; Aimi, N.; Ponglux, D.; Watanabe, K. Antinociceptive effect of 7-hydroxymitragynine in mice: Discovery of an orally active opioid analgesic from the Thai medicinal herb Mitragyna speciosa. *Life Sci.* **2004**, *74*, 2143–2155. [CrossRef] [PubMed]
44. Matsumoto, K.; Horie, S.; Takayama, H.; Ishikawa, H.; Aimi, N.; Ponglux, D.; Murayama, T.; Watanabe, K. Antinociception, tolerance and withdrawal symptoms induced by 7-hydroxymitragynine, an alkaloid from the Thai medicinal herb Mitragyna speciosa. *Life Sci.* **2005**, *78*, 2–7. [CrossRef] [PubMed]
45. Matsumoto, K.; Hatori, Y.; Murayama, T.; Tashima, K.; Wongseripipatana, S.; Misawa, K.; Kitajima, M.; Takayama, H.; Horie, S. Involvement of μ-opioid receptors in antinociception and inhibition of gastrointestinal transit induced by 7-hydroxymitragynine, isolated from Thai herbal medicine Mitragyna speciosa. *Eur. J. Pharmacol.* **2006**, *549*, 63–70. [CrossRef] [PubMed]
46. Kruegel, A.C.; Uprety, R.; Grinnell, S.G.; Langreck, C.; Pekarskaya, E.A.; Le Rouzic, V.; Ansonoff, M.; Gassaway, M.M.; Pintar, J.E.; Pasternak, G.W.; et al. 7-Hydroxymitragynine Is an Active Metabolite of Mitragynine and a Key Mediator of Its Analgesic Effects. *ACS Cent. Sci.* **2019**, *5*, 992–1001. [CrossRef] [PubMed]
47. Hemby, S.E.; McIntosh, S.; Leon, F.; Cutler, S.J.; McCurdy, C.R. Abuse liability and therapeutic potential of the *Mitragyna speciosa* (kratom) alkaloids mitragynine and 7-hydroxymitragynine: Kratom abuse liability. *Addict. Biol.* **2018**. [CrossRef]
48. Groer, C.E.; Tidgewell, K.; Moyer, R.A.; Harding, W.W.; Rothman, R.B.; Prisinzano, T.E.; Bohn, L.M. An Opioid Agonist that Does Not Induce μ-Opioid Receptor—Arrestin Interactions or Receptor Internalization. *Mol. Pharmacol.* **2007**, *71*, 549–557. [CrossRef]
49. Butelman, E.R.; Kreek, M.J. Salvinorin A, a kappa-opioid receptor agonist hallucinogen: Pharmacology and potential template for novel pharmacotherapeutic agents in neuropsychiatric disorders. *Front. Pharmacol.* **2015**, *6*, 190. [CrossRef]
50. Wu, Z.; Hruby, V.J. Toward a Universal μ-Agonist Template for Template-Based Alignment Modeling of Opioid Ligands. *ACS Omega* **2019**, *4*, 17457–17476. [CrossRef]
51. Majumdar, S.; Devi, L.A. Strategy for making safer opioids bolstered. *Nature* **2018**, *553*, 286–288. [CrossRef]
52. Váradi, A.; Palmer, T.C.; Haselton, N.; Afonin, D.; Subrath, J.J.; Le Rouzic, V.; Hunkele, A.; Pasternak, G.W.; Marrone, G.F.; Borics, A.; et al. Synthesis of Carfentanil Amide Opioids Using the Ugi Multicomponent Reaction. *ACS Chem. Neurosci.* **2015**, *6*, 1570–1577. [CrossRef]
53. Kliewer, A.; Schmiedel, F.; Sianati, S.; Bailey, A.; Bateman, J.T.; Levitt, E.S.; Williams, J.T.; Christie, M.J.; Schulz, S. Phosphorylation-deficient G-protein-biased μ-opioid receptors improve analgesia and diminish tolerance but worsen opioid side effects. *Nat. Commun.* **2019**, *10*, 367. [CrossRef] [PubMed]
54. Kliewer, A.; Gillis, A.; Hill, R.; Schmiedel, F.; Bailey, C.; Kelly, E.; Henderson, G.; Christie, M.J.; Schulz, S. Morphine-induced respiratory depression is independent of β-arrestin2 signalling. *Br. J. Pharmacol.* **2020**, *177*, 2923–2931. [CrossRef] [PubMed]
55. Beck, T.C.; Hapstack, M.A.; Beck, K.R.; Dix, T.A. Therapeutic Potential of Kappa Opioid Agonists. *Pharmaceuticals* **2019**, *12*, 95. [CrossRef] [PubMed]
56. Carr, G.V.; Mague, S.D. p38: The Link between the κ-Opioid Receptor and Dysphoria. *J. Neurosci.* **2008**, *28*, 2299–2300. [CrossRef] [PubMed]

57. Ehrich, J.M.; Messinger, D.I.; Knakal, C.R.; Kuhar, J.R.; Schattauer, S.S.; Bruchas, M.R.; Zweifel, L.S.; Kieffer, B.L.; Phillips, P.E.M.; Chavkin, C. Kappa Opioid Receptor-Induced Aversion Requires p38 MAPK Activation in VTA Dopamine Neurons. *J. Neurosci.* **2015**, *35*, 12917–12931. [CrossRef] [PubMed]
58. Phan, N.; Lotts, T.; Antal, A.; Bernhard, J.; Ständer, S. Systemic Kappa Opioid Receptor Agonists in the Treatment of Chronic Pruritus: A Literature Review. *Acta Derm. Venereol.* **2012**, *92*, 555–560. [CrossRef]
59. White, K.L.; Robinson, J.E.; Zhu, H.; DiBerto, J.F.; Polepally, P.R.; Zjawiony, J.K.; Nichols, D.E.; Malanga, C.J.; Roth, B.L. The G Protein-Biased κ-Opioid Receptor Agonist RB-64 is Analgesic with a Unique Spectrum of Activities In Vivo. *J. Pharmacol. Exp. Ther.* **2014**, *352*, 98–109. [CrossRef]
60. Kivell, B.; Paton, K.; Kumar, N.; Morani, A.; Culverhouse, A.; Shepherd, A.; Welsh, S.; Biggerstaff, A.; Crowley, R.; Prisinzano, T. Kappa Opioid Receptor Agonist Mesyl Sal B Attenuates Behavioral Sensitization to Cocaine with Fewer Aversive Side effects than Salvinorin A in Rodents. *Molecules* **2018**, *23*, 2602. [CrossRef]
61. Brust, T.F.; Morgenweck, J.; Kim, S.A.; Rose, J.H.; Locke, J.L.; Schmid, C.L.; Zhou, L.; Stahl, E.L.; Cameron, M.D.; Scarry, S.M.; et al. Biased agonists of the kappa opioid receptor suppress pain and itch without causing sedation or dysphoria. *Sci. Signal.* **2016**, *9*, ra117. [CrossRef]
62. Spetea, M.; Eans, S.O.; Ganno, M.L.; Lantero, A.; Mairegger, M.; Toll, L.; Schmidhammer, H.; McLaughlin, J.P. Selective κ receptor partial agonist HS666 produces potent antinociception without inducing aversion after i.c.v. administration in mice: HS666 produces analgesia without causing aversion. *Br. J. Pharmacol.* **2017**, *174*, 2444–2456. [CrossRef]
63. Rives, M.-L.; Rossillo, M.; Liu-Chen, L.-Y.; Javitch, J.A. 6′-Guanidinonaltrindole (6′-GNTI) Is a G Protein-biased κ-Opioid Receptor Agonist That Inhibits Arrestin Recruitment. *J. Biol. Chem.* **2012**, *287*, 27050–27054. [CrossRef] [PubMed]
64. Schmid, C.L.; Streicher, J.M.; Groer, C.E.; Munro, T.A.; Zhou, L.; Bohn, L.M. Functional Selectivity of 6′-Guanidinonaltrindole (6′-GNTI) at κ-Opioid Receptors in Striatal Neurons. *J. Biol. Chem.* **2013**, *288*, 22387–22398. [CrossRef] [PubMed]
65. Zhou, L.; Lovell, K.M.; Frankowski, K.J.; Slauson, S.R.; Phillips, A.M.; Streicher, J.M.; Stahl, E.; Schmid, C.L.; Hodder, P.; Madoux, F.; et al. Development of Functionally Selective, Small Molecule Agonists at Kappa Opioid Receptors. *J. Biol. Chem.* **2013**, *288*, 36703–36716. [CrossRef]
66. Gupta, A.; Gomes, I.; Bobeck, E.N.; Fakira, A.K.; Massaro, N.P.; Sharma, I.; Cavé, A.; Hamm, H.E.; Parello, J.; Devi, L.A. Collybolide is a novel biased agonist of κ-opioid receptors with potent antipruritic activity. *Proc. Natl. Acad. Sci. USA* **2016**, *113*, 6041–6046. [CrossRef] [PubMed]
67. Zhou, Y.; Crowley, R.; Prisinzano, T.; Kreek, M.J. Effects of mesyl salvinorin B alone and in combination with naltrexone on alcohol deprivation effect in male and female mice. *Neurosci. Lett.* **2018**, *673*, 19–23. [CrossRef]
68. Lovell, K.M.; Frankowski, K.J.; Stahl, E.L.; Slauson, S.R.; Yoo, E.; Prisinzano, T.E.; Aubé, J.; Bohn, L.M. Structure–Activity Relationship Studies of Functionally Selective Kappa Opioid Receptor Agonists that Modulate ERK 1/2 Phosphorylation While Preserving G Protein Over βArrestin2 Signaling Bias. *ACS Chem. Neurosci.* **2015**, *6*, 1411–1419. [CrossRef]
69. Shim, W.-S.; Oh, U. Histamine-Induced Itch and its Relationship with Pain. *Mol. Pain* **2008**, *4*. [CrossRef]
70. Huskinson, S.L.; Platt, D.M.; Brasfield, M.; Follett, M.E.; Prisinzano, T.E.; Blough, B.E.; Freeman, K.B. Quantification of observable behaviors induced by typical and atypical kappa-opioid receptor agonists in male rhesus monkeys. *Psychopharmacology* **2020**, *237*, 2075–2087. [CrossRef]
71. Spetea, M.; Berzetei-Gurske, I.P.; Guerrieri, E.; Schmidhammer, H. Discovery and Pharmacological Evaluation of a Diphenethylamine Derivative (HS665), a Highly Potent and Selective κ Opioid Receptor Agonist. *J. Med. Chem.* **2012**, *55*, 10302–10306. [CrossRef]
72. Fortin, M.; Degryse, M.; Petit, F.; Hunt, P.F. The dopamine D2 agonists RU 24213 and RU 24926 are also KAPPA-opioid receptor antagonists. *Neuropharmacology* **1991**, *30*, 409–412. [CrossRef]
73. Erli, F.; Guerrieri, E.; Ben Haddou, T.; Lantero, A.; Mairegger, M.; Schmidhammer, H.; Spetea, M. Highly Potent and Selective New Diphenethylamines Interacting with the κ-Opioid Receptor: Synthesis, Pharmacology, and Structure–Activity Relationships. *J. Med. Chem.* **2017**, *60*, 7579–7590. [CrossRef] [PubMed]
74. Dunn, A.; Reed, B.; Erazo, J.; Ben-Ezra, A.; Kreek, M.J. Signaling properties of structurally diverse kappa opioid receptor ligands: Towards in vitro models of in vivo responses. *ACS Chem. Neurosci.* **2019**, 9b00195. [CrossRef] [PubMed]

75. Waldhoer, M.; Fong, J.; Jones, R.M.; Lunzer, M.M.; Sharma, S.K.; Kostenis, E.; Portoghese, P.S.; Whistler, J.L. A heterodimer-selective agonist shows in vivo relevance of G protein-coupled receptor dimers. *Proc. Natl. Acad. Sci. USA* **2005**, *102*, 9050–9055. [CrossRef] [PubMed]
76. White, K.L.; Scopton, A.P.; Rives, M.-L.; Bikbulatov, R.V.; Polepally, P.R.; Brown, P.J.; Kenakin, T.; Javitch, J.A.; Zjawiony, J.K.; Roth, B.L. Identification of Novel Functionally Selective κ-Opioid Receptor Scaffolds. *Mol. Pharmacol.* **2014**, *85*, 83–90. [CrossRef] [PubMed]
77. Zangrandi, L.; Burtscher, J.; MacKay, J.P.; Colmers, W.F.; Schwarzer, C. The G-protein biased partial κ opioid receptor agonist 6′-GNTI blocks hippocampal paroxysmal discharges without inducing aversion: G-protein biased κ-receptor agonists in epilepsy. *Br. J. Pharmacol.* **2016**, *173*, 1756–1767. [CrossRef]
78. Lu, K.; Luo, T.; Xiang, Z.; You, Z.; Fathi, R.; Chen, J.; Yang, Z. A Concise and Diversity-Oriented Strategy for the Synthesis of Benzofurans and Indoles via Ugi and Diels−Alder Reactions. *J. Comb. Chem.* **2005**, *7*, 958–967. [CrossRef]
79. Frankowski, K.J.; Ghosh, P.; Setola, V.; Tran, T.B.; Roth, B.L.; Aubé, J. N-Alkyl-octahydroisoquinolin-1-one-8-carboxamides: Selective and Nonbasic κ-Opioid Receptor Ligands. *ACS Med. Chem. Lett.* **2010**, *1*, 189–193. [CrossRef]
80. Bui, A.-M.; Cavé, A.; Janot, M.-M.; Parello, J.; Potier, P.; Scheidegger, U. Isolement et analyse structurale du collybolide, nouveau sesquiterpene extrait de Collybia maculata alb. et sch. ex fries (basidiomycetes). *Tetrahedron* **1974**, *30*, 1327–1336. [CrossRef]
81. Erspamer, V.; Melchiorri, P.; Falconieri-Erspamer, G.; Negri, L.; Corsi, R.; Severini, C.; Barra, D.; Simmaco, M.; Kreil, G. Deltorphins: A family of naturally occurring peptides with high affinity and selectivity for δ opioid binding sites. *Proc. Natl. Acad. Sci. USA* **1989**, *86*, 5188–5192. [CrossRef]
82. Gavériaux-Ruff, C.; Karchewski, L.A.; Hever, X.; Matifas, A.; Kieffer, B.L. Inflammatory pain is enhanced in delta opioid receptor-knockout mice. *Eur. J. Neurosci.* **2008**, *27*, 2558–2567. [CrossRef]
83. Pradhan, A.A.A.; Walwyn, W.; Nozaki, C.; Filliol, D.; Erbs, E.; Matifas, A.; Evans, C.; Kieffer, B.L. Ligand-Directed Trafficking of the δ-Opioid Receptor *In Vivo*: Two Paths Toward Analgesic Tolerance. *J. Neurosci.* **2010**, *30*, 16459–16468. [CrossRef] [PubMed]
84. Filliol, D.; Ghozland, S.; Chluba, J.; Martin, M.; Matthes, H.W.D.; Simonin, F.; Befort, K.; Gavériaux-Ruff, C.; Dierich, A.; LeMeur, M.; et al. Mice deficient for δ- and μ-opioid receptors exhibit opposing alterations of emotional responses. *Nat. Genet.* **2000**, *25*, 195–200. [CrossRef] [PubMed]
85. Pradhan, A.A.; Befort, K.; Nozaki, C.; Gavériaux-Ruff, C.; Kieffer, B.L. The delta opioid receptor: An evolving target for the treatment of brain disorders. *Trends Pharmacol. Sci.* **2011**, *32*, 581–590. [CrossRef]
86. Cahill, C.M.; Morinville, A.; Hoffert, C.; O'Donnell, D.; Beaudet, A. Up-regulation and trafficking of δ opioid receptor in a model of chronic inflammation: Implications for pain control. *Pain* **2003**, *101*, 199–208. [CrossRef]
87. Henry, A.G.; White, I.J.; Marsh, M.; von Zastrow, M.; Hislop, J.N. The Role of Ubiquitination in Lysosomal Trafficking of δ-Opioid Receptors. *Traffic* **2011**, *12*, 170–184. [CrossRef] [PubMed]
88. Codd, E.E.; Carson, J.R.; Colburn, R.W.; Stone, D.J.; Van Besien, C.R.; Zhang, S.-P.; Wade, P.R.; Gallantine, E.L.; Meert, T.F.; Molino, L.; et al. JNJ-20788560 [9-(8-Azabicyclo[3.2.1]oct-3-ylidene)-9 H-xanthene-3-carboxylic Acid Diethylamide], a Selective Delta Opioid Receptor Agonist, is a Potent and Efficacious Antihyperalgesic Agent That Does Not Produce Respiratory Depression, Pharmacologic Tolerance, or Physical Dependence. *J. Pharmacol. Exp. Ther.* **2009**, *329*, 241–251. [CrossRef]
89. Broom, D.; Jutkiewicz, E.; Folk, J.; Traynor, J.; Rice, K.; Woods, J. Convulsant activity of a non-peptidic δ-opioid receptor agonist is not required for its antidepressant-like effects in Sprague-Dawley rats. *Psychopharmacology* **2002**, *164*, 42–48. [CrossRef]
90. Nozaki, C.; Nagase, H.; Nemoto, T.; Matifas, A.; Kieffer, B.L.; Gaveriaux-Ruff, C. In vivo properties of KNT-127, a novel δ opioid receptor agonist: Receptor internalization, antihyperalgesia and antidepressant effects in mice: KNT-127 ligand-biased agonism at δ opioid receptor. *Br. J. Pharmacol.* **2014**, *171*, 5376–5386. [CrossRef]
91. Gendron, L.; Cahill, C.M.; von Zastrow, M.; Schiller, P.W.; Pineyro, G. Molecular Pharmacology of δ-Opioid Receptors. *Pharmacol. Rev.* **2016**, *68*, 631–700. [CrossRef]
92. Tian, X.; Guo, J.; Zhu, M.; Li, M.; Wu, G.; Xia, Y. δ-Opioid Receptor Activation Rescues the Functional TrkB Receptor and Protects the Brain from Ischemia-Reperfusion Injury in the Rat. *PLoS ONE* **2013**, *8*, e69252. [CrossRef]

93. Fenalti, G.; Giguere, P.M.; Katritch, V.; Huang, X.-P.; Thompson, A.A.; Cherezov, V.; Roth, B.L.; Stevens, R.C. Molecular control of δ-opioid receptor signalling. *Nature* **2014**, *506*, 191–196. [CrossRef] [PubMed]
94. Claff, T.; Yu, J.; Blais, V.; Patel, N.; Martin, C.; Wu, L.; Han, G.W.; Holleran, B.J.; Van der Poorten, O.; White, K.L.; et al. Elucidating the active δ-opioid receptor crystal structure with peptide and small-molecule agonists. *Sci. Adv.* **2019**, *5*, eaax9115. [CrossRef] [PubMed]
95. Bradbury, F.A.; Zelnik, J.C.; Traynor, J.R. G Protein independent phosphorylation and internalization of the δ-opioid receptor. *J. Neurochem.* **2009**, *109*, 1526–1535. [CrossRef]
96. Xu, C.; Hong, M.-H.; Zhang, L.-S.; Hou, Y.-Y.; Wang, Y.-H.; Wang, F.-F.; Chen, Y.-J.; Xu, X.-J.; Chen, J.; Xie, X.; et al. Serine 363 of the δ-opioid receptor is crucial for adopting distinct pathways to activate ERK1/2 in response to stimulation with different ligands. *J. Cell Sci.* **2010**, *123*, 4259–4270. [CrossRef] [PubMed]
97. Qiu, Y.; Loh, H.H.; Law, P.-Y. Phosphorylation of the δ-Opioid Receptor Regulates Its β-Arrestins Selectivity and Subsequent Receptor Internalization and Adenylyl Cyclase Desensitization. *J. Biol. Chem.* **2007**, *282*, 22315–22323. [CrossRef]
98. Aguila, B.; Coulbault, L.; Davis, A.; Marie, N.; Hasbi, A.; Le bras, F.; Tóth, G.; Borsodi, A.; Gurevich, V.V.; Jauzac, P.; et al. ßarrestin1-biased agonism at human δ-opioid receptor by peptidic and alkaloid ligands. *Cell. Signal.* **2012**, *24*, 699–707. [CrossRef]
99. Cen, B.; Xiong, Y.; Ma, L.; Pei, G. Direct and differential interaction of beta-arrestins with the intracellular domains of different opioid receptors. *Mol. Pharmacol.* **2001**, *59*, 758–764. [CrossRef] [PubMed]
100. Pradhan, A.A.; Perroy, J.; Walwyn, W.M.; Smith, M.L.; Vicente-Sanchez, A.; Segura, L.; Bana, A.; Kieffer, B.L.; Evans, C.J. Agonist-Specific Recruitment of Arrestin Isoforms Differentially Modify Delta Opioid Receptor Function. *J. Neurosci.* **2016**, *36*, 3541–3551. [CrossRef]
101. Vicente-Sanchez, A.; Dripps, I.J.; Tipton, A.F.; Akbari, H.; Akbari, A.; Jutkiewicz, E.M.; Pradhan, A.A. Tolerance to high-internalizing δ opioid receptor agonist is critically mediated by arrestin 2. *Br. J. Pharmacol.* **2018**, *175*, 3050–3059. [CrossRef]
102. Dripps, I.J.; Boyer, D.T.; Neubig, R.R.; Rice, K.C.; Traynor, J.R.; Jutkiewicz, E.M. Role of signalling molecules in behaviours mediated by the δ opioid receptor agonist SNC80: Signalling bias and δ-receptor activity. *In Vivo Br. J. Pharmacol.* **2018**, *175*, 891–901. [CrossRef]
103. Pradhan, A.A.; Smith, M.L.; Kieffer, B.L.; Evans, C.J. Ligand-directed signalling within the opioid receptor family: Ligand-directed signalling at opioid receptors. *Br. J. Pharmacol.* **2012**, *167*, 960–969. [CrossRef] [PubMed]
104. Jimenez-Vargas, N.N.; Gong, J.; Wisdom, M.J.; Jensen, D.D.; Latorre, R.; Hegron, A.; Teng, S.; DiCello, J.J.; Rajasekhar, P.; Veldhuis, N.A.; et al. Endosomal signaling of delta opioid receptors is an endogenous mechanism and therapeutic target for relief from inflammatory pain. *Proc. Natl. Acad. Sci. USA* **2020**, *117*, 15281–15292. [CrossRef] [PubMed]
105. Conibear, A.E.; Asghar, J.; Hill, R.; Henderson, G.; Borbely, E.; Tekus, V.; Helyes, Z.; Palandri, J.; Bailey, C.; Starke, I.; et al. A Novel G Protein–Biased Agonist at the δ Opioid Receptor with Analgesic Efficacy in Models of Chronic Pain. *J. Pharmacol. Exp. Ther.* **2020**, *372*, 224–236. [CrossRef]
106. Pasquinucci, L.; Turnaturi, R.; Calò, G.; Pappalardo, F.; Ferrari, F.; Russo, G.; Arena, E.; Montenegro, L.; Chiechio, S.; Prezzavento, O.; et al. (2S)-N-2-methoxy-2-phenylethyl-6,7-benzomorphan compound (2S-LP2): Discovery of a biased mu/delta opioid receptor agonist. *Eur. J. Med. Chem.* **2019**, *168*, 189–198. [CrossRef]
107. Chiang, T.; Sansuk, K.; van Rijn, R.M. β-Arrestin 2 dependence of δ opioid receptor agonists is correlated with alcohol intake: Biased δ receptor agonists for treating alcohol use disorders. *Br. J. Pharmacol.* **2016**, *173*, 332–343. [CrossRef]
108. Nagase, H.; Yajima, Y.; Fujii, H.; Kawamura, K.; Narita, M.; Kamei, J.; Suzuki, T. The pharmacological profile of delta opioid receptor ligands, (+) and (-) TAN-67 on pain modulation. *Life Sci.* **2001**, *68*, 2227–2231. [CrossRef]
109. van Rijn, R.M.; Brissett, D.I.; Whistler, J.L. Dual Efficacy of Delta Opioid Receptor-Selective Ligands for Ethanol Drinking and Anxiety. *J. Pharmacol. Exp. Ther.* **2010**, *335*, 133–139. [CrossRef]
110. Nagase, H.; Nemoto, T.; Matsubara, A.; Saito, M.; Yamamoto, N.; Osa, Y.; Hirayama, S.; Nakajima, M.; Nakao, K.; Mochizuki, H.; et al. Design and synthesis of KNT-127, a δ-opioid receptor agonist effective by systemic administration. *Bioorg. Med. Chem. Lett.* **2010**, *20*, 6302–6305. [CrossRef]

111. Saitoh, A.; Sugiyama, A.; Nemoto, T.; Fujii, H.; Wada, K.; Oka, J.-I.; Nagase, H.; Yamada, M. The novel δ opioid receptor agonist KNT-127 produces antidepressant-like and antinociceptive effects in mice without producing convulsions. *Behav. Brain Res.* **2011**, *223*, 271–279. [CrossRef]
112. Saitoh, A.; Yamada, M. Antidepressant-like Effects of δ Opioid Receptor Agonists in Animal Models. *Curr. Neuropharmacol.* **2012**, *10*, 231–238. [CrossRef]
113. Pradhan, A.A.A.; Becker, J.A.J.; Scherrer, G.; Tryoen-Toth, P.; Filliol, D.; Matifas, A.; Massotte, D.; Gavériaux-Ruff, C.; Kieffer, B.L. In Vivo Delta Opioid Receptor Internalization Controls Behavioral Effects of Agonists. *PLoS ONE* **2009**, *4*, e5425. [CrossRef] [PubMed]
114. Marie, N.; Lecoq, I.; Jauzac, P.; Allouche, S. Differential Sorting of Human δ-Opioid Receptors after Internalization by Peptide and Alkaloid Agonists. *J. Biol. Chem.* **2003**, *278*, 22795–22804. [CrossRef] [PubMed]
115. Witkin, J.M.; Statnick, M.A.; Rorick-Kehn, L.M.; Pintar, J.E.; Ansonoff, M.; Chen, Y.; Tucker, R.C.; Ciccocioppo, R. The biology of Nociceptin/Orphanin FQ (N/OFQ) related to obesity, stress, anxiety, mood, and drug dependence. *Pharmacol. Ther.* **2014**, *141*, 283–299. [CrossRef] [PubMed]
116. Schröder, W.; Lambert, D.G.; Ko, M.C.; Koch, T. Functional plasticity of the N/OFQ-NOP receptor system determines analgesic properties of NOP receptor agonists: The N/OFQ-NOP receptor system in analgesia. *Br. J. Pharmacol.* **2014**, *171*, 3777–3800. [CrossRef] [PubMed]
117. Byford, A.J.; Anderson, A.; Jones, P.S.; Palin, R.; Houghton, A.K. The Hypnotic, Electroencephalographic, and Antinociceptive Properties of Nonpeptide ORL1 Receptor Agonists after Intravenous Injection in Rodents. *Anesth. Analg.* **2007**, *104*, 174–179. [CrossRef]
118. Linz, K.; Schröder, W.; Frosch, S.; Christoph, T. Opioid-type Respiratory Depressant Side Effects of Cebranopadol in Rats Are Limited by Its Nociceptin/Orphanin FQ Peptide Receptor Agonist Activity. *Anesthesiology* **2017**, *126*, 708–715. [CrossRef]
119. Ding, H.; Kiguchi, N.; Yasuda, D.; Daga, P.R.; Polgar, W.E.; Lu, J.J.; Czoty, P.W.; Kishioka, S.; Zaveri, N.T.; Ko, M.-C. A bifunctional nociceptin and mu opioid receptor agonist is analgesic without opioid side effects in nonhuman primates. *Sci. Transl. Med.* **2018**, *10*, eaar3483. [CrossRef]
120. Shoblock, J.R. The Pharmacology of Ro 64-6198, a Systemically Active, Nonpeptide NOP Receptor (Opiate Receptor-Like 1, ORL-1) Agonist with Diverse Preclinical Therapeutic Activity. *CNS Drug Rev.* **2007**, *13*, 107–136. [CrossRef]
121. Gavioli, E.C.; Calo', G. Nociceptin/orphanin FQ receptor antagonists as innovative antidepressant drugs. *Pharmacol. Ther.* **2013**, *140*, 10–25. [CrossRef]
122. Vitale, G.; Filaferro, M.; Micioni Di Bonaventura, M.V.; Ruggieri, V.; Cifani, C.; Guerrini, R.; Simonato, M.; Zucchini, S. Effects of [Nphe^1, Arg^{14}, Lys^{15}] N/OFQ-NH$_2$ (UFP-101), a potent NOP receptor antagonist, on molecular, cellular and behavioural alterations associated with chronic mild stress. *J. Psychopharmacol.* **2017**, *31*, 691–703. [CrossRef]
123. Asth, L.; Ruzza, C.; Malfacini, D.; Medeiros, I.; Guerrini, R.; Zaveri, N.T.; Gavioli, E.C.; Calo', G. Beta-arrestin 2 rather than G protein efficacy determines the anxiolytic-versus antidepressant-like effects of nociceptin/orphanin FQ receptor ligands. *Neuropharmacology* **2016**, *105*, 434–442. [CrossRef] [PubMed]
124. Ciccocioppo, R.; Angeletti, S.; Sanna, P.P.; Weiss, F.; Massi, M. Effect of nociceptin/orphanin FQ on the rewarding properties of morphine. *Eur. J. Pharmacol.* **2000**, *404*, 153–159. [CrossRef]
125. Di Giannuario, A.; Pieretti, S. Nociceptin differentially affects morphine-induced dopamine release from the nucleus accumbens and nucleus caudate in rats. *Peptides* **2000**, *21*, 1125–1130. [CrossRef]
126. Ko, M.-C.; Caló, G. (Eds.) The Nociceptin/Orphanin FQ Peptide Receptor. In *Handbook of Experimental Pharmacology*; Springer International Publishing: Cham, Switzerland, 2019; Volume 254, ISBN 978-3-030-20185-2.
127. Chang, S.D.; Mascarella, S.W.; Spangler, S.M.; Gurevich, V.V.; Navarro, H.A.; Carroll, F.I.; Bruchas, M.R. Quantitative Signaling and Structure-Activity Analyses Demonstrate Functional Selectivity at the Nociceptin/Orphanin FQ Opioid Receptor. *Mol. Pharmacol.* **2015**, *88*, 502–511. [CrossRef]
128. Zhang, N.R.; Planer, W.; Siuda, E.R.; Zhao, H.-C.; Stickler, L.; Chang, S.D.; Baird, M.A.; Cao, Y.-Q.; Bruchas, M.R. Serine 363 Is Required for Nociceptin/Orphanin FQ Opioid Receptor (NOPR) Desensitization, Internalization, and Arrestin Signaling. *J. Biol. Chem.* **2012**, *287*, 42019–42030. [CrossRef]

129. Mann, A.; Moulédous, L.; Froment, C.; O'Neill, P.R.; Dasgupta, P.; Günther, T.; Brunori, G.; Kieffer, B.L.; Toll, L.; Bruchas, M.R.; et al. Agonist-selective NOP receptor phosphorylation correlates in vitro and in vivo and reveals differential post-activation signaling by chemically diverse agonists. *Sci. Signal.* **2019**, *12*, eaau8072. [CrossRef]
130. Malfacini, D.; Ambrosio, C.; Gro', M.C.; Sbraccia, M.; Trapella, C.; Guerrini, R.; Bonora, M.; Pinton, P.; Costa, T.; Calo', G. Pharmacological Profile of Nociceptin/Orphanin FQ Receptors Interacting with G-Proteins and β-Arrestins 2. *PLoS ONE* **2015**, *10*, e0132565. [CrossRef]
131. Donica, C.L.; Awwad, H.O.; Thakker, D.R.; Standifer, K.M. Cellular Mechanisms of Nociceptin/Orphanin FQ (N/OFQ) Peptide (NOP) Receptor Regulation and Heterologous Regulation by N/OFQ. *Mol. Pharmacol.* **2013**, *83*, 907–918. [CrossRef]
132. Vezzi, V.; Onaran, H.O.; Molinari, P.; Guerrini, R.; Balboni, G.; Calò, G.; Costa, T. Ligands Raise the Constraint That Limits Constitutive Activation in G Protein-coupled Opioid Receptors. *J. Biol. Chem.* **2013**, *288*, 23964–23978. [CrossRef]
133. Rizzi, A.; Cerlesi, M.C.; Ruzza, C.; Malfacini, D.; Ferrari, F.; Bianco, S.; Costa, T.; Guerrini, R.; Trapella, C.; Calo', G. Pharmacological characterization of cebranopadol a novel analgesic acting as mixed nociceptin/orphanin FQ and opioid receptor agonist. *Pharmacol. Res. Perspect.* **2016**, *4*, e00247. [CrossRef]
134. Chao, P.-K.; Chang, H.-F.; Chang, W.-T.; Yeh, T.-K.; Ou, L.-C.; Chuang, J.-Y.; Tsu-An Hsu, J.; Tao, P.-L.; Loh, H.H.; Shih, C.; et al. BPR1M97, a dual mu opioid receptor/nociceptin-orphanin FQ peptide receptor agonist, produces potent antinociceptive effects with safer properties than morphine. *Neuropharmacology* **2020**, *166*, 107678. [CrossRef] [PubMed]
135. Chen, S.-R.; Ke, Y.-Y.; Yeh, T.-K.; Lin, S.-Y.; Ou, L.-C.; Chen, S.-C.; Chang, W.-T.; Chang, H.-F.; Wu, Z.-H.; Hsieh, C.-C.; et al. Discovery, structure-activity relationship studies, and anti-nociceptive effects of N-(1,2,3,4-tetrahydro-1-isoquinolinylmethyl)benzamides as novel opioid receptor agonists. *Eur. J. Med. Chem.* **2017**, *126*, 202–217. [CrossRef] [PubMed]
136. Wichmann, J.; Adam, G.; Röver, S.; Cesura, A.M.; Dautzenberg, F.M.; Jenck, F. 8-Acenaphthen-1-yl-1-phenyl-1,3,8-triaza-spiro[4.5]decan-4-one derivatives as orphanin FQ receptor agonists. *Bioorg. Med. Chem. Lett.* **1999**, *9*, 2343–2348. [CrossRef]
137. Holanda, V.A.D.; Pacifico, S.; Azevedo Neto, J.; Finetti, L.; Lobão-Soares, B.; Calo, G.; Gavioli, E.C.; Ruzza, C. Modulation of the NOP receptor signaling affects resilience to acute stress. *J. Psychopharmacol.* **2019**, *33*, 1540–1549. [CrossRef] [PubMed]
138. Kotlińska, J.; Wichmann, J.; Legowska, A.; Rolka, K.; Silberring, J. Orphanin FQ/nociceptin but not Ro 65-6570 inhibits the expression of cocaine-induced conditioned place preference. *Behav. Pharmacol.* **2002**, *13*, 229–235. [CrossRef]
139. Rutten, K.; De Vry, J.; Bruckmann, W.; Tzschentke, T.M. Effects of the NOP receptor agonist Ro65-6570 on the acquisition of opiate- and psychostimulant-induced conditioned place preference in rats. *Eur. J. Pharmacol.* **2010**, *645*, 119–126. [CrossRef]
140. Varty, G.B.; Lu, S.X.; Morgan, C.A.; Cohen-Williams, M.E.; Hodgson, R.A.; Smith-Torhan, A.; Zhang, H.; Fawzi, A.B.; Graziano, M.P.; Ho, G.D.; et al. The Anxiolytic-Like Effects of the Novel, Orally Active Nociceptin Opioid Receptor Agonist 8-[bis(2-Methylphenyl)methyl]-3-phenyl-8-azabicyclo[3.2.1]octan-3-ol (SCH 221510). *J. Pharmacol. Exp. Ther.* **2008**, *326*, 672–682. [CrossRef]
141. Tzschentke, T.M.; Kögel, B.Y.; Frosch, S.; Linz, K. Limited potential of cebranopadol to produce opioid-type physical dependence in rodents: Weak cebranopadol dependence. *Addict. Biol.* **2018**, *23*, 1010–1019. [CrossRef]
142. Tzschentke, T.M.; Linz, K.; Frosch, S.; Christoph, T. Antihyperalgesic, Antiallodynic, and Antinociceptive Effects of Cebranopadol, a Novel Potent Nociceptin/Orphanin FQ and Opioid Receptor Agonist, after Peripheral and Central Administration in Rodent Models of Neuropathic Pain. *Pain Pract.* **2017**, *17*, 1032–1041. [CrossRef]
143. Hirao, A.; Imai, A.; Sugie, Y.; Yamada, Y.; Hayashi, S.; Toide, K. Pharmacological Characterization of the Newly Synthesized Nociceptin/Orphanin FQ–Receptor Agonist 1-[1-(1-Methylcyclooctyl)-4-piperidinyl]-2-[(3R)-3-piperidinyl]-1H-benzimidazole as an Anxiolytic Agent. *J. Pharmacol. Sci.* **2008**, *106*, 361–368. [CrossRef]
144. Thomsen, C.; Hohlweg, R. (8-Naphthalen-1-ylmethyl-4-oxo-1-phenyl-1,3,8-triaza-spiro[4.5]dec-3-yl)-acetic acid methyl ester (NNC 63-0532) is a novel potent nociceptin receptor agonist. *Br. J. Pharmacol.* **2000**, *131*, 903–908. [CrossRef] [PubMed]

145. Gillis, A.; Sreenivasan, V.; Christie, M.J. Intrinsic efficacy of opioid ligands and its importance for apparent bias, operational analysis and therapeutic window. *Mol. Pharmacol.* **2020**, mol.119.119214. [CrossRef] [PubMed]
146. Grim, T.W.; Acevedo-Canabal, A.; Bohn, L.M. Toward Directing Opioid Receptor Signaling to Refine Opioid Therapeutics. *Biol. Psychiatry* **2020**, *87*, 15–21. [CrossRef] [PubMed]
147. Che, T.; Majumdar, S.; Zaidi, S.A.; Ondachi, P.; McCorvy, J.D.; Wang, S.; Mosier, P.D.; Uprety, R.; Vardy, E.; Krumm, B.E.; et al. Structure of the Nanobody-Stabilized Active State of the Kappa Opioid Receptor. *Cell* **2018**, *172*, 55–67.e15. [CrossRef] [PubMed]
148. Majumdar, S.; Burgman, M.; Haselton, N.; Grinnell, S.; Ocampo, J.; Pasternak, A.R.; Pasternak, G.W. Generation of novel radiolabeled opiates through site-selective iodination. *Bioorg. Med. Chem. Lett.* **2011**, *21*, 4001–4004. [CrossRef]
149. Xu, J.; Lu, Z.; Narayan, A.; Le Rouzic, V.P.; Xu, M.; Hunkele, A.; Brown, T.G.; Hoefer, W.F.; Rossi, G.C.; Rice, R.C.; et al. Alternatively spliced mu opioid receptor C termini impact the diverse actions of morphine. *J. Clin. Investig.* **2017**, *127*, 1561–1573. [CrossRef]

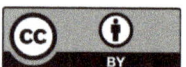

© 2020 by the authors. Licensee MDPI, Basel, Switzerland. This article is an open access article distributed under the terms and conditions of the Creative Commons Attribution (CC BY) license (http://creativecommons.org/licenses/by/4.0/).

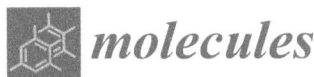

Review

Biased versus Partial Agonism in the Search for Safer Opioid Analgesics

Joaquim Azevedo Neto [1], Anna Costanzini [2], Roberto De Giorgio [2], David G. Lambert [3], Chiara Ruzza [1,4,*] and Girolamo Calò [1]

[1] Department of Biomedical and Specialty Surgical Sciences, Section of Pharmacology, University of Ferrara, 44121 Ferrara, Italy; zvdjmg@unife.it (J.A.N.); g.calo@unife.it (G.C.)
[2] Department of Morphology, Surgery, Experimental Medicine, University of Ferrara, 44121 Ferrara, Italy; anna.costanzini@unife.it (A.C.); dgrrrt@unife.it (R.D.G.)
[3] Department of Cardiovascular Sciences, Anesthesia, Critical Care and Pain Management, University of Leicester, Leicester LE1 7RH, UK; dgl3@leicester.ac.uk
[4] Technopole of Ferrara, LTTA Laboratory for Advanced Therapies, 44122 Ferrara, Italy
* Correspondence: chiara.ruzza@unife.it

Academic Editor: Helmut Schmidhammer
Received: 23 July 2020; Accepted: 23 August 2020; Published: 25 August 2020

Abstract: Opioids such as morphine—acting at the mu opioid receptor—are the mainstay for treatment of moderate to severe pain and have good efficacy in these indications. However, these drugs produce a plethora of unwanted adverse effects including respiratory depression, constipation, immune suppression and with prolonged treatment, tolerance, dependence and abuse liability. Studies in β-arrestin 2 gene knockout (βarr2(−/−)) animals indicate that morphine analgesia is potentiated while side effects are reduced, suggesting that drugs biased away from arrestin may manifest with a reduced-side-effect profile. However, there is controversy in this area with improvement of morphine-induced constipation and reduced respiratory effects in βarr2(−/−) mice. Moreover, studies performed with mice genetically engineered with G-protein-biased mu receptors suggested increased sensitivity of these animals to both analgesic actions and side effects of opioid drugs. Several new molecules have been identified as mu receptor G-protein-biased agonists, including oliceridine (TRV130), PZM21 and SR–17018. These compounds have provided preclinical data with apparent support for bias toward G proteins and the genetic premise of effective and safer analgesics. There are clinical data for oliceridine that have been very recently approved for short term intravenous use in hospitals and other controlled settings. While these data are compelling and provide a potential new pathway-based target for drug discovery, a simpler explanation for the behavior of these biased agonists revolves around differences in intrinsic activity. A highly detailed study comparing oliceridine, PZM21 and SR–17018 (among others) in a range of assays showed that these molecules behave as partial agonists. Moreover, there was a correlation between their therapeutic indices and their efficacies, but not their bias factors. If there is amplification of G-protein, but not arrestin pathways, then agonists with reduced efficacy would show high levels of activity at G-protein and low or absent activity at arrestin; offering analgesia with reduced side effects or 'apparent bias'. Overall, the current data suggests—and we support—caution in ascribing biased agonism to reduced-side-effect profiles for mu-agonist analgesics.

Keywords: opioids; mu receptor; analgesia; opioid side effects; biased agonism; partial agonism

1. Introduction

Opioid analgesics remain the gold standard for the treatment of moderate to severe pain. This is due to their unique mechanism of action; a powerful inhibitory effect both on nociception and on the emotional, cognitive and behavioral responses to pain states. However, the use of opioid analgesics is limited by their significant side effects, which include respiratory depression, constipation and, with prolonged treatment, tolerance, dependence and abuse liability. The right balance between control of pain and the risks associated with opioid drug treatment (particularly with long term treatments) is not easy to achieve. There are countries in which health systems overestimate the risks associated with opioid drug therapies often causing unsatisfactory management of pain (e.g., Italy [1]), whereas the health systems of other countries (e.g., USA) underestimated the risks associated with opioid drug prescription contributing to the opioid epidemic [2] that caused a 4-fold increase of fatal overdoses in the last two decades. This underscores the need for novel drugs that maintain the analgesic effectiveness of classical opioids, but with improved side effect profile.

Different strategies have been developed in the search for safer opioid analgesics, including increasing endogenous opioid signaling with enkephalinase inhibitors [3,4] use of mu opioid receptor positive allosteric modulators [5,6] peripherally restricted opioids [7] or pH-dependent mu-receptor agonists [8,9] and mixed opioid receptor agonists [10,11]. In addition, mixed agonists for mu and nociceptin/orphanin FQ receptors, showing promising profiles in preclinical studies, have been recently reported in the literature (reviewed in [12]). The most advanced among these compounds, cebranopadol [13] is now in advanced clinical development as an analgesic [14,15].

Another potential strategy for the development of safer opioid analgesics is based on the concept of functional selectivity or biased agonism, which is the ability of some receptor ligands to selectively stimulate one signaling pathway (e.g., selectivity for G protein or arrestin) [16]. This phenomenon has great potential in terms of drug discovery since it can be exploited to dissect the various responses associated with the activation of a given receptor. This would facilitate the discovery of ligands able to activate the signaling pathways associated with beneficial effects while avoiding those pathways associated with side effects, thus generating safer drugs [16]. In recent years, biased ligands were identified and characterized for several different G protein coupled receptors (GPCR) [17] including the mu opioid receptor. The aim of this short review is the critical analysis of the available literature regarding the potential of mu-receptor-biased agonists for development as innovative analgesics.

2. Genetic Studies

The first indication of a role of β-arrestin 2 in the in vivo regulation of the analgesic response to opioids was provided by Bohn and collaborators with the use of mice knockout for the βarrestin 2 gene (βarr2(−/−)) [18]. In these mice the analgesic effects of morphine are not only preserved, but potentiated; in fact, the ED_{50} of morphine is 10 and 6 mg/kg in βarr2(+/+) and βarr2(−/−) mice, respectively. Moreover, the effects of a single dose of morphine were prolonged in βarr2(−/−) mice. Naloxone prevented the analgesic response to morphine in both genotypes. Finally, no changes in [^{3}H]naloxone binding in various brain regions were evident between βarr2(+/+) and βarr2(−/−) mice [18]. Another study [19] demonstrated that βarr2(−/−) mice do not develop tolerance to the analgesic effect of morphine while they were similar to wild type animals in terms of morphine physical dependence, as demonstrated behaviorally by naloxone precipitated withdrawal syndrome and biochemically by upregulation of adenylyl cyclase activity [19]. In addition, the rewarding properties of morphine (but not of cocaine), assessed using the conditioned place preference test, were larger in βarr2(−/−) than βarr2(+/+) mice [20]. The logical next step of the investigation of morphine responses in βarr2(−/−) mice was to study the most common acute side effects of opioid drugs; constipation [21] and respiratory depression [22,23]. As far as opioid-induced constipation is concerned the effects of morphine were investigated in βarr2(−/−) and βarr2(+/+) mice by measuring accumulated fecal boli and bead expulsion time. In both the assays βarr2(−/−) animals were less sensitive to morphine than βarr2(+/+) mice [24]. Similar results were obtained investigating morphine-induced respiratory depression in whole-body plethysmography studies; the results of these experiments demonstrated that morphine produces significantly less suppression of respiratory frequency in βarr2(−/−) mice [24]. These findings were interpreted assuming that βarr2 acts (as expected) as a desensitizing element of morphine analgesia, while it significantly contributes to the cellular signaling relevant for the respiratory and gastrointestinal side effects of morphine [24]. Of note is that these findings contrast with more recent observations demonstrating that opioid-induced respiratory depression is due to mu receptor/G_i/G protein-coupled inwardly rectifying potassium (GIRK) channels signaling in neurons of the respiratory center [25,26].

Collectively the studies by the Bohn group suggested that eliminating βarr2 increased morphine analgesic potency while decreasing its ability to induce constipation and respiratory depression; this makes morphine a safer analgesic. These studies led to the very attractive hypothesis that drugs able to promote mu receptor interaction with G protein, but not βarr2 (i.e., mu receptor G protein-biased agonists, see next section), should mimic the profile of morphine in βarr2(−/−) mice and could be developed as an innovative class of safer opioid analgesics [27,28].

However recent research findings obtained with genetic tools questioned the above hypothesis. In fact a consortium of three different laboratories in Sydney, Bristol and Jena reexamined opioid side effects in βarr2(−/−) mice [29]. In these studies, three independent groups investigated the respiratory depressant effects of morphine using different plethysmography systems in independently bred βarr2(−/−) and βarr2(+/+) mice. In all three sets of results morphine, in the range of doses 3–30 mg/kg, produced a dose dependent reduction of respiratory rate which was virtually superimposable in βarr2(−/−) and βarr2(+/+) animals. Similar results were obtained by the group in Jena using fentanyl (0.05–3 mg/kg) as the mu-receptor agonist. In addition, the same group also reinvestigated opioid-induced constipation in βarr2(−/−) and βarr2(+/+) mice. Both morphine and fentanyl elicited a dose dependent reduction of accumulated fecal boli with similar potency and maximal effects in βarr2(−/−) and wild type animals [29]. We have performed similar experiments and our findings are summarized in Figures 1 and 2. In line with Bohn's original findings [18], morphine (0.1–10 mg/kg) and fentanyl (0.01–1 mg/kg) elicited dose dependent antinociceptive effects in the mouse tail withdrawal assay being approximately two-fold more potent in βarr2(−/−) than βarr2(+/+) mice (Figure 2). In accumulated fecal boli experiments, morphine (3–30 mg/kg) and fentanyl (0.1–1 mg/kg) dose dependently inhibited gastrointestinal functions with no major differences in βarr2(−/−) compared to βarr2(+/+) mice (Figure 1), which is in agreement with the findings obtained by the group in Jena [29]. The reason for the discrepancy between the results obtained with βarr2(−/−) mice by different research groups is not known; it has been suggested [29] that mixed genetic backgrounds may have a role in the discrepancy. However, in all studies, this possible confounding factor was considered and minimized using littermates or backcrossed animals.

In a recent very elegant study novel genetic tools have been generated and investigated in order to shed light on the relationship between arrestins and morphine analgesia and side effects [30]. As described for virtually all GPCR [31], the activated mu receptor is recognized by G protein–receptor kinases (GRKs) that phosphorylate several serine and threonine residues located in the cytoplasmic loops and carboxyl-terminal; the phosphorylated receptor can then bind arrestins. To prevent this phenomenon three lines of mutant mice were generated by knocking in mu receptor genes with serine- and threonine-to-alanine mutations in the carboxyl-terminus of the protein that render the receptor increasingly unable to recruit β-arrestins. Thus, these mutant mice express G-protein-biased mu receptors. Importantly, autoradiographic studies demonstrated no differences between the knock-in lines and wild type animals in terms of mu receptor density in different brain areas. The phosphorylation-deficient mu knock-in mice displayed; (i) enhanced opioid-mediated analgesia in the hot-plate test, (ii) reduced liability to develop tolerance to the analgesic effects of opioid drugs after a seven-day chronic treatment with osmotic pumps and (iii) similar signs of withdrawal in response to the administration of naloxone after chronic treatment with morphine or fentanyl, all compared to wild type animals. With respect to these opioid related actions, these knock-in mice displayed a phenotype similar to that of βarr2(−/−) mice [18,19]. These data demonstrated that mu receptor carboxyl-terminal multisite phosphorylation and mu receptor/βarr2 interaction are crucial regulators of opioid analgesia and tolerance, but not physical dependence. As far as the respiratory and gastrointestinal side effects of opioids are concerned, all genotypes of phosphorylation-deficient G protein-biased mu knock-in mice responded to equianalgesic doses of morphine and fentanyl with profound respiratory depression and constipation. Moreover, a detailed analysis of morphine and fentanyl ED_{50} values for analgesia versus their ED_{50} for respiratory depression and constipation yielded highly significant correlation coefficients. Collectively these findings suggest that the lack of mu receptor phosphorylation promotes enhanced analgesia and a proportional increase in respiratory depression and constipation thus not supporting a role for β-arrestin signaling in opioid side effects [30]. Clearly these results argue against the hypothesis that mu agonists biased toward G proteins may act as safer analgesics.

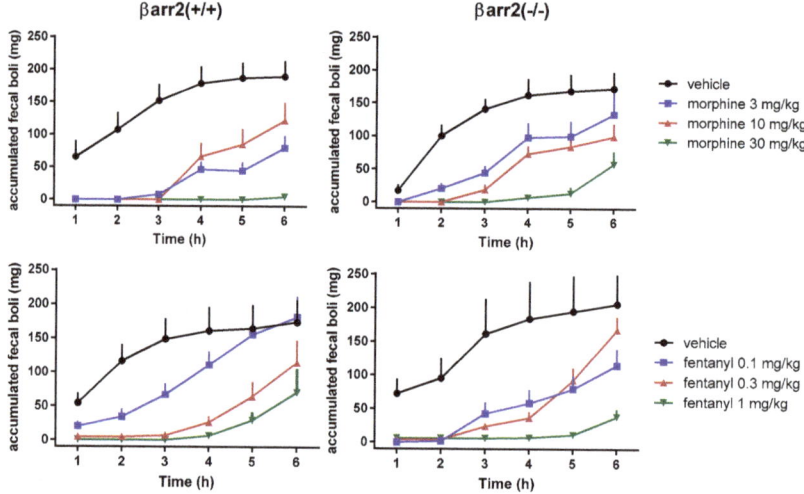

Figure 1. Mouse accumulated fecal boli assay. Dose response curves to morphine (**top** panels) and fentanyl (**bottom** panels) in βarr2(+/+) (**left** panels) and βarr2(−/−) (**right** panels) mice. Data are mean ± SEM of 7 animals for each treatment. Experiments were performed as described in [24].

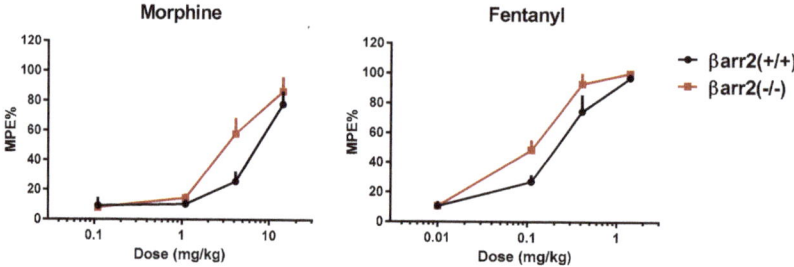

Figure 2. Mouse tail withdrawal assay. Dose response curves to morphine (**left** panel) and fentanyl (**right** panel) in βarr2(+/+) and βarr2(−/−) mice. Data are mean ± SEM of 6 animals for each treatment. Experiments were performed as described in [32].

3. Pharmacological Studies—Are Mu-Receptor Agonists Biased Toward G Proteins Safer Analgesics?

Based on the original findings obtained in βarr2(−/−) animals [18,19,24] and on the hypothesis that mu receptor/βarr2 signaling is involved in opioid acute side effects, several groups developed projects aimed at the identification and pharmacological characterization of mu receptor G protein-biased agonists as innovative analgesics.

The first and most widely studied molecule of this class is oliceridine (aka TRV130) [33] (see chemical structure in Figure 3). The structure–activity relationship study that led to its identification is described by Chen and colleagues [34]. Oliceridine binds to the human, rat and mouse mu receptor with low nanomolar affinities and inhibits cAMP accumulation in HEK293 cells expressing the human recombinant mu receptor with similar maximal effects but higher potency than morphine. However, oliceridine displayed a lower efficacy than morphine for stimulating mu receptor phosphorylation and internalization and for recruiting βarr2. Moreover, the inhibitory effects of oliceridine in the cAMP assay were competitively antagonized by naloxone while oliceridine competitively antagonized DAMGO-induced βarr2 recruitment. Of note the agonist potency of oliceridine in the cAMP assay (pEC_{50} 8.2) is similar to its antagonist potency (pA_2 7.7) in βarr2 recruitment experiments. Thus, in vitro studies suggested that oliceridine behaves as a mu-receptor agonist biased toward G proteins [35]. In the same study DeWire et al. investigated the in vivo actions of oliceridine. This compound elicited dose dependent and robust antinociceptive effects in various analgesiometric assays in mice and rats producing similar maximal effects to morphine but with approximately 10-fold higher potency. Interestingly, in experiments investigating the gastrointestinal (fecal boli accumulation and glass bead expulsion in mice) and respiratory (blood pCO_2 and pO_2 in rats) side effects of opioids, oliceridine was less potent and effective than morphine [35]. Thus, compared to morphine, the G protein-biased mu receptor agonist oliceridine displayed a larger therapeutic index; this finding corroborates the hypothesis based on the original studies in βarr2(−/−) animals [18,24] that βarr2 signaling is involved in the acute side effects of opioid analgesics. The G protein-biased mu receptor agonist activity of oliceridine as well as its antinociceptive activity were later confirmed by Mori et al. [36]. In this study, the authors also demonstrated that the antinociceptive effects of oliceridine in the mouse sciatic nerve ligation model are associated with lower tolerance liability than fentanyl [36]. This latter finding was independently confirmed by a different group that compared the antinociceptive effects of morphine and oliceridine after a 4-day treatment with the mouse tail withdrawal assay [37]. Interestingly these authors also reported that mice treated chronically with oliceridine display, in response to an injection of naloxone, a withdrawal syndrome similar to that observed in morphine treated mice. Again, these findings are in line with the original hypothesis of the Bohn group [19] that βarr2 signaling is involved in opioid tolerance, but not dependence.

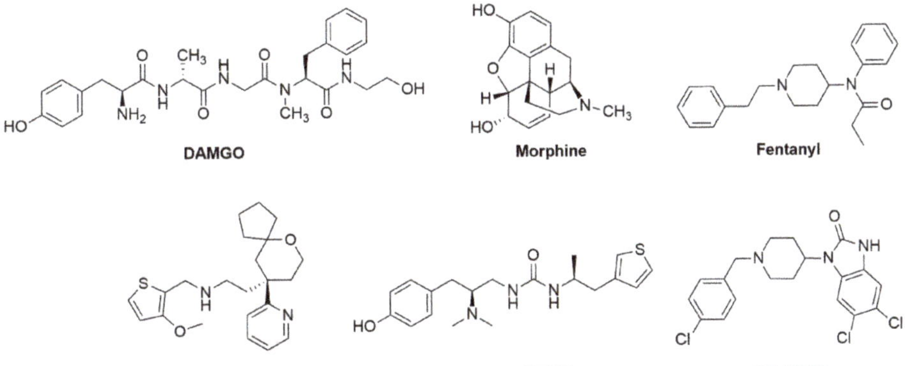

Figure 3. Chemical structures of DAMGO, morphine, fentanyl, oliceridine, PZM21 and SR–17018.

As far as abuse liability is concerned, oliceridine has been investigated in rats self-administering drugs under a progressive-ratio schedule of reinforcement. Compared to oxycodone, oliceridine was found to be equipotent and equieffective in self-administration and thermal antinociception experiments [38]. Similar results were reported in rat fentanyl discrimination studies where oliceridine was approximately two-fold more potent in producing fentanyl stimulus effects versus antinociception [39]. The abuse liability of oliceridine was also reported by Altarifi et al. [40] using an intracranial self-stimulation procedure in rats. This study also questioned the increased therapeutic index of oliceridine when compared to morphine. Indeed, the effects of oliceridine were the same as morphine both in the mouse tail withdrawal assay and in the mouse accumulated fecal boli test [40].

Oliceridine was also used in comparison with morphine [41,42], or other mu ligands [43,44] in molecular dynamics studies aimed at investigating the active structure of mu receptor interacting with G protein and arrestin. However, the detailed analysis of these studies goes beyond the scope of this article.

Oliceridine has been investigated in the clinic. A first-in-human study was conducted with ascending doses of oliceridine administered intravenously over the dose range of 0.15–7 mg [45]. Oliceridine caused dose-related pupil constriction confirming mu receptor engagement. Nausea and vomiting observed at the 7 mg dose limited further dose escalation. Collectively this study suggests that oliceridine may have a broad margin between doses causing mu receptor-mediated pharmacology and doses causing mu opioid receptor-mediated intolerance [45]. Another study investigated the effects of oliceridine and morphine after single intravenous injections in thirty healthy men; oliceridine produced greater analgesia than morphine with less reduction in respiratory drive and less severe nausea [46]. The efficacy and tolerability of oliceridine in acute pain management after bunionectomy has been investigated in a Phase II, randomized and placebo- and active-controlled study. The results demonstrated that oliceridine rapidly produces profound analgesia in moderate to severe acute pain, with a profile of tolerability like morphine [47]. Similar results were obtained in a Phase IIb study in patients with moderate to severe acute pain following abdominoplasty. These clinical results suggest that oliceridine promotes effective, rapid analgesia in patients with postoperative pain, with acceptable safety/tolerability profiles and a potentially wider therapeutic window than morphine [48]. Moreover, favorable analgesia over respiratory depression has been reported for oliceridine, but not morphine in a recent study that reanalyzed data obtained from healthy volunteers and postoperative patients [49] Finally, the analgesic effectiveness and favorable safety/tolerability profiles of oliceridine regarding respiratory and gastrointestinal adverse effects compared to morphine have been confirmed in different Phase III studies [50–52]. In October 2018, the FDA Advisory Committee voted 8 against and 7 in favor of the approval of oliceridine for the management of moderate to severe acute pain. A new application was submitted and on the seventh August 2020 the FDA approved oliceridine with the name Olinvyk™ for short term intravenous use in "hospitals and other controlled settings". Oliceridine will soon be available in the market and larger studies will more thoroughly define its analgesic effectiveness and tolerability profiles in clinical practice.

Another interesting molecule acting as G-protein-biased mu-receptor agonist is PZM21 [53] (see chemical structure in Figure 3). This molecule was identified by docking over three million commercially available lead-like compounds with the orthosteric pocket of the 3D crystal structure of the mu receptor; solved in its inactive state in 2012 [54]. In receptor binding studies PZM21 displayed high affinity (pK_i 9) and selectivity for the mu opioid receptor. In functional studies PZM21 behaved as a potent agonist in different Gi/o-mediated signaling assays while it was virtually inactive in recruiting βarr2. Agonist activity of PZM21 in the βarr2 recruitment assay can be detected after transfecting cells with GRK2. However, under these conditions, the efficacy of PZM21 (0.32) was a fraction of that of DAMGO (1.00) and even morphine (0.52) [53]. Thus, these results suggest that PZM21 behaves as a mu receptor agonist biased toward G protein signaling. Of note in all these experiments oliceridine has been also assayed, producing results similar to those obtained with PZM21. When tested in mice, PZM21 (10–40 mg/kg) elicited antinociceptive effects in the hotplate and formalin test, but not in the mouse tail flick assay. The reason for these assay-specific effects of PZM21 are presently unknown. More important, the analgesic effects of PZM21 (as well as those of morphine) in the hotplate test were absent in mu receptor gene knockout mice. When tested in the mouse accumulated fecal boli assay at equianalgesic doses PZM21 elicited constipation that was less than that produced by morphine. Concerning respiratory effects, whole-body plethysmography studies demonstrated that while morphine profoundly depressed respiration, the effects of PZM21 was indistinguishable from vehicle [53]; however it should be noted that in these experiments the vehicle injection produced a respiratory depressant effect. Collectively, the results obtained with PZM21 confirm findings with oliceridine suggesting that mu receptor agonists biased toward G protein signaling elicit robust analgesia associated with less respiratory and gastrointestinal side effects.

However, some PZM21 findings were not confirmed in other studies. In bioluminescence resonance energy transfer (BRET) studies PZM21 behaved as a low efficacy partial agonist in promoting mu receptor interaction with both G protein and βarr2 [55]. The analgesic effect of PZM21 in the hot plate assay has been confirmed but this was associated with a clear inhibition of respiratory function. In mice receiving twice-daily doses of PZM21 for four days, complete tolerance developed to the antinociceptive but not respiratory depressant effects [55]. Similar findings were previously obtained with morphine in a study performed under the same experimental conditions [56]. Thus, in this latter study, no major differences were found between the pharmacological profile of PZM21 and that of the standard opioid analgesic morphine. PZM21 caused dose-dependent antinociception after systemic and spinal administration; after repeated administration tolerance developed to the antinociceptive actions of PZM21 and animals became physically dependent as demonstrated by naloxone-precipitated withdrawal syndrome [57]. Recently the actions of PZM21 were compared with those of morphine and oxycodone in non-human primates [58]. After systemic administration, PZM21-induced dose-dependent thermal antinociceptive effects being 10-fold less potent than oxycodone. In self-administration studies PZM21 exerted reinforcing effects similar to oxycodone. After intrathecal administration, PZM21 mimicked morphine, producing naltrexone sensitive antiallodynic effects associated with long-lasting scratching [58]. The chemical template of PZM21 has been used for structure activity relationship studies that led to the identification of novel G-protein-biased mu-receptor agonists [59,60].

Other compounds acting as selective mu-receptor agonists with different degrees of bias toward G protein signaling have been discovered in a study specifically aimed at investigating whether the magnitude of the bias factor of a mu agonist will impact its therapeutic index (analgesia versus respiratory depression) [61]. A series of compounds with a piperidine core structure were generated and demonstrated to act as high affinity and selective mu ligands in receptor binding studies. These novel compounds were investigated using the human recombinant mu receptor in functional assays including agonist stimulated GTPγ[^{35}S] binding, cAMP accumulation and βarr2 recruitment using the operational model [62] to estimate their bias factors. The pharmacological effects of these compounds were systematically compared to those of DAMGO as a reference agonist and of morphine and fentanyl as clinically relevant drugs. Results of these studies suggest that fentanyl and SR-11501 behave as mu receptor βarr2-biased agonists, morphine, SR-14968 and SR-14969 behave as unbiased agonists, SR-15098, SR-15099 and SR-17018 (see chemical structure in Figure 3) behave as G protein-biased agonists [61]. Importantly this rank order of bias remains the same when compounds were tested in preparations expressing the mouse mu opioid receptor. Pharmacokinetic studies demonstrated that these SR compounds are able to cross the blood–brain barrier after systemic administration. In the hot plate and tail withdrawal assays SR compounds elicited antinociceptive effects in wild type mice but not in mu receptor gene knockout mice, confirming their high selectivity of action in vivo. When tested for respiratory depressant effects (oxygen saturation and respiratory rate) at morphine equianalgesic doses SR-15098, SR-15099 and SR-17018 (i.e., those molecules showing the higher bias toward G proteins), produced the least respiratory suppression. To carefully estimate the therapeutic index of these molecules dose response studies were performed and ED_{50} values calculated for the analgesiometric assays (hot plate and tail withdrawal tests) and for respiratory depressant effects (oxygen saturation and respiratory rate). A robust correlation between bias factor and therapeutic index was found: the higher the bias toward G protein signaling, the higher the therapeutic index. In a recent study the effects of chronic treatment with SR–17018 via subcutaneous osmotic minipumps was investigated [63]. In contrast to morphine, SR–17018 does not produce tolerance in the hot plate test. However, after minipump removal, mice treated with SR–17018 displayed significant signs of withdrawal, similar to morphine [63].

Collectively the results of these studies appear to confirm the original hypothesis, based on work with βarr2(−/−) mice [18,19,24], that mu-receptor agonists that do not recruit βarr2 display reduced tolerance liability and, more important, are safer analgesics.

4. Pharmacological Studies—Are Mu Receptors Partial Agonists Safer Analgesics?

Direct comparison of the pharmacological features of novel molecules investigated in different laboratories, with different in vitro assays and protocols and diverse in vivo models is always difficult. Gillis et al. [64] reexamined the pharmacological profiles of the G protein-biased agonists oliceridine, PZM21 and SR–17018 in parallel experiments and compared the profiles with those of DAMGO and the clinically viable drugs fentanyl, methadone, morphine, oxycodone and buprenorphine. The mu agonist properties of this panel of ligands were carefully examined using rigorous pharmacological approaches, which consisted of using the same cell line (HEK293 cells expressing the human recombinant mu receptor) and a large panel of assays. To investigate mu/G protein pathways BRET-based assays were used to measure mu receptor interaction with a conformationally selective nanobody, with a truncated, soluble "mini" G_i protein and with $G\alpha_{i2}$. Moreover, mu receptor inhibition of cAMP levels via G_i was also studied with a BRET assay. In addition, Gβγ-mediated activation of GIRK channels was investigated with a membrane potential-sensitive dye. To investigate mu receptor regulatory pathways BRET-based assays were used to measure mu receptor interaction with GRK2 and βarr2 and also mu receptor internalization. Finally using phosphosite-specific antibodies, agonist-induced C-terminal phosphorylation of the mu receptor was studied. Importantly, in order to obtain robust and consistent concentration–response curves that allow a precise assessment of ligand potency and efficacy, manipulations were performed with the aim of avoiding conditions characterized by an extremely low or extremely high efficiency of the stimulus–response coupling. Thus, GIRK experiments were performed in the absence and presence of an irreversible mu antagonist, βarr2 recruitment and receptor internalization studies were performed in the absence and presence of overexpressed GRK2 and nanobody and mini G_i protein recruitment experiments were performed with an excess of reporter probes.

The results obtained in G protein assay demonstrated that oliceridine, PZM21 and SR–17018 are indeed mu receptor partial agonists. In particular the following rank order of maximal effects was determined: DAMGO = fentanyl = methadone > morphine = oxycodone > oliceridine = PZM21 ≥ SR–17018 ≥ buprenorphine which was highly conserved in all the assays (r^2 always ≥ 0.79) including ligand-induced C-terminal phosphorylation of the mu receptor. Of note is that the partial agonist behavior of PZM21 and oliceridine at the mu receptor has already been reported for ion channel signaling using electrophysiological and Ca^{2+} imaging techniques [65] and in biochemical assays (Azzam et al. personal communication). Surprisingly, this same rank order of maximal effects was measured in receptor regulatory pathway assays (GRK2 and βarr2 and receptor internalization) for all compounds; thus, suggesting that they have similar activity in both G protein and receptor regulatory pathways. These results were confirmed by operational model analysis that demonstrated across the different assays no significant bias factors for all ligands, including, the putative G-protein-biased-agonists oliceridine, PZM21 and SR–17018. For a comprehensive discussion of the possible reasons that may explain the discrepant results obtained by Gillis et al. [64] compared to previously published findings [35,53,61], the reader is referred to Gillis et al. [66].

In order to compare their analgesic and respiratory depressant effects, fentanyl, morphine, oliceridine, PZM21, SR–17018 and buprenorphine were evaluated in dose–response studies in the hot plate and whole-body plethysmography assays [64]. All compounds evoked robust and dose-dependent antinociceptive effects in the hot plate test with kinetics of action in line with previously published findings. However, the dose–response curve for SR–17018 could not be completed due to solubility issues. In whole-body plethysmography dose–response studies, all compound produced a statistically significant reduction in respiratory frequency, but the effects of buprenorphine, oliceridine, PZM21 and SR–17018 were lower than those of morphine or fentanyl. The results of in vivo experiments were then used to calculate the therapeutic index of these mu agonists (of note the therapeutic index of SR–17018 could only be roughly estimated due to incomplete dose–response curve data). The rank order of therapeutic indices was buprenorphine > SR–17018 = PZM21 ≥ oliceridine ≥ morphine ≥ fentanyl. There was no correlation between therapeutic index and bias factor while there was a clear inverse relationship between therapeutic index and ligand efficacy [64]. Importantly the above mentioned rank order of therapeutic index is in line with clinical studies suggesting the following rank order of tolerability for the treatment of moderate to severe pain buprenorphine > morphine ≥ fentanyl [67,68].

Collectively this study demonstrated that putative G-protein-biased agonists behave as low efficacy partial agonists. Moreover, this study confirmed the higher therapeutic index (analgesia versus respiratory depression) of oliceridine, PZM21 and SR–17018 (as well as buprenorphine) compared to classical opioid analgesics (morphine and fentanyl) and provides robust evidence that these actions are likely due to and can be predicted by, partial rather than biased agonism.

5. Conclusions

Early studies performed with βarr2(−/−) mice suggested that mu receptor interaction with βarr2 is involved in morphine gastrointestinal and respiratory side effects [24] but not its analgesic action [18]. This observation led to the hypothesis that mu-receptor agonists biased toward G protein may offer safety advantages as analgesics. This hypothesis was later confirmed in preclinical studies demonstrating that the mu receptor G protein-biased agonists oliceridine [35], PZM21 [53] and SR-17018 [61] displayed an improved therapeutic index compared to morphine. For oliceridine this improved therapeutic index has been confirmed in a large series of clinical studies [33]. However this general supposition of improved side effect profile has recently been questioned by the following data: different laboratories did not replicate the original findings regarding the improved therapeutic index of morphine in βarr2(−/−) mice [29], the therapeutic index of morphine is not improved in genetically engineered mice expressing G protein-biased mu receptors [30]. In addition, a recent study in which oliceridine, PZM21 and SR-17018 were tested in parallel in vitro and in vivo experiments confirmed the improved therapeutic indices of these mu ligands but demonstrated that their improved safety profile is likely attributable to low efficacy partial agonism rather than G protein-bias [64]. Based on the available evidence it is reasonable to suggest that the biased agonism as a strategy is unlikely to produce safer opioid analgesics. We close with the following statement from T Kenakin [16]: "biased signaling still has the potential to justify revisiting of receptor targets previously thought to be intractable and also furnishes the means to pursue targets previously thought to be forbidden due to deleterious physiology". Increasing the rate of success in drug discovery programs based on biased agonism requires rigorous pharmacological approaches to both assay development and data analysis. Moreover, knowledge of cell types responsible for specific pathologies and the associated signaling pathways activated during that pathological insult also require careful study, as discussed by Michel et al. [69].

Funding: This research was funded by the Italian Ministry of University (2015WX8Y5BB PRIN grant to GC) and from the University of Ferrara (FAR grant to GC, CR and RDG; FIR grant to CR). Work on opioids in the laboratory of DGL is funded by British Journal of Anesthesia and British Heart Foundation.

Conflicts of Interest: The authors declare no conflict of interest.

References

1. Leone, R.; Magro, L. In a Pharmaco-Vigillance.eu, Opioids: The Real Concern is That They are Not Used in Pain. 2015. Available online: https://www.farmacovigilanza.eu/content/oppioidi-la-vera-preoccupazione-%C3%A8-che-non-si-usano-nel-dolore (accessed on 22 July 2020).
2. Volkow, N.D.; Blanco, C. The changing opioid crisis: Development, challenges and opportunities. *Mol. Psychiatry* **2020**. [CrossRef]

3. Raffa, R.B.; Pergolizzi, J.V.; Taylor, R.; Ossipov, M.H. Indirect-acting strategy of opioid action instead of direct receptor activation: Dual-acting enkephalinase inhibitors (DENKIs). *J. Clin. Pharm. Ther.* **2018**, *43*, 443–449. [CrossRef] [PubMed]
4. Roques, B.P.; Fournié-Zaluski, M.C.; Wurm, M. Inhibiting the breakdown of endogenous opioids and cannabinoids to alleviate pain. *Nat. Rev. Drug Discov.* **2012**, *11*, 292–310. [CrossRef] [PubMed]
5. Remesic, M.; Hruby, V.J.; Porreca, F.; Lee, Y.S. Recent Advances in the Realm of Allosteric Modulators for Opioid Receptors for Future Therapeutics. *ACS Chem. Neurosci.* **2017**, *8*, 1147–1158. [CrossRef] [PubMed]
6. Livingston, K.E.; Traynor, J.R. Allostery at opioid receptors: Modulation with small molecule ligands. *Br. J. Pharmacol.* **2018**, *175*, 2846–2856. [CrossRef]
7. Sehgal, N.; Smith, H.; Manchikanti, L. Narrative Review Peripherally Acting Opioids and Clinical Implications for Pain Control. *Pain Physician* **2011**, *14*, 249–258.
8. Spahn, V.; Del Vecchio, G.; Rodriguez-Gaztelumendi, A.; Temp, J.; Labuz, D.; Kloner, M.; Reidelbach, M.; Machelska, H.; Weber, M.; Stein, C. Opioid receptor signaling, analgesic and side effects induced by a computationally designed pH-dependent agonist. *Sci. Rep.* **2018**, *8*, 8965. [CrossRef]
9. Rodriguez-Gaztelumendi, A.; Spahn, V.; Labuz, D.; MacHelska, H.; Stein, C. Analgesic effects of a novel pH-dependent m-opioid receptor agonist in models of neuropathic and abdominal pain. *Pain* **2018**, *159*, 2277–2284. [CrossRef]
10. Dietis, N.; Guerrini, R.; Calo, G.; Salvadori, S.; Rowbotham, D.; Lambert, D.G. Simultaneous targeting of multiple opioid receptors: A strategy to improve side-effect profil. *Br. J. Anaesth.* **2009**, *103*, 38–49. [CrossRef]
11. Azzam, A.A.H.; McDonald, J.; Lambert, D.G. Hot topics in opioid pharmacology: Mixed and biased opioids. *Br. J. Anaesth.* **2019**, *122*, e136–e145. [CrossRef]
12. Kiguchi, N.; Ding, H.; Ko, M.C. Therapeutic potentials of NOP and MOP receptor coactivation for the treatment of pain and opioid abuse. *J. Neurosci. Res.* **2020**. [CrossRef] [PubMed]
13. Linz, K.; Christoph, T.; Tzschentke, T.M.; Koch, T.; Schiene, K.; Gautrois, M.; Schröder, W.; Kögel, B.Y.; Beier, H.; Englberger, W.; et al. Cebranopadol: A novel potent analgesic nociceptin/orphanin FQ peptide and opioid receptor agonist. *J. Pharmacol. Exp. Ther.* **2014**, *349*, 535–548. [CrossRef] [PubMed]
14. Tzschentke, T.M.; Linz, K.; Koch, T.; Christoph, T. Cebranopadol: A novel first-in-class potent analgesic acting via NOP and opioid receptors. In *Handbook of Experimental Pharmacology*; Springer: New York, NY, USA, 2019; Volume 254, pp. 367–398. [CrossRef]
15. Calo, G.; Lambert, D.G. Nociceptin/orphanin FQ receptor ligands and translational challenges: Focus on cebranopadol as an innovative analgesic. *Br. J. Anaesth.* **2018**, *121*, 1105–1114. [CrossRef]
16. Kenakin, T. Biased receptor signaling in drug discovery. *Pharmacol. Rev.* **2019**, *71*, 267–315. [CrossRef] [PubMed]
17. Tan, L.; Yan, W.; McCorvy, J.D.; Cheng, J. Biased Ligands of G Protein-Coupled Receptors (GPCRs): Structure-Functional Selectivity Relationships (SFSRs) and Therapeutic Potential. *J. Med. Chem.* **2018**, *61*, 9841–9878. [CrossRef] [PubMed]
18. Bohn, L.M.; Lefkowitz, R.J.; Gainetdinov, R.R.; Peppel, K.; Caron, M.G.; Lin, F.T. Enhanced morphine analgesia in mice lacking β-arrestin 2. *Science* **1999**, *286*, 2495–2498. [CrossRef]
19. Bohn, L.M.; Gainetdinov, R.R.; Lin, F.T.; Lefkowitz, R.J.; Caron, M.G. µ-opioid receptor desensitization by β-arrestin-2 determines morphine tolerance but not dependence. *Nature* **2000**, *408*, 720–723. [CrossRef]
20. Bohn, L.M.; Gainetdinov, R.R.; Sotnikova, T.D.; Medvedev, I.O.; Lefkowitz, R.J.; Dykstra, L.A.; Caron, M.G. Enhanced Rewarding Properties of Morphine, but not Cocaine, in βarrestin-2 Knock-Out Mice. *J. Neurosci.* **2003**, *23*, 10265–10273. [CrossRef]
21. Farmer, A.D.; Drewes, A.M.; Chiarioni, G.; De Giorgio, R.; O'Brien, T.; Morlion, B.; Tack, J. Pathophysiology and management of opioid-induced constipation: European expert consensus statement. *United Eur. Gastroenterol. J.* **2019**, *7*, 7–20. [CrossRef]
22. Algera, M.H.; Kamp, J.; van der Schrier, R.; van Velzen, M.; Niesters, M.; Aarts, L.; Dahan, A.; Olofsen, E. Opioid-induced respiratory depression in humans: A review of pharmacokinetic–pharmacodynamic modelling of reversal. *Br. J. Anaesth.* **2019**, *122*, e168–e179. [CrossRef]
23. Kiyatkin, E.A. Respiratory depression and brain hypoxia induced by opioid drugs: Morphine, oxycodone, heroin, and fentanyl. *Neuropharmacology* **2019**, *151*, 219–226. [CrossRef] [PubMed]
24. Raehal, K.M.; Walker, J.K.L.; Bohn, L.M. Morphine side effects in β-arrestin 2 knockout mice. *J. Pharmacol. Exp. Ther.* **2005**, *314*, 1195–1201. [CrossRef] [PubMed]

25. Montandon, G.; Ren, J.; Victoria, N.C.; Liu, H.; Wickman, K.; Greer, J.J.; Horner, R.L. G-protein-gated inwardly rectifying potassium channels modulate respiratory depression by Opioids. *Anesthesiology* **2016**, *124*, 641–650. [CrossRef] [PubMed]
26. Levitt, E.S.; Abdala, A.P.; Paton, J.F.R.; Bissonnette, J.M.; Williams, J.T. μ opioid receptor activation hyperpolarizes respiratory-controlling Kölliker-Fuse neurons and suppresses post-inspiratory drive. *J. Physiol.* **2015**, *593*, 4453–4469. [CrossRef]
27. Madariaga-Mazón, A.; Marmolejo-Valencia, A.F.; Li, Y.; Toll, L.; Houghten, R.A.; Martinez-Mayorga, K. Mu-Opioid receptor biased ligands: A safer and painless discovery of analgesics? *Drug Discov. Today* **2017**, *22*, 1719–1729. [CrossRef]
28. Grim, T.W.; Acevedo-Canabal, A.; Bohn, L.M. Toward Directing Opioid Receptor Signaling to Refine Opioid Therapeutics. *Biol. Psychiatry* **2020**, *87*, 15–21. [CrossRef]
29. Kliewer, A.; Gillis, A.; Hill, R.; Schmiedel, F.; Bailey, C.; Kelly, E.; Henderson, G.; Christie, M.J.; Schulz, S. Morphine-induced respiratory depression is independent of β-arrestin2 signalling. *Br. J. Pharmacol.* **2020**, *177*, 2923–2931. [CrossRef]
30. Kliewer, A.; Schmiedel, F.; Sianati, S.; Bailey, A.; Bateman, J.T.; Levitt, E.S.; Williams, J.T.; Christie, M.J.; Schulz, S. Phosphorylation-deficient G-protein-biased μ-opioid receptors improve analgesia and diminish tolerance but worsen opioid side effects. *Nat. Commun.* **2019**, *10*, 367. [CrossRef]
31. Gurevich, V.V.; Gurevich, E.V. GPCR signaling regulation: The role of GRKs and arrestins. *Front. Pharmacol.* **2019**, *10*, 125. [CrossRef]
32. Rizzi, A.; Cerlesi, M.C.; Ruzza, C.; Malfacini, D.; Ferrari, F.; Bianco, S.; Costa, T.; Guerrini, R.; Trapella, C.; Calo', G. Pharmacological characterization of cebranopadol a novel analgesic acting as mixed nociceptin/orphanin FQ and opioid receptor agonist. *Pharmacol. Res. Perspect.* **2016**, *4*, e00247. [CrossRef]
33. Gan, T.J.; Wase, L. Oliceridine, a G protein-selective ligand at the μ-opioid receptor, for the management of moderate to severe acute pain. *Drugs Today* **2020**, *56*, 269–286. [CrossRef] [PubMed]
34. Chen, X.T.; Pitis, P.; Liu, G.; Yuan, C.; Gotchev, D.; Cowan, C.L.; Rominger, D.H.; Koblish, M.; Dewire, S.M.; Crombie, A.L.; et al. Structure-activity relationships and discovery of a g protein biased μ opioid receptor ligand, [(3-methoxythiophen-2-yl)methyl]({2-[(9 r)-9-(pyridin-2-yl)-6-oxaspiro-[4.5]decan-9-yl]ethyl})amine (TRV130), for the treatment of acute severe pain. *J. Med. Chem.* **2013**, *56*, 8019–8031. [CrossRef]
35. DeWire, S.M.; Yamashita, D.S.; Rominger, D.H.; Liu, G.; Cowan, C.L.; Graczyk, T.M.; Chen, X.T.; Pitis, P.M.; Gotchev, D.; Yuan, C.; et al. A G protein-biased ligand at the μ-opioid receptor is potently analgesic with reduced gastrointestinal and respiratory dysfunction compared with morphines. *J. Pharmacol. Exp. Ther.* **2013**, *344*, 708–717. [CrossRef] [PubMed]
36. Mori, T.; Kuzumaki, N.; Arima, T.; Narita, M.M.; Tateishi, R.; Kondo, T.; Hamada, Y.; Kuwata, H.; Kawata, M.; Yamazaki, M.; et al. Usefulness for the combination of G protein- and β-arrestin-biased ligands of μ-opioid receptors: Prevention of antinociceptive tolerance. *Mol. Pain* **2017**, *13*, 1744806917740030. [CrossRef] [PubMed]
37. Liang, D.Y.; Li, W.W.; Nwaneshiudu, C.; Irvine, K.A.; Clark, J.D. Pharmacological Characters of Oliceridine, a μ-Opioid Receptor G-Protein-Biased Ligand in Mice. *Anesth. Analg.* **2019**, *129*, 1414–1421. [CrossRef]
38. Austin Zamarripa, C.; Edwards, S.R.; Qureshi, H.N.; Yi, J.N.; Blough, B.E.; Freeman, K.B. The G-protein biased mu-opioid agonist, TRV130, produces reinforcing and antinociceptive effects that are comparable to oxycodone in rats. *Drug Alcohol Depend.* **2018**, *192*, 158–162. [CrossRef]
39. Schwienteck, K.L.; Faunce, K.E.; Rice, K.C.; Obeng, S.; Zhang, Y.; Blough, B.E.; Grim, T.W.; Negus, S.S.; Banks, M.L. Effectiveness comparisons of G-protein biased and unbiased mu opioid receptor ligands in warm water tail-withdrawal and drug discrimination in male and female rats. *Neuropharmacology* **2019**, *150*, 200–209. [CrossRef]
40. Altarifi, A.A.; David, B.; Muchhala, K.H.; Blough, B.E.; Akbarali, H.; Negus, S.S. Effects of acute and repeated treatment with the biased mu opioid receptor agonist TRV130 (oliceridine) on measures of antinociception, gastrointestinal function, and abuse liability in rodents. *J. Psychopharmacol.* **2017**, *31*, 730–739. [CrossRef]
41. Granier, S.; Manglik, A.; Kruse, A.C.; Kobilka, T.S.; Thian, F.S.; Weis, W.I.; Kobilka, B.K. Structure of the δ-opioid receptor bound to naltrindole. *Nature* **2012**, *485*, 400–404. [CrossRef]
42. Schneider, S.; Provasi, D.; Filizola, M. How oliceridine (TRV-130) binds and stabilizes a μ-opioid receptor conformational state that selectively triggers G protein signaling pathways. *Biochemistry* **2016**, *55*, 6456–6466. [CrossRef]

43. Cheng, J.X.; Cheng, T.; Li, W.H.; Liu, G.X.; Zhu, W.L.; Tang, Y. Computational insights into the G-protein-biased activation and inactivation mechanisms of the μ opioid receptor. *Acta Pharmacol. Sin.* **2018**, *39*, 154–164. [CrossRef]
44. Mafi, A.; Kim, S.-K.; Goddard, W.A. Mechanism of β-arrestin recruitment by the μ-opioid G protein-coupled receptor. *Proc. Natl. Acad. Sci. USA* **2020**, *117*, 16346–16355. [CrossRef]
45. Soergel, D.G.; Ann Subach, R.; Sadler, B.; Connell, J.; Marion, A.S.; Cowan, C.L.; Violin, J.D.; Lark, M.W. First clinical experience with TRV130: Pharmacokinetics and pharmacodynamics in healthy volunteers. *J. Clin. Pharmacol.* **2014**, *54*, 351–357. [CrossRef]
46. Soergel, D.G.; Subach, R.A.; Burnham, N.; Lark, M.W.; James, I.E.; Sadler, B.M.; Skobieranda, F.; Violin, J.D.; Webster, L.R. Biased agonism of the l-opioid receptor by TRV130 increases analgesia and reduces on-target adverse effects versus morphine: A randomized, double-blind, placebo-controlled, crossover study in healthy volunteers. *Pain* **2014**, *155*, 1829–1835. [CrossRef]
47. Viscusi, E.R.; Webster, L.; Kuss, M.; Daniels, S.; Bolognese, J.A.; Zuckerman, S.; Soergel, D.G.; Subach, R.A.; Cook, E.; Skobieranda, F. A randomized, phase 2 study investigating TRV130, a biased ligand of the -opioid receptor, for the intravenous treatment of acute pain. *Pain* **2016**, *157*, 264–272. [CrossRef]
48. Singla, N.; Minkowitz, H.S.; Soergel, D.G.; Burt, D.A.; Subach, R.A.; Salamea, M.Y.; Fossler, M.J.; Skobieranda, F. A randomized, phase IIb study investigating oliceridine (TRV130), a novel μ-receptor G-protein pathway selective (μ-GPS) modulator, for the management of moderate to severe acute pain following abdominoplasty. *J. Pain Res.* **2017**, *10*, 2413–2424. [CrossRef]
49. Dahan, A.; van Dam, C.J.; Niesters, M.; van Velzen, M.; Fossler, M.J.; Demitrack, M.A.; Olofsen, E. Benefit and Risk Evaluation of Biased μ-Receptor Agonist Oliceridine versus Morphine. *Anesthesiology* **2020**, *133*, 559–568. [CrossRef]
50. Singla, N.K.; Skobieranda, F.; Soergel, D.G.; Salamea, M.; Burt, D.A.; Demitrack, M.A.; Viscusi, E.R. APOLLO-2: A Randomized, Placebo and Active-Controlled Phase III Study Investigating Oliceridine (TRV130), a G Protein–Biased Ligand at the μ-Opioid Receptor, for Management of Moderate to Severe Acute Pain Following Abdominoplasty. *Pain Pract.* **2019**, *19*, 715–731. [CrossRef]
51. Viscusi, E.R.; Skobieranda, F.; Soergel, D.G.; Cook, E.; Burt, D.A.; Singla, N. APOLLO-1: A randomized placebo and activecontrolled phase iii study investigating oliceridine (TRV130), a G protein-biased ligand at the μ-opioid receptor, for management of moderateto-severe acute pain following bunionectomy. *J. Pain Res.* **2019**, *12*, 927–943. [CrossRef]
52. Bergese, S.D.; Brzezinski, M.; Hammer, G.B.; Beard, T.L.; Pan, P.H.; Mace, S.E.; Berkowitz, R.D.; Cochrane, K.; Wase, L.; Minkowitz, H.S.; et al. ATHENA: A phase 3, open-label study of the safety and effectiveness of oliceridine (TRV130), a g-protein selective agonist at the μ-opioid receptor, in patients with moderate to severe acute pain requiring parenteral opioid therapy. *J. Pain Res.* **2019**, *12*, 3113–3126. [CrossRef]
53. Manglik, A.; Lin, H.; Aryal, D.K.; McCorvy, J.D.; Dengler, D.; Corder, G.; Levit, A.; Kling, R.C.; Bernat, V.; Hübner, H.; et al. Structure-based discovery of opioid analgesics with reduced side effects. *Nature* **2016**, *537*, 185–190. [CrossRef] [PubMed]
54. Manglik, A.; Kruse, A.C.; Kobilka, T.S.; Thian, F.S.; Mathiesen, J.M.; Sunahara, R.K.; Pardo, L.; Weis, W.I.; Kobilka, B.K.; Granier, S. Crystal structure of the μ-opioid receptor bound to a morphinan antagonist. *Nature* **2012**, *485*, 321–326. [CrossRef] [PubMed]
55. Hill, R.; Disney, A.; Conibear, A.; Sutcliffe, K.; Dewey, W.; Husbands, S.; Bailey, C.; Kelly, E.; Henderson, G. The novel μ-opioid receptor agonist PZM21 depresses respiration and induces tolerance to antinociception. *Br. J. Pharmacol.* **2018**, *175*, 2653–2661. [CrossRef]
56. Hill, R.; Lyndon, A.; Withey, S.; Roberts, J.; Kershaw, Y.; Maclachlan, J.; Lingford-Hughes, A.; Kelly, E.; Bailey, C.; Hickman, M.; et al. Ethanol reversal of tolerance to the respiratory depressant effects of morphine. *Neuropsychopharmacology* **2016**, *41*, 762–773. [CrossRef]
57. Kudla, L.; Bugno, R.; Skupio, U.; Wiktorowska, L.; Solecki, W.; Wojtas, A.; Golembiowska, K.; Zádor, F.; Benyhe, S.; Buda, S.; et al. Functional characterization of a novel opioid, PZM21, and its effects on the behavioural responses to morphine. *Br. J. Pharmacol.* **2019**, *176*, 4434–4445. [CrossRef]
58. Ding, H.; Kiguchi, N.; Perrey, D.; Nguyen, T.; Czoty, P.; Hsu, F.-C.; Zhang, Y.; Ko, M.C. Antinociceptive, Reinforcing, and Pruritic Effects of a G-Protein Signalling-Biased Mu Opioid Receptor Agonist, PZM21, in Nonhuman Primates. *Br. J. Anaesth.* **2020**, in press. [CrossRef]

59. Ma, M.; Sun, J.; Li, M.; Yu, Z.; Cheng, J.; Zhong, B.; Shi, W. Synthesis and evaluation of novel biased μ-opioid-receptor (μOR) agonists. *Molecules* **2019**, *24*, 259. [CrossRef]
60. Ma, M.; Li, X.; Tong, K.; Cheng, J.; Yu, Z.; Ren, F.; Zhong, B.; Shi, W. Discovery of Biased Mu-Opioid Receptor Agonists for the Treatment of Pain. *ChemMedChem* **2020**, *15*, 155–161. [CrossRef]
61. Schmid, C.L.; Kennedy, N.M.; Ross, N.C.; Lovell, K.M.; Yue, Z.; Morgenweck, J.; Cameron, M.D.; Bannister, T.D.; Bohn, L.M. Bias Factor and Therapeutic Window Correlate to Predict Safer Opioid Analgesics. *Cell* **2017**, *171*, 1165.e13–1175.e13. [CrossRef]
62. Black, J.W.; Leff, P. Operational models of pharmacological agonism. *Proc. R. Soc. Biol. Sci.* **1983**, *220*, 141–162. [CrossRef]
63. Grim, T.W.; Schmid, C.L.; Stahl, E.L.; Pantouli, F.; Ho, J.H.; Acevedo-Canabal, A.; Kennedy, N.M.; Cameron, M.D.; Bannister, T.D.; Bohn, L.M. A G protein signaling-biased agonist at the μ-opioid receptor reverses morphine tolerance while preventing morphine withdrawal. *Neuropsychopharmacology* **2020**, *45*, 416–425. [CrossRef] [PubMed]
64. Gillis, A.; Gondin, A.B.; Kliewer, A.; Sanchez, J.; Lim, H.D.; Alamein, C.; Manandhar, P.; Santiago, M.; Fritzwanker, S.; Schmiedel, F.; et al. Low intrinsic efficacy for G protein activation can explain the improved side effect profiles of new opioid agonists. *Sci. Signal.* **2020**, *13*, eaaz3140. [CrossRef] [PubMed]
65. Yudin, Y.; Rohacs, T. The G-protein-biased agents PZM21 and TRV130 are partial agonists of μ-opioid receptor-mediated signalling to ion channels. *Br. J. Pharmacol.* **2019**, *176*, 3110–3125. [CrossRef]
66. Gillis, A.; Sreenivasan, V.; Christie, M.J. Intrinsic efficacy of opioid ligands and its importance for apparent bias, operational analysis and therapeutic window. *Mol. Pharmacol.* **2020**, *14*, mol.119.119214. [CrossRef]
67. Dahan, A. Opioid-induced respiratory effects: New data on buprenorphine. *Palliat. Med.* **2006**, *20*, s3–s8.
68. Wolff, R.F.; Aune, D.; Truyers, C.; Hernandez, A.V.; Misso, K.; Riemsma, R.; Kleijnen, J. Systematic review of efficacy and safety of buprenorphine versus fentanyl or morphine in patients with chronic moderate to severe pain. *Curr. Med. Res. Opin.* **2012**, *28*, 833–845. [CrossRef]
69. Michel, M.C.; Charlton, S.J. Biased agonism in drug discovery-is it too soon to choose a path? *Mol. Pharmacol.* **2018**, *93*, 259–265. [CrossRef]

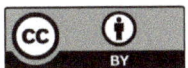

© 2020 by the authors. Licensee MDPI, Basel, Switzerland. This article is an open access article distributed under the terms and conditions of the Creative Commons Attribution (CC BY) license (http://creativecommons.org/licenses/by/4.0/).

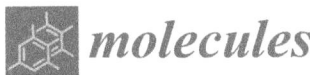

Review

Biased Opioid Antagonists as Modulators of Opioid Dependence: Opportunities to Improve Pain Therapy and Opioid Use Management

Wolfgang Sadee [1,2,3,*], John Oberdick [4] and Zaijie Wang [5]

1. Department of Cancer Biology and Genetics, College of Medicine, The Ohio State University, Columbus, OH 43210, USA
2. Aether Therapeutics Inc., 4200 Marathon Blvd. Austin, TX 78756, USA
3. Pain and Addiction Research Center, University of California San Francisco, San Francisco, CA 94158, USA
4. Department of Neuroscience, College of Medicine, The Ohio State University Wexner Medical Center, Columbus, OH 43210, USA; John.Oberdick@osumc.edu
5. Departments of Pharmaceutical Sciences and Neurology, University of Illinois at Chicago. Chicago, IL 60612, USA; zjwang@uic.edu
* Correspondence: wolfgang.sadee@osumc.edu

Academic Editor: Mariana Spetea
Received: 31 July 2020; Accepted: 4 September 2020; Published: 11 September 2020

Abstract: Opioid analgesics are effective pain therapeutics but they cause various adverse effects and addiction. For safer pain therapy, biased opioid agonists selectively target distinct μ opioid receptor (MOR) conformations, while the potential of biased opioid antagonists has been neglected. Agonists convert a dormant receptor form (MOR-μ) to a ligand-free active form (MOR-μ*), which mediates MOR signaling. Moreover, MOR-μ converts spontaneously to MOR-μ* (basal signaling). Persistent upregulation of MOR-μ* has been invoked as a hallmark of opioid dependence. Contrasting interactions with both MOR-μ and MOR-μ* can account for distinct pharmacological characteristics of inverse agonists (naltrexone), neutral antagonists (6β-naltrexol), and mixed opioid agonist-antagonists (buprenorphine). Upon binding to MOR-μ*, naltrexone but not 6β-naltrexol suppresses MOR-μ*signaling. Naltrexone blocks opioid analgesia non-competitively at MOR-μ*with high potency, whereas 6β-naltrexol must compete with agonists at MOR-μ, accounting for ~100-fold lower in vivo potency. Buprenorphine's bell-shaped dose–response curve may also result from opposing effects on MOR-μ and MOR-μ*. In contrast, we find that 6β-naltrexol potently prevents dependence, below doses affecting analgesia or causing withdrawal, possibly binding to MOR conformations relevant to opioid dependence. We propose that 6β-naltrexol is a biased opioid antagonist modulating opioid dependence at low doses, opening novel avenues for opioid pain therapy and use management.

Keywords: μ opioid receptor; receptor model; biased ligands; dependence; pain therapy; neonatal opioid withdrawal syndrome; naltrexone; 6β-naltrexol; buprenorphine

1. Introduction

The μ opioid receptor (MOR) is the main target of opioid analgesics, providing strong pain relief but also causing multiple adverse effects and addiction. Documented to exist in multiple forms with distinct functions, MOR and its ligands elicit a perplexingly broad spectrum of effects—opening the opportunity for discovering opioid analgesics with reduced adverse effects. Among these, biased agonist ligands can be directed to stimulate optimal MOR signaling properties [1]. On the other hand, biased MOR antagonists capable of blocking deleterious signaling or regulatory pathways have received less attention. Reviewing documented opioid drug effects, we propose a novel receptor model that can account for diverse pharmacological effects of MOR ligands, including biased antagonists. The type of ligand considered here is thought to differ from allosteric modulators of MOR [2,3] by interacting with the orthosteric site of agonist binding. Biased MOR antagonists could serve as modulators of opioid dependence, for improved pain therapy and opioid use management.

2. Evidence for Multiple Receptor Conformations with Distinct Signaling Pathways, and the Potential of Biased Agonists

G protein coupled receptors (GPCRs) are flexible membrane proteins that require lipids, signaling proteins, and co-factors or ligands to attain conformational stability. As a result, GPCRs exist in various conformations as a function of cellular environment, each accepting a distinct spectrum of ligands associated with distinct signaling or regulatory pathways [1,4–6]. These properties of GPCRs have triggered a search for biased agonists that selectively activate one pathway over the other, to enhance desired pharmacological outcomes relative to adverse effects [6–10]. MOR indeed appears to exist in multiple forms with distinct signaling and regulatory pathways [1]. Focus in the opioid field has been on creating efficacious pain therapies without unwanted side effects, including tolerance, dependence, and drug craving—hallmarks of addiction—respiratory depression, and various adverse effects (constipation and opioid-induced bowel dysfunction, bone loss, immune dysregulation, nausea, and more) [1–3,11]. MOR is considered a main mediator of these actions. Separating desirable from adverse effects is a central goal of current opioid research.

Biased agonists binding to receptors either coupled to G proteins or interacting with other scaffolding proteins including beta-arrestins have taken center stage in the search for opioid analgesics with less tolerance and withdrawal effects [1,12] and low respiratory depression potential [9]—The latter is a cause of countless overdose deaths. While beta-arrestins are thought mainly to orchestrate receptor desensitization, they can also activate tyrosine kinases and downstream signaling [13]. Results with biased opioid agonists are promising but must still be viewed with caution, as none are as of yet approved for general use.

Some reports propose that opioid receptors and specifically MOR exist in different forms in peripheral versus central neurons [13]. Peripheral and central opioid receptor systems could interact dynamically, for example in the induction of opioid induced hyperalgesia, reported to be mediated both centrally and peripherally [14,15]. Peripheral MOR sites could have relevance to inflammation induced neuropathic pain, invoking beta-arestin-2 silenced MOR sites in afferent nociceptors [14,16], that get activated upon inflammatory stimuli. MOR activation could then suppress pain sensation, but also lead to a vicious circle of sustained neuropathic pain [14,16]. While an attractive model to account for the presence of 'silent' MOR sites, the evidence is still missing how the activation occurs and whether these silent MOR sites perform signaling not measured by conventional means.

All extant MOR signaling models can account for only part of the astounding diversity of pharmacological effects observed in countless published studies, including unexpected opioid antagonist effects—the focus of this article to explore opportunities for developing safer opioid analgesics.

3. A Basally Active Receptor Mediating MOR Signaling (MOR-μ*)

Capable of signaling spontaneously, GPCRs are restrained in an inactive ground state consisting of large complexes with lipids, proteins, and co-factors. Upon binding to this ground state, agonists trigger a change in receptor conformation sufficient to release constraints keeping the receptor silent, thereby, initiating the signaling cascade. Hence, ground and activated receptor states of the μ opioid receptor, designated here as MOR-μ and MOR-μ*, respectively, assume distinct conformations, often leading to reduced agonist binding affinity to MOR-μ* (Figure 1) [17–19]. Typical opioid drugs such as morphine and etorphine potently bind to the ground state MOR-μ but rapidly dissociate from MOR-μ* [20]. However, continued association of the agonist with the activated receptor is also possible and could contribute to biased agonist signaling for some GPCRs [9]. We have shown that the ultra-potent etorphine enters the rat brain and occupies only 1% of MOR sites at its antinociceptive EC50 (<0.001 mg/kg) [20], previously suggested to indicate a 'receptor reserve' [21]. It appears more likely that etorphine binds with high affinity to MOR-µ and upon rapid activation dissociates from MOR-µ*, which carries out the signaling process in the absence of agonist ligand. Consistent with this hypothesis, we had shown that the etorphine off-rate has a dissociation half-life (t1/2) less than 1 min in vivo (rat brain), whereas, after sacrifice and tissue homogenization, the dissociation t1/2 increases to ~40 min [20]—the in vivo activation state no longer remains intact. Therefore, it is important to consider the relative affinities and effects of ligands at both MOR-µ and MOR-µ* in life tissues, to understand opioid effects.

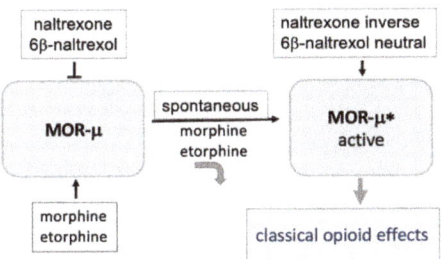

Figure 1. Model of the µ opioid receptor, invoking a silent ground state MOR-µ and a ligand-free activated state µ opioid receptor (MOR)-µ*. Most opioid agonists have low affinity for MOR-µ*, and therefore, dissociate from the receptor, with MOR-µ* responsible for the signaling process. The antagonists naltrexone and 6b-naltrexol (6BN) are proposed to have high affinity for both MOR-µ and MOR-µ*, blocking agonist-mediated activation of MOR-µ in a competitive fashion. Naltrexone potently blocks MOR-µ* activity as an inverse agonist, whereas the neutral antagonist 6BN binds to MOR-µ* but does not prevent signaling—both acting in a non-competitive fashion at the ligand-free MOR-µ.

We and others had further demonstrated that the ground state MOR-µ receptor can spontaneously convert to active MOR-µ*, in the absence of any ligand (Figure 1) [17–19,22], as demonstrated for numerous GPCRs. Moreover, basal MOR-µ* activity increases upon sustained opioid agonist exposure and appears to play a role in opioid dependence [17–19,22]—the mechanism by which elevated MOR-µ* signaling is maintained over time remains elusive. Enhanced MOR-µ* activity results in high sensitivity to inverse opioid antagonists such as naloxone and naltrexone, apparently acting at the ligand-free MOR-µ* in a non-competitive fashion, with as little as 50–100 microgram naloxone given iv causing aversive reactions in methadone-managed opioid use patients (typically receiving 50–100 mg/day methadone). We propose that pharmacological MOR antagonist effects reflect binding affinity and efficacy at both MOR-µ and MOR-µ*. Three opioid drugs serve to illustrate these interactions.

Naltrexone: Naltrexone is clinically used to prevent opioid relapse and reduce alcohol binge drinking [23–25]. An inverse antagonist, naltrexone suppresses basal MOR-µ* activity and thereby potently causes withdrawal symptoms in dependent subjects [19,26–29]. In addition, naltrexone antagonizes antinociception of 30 mg/kg morphine with an IC50 of 0.007 mg/kg in mice [26] (Table 1). This extraordinary potency against a high agonist dose can be accounted for by non-competitive binding of naltrexone to morphine-generated ligand-free MOR-µ*, thereby suppressing signaling activity. Similar high naltrexone potency has been reported in rhesus monkeys against both fentanyl analgesia and in causing withdrawal in dependent animals (pA2 8.5 mg/kg) [29] (Table 1). Because strong naltrexone-induced withdrawal reactions continue in dependent subjects even after the opioid drug has been fully excreted, naltrexone therapy to prevent relapse is started only 1–2 weeks after complete opioid withdrawal [30].

Table 1. Relative potency of naltrexone and 6BN in vivo. Data are from publications that compare naltrexone with 6BN, with regards to opioid antinociception or causing withdrawal in opioid-dependent animals, and in vitro MOR binding in rhesus monkey cortical brain homogenates.

Species	Test	Agonist (Dose, Route)	Antagonist ID50, or pA2, KI Binding (Rote)		Ref.
			Naltrexone	6β-Naltrexol	
mouse	hotplate	morphine (30 mg/kg, i.p.)	0.007 mg/kg (i.p.)	1.3 mg/kg (i.p.)	[26]
mouse	withdrawal jumping	morphine (73 mg pellet, s.c., 3d)	0.09 mg/kg (i.p.)	6.9 mg/kg (i.p.)	[27]
mouse	tail-flick	hydrocodone (3.2 mg/kg, i.v.)	0.53 mg/kg (p.o.) *	2.4 mg/kg (p.o.) *	[31]
rhesus monkey	tail-withdrawal	alfentanil (0.01–5 mg/kg, s.c.)	pA2 8.5 * (0.0032–0.32 mg/kg, s.c.)	pA2 6.5* (0.32–3.2 mg/kg, s.c.)	[29]
rhesus monkey	precipitated withdrawal	morphine (6.4 mg/kg, i.m. for 3d) (respiratory functions)	0.004 mg/kg (i.m. for 3d)	0.33 mg/kg (i.m. for 3d)	[29]
rhesus monkey	MOR binding,	^{3}H-DAMGO (1 nM, in vitro) ^{3}H-diprenorphine (0.2 nM)	0.31 nM, Ki = 1.7 nM	Ki = 0.74 nM KI = 3.2 nM	[29]

* pA2 values are—log measures; i.e., 6BN is 100-fold less potent than naltrexone.

6β-naltrexol (6BN): Naltrexone is converted to its main metabolite 6BN, a neutral antagonist (Figure 2) [19,27,28]. With the hypothesis that 6BN binds potently to MOR-µ* without suppressing signaling, we propose that 6BN blocks opioid analgesia or causes withdrawal only at much higher doses (Table 1) because it needs to compete with the opioid agonist at MOR-µ (Figure 1). Even though in vitro MOR binding affinity is nearly equal to that of naltrexone (Ki 3.2 nM vs. 1.7 nM, respectively, in rhesus monkeys [29]), 6BN is >100-fold less potent than naltrexone in blocking antinociception and causing withdrawal, in mice, guinea pigs, and rhesus monkeys [26–29] (Table 1). For example 6BN has an ID50 of 1.3 mg/kg in reversing morphine antinociception in mice vs. 0.007 mg/kg naltrexone [26]. In view of near equal binding affinity at MOR (Table 1), these results cannot be fully accounted for by slower access of 6BN to the brain (see below), but are resolved if 6BN indeed binds potently to MOR-µ* while not preventing MOR-µ* signaling, acting as a neutral antagonist. At higher doses only, 6BN is capable of competing with the opioid agonist at MOR-µ, preemptively preventing its activation to MOR-µ* by an agonist. As a result, 6BN blocks opioid analgesia only at high doses, or requires high doses to cause withdrawal in a dependent subject present [18,31]. After withdrawal when the opioid is excreted, for example 24 h after the last morphine dose in mice, 6BN no longer causes withdrawal. In contrast, naloxone and naltrexone still elicit substantial withdrawal at 24 h and later by blocking MOR-µ* activity, which is sustained and thereby also maintains the dependent state [27].

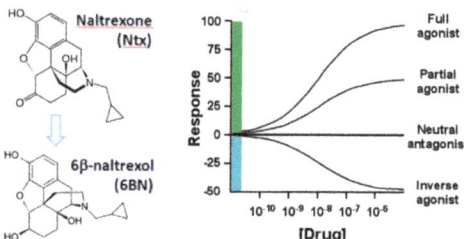

Figure 2. Metabolic conversion of naltrexone to 6BN, and hypothetical dose–response curves for agonists and antagonists. Etorphine is considered a full agonist and morphine a partial agonist, while 6BN is a neutral antagonist, and naltrexone an inverse agonist–the efficacy as an inverse agonist remains to be determined–measured against BTNX considered a full antagonist. Naltrexone and naloxone are near neutral antagonists in an opioid-naïve state, possibly because basal MOR-µ* activity is low in brain regions involved in withdrawal activity.

These properties of neutral MOR antagonists such as 6BN, naloxol, and naltrexamine, and their derivatives [31], offer new approaches to the management of drug use disorder. Similar receptor models may also apply to other opioid receptors (DOR and KOR), and more broadly to other GPCR families. 6BN and its analogues bind to MOR, DOR, and KOR, but inverse and neutral efficacy may differ between receptors; for example, 6BN acts as an inverse agonist at KOR after agonist pretreatment in tissue culture, whereas naltrexone appears to be neutral [32]. The influence of 6BN interactions with DOR and KOR remain to be studied.

Buprenorphine. For treatment of opioid use disorder, buprenorphine has been adopted broadly as it has only intermediate efficacy at MOR, but suppresses drug craving [33]. Mixed agonists–antagonists are less efficacious analgesics that can cause withdrawal in highly dependent subjects if they fail to elicit the level of MOR signaling needed in profound dependence [34]. Partial opioid agonists and mixed agonists–antagonists may stay engaged with MOR-μ for a longer time period before activation to MOR-μ*, and they also could retain some affinity for MOR-μ*. In animal studies, buprenorphine displays an unusual inverse bell-shaped dose–response curve in antinociceptive tests and in drug seeking behavior [35,36], antagonizing its own action at very high doses. We had observed that administration of high buprenorphine doses to rats first leads to sedation and catatonia, but when more buprenorphine floods into the brain, the animals wake up and behave normally, only to revert to a catatonic state when drug levels begin to decrease again before returning to normal activity (unpublished observations). Several hypotheses have been proposed to account for this pharmacological effect, but the answer has remained delusive. Considering the MOR model shown in Figure 1, a parsimonious solution offers itself: assume buprenorphine activates MOR-μ to an intermediate level, it then dissociates and enables MOR-μ* signaling to occur. However, buprenorphine could have residual and sufficient affinity to MOR-μ* to bind to it when given at higher doses, but then acting as an inverse agonist at MOR-μ*. In this fashion, buprenorphine can indeed antagonize its own action at high doses. While this hypothesis requires further testing, it can serve as a conceptual template for new drug development.

4. Peripherally Active μ Opioid Receptor Antagonists (PAMORA) and 6β-Naltrexol

The peripheral opioid system plays multiple roles, for example in the g.i. tract and in nociceptor neurons, the latter involved in peripheral analgesia [37]. PAMORAs including methylnaltrexone, naloxegol, alvimopan, and naldemdine are in clinical use to treat opioid-induced bowel dysfunction and constipation [15,38]. Peripheral selectivity is thought to depend on limited access to the CNS through the blood–brain-barrier (BBB), either because of high polarity or by extrusion via export transporters [39]. Similarly, 6BN has somewhat restricted access to the CNS, in part accounting for its peripheral selectivity. This leads to 5–10 fold higher 6BN blood over brain levels, and higher potency in blocking opioid effects on the g.i. tract in mice compared to centrally mediated opioid antinociception [40]. In opioid-naïve human volunteers, 6BN blocks morphine-induced slowing of bowel movements with an IC50 of ~3 mg (both drugs given i.v.), whereas analgesia measured in a cold pressure assay was unaffected by the highest tested dose of 20 mg 6BN [41].

Recent results indicate that 6BN's peripheral selectivity is not solely due to slow penetration of the BBB. Whereas, we have found higher blood than brain 6BN levels in mice [42] and guinea pigs [43], 6BN enters the brain of rhesus monkeys with less restriction, resulting in equal blood and brain levels (Figure 3). Yet, 6BN is >100-fold less potent than naltrexone in blocking fentanyl antinociception and in causing withdrawal in rhesus monkeys [29], similar to what is found in mice and guinea pigs. Testing the potency of naltrexone and 6BN in antagonizing the fentanyl-induced suppression of electrically stimulated peristalsis in the guinea pig ileum, Porter et al. [26] reported IC50 concentrations of 0.26 and 0.09 nM, respectively, showing that 6BN was not only highly potent in this assay, but also more potent than naltrexone, in contrast to its slightly lower affinity to MOR measured in vitro. These results are inconsistent with canonical MOR receptor models, but rather suggests the presence of additional MOR conformations of yet unknown structure and function, with high 6BN affinity.

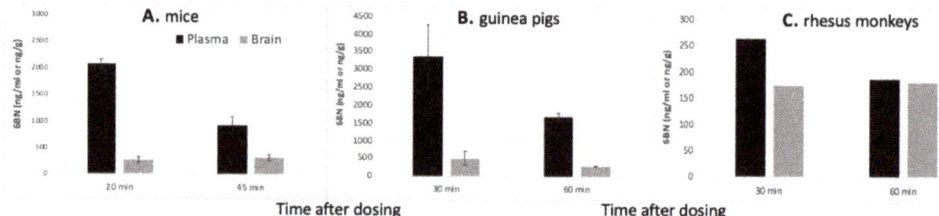

Figure 3. Maternal plasma and brain levels of 6BN in adult female pregnant mice, guinea pigs, and rhesus monkeys. (**A**) 6BN levels in mice at 20 and 45 min after injection (10 mg/kg, s.c.) (data from [42]). (**B**) 6BN levels in guinea pigs at 30 and 60 min after injection (10/mg/kg, s.c.) (data from [43]). (**C**) 6BN levels in rhesus monkeys at 30 and 60 min after injection (2 mg/kg, i.v.) (J. Oberdick, unpublished; n = 1 at each time point; a range of 6BN doses and regimen gave similar results).

The possible presence of distinct MOR conformations, or varying relative abundance between conformations as a function of cellular environment, and in the periphery compared to the CNS, has been reviewed by Jeske [13], suggesting that beta-arrestin coupled MOR sites in afferent nociceptors account for their silent status, being activated only upon inflammatory stimuli. MOR-μ* basal activity appears also to be absent in peripheral afferent nociceptor neurons, but emerges upon nociceptive stimuli as a physiological countermeasure leading to abatement of neuropathic pain [16,44]. However, if such basal MOR activity fails to be reversed, it can contribute to chronic neuropathic pain. Only 6BN, but not naltrexone, can facilitate the reversal of chronic neuropathic pain, revealing the biological relevance of MOR-μ* basal activity [16,44]. Whether such MOR sites also exist in the g.i. tract remains to be determined. The finding of extreme 6BN potency in the guinea pig ileum indicates the existence of MOR sites at which 6BN may act with high potency in a non-competitive manner.

We have observed that 6BN becomes more potent in blocking gastrointestinal effects of morphine in mice when pre-administered, with maximum potency reached at ~100 min before morphine [26]. This result supports a model in which MOR exists in two different conformations, namely MOR-μ and a novel MOR form of yet unknown function. We hypothesize that this MOR state is in equilibrium with MOR-μ and is stabilized by 6BN binding, shifting the equilibrium away from MOR-μ, thereby preventing activation to MOR-μ*. Such equilibrium between receptor states could exist in the CNS as well, but with tissue specific preference for one form or the other—a potential mechanism for peripheral selectivity of some opioid ligands. This MOR model also predicts novel actions of ligands such as 6BN in modulating MOR signaling—for example affecting opioid dependence.

5. 6BN Prevents Development of Opioid Dependence with High Potency

Repeated use of opioid analgesics leads to tolerance, dependence, hyperalgesia, and drug seeking behavior. All these effects underlie distinct processes while common mechanisms may also exist leading to opioid addiction. We have postulated that increased and sustained formation of MOR-μ* characterizes the dependent state, accounting for the high potency of inverse agonists to elicit withdrawal behavior [17–19,22]. Here, we address the novel hypothesis that an as yet poorly defined receptor conformation may be involved in dependence, possibly with high affinity for 6BN.

In a first set of experiments, we tested whether 6BN given together with daily doses of morphine (10–20 mg/kg) for 6 days prevents naloxone-induced withdrawal behavior in juvenile mice (5–15 days old)—with the goal of developing a model for preventive therapy for neonatal opioid withdrawal syndrome (NOWS). In juvenile mice, 6BN readily enters the brain as the BBB remains underdeveloped until day 20 post-partum, while naloxone-induced opioid dependence can be readily measured at 10–18 days after birth [42]. Co-administration of 6BN with morphine potently prevents naloxone-induced withdrawal, tested 3 h after the last dose. 6BN displayed an IC50 of ~0.03 mg/kg (Figure 4) [42], substantially below the expected antinociceptive IC50 in adult mice [27]. In this experimental design, morphine is not yet completely eliminated from the circulation at time of testing, yielding a rather shallow dose–response curve as naloxone acts by both blocking MOR-μ* and antagonizing morphine at MOR-μ, the latter process not expected to be affected by 6BN. In addition, we had observed that naloxone-induced withdrawal jumping was delayed even at the lowest dose of 6BN tested (0.0067 mg/kg) [42]. These results suggest that 6BN reduces or prevents dependence at exceedingly low doses that do not block antinociceptive effects nor cause immediate withdrawal.

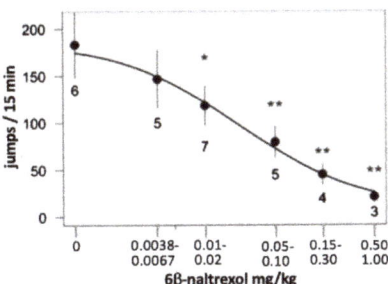

Figure 4. Co-administration (s.c.) of 6BN with morphine daily over 5 days to juvenile mice potently reduces naloxone-induced withdrawal behavior. Morphine injections were started on postnatal day 12 at 10 mg/kg for 3 days, followed by 3 days of 20 mg/kg. Increasing doses of 6BN were co-administered, with the dose doubled when morphine was doubled. On day 6, 30 mg/kg naloxone was injected s.c., and withdrawal jumping was measured. * p, 0.05; and ** p, 0.01 compared to no 6BN (adapted from [42]).

Encouraged by these results, we subsequently tested co-administration to adult guinea pigs of 6BN with methadone (10 mg/kg) for 3 days, with withdrawal testing on day 4, finding an IC50 6BN dose of ~0.01 mg/kg to block naloxone-induced locomotion [43], two orders of magnitude below the dose required to block antinociception [26]. Similarly, co-administration of an s.c. dose as low as 0.03 mg/kg 6BN completely suppresses naloxone-induced withdrawal jumping in adult mice made dependent on morphine (10 mg/kg for 5 days) (Z. Wang; unpublished data). Lastly, Oberdick et al. have tested daily 6BN co-treatment with methadone (5–7 mg/kg, s.c.) in pregnant guinea pig dams, starting at gestational day 50 until delivery (GD~60), to prevent withdrawal behavior in guinea pig pups measured one day after birth. Even though placental 6BN transfer is slower in pregnant guinea pigs compared to mice and rhesus monkeys, the IC50 of 6BN is ~0.025 mg/kg, again displaying unexpected potency [43].

Taken together, these results demonstrate that 6BN possesses high potency in preventing the development of dependence during repeated opioid drug exposure, at doses that do not affect antinociception nor cause overt withdrawal. The high potency of 6BN in preventing dependence cannot be accounted for by classical opioid receptor models, even when 6BN access to the brain is limited. It is possible that the distribution of potent receptor ligands between blood and brain is non-linear at very low concentrations, since potent opioid antagonists tend to accumulate at the receptor and are retained in the brain—with a large portion of the total drug level in the brain bound to the receptor [45]. Such a receptor retention mechanism, assuming a discrete receptor micro-compartment where the drug is sequestered, can counteract the slow access of 6BN to the brain and enhance CNS potency for drugs with high receptor affinity.

Repeated priming with opioids can lead to hyperalgesia, at least in part mediated by peripheral afferent nociceptors [46]. Blocking MOR sites in peripheral nociceptive afferent neurons with a peripheral antagonist, methylnaltrexone, was shown to suppress development of tolerance and opioid-induced hyperalgesia (OIH) [14]. Preliminary evidence indicates that 6BN is similarly effective against OIH, again with high potency (Z. Wang, unpublished). Possibly, the same mechanisms underlie prevention of dependence and OIH with 6BN.

6. Hypothesis: A Novel MOR Receptor Model Relevant to Opioid Dependence Invoking a Site with High Affinity to 6BN

Our results demonstrate that 6BN prevents opioid dependence with higher potency compared to blocking antinociception or causing withdrawal. Its potency in this regard is similar to the high potency of naltrexone in blocking antinociception or causing withdrawal, whereas 6BN is two orders of magnitude less potent than naltrexone in these measures. We, therefore, propose that 6BN is a biased opioid ligand binding potently to a distinct MOR site in a non-competitive fashion and modulating dependence, expanding the concept of multiple receptor conformations with distinct ligand affinities that has enabled development of biased agonists.

How can 6BN prevent or reverse opioid dependence caused by MOR agonists? We propose a model of interacting MOR conformations that can account for the observed results with 6BN (Figure 5), in view of dynamic regulation of peripheral opioid receptors [13]. Assume a distinct MOR site (MOR-μ^x) in equilibrium with MOR-μ, reminiscent of previously postulated 'receptor reserve'. MOR-μ^x could comprise multiple receptor states, including the beta-arrestin coupled site proposed to be more prevalent in peripheral neurons [13], with each MOR conformation dependent on interacting proteins and factors in target tissues. While the proposed MOR-μ- MOR-μ^x equilibrium could vary as a function of cell type and could favor MOR-μ^x in the opioid-naïve state, in this model agonist treatment shifts the balance towards MOR-μ together with lasting enhanced spontaneous MOR-μ^* activity, a hallmark of the dependent state. Assuming 6BN had high affinity for MOR-μ^x than for MOR-μ, higher than other opioid ligands including naltrexone, thereby stabilizing this conformation, even small doses of 6BN could reverse the MOR-μ- MOR-μ^x equilibrium towards the opioid-naïve state characterized by more prevalent MOR-μ^x. In support of this hypothesis, we had observed that 6BN becomes more potent in blocking morphine's inhibition of peristaltic motility in mice when injected before morphine, with maximum potency reached at ~100 min before morphine [40]. This long delay is not accounted for the by the rapid peak of 6BN levels reaching the circulation, but rather is consistent with gradual depletion of MOR-μ sites towards MOR-μ^x sites. Similarly, the ability of 6BN, but not naltrexone, to reverse elevated MOR-μ^* basal activity in chronic neuropathic pain is consistent with the model's predictions [16,44].

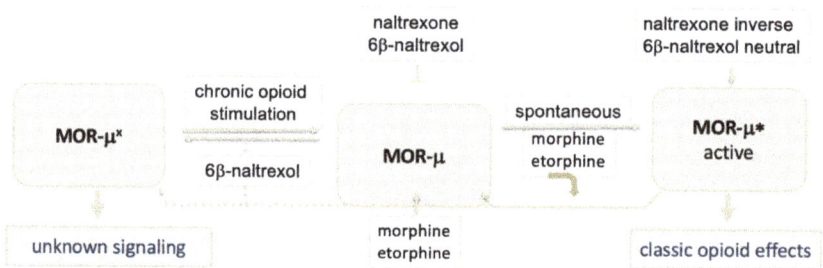

Figure 5. Extended model of the μ opioid receptor (MOR). Starting with the model shown in Figure 1, we add an additional receptor conformation termed MOR-μ^x, which could exist in multiple states. We hypothesize that MOR-μ^x is in equilibrium with MOR-μ, and that chronic activation of MOR-μ shifts the equilibrium and depletes MOR-μ^x, leading to elevated to MOR-μ^* activity, a hallmark of the dependent state. BN is proposed to bind with high affinity to MOR-μ^x and stabilize this conformation, preserving the MOR-μ^x - MOR-μ^* equilibrium of the opioid-naïve non-dependent state. It is also feasible that 6BN could facilitate conversion of MOR-μ^* to MOR-μ^x, suggested by the dotted line. This model can account for high potency of 6BN to prevent or reverse the opioid dependent state in a non-competitive fashion with opioid agonists.

The nature of the postulated MOR-μ^x site remains elusive but parallels the two-state model proposed for MOR in peripheral afferent nociceptors [13]. Multiple forms are likely to exist, including hetero-dimeric MOR–GPCR complexes [47,48], some forms with signaling pathways opposing canonical MOR pathways. A MOR–DOR dimer was found to stimulate intracellular calcium release via Gi proteins, an effect opposing the canonical inhibition of influx calcium channels by MOR [49]. Moreover, MOR had been shown to activate calcium influx channels including TRPV1, via G proteins [50]. We had identified a MOR site in transfected HEK293 cells that stimulates calcium influx over the first 10 s of morphine exposure, followed by separate intracellular calcium release, with selectivity for epoxymorphinans (e.g., morphine, naloxone, and naltrexone) but very low affinity to other opioids (e.g., etorphine, diprenorphine, levorphanol, and fentanyl) [51]. While opposite to the well-established MOR-mediated inhibition of calcium influx channels and activation of potassium channels, this stimulatory signaling pathway is also mediated by pertussis toxin-sensitive G proteins. Its ligand binding affinities are similar to those of a labile MOR site we had identified in rat brain tissues (MOR-λ) that rapidly decays upon tissue homogenization but accounts for ~40% of all labeled ^{3}H-naloxone binding sites in rat brain [52]. It is too early to speculate on the identity of the postulated MOR-μ^x site, whether the observed MOR-λ sites account at least in part for MOR-μ^x, and whether it is silent or coupled to an unorthodox signaling pathway. We are now embarking on the characterization of this hypothesized high affinity 6BN site.

7. Potential Clinical Applications

As peripherally selective neutral opioid antagonists, 6BN and its congeners can serve as PAMORAs, treating constipation and opioid induced bowel dysfunction. Exploratory Phase I clinical trials have shown that 6BN given ci potently blocks morphine (10 mg/kg) induced slowing of bowel movements at doses that do not prevent opioid analgesia [40]. In a small e-IND study of methadone maintenance patients ($n = 4$), 6BN at doses up to 1mg iv caused bowel movements and limited peripheral withdrawal but no central withdrawal symptoms [53]. Its potency may be similar to that of naldemedine (0.5 mg effective dose) in treating constipation [39]. On the other hand, acting with high potency as a modulator of opioid dependence, compounds like 6BN offer multiple additional therapeutic opportunities. Among these, pharmaceutical formulations combining any opioid analgesic with low-dose 6BN could result in safer pain therapeutics, avoiding opioid dependence without precipitating withdrawal, and possibly also opioid induced hyperalgesia, an element affecting tolerance. In addition, 6BN has a longer half-life (~12 h) than typical opioid analgesics (~4 h), thereby accumulating upon frequent dosing in opioid use disorder subjects, and reaching the brain in sufficient amounts to blunt the opioid effect (Figure 6). Lastly, 6BN might facilitate opioid withdrawal under weaning protocols, followed by continued dosing at a higher dose level to prevent recidivism.

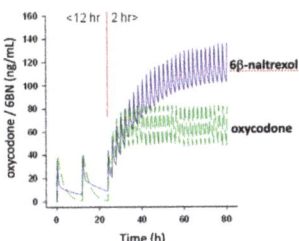

Figure 6. Simulated plasma levels of oxycodone (20 mg) co-administered s.c. with 6BN (15 mg). The pharmacokinetic model is based on published human blood level data for both compounds, assuming 4 and 12 h half-lives, respectively. Over the first 24 h, dosing occurs every 12 h, with low accumulation for either drug. Then, dosing continues every 2 h, simulating abuse conditions, leading to substantial accumulation of 6BN. Whereas, 15 mg 6BN is not expected to interfere with analgesia, with rapid dosing 6BN can reach levels that blunt CNS effects of the agonist, thereby reducing addiction risk.

The high potency of 6BN to prevent neonatal withdrawal behavior in guinea pig pups exposed to methadone in utero [43] promises a novel preventive therapy for neonatal opioid withdrawal syndrome (NOWS), a severe form of opioid withdrawal requiring prolonged stay in neonatal intensive care units, with only palliative therapy available [54–57]. Low-dose 6BN given to pregnant women in need of opioid pain therapy or in management protocols for opioid use disorder (e.g., with methadone or buprenorphine [55,58]) has the potential to prevent NOWS without causing substantial withdrawal in both mother and fetus. Efforts are ongoing to bring 6BN into the clinic for this purpose.

Naltrexone is currently the treatment of choice for preventing relapse, but cannot be given until one to two weeks after complete weaning to avoid strong drug-induced withdrawal, which can be avoided with staggered 6BN dosing schedules. Naltrexone administration leads to higher 6BN levels compared to the parent drug, but 6BN has low potency as an antagonist against centrally mediated analgesia, and the 6BN/naltrexone ratios are quite variable between subjects—leading to the common assumption that 6BN does not contribute to naltrexone's effects. Ultra-low naltrexone doses combined with opioid analgesics have been proposed to enhance efficacy and reduce tolerance [59,60]. However, the theoretical underpinnings for these observations remain poorly understood. Our MOR model suggests that 6BN generated as a metabolite of naltrexone can have potent effects per se, but is counteracted by naltrexone which has high affinity for MOR-μ and MOR-μ*. It is critical that these questions are resolved to enable development of optimal pain therapies and management strategies for opioid use disorder.

MOR has also been implicated in other drug use disorders, most prominently in reducing binge drinking in alcoholics [25]. While effective in a portion of subjects with alcohol use disorder, naltrexone causes aversion in some subjects leading to low compliance and cessation of therapy. It is possible that the opioid receptor is activated in alcohol use disorder, leading to elevated MOR-μ*, with naltrexone triggering opioid-like withdrawal symptoms. Selecting 6BN as an alternative to naltrexone could avoid aversive effects while maintaining efficacy.

8. Biased Antagonism at GPCRs and Future Studies

A review of the literature reveals overwhelming evidence towards biased agonists that engage differential receptor conformations and signaling pathways, whereas biased antagonists remain neglected [10,61]. Violin et al. [10] mention specifically the potential for both biased agonists and antagonists as it is apparent that both can bind differentially to various receptor conformations with distinct effects, but discuss only agonists in detail. Among the few specific examples of biased antagonism, a biased CCR3 antagonist was reported to prevent receptor internalization via a β-arrestin pathway while still allowing G protein coupling, thereby effectively blocking eosinophil recruitment in vivo [62]—showing that an agonist can be rendered biased by simultaneously blocking one of two pathways. Similar dual ligand effects have been reported for adrenergic [63] and dopamine receptors (aripiprazole) [61]. The opioid literature almost entirely focuses on biased agonism. Recent studies have shown that the numerous endogenous opioid peptides differ among each other in stimulating distinct signaling, as reported for opioid drugs [64,65], but all considered to act as agonists—An area worthy of further study.

The ability of low-dose 6BN selectively to block a pathway relevant to dependence adds a new dimension to biased opioid ligands. Future molecular studies need to focus on characterization of the proposed novel MOR-μ^x site. We have already detected longer retention of 6BN in guinea pig brain at low levels than expected from its short half-life, likely mediated by retention at the receptor with high affinity (unpublished). This finding opens an experimental approach to study properties of a MOR-μ^x with high affinity for 6BN.

In conclusion, we propose a novel MOR model with multiple interconverting receptor forms. Exploiting distinct ligand affinities and functions for both agonists and antagonists promises novel strategies for management of opioid use disorder and improved opioid pain therapies.

9. Patents

The following patents are relevant to this paper: "Combination analgesic employing opioid and neutral antagonist". W. Sadee, E.J. Bilsky, and J. Yancey-Wrona. U.S. patent number 8,748,448 B2. Date filed November 28, 2012; and patent related patents: US6713488 B2, US8883817B2, US9061024B2, and EP2214672.

Author Contributions: W.S. formulated the receptor model and wrote the manuscript. J.O. contributed to the modal's concept, carried out key studies in mice and guinea pigs, and edited the manuscript. Z.W. designed and supervised experiments in mice yielding results that informed model development and edited the manuscript. All authors have read and agreed to the published version of the manuscript.

Funding: This work was supported by NIH research grants NIH R21-HD092011 to J.O. and NIH R44-DA045414 to W.S.

Conflicts of Interest: WS is Chief Scientific Officer of Aether Therapeutics and holds shares in Aether.

References

1. Valentino, R.J.; Volkow, N.D. Untangling the complexity of opioid receptor function. *Neuropsychopharm* **2018**, *43*, 2514–2520. [CrossRef] [PubMed]
2. Shang, Y.; Filizola, M. Opioid receptors: Structural and mechanistic insights into pharmacology and signaling. *Eur. J. Pharmacol.* **2015**, *763*, 206–213. [CrossRef] [PubMed]
3. Burford, N.T.; Traynor, J.R.; Alt, A. Positive allosteric modulators of the μ-opioid receptor: A novel approach for future pain medications. *Br. J. Pharmacol.* **2015**, *172*, 277–286. [CrossRef] [PubMed]
4. Du, Y.; Duc, N.M.; Rasmussen, S.G.F.; Hilger, D.; Kubiak, X.; Wang, L.; Bohon, J.; Kim, H.R.; Wegrecki, M.; Asuru, A.; et al. Assembly of a GPCR-G Protein Complex. *Cell* **2019**, *177*, 1232–1242. [CrossRef] [PubMed]
5. Park, P.S. Ensemble of G protein-coupled receptor active states. *Curr. Med. Chem.* **2012**, *19*, 1146–1154. [CrossRef] [PubMed]
6. Hauser, A.S.; Attwood, M.M.; Rask-Andersen, M.; Schiöth, H.B.; Gloriam, D.E. Trends in GPCR drug discovery: New agents, targets and indications. *Nat. Rev. Drug Discov.* **2017**, *6*, 829–842. [CrossRef] [PubMed]
7. Seyedabadi, M.; Ghahremani, M.H.; Albert, P.R. Biased signaling of G protein coupled receptors (GPCRs): Molecular determinants of GPCR/transducer selectivity and therapeutic potential. *Pharmacol. Ther.* **2019**, *200*, 148–178. [CrossRef] [PubMed]
8. Wootten, D.; Christopoulos, A.; Marti-Solano, M.; Babu, M.M.; Sexton, P.M. Mechanisms of signalling and biased agonism in G protein-coupled receptors. *Nat. Rev. Mol. Cell Biol.* **2018**, *19*, 638–653. [CrossRef] [PubMed]
9. Schmid, C.L.; Kennedy, N.M.; Ross, N.C.; Lovell, K.M.; Yue, Z.; Morgenweck, J.; Cameron, M.D.; Bannister, T.D.; Bohn, L.M. Bias factor and therapeutic window correlate to predict safer opioid analgesics. *Cell* **2017**, *171*, 1165–1175. [CrossRef] [PubMed]
10. Violin, J.D.; Crombie, A.L.; Soergel, D.G.; Lark, M.W. Biased ligands at G-protein-coupled receptors: Promise and progress. *Trends Pharmacol. Sci.* **2014**, *35*, 308–316. [CrossRef]
11. Chan, H.C.S.; McCarthy, D.; Li, J.; Palczewski, K.; Yuan, S. Designing safer analgesics via μ-opioid receptor pathways. *Trends Pharmacol. Sci.* **2017**, *38*, 1016–1037. [CrossRef] [PubMed]
12. Grim, T.W.; Schmid, C.L.; Stahl, E.L.; Pantouli, P.; Ho, J.-H.; Acevedo-Canabal, A.; Kennedy, N.M.; Cameron, M.D.; Bannister, T.D.; Bohn, L.M. A G protein signaling-biased agonist at the μ-opioid receptor reverses morphine tolerance while preventing morphine withdrawal. *Neuropsychopharm* **2019**, *45*, 416–425. [CrossRef] [PubMed]
13. Jeske, N.A. Dynamic Opioid Receptor Regulation in the Periphery. *Mol. Pharmacol.* **2019**, *95*, 463–467. [CrossRef] [PubMed]
14. Corder, G.; Tawfik, V.L.; Wang, D.; Sypek, E.I.; Low, S.A.; Dickinson, J.R.; Sotoudeh, C.; Clark, J.D.; Barres, B.A.; Bohlen, C.J.; et al. Loss of μ opioid receptor signaling in nociceptors, but not microglia, abrogates morphine tolerance without disrupting analgesia. *Nat. Med.* **2017**, *23*, 164–173.

15. Streicher, J.M.; Bilsky, E.J. Peripherally acting mu-opioid receptor antagonists for the treatment of opioid-related side effects: Mechanism of action and clinical implications. *J. Pharm. Pract.* **2017**, *31*, 658–669. [CrossRef] [PubMed]
16. Sullivan, L.C.; Chavera, T.S.; Jamshidi, R.J.; Berg, K.A.; Clarke, W.P. Constitutive Desensitization of Opioid Receptors in Peripheral Sensory Neurons. *J. Pharmacol. Exp. Ther.* **2016**, *359*, 411–419. [CrossRef]
17. Wang, Z.; Bilsky, E.J.; Porreca, F.; Sadée, W. Constitutive µ Receptor Activation as a Regulatory Mechanism Underlying Narcotic Tolerance and Dependence. *Life Sci.* **1994**, *54*, PL339–PL350. [CrossRef]
18. Sadee, W.; Wang, D.; Bilsky, E.J. Basal opioid receptor activity, neutral antagonists, and therapeutic opportunities. *Life Sci.* **2005**, *76*, 1427–1437. [CrossRef]
19. Wang, D.; Raehal, K.M.; Lin, E.T.; Lowery, J.J.; Kieffer, B.L.; Bilsky, E.J.; Sadée, W. Basal signaling mu opioid receptor in mouse brain: Role in narcotic dependence. *J. Pharm. Exp. Ther.* **2004**, *308*, 512–520. [CrossRef]
20. Perry, D.C.; Rosenbaum, J.S.; Kurowski, M.; Sadée, W. ^{3}H-Etorphine Receptor Binding *In Vivo*: Small Fractional Occupancy Elicits Analgesia. *Molec. Pharmacol.* **1982**, *21*, 272–279.
21. Hoare, S.R.J.; Pierre, N.; Moya, A.G.; Larson, B. Kinetic operational models of agonism for G-protein-coupled receptors. *J. Theor. Biol.* **2018**, *446*, 168–204. [CrossRef] [PubMed]
22. Corder, G.; Doolen, S.; Donahue, R.R.; Winter, M.K.; Jutras, B.K.L.; He, Y.; Hu, X.; Wieskopf, J.S.; Mogil, J.S.; Storm, D.R.; et al. Constitutive µ-opioid receptor activity leads to long-term endogenous analgesia and dependence. *Science* **2013**, *341*, 1394–1399. [CrossRef] [PubMed]
23. Blanco, C.; Volkow, N.D. Management of opioid use disorder in the USA: Present status and future directions. *Lancet* **2019**, *393*, 1760–1772. [CrossRef] [PubMed]
24. Wachman, E.M.; Saia, K.; Miller, M.; Valle, E.; Shrestha, H.; Carter, G.; Werler, M.; Jones, H. Naltrexone Treatment for Pregnant Women with Opioid Use Disorder Compared with Matched Buprenorphine Control Subjects. *Clin. Ther.* **2019**, *41*, 1681–1689. [CrossRef]
25. Dunbar, J.L.; Turncliff, R.Z.; Dong, Q.; Silverman, B.L.; Ehrich, E.W.; Lasseter, K.C. Single-and multiple-dose pharmacokinetics of long-acting injectable naltrexone. *Alcoholism Clin. Exper. Res.* **2006**, *30*, 480–490. [CrossRef]
26. Porter, S.J.; Somogyi, A.A.; White, J.M. In vivo and in vitro potency studies of 6β-naltrexol, the major human metabolite of naltrexone. *Addict. Biol.* **2002**, *7*, 219–225. [CrossRef]
27. Raehal, K.M.; Lowery, J.J.; Bhamidipati, C.M.; Paolino, R.M.; Blair, J.R.; Wang, D.; Sadée, W.; Bilsky, E.J. In vivo characterization of 6β-naltrexol, an opioid ligand with less inverse agonist activity compared with naltrexone and naloxone in opioid-dependent mice. *J. Pharmacol. Exp. Ther.* **2005**, *313*, 1150–1162. [CrossRef]
28. Sirohi, S.; Dighe, S.V.; Madia, P.A.; Yoburn, B.C. The relative potency of inverse opioid agonists and a neutral opioid antagonist in precipitated withdrawal and antagonism of analgesia and toxicity. *J. Pharmacol. Exp. Ther.* **2009**, *330*, 513–519. [CrossRef]
29. Yancey-Wrona, J.E.; Raymond, T.J.; Mercer, H.K.; Sadee, W.; Bilsky, E.J. 6β-Naltrexol preferentially antagonizes opioid effects on gastrointestinal transit compared to antinociception in mice. *Life Sci.* **2009**, *85*, 413–420. [CrossRef]
30. Ko, M.C.; Divin, M.F.; Lee, H.; Woods, J.H.; Traynor, J.R. Differential in Vivo Potencies of Naltrexone and 6β-Naltrexol in the Monkey. *J. Pharmacol. Exp. Ther.* **2006**, *316*, 772–779. [CrossRef]
31. Wang, D.; Raehal, K.M.; Bilsky, E.J.; Sadee, W. Inverse agonists and neutral antagonists at µ opioid receptor (MOR): Possible role of basal receptor signaling in narcotic dependence. *J. Neurochem.* **2001**, *77*, 1590–1600. [CrossRef] [PubMed]
32. Wang, D.; Sun, X.; Sadee, W. Different effects of opioid antagonists on mu, delta, and kappa opioid receptors with and without agonist pretreatment. *J. Pharmacol. Exp. Ther.* **2007**, *321*, 544–552. [CrossRef] [PubMed]
33. Dunlop, A.J.; Brown, A.L.; Oldmeadow, C.; Harris, A.; Gill, A.; Sadler, C.; Ribbons, K.; Attia, J.; Barker, D.; Ghijben, P.; et al. Effectiveness and cost-effectiveness of unsupervised buprenorphine-naloxone for the treatment of heroin dependence in a randomized waitlist-controlled trial. *Drug Alcohol Depend.* **2017**, *174*, 181–191. [CrossRef] [PubMed]
34. Rosado, J.; Walsh, S.L.; Bigelow, G.E.; Strain, E.C. Sublingual buprenorphine/naloxone precipitated withdrawal in subjects maintained on 100 mg of daily methadone. *Drug Alcohol Depend.* **2007**, *90*, 261–269. [CrossRef] [PubMed]
35. Cowen, A.; Lewis, J.W.; MacFarlane, I.R. Agonist and antagonist properties of buprenorphine, a new antinociceptive agent. *Brit. J. Pharmacol.* **1977**, *60*, 537–545. [CrossRef] [PubMed]

36. Tzschentke, T.M. Reassessment of buprenorphine in conditioned place preference: Temporal and pharmacological considerations. *Psychopharmacology* **2004**, *172*, 58–67. [CrossRef]
37. Fürst, S.; Zádori, Z.S.; Zádor, F.; Király, K.; Balogh, M.; László, S.B.; Hutka, B.; Mohammadzadeh, A.; Calabrese, C.; Galambos, A.R.; et al. On the Role of Peripheral Sensory and Gut Mu Opioid Receptors: Peripheral Analgesia and Tolerance. *Molecules* **2020**, *25*, 2473. [CrossRef]
38. Song, X.; Wang, D.; Qu, X.; Dong, N.; Teng, S. A meta-analysis of naldemedine for the treatment of opioid-induced constipation. *Expert Rev. Clin. Pharmacol.* **2019**, *12*, 121–128. [CrossRef] [PubMed]
39. Kalvass, J.C.; Olson, E.R.; Cassidy, M.P.; Selley, D.E.; Pollack, G.M. Pharmacokinetics and pharmacodynamics of seven opioids in P-glycoprotein-competent mice: Assessment of unbound brain EC50,u and correlation of in vitro, preclinical, and clinical data. *J. Pharmacol. Exp. Ther.* **2007**, *323*, 346–355. [CrossRef]
40. Farid, W.O.; Dunlop, S.A.; Tait, R.J.; Hulse, G.K. The effects of maternally administered methadone, buprenorphine and naltrexone on offspring: Review of human and animal data. *Curr. Neuropharmacol.* **2008**, *6*, 125–150. [CrossRef]
41. Yancey-Wrona, J.; Dallaire, B.; Bilsky, E.; Bath, B.; Burkart, J.; Wenster, L.; Magiera, D.; Yang, X.; Phelps, M.; Sadee, W. 6β-naltrexol, a peripherally selective opioid antagonist that inhibits morphine- induced slowing of gastrointestinal transit: An exploratory study. *Pain Medicine* **2011**, *12*, 1727–1737. [CrossRef] [PubMed]
42. Oberdick, J.; Ling, Y.; Phelps, M.A.; Yudovich, M.S.; Schilling, K.; Sadee, W. Preferential delivery of an opioid antagonist to the fetal brain in pregnant mice. *J. Pharmacol. Exp. Ther.* **2016**, *358*, 22–30. [CrossRef] [PubMed]
43. Safa, A.; Lau, A.R.; Aten, S.; Schilling, K.; Bales, K.L.; Miller, V.; Fitzgerald, J.; Chen, M.; Hill, K.; Dzwigalski, K.; et al. Pharmacological prevention of neonatal opioid withdrawal in a pregnant guinea pig model. *bioRxiv* **2020**. [CrossRef]
44. Walwyn, W.M.; Chen, C.; Kim, H.; Minasyan, A.; Ennes, H.S.; McRoberts, J.A.; Marvizon, J.C.G. Sustained suppression of hyperalgesia during latent sensitization by mu-, delta-, and kappa-opioid receptors and 2A-adrenergic receptors: Role of constitutive activity. *Neurobiol. Dis.* **2016**, *36*, 204–221.
45. Perry, D.C.; Mullis, K.B.; Oie, S.; Sadée, W. Opiate Antagonist Receptor Binding In Vivo: Evidence for a New Receptor Binding Model. *Brain Research* **1980**, *199*, 49–61. [CrossRef]
46. Araldi, D.; Ferrari, L.F.; Levine, J.D. Hyperalgesic priming (type II) induced by repeated opioid exposure: Maintenance mechanisms. *Pain* **2017**, *158*, 1204–1216. [CrossRef] [PubMed]
47. Wang, D.; Sun, X.; Bohn, L.M.; Sadée, W. Opioid receptor homo- and hetero-dimerization in living cells by quantitative bioluminescence resonance energy transfer. *Molec. Pharmacol.* **2005**, *67*, 2173–2184. [CrossRef]
48. Gupta, A.; Décaillot, F.M.; Devi, L.A. Targeting opioid receptor heterodimers: Strategies for screening and drug development. *AAPS J.* **2006**, *8*, E153–E159. [CrossRef] [PubMed]
49. Charles, A.C.; Mostovskaya, N.; Asas, K.; Evans, C.J.; Dankovich, M.L.; Hales, T.G. Coexpression of delta-opioid receptors with mu receptors in GH3 cells changes the functional response to micro agonists from inhibitory to excitatory. *Mol. Pharmacol.* **2003**, *63*, 89–95. [CrossRef]
50. Scherer, P.C.; Zaccor, N.W.; Neumann, N.M.; Vasavda, C.; Barrow, R.; Ewald, A.J.; Rao, F.; Sumner, C.J.; Snyder, S.H. TRPV1 is a physiological regulator of μ-opioid receptors. *Proc. Natl. Acad. Sci. USA* **2017**, *114*, 13561–13566. [CrossRef]
51. Quillan, J.M.; Carlson, K.W.; Song, C.; Wang, D.; Sadée, W. Differential Effects of μ Opioid Receptor (MOR) Ligands on Ca^{2+} Signaling. *J. Pharmacol. Exp. Ther.* **2002**, *302*, 1002–1012. [CrossRef] [PubMed]
52. Grevel, J.; Sadée, W. An Opiate Binding Site in Rat Brain is Highly Selective for 4,5-Epoxymorphinans. *Science* **1983**, *221*, 1198–1201. [CrossRef] [PubMed]
53. AIKO Biotechnology. A Phase-I, Two-Stage, Double-Blind, Placebo-Controlled, Pharmacokinetic and Pharmacodynamic Trial of Low Doses of Intravenous 6β-Naltrexol (AIKO-150) in Opioid-Dependent Subjects. ClinicalTrials.gov. Available online: https://clinicaltrials.gov/ct2/show/NCT00829777?term=AIKO&rank=1 (accessed on 31 August 2020).
54. Kocherlakota, P. Neonatal abstinence syndrome. *Pediatrics* **2004**, *134*, e547–e561. [CrossRef] [PubMed]
55. Jones, H.E.; Kaltenbach, K.; Heil, S.H.; Stine, S.M.; Coyle, M.G.; Arria, A.M.; O'Grady, K.E.; Selby, P.; Martin, P.R.; Fischer, G. Neonatal abstinence syndrome after methadone or buprenorphine exposure. *N. Engl. J. Med.* **2010**, *363*, 2320–2331. [CrossRef] [PubMed]
56. Walsh, M.C.; Crowley, M.; Wexelblatt, S.; Ford, S.; Kuhnell, P.; Kaplan, H.C.; McClead, R.; Macaluso, M.; Lannon, C. Ohio perinatal quality collaborative improves care of neonatal narcotic abstinence syndrome. *Pediatrics* **2018**, *141*, e20170900. [CrossRef]

57. Conradt, E.; Crowell, S.E.; Lester, B.M. Early life stress and environmental influences on the neurodevelopment of children with prenatal opioid exposure. *Neurobiol. Stress* **2018**, *9*, 48–54. [CrossRef]
58. Arlettaz, R.; Kashiwagi, M.; Das-Kundu, S.; Fauchere, J.C.; Lang, A.; Bucher, H.U. Methadone maintenance program in pregnancy in a swiss perinatal center (II): Neonatal outcome and social resources. *Acta Obstet. Gynecol. Scand.* **2005**, *84*, 145–150. [CrossRef]
59. Leri, F.; Burns, L.H. Ultra-low-dose naltrexone reduces the rewarding potency of oxycodone and relapse vulnerability in rats. *Pharmacol. Biochem. Behav.* **2005**, *82*, 252–262. [CrossRef]
60. Tompkins, D.A.; Lanier, R.K.; Harrison, J.A.; Strain, E.C.; Bigelow, G.E. Human abuse liability assessment of oxycodone combined with ultra-low-dose naltrexone. *Psychopharmacology* **2010**, *210*, 471–480. [CrossRef]
61. Stott, L.A.; Hall, D.A.; Holliday, N.D. Unravelling intrinsic efficacy and ligand bias at G protein coupled receptors: A practical guide to assessing functional data. *Biochem. Pharmacol.* **2016**, *101*, 1–12. [CrossRef]
62. Grozdanovic, M.; Laffey, K.G.; Abdelkarim, H.; Hitchinson, B.; Harijith, A.; Moon, H.G.; Park, G.Y.; Rousslang, L.K.; Masterson, J.C.; Furuta, G.T.; et al. Novel peptide nanoparticle-biased antagonist of CCR3 blocks eosinophil recruitment and airway hyperresponsiveness. *J. Allergy Clin. Immunol.* **2019**, *143*, 669.e12–680.e12. [CrossRef] [PubMed]
63. Desimine, V.L.; McCrink, K.A.; Parker, B.M.; Wertz, S.L.; Maning, J.; Lymperopoulos, A. Biased agonism/antagonism of cardiovascular GPCRs for heart failure therapy. *Int. Rev. Cell Mol. Biol.* **2018**, *339*, 41–61. [PubMed]
64. Gomes, I.; Sierra, S.; Lueptow, L.; Gupta, A.; Gouty, S.; Margolis, E.B.; Cox, B.M.; Devi, L.A. Biased signaling by endogenous opioid peptides. *Proc. Natl. Acad. Sci. USA* **2020**, *117*, 11820–11828. [CrossRef] [PubMed]
65. Thompson, G.L.; Lane, J.R.; Coudrat, T.; Sexton, P.M.; Christopoulos, A.; Canals, M. Biased agonism of endogenous opioid peptides at the μ-opioid receptor. *Mol. Pharmacol.* **2015**, *88*, 335–346. [CrossRef] [PubMed]

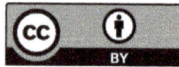

© 2020 by the authors. Licensee MDPI, Basel, Switzerland. This article is an open access article distributed under the terms and conditions of the Creative Commons Attribution (CC BY) license (http://creativecommons.org/licenses/by/4.0/).

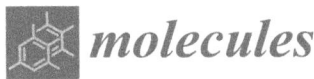 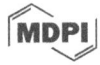

Article

Molecular Modeling of µ Opioid Receptor Ligands with Various Functional Properties: PZM21, SR-17018, Morphine, and Fentanyl—Simulated Interaction Patterns Confronted with Experimental Data

Sabina Podlewska [1,2], Ryszard Bugno [2], Lucja Kudla [2], Andrzej J. Bojarski [2] and Ryszard Przewlocki [2,*]

[1] Department of Technology and Biotechnology of Drugs, Jagiellonian University Medical College, 9 Medyczna Street, 30-688 Cracow, Poland; smusz@if-pan.krakow.pl
[2] Maj Institute of Pharmacology, Polish Academy of Sciences, 12 Smętna Street, 31-343 Cracow, Poland; bugno@if-pan.krakow.pl (R.B.); kudla@if-pan.krakow.pl (L.K.); bojarski@if-pan.krakow.pl (A.J.B.)
* Correspondence: nfprzewl@cyf-kr.edu.pl; Tel.: +48-12662-32-38

Academic Editor: Helmut Schmidhammer
Received: 31 July 2020; Accepted: 6 October 2020; Published: 12 October 2020

Abstract: Molecular modeling approaches are an indispensable part of the drug design process. They not only support the process of searching for new ligands of a given receptor, but they also play an important role in explaining particular activity pathways of a compound. In this study, a comprehensive molecular modeling protocol was developed to explain the observed activity profiles of selected µ opioid receptor agents: two G protein-biased µ opioid receptor agonists (PZM21 and SR-17018), unbiased morphine, and the β-arrestin-2-biased agonist, fentanyl. The study involved docking and molecular dynamics simulations carried out for three crystal structures of the target at a microsecond scale, followed by the statistical analysis of ligand–protein contacts. The interaction frequency between the modeled compounds and the subsequent residues of a protein during the simulation was also correlated with the output of in vitro and in vivo tests, resulting in the set of amino acids with the highest Pearson correlation coefficient values. Such indicated positions may serve as a guide for designing new G protein-biased ligands of the µ opioid receptor.

Keywords: µ opioid receptor; molecular dynamics; docking; interaction fingerprints; biased agonists; SR-17018; PZM21; morphine; fentanyl

1. Introduction

Opioids are effective analgesics widely used for severe pain treatment. However, the majority of them, including morphine, produce side effects limiting their use, such as respiratory depression, constipation, and addiction. An epidemic in both western and developing countries of opioid use disorder and overdose deaths from prescription opioids has led recently to the search for new painkillers deprived of this action or with limited effects—in particular, respiratory depression. One of the most interesting approaches is based on the observation that an opioid acting via the µ opioid receptor may activate intracellular signal pathways with varying strength. These ideas of so-called biased signaling or functional selectivity suggest that some opioids may activate the G protein signal pathway and mediate the analgesic effect via the µ opioid receptor and avoid stimulation of the β-arrestin-2 pathway (which seems to be involved in the observed side effects [1]) at the same time. Therefore, the main interest in the case of the µ opioid receptor ligands is focused on the synthesis of opioid G protein-biased agonists that preferentially activate the G protein but not the β-arrestin-2 pathway. Identification of the crystal structure of µ opioid receptors has opened up, on the one hand, a better understanding of the structure of opioid receptors and, on the other, the development of new computer modeling technologies that have enabled the identification and synthesis of new biased opioids. One of them was PZM21, selected by molecular docking after virtual testing for selective bias activation of the μ opioid receptor [2]. This substance is in fact characterized by functional selectivity because it activates the G protein but not β-arrestins. In preclinical studies, PZM21 has been shown to be analgesic, with no conditioned place preference (CPP) production or locomotor stimulation observed [2,3]; on the other hand, it led to the development of rapid analgesic tolerance in the hot plate and tail-flick tests in mice [3,4] and caused respiratory depression [4]. Bohn's group [5] recently identified a series of biased μ opioid receptor agonists. Among them, SR-17018 appears to be of great interest because it displays the highest bias towards G protein signaling compared to β-arrestin-2 recruitment [5] and shows antinociceptive activity and a very little respiratory suppression in mice [6]. In addition, long-term oral administration of SR-17018 did not lead to antinociceptive tolerance, prevented morphine withdrawal, and restored morphine antinociception in morphine-tolerant animals [6].

The emergence of new G protein-biased ligands has stimulated studies aimed at developing new ligands of this type, as well as research on the detailed mode of action of the already developed biased compounds. This research involves both experimental and computational studies of various types. In silico methods support the design and development of new drugs at different levels, starting from searching for drug candidates, via optimization of their activity and physicochemical properties, to support in the analysis of their efficiency after introduction to the market [7–9]. Computational approaches also help in understanding the mechanisms of compound action and simulate processes occurring during receptor activation [10–12].

Molecular modeling approaches use various data types to derive predictions of compound activity. Ligand-based methods use information only on the structure of compounds [13–16], whereas structure-based tools rely on the spatial orientation of atoms of the target protein and use docking to predict ligand fitting in the respective binding site [17,18]. One ligand–receptor complex returned by a docking program captures just one moment of the mutual orientation of a compound and protein. More computationally demanding but also much more informative method is molecular dynamics (MD), which enables simulation of the behavior of the modeled system (e.g., ligand–protein complex) in time [19,20].

In this study, we apply docking and MD simulations to explain the activity profiles of selected μ opioid receptor agents. We compare and analyze using molecular modeling methods, docking and MD simulations, four selected opioids targeting the μ opioid receptor: novel G protein-biased μ opioid receptor agonists, PZM21 and SR-17018 [2,5], unbiased morphine, and the β-arrestin-2-biased agonist, fentanyl. Extensive in silico examination of these ligands with reference to their μ opioid receptor activity involved docking to three μ opioid receptor crystal structures, MD simulations carried out at a microsecond scale (2 μs), and the statistical analysis of ligand–protein contacts during simulations. The interaction frequencies of a compound with the subsequent amino acids were confronted with the outcome of the selected in vitro and in vivo tests and positions with the highest correlation were identified. The set of such selected residues should be of particular interest when designing new G protein-biased μ opioid receptor agents. In addition, the orientation of W293^{6x48} (residue important for μ opioid receptor activation) during simulation was examined and confronted with the ligand activity profiles. The residue numbering provided in superscripts follows the GPCRdb [21] numbering scheme.

2. Results and Discussion

2.1. Comparison of Modeled Ligands and μ Opioid Receptor Crystal Structures

The modeled compounds were compared in terms of their structures and selected physicochemical properties, which were determined using InstantJChem [22] (Table 1).

Table 1. Structure and properties of the μ opioid receptor ligands examined in the study.

Compound Symbol	Compound Structure	μ Opioid Receptor Activity	Molecular Weight *	LogP **	# H Bond Acceptors	# H Bond Donors	# Rotatable Bonds
PZM21		G protein-biased agonist	361.50	2.85	3	3	8
SR-17018		G protein-biased agonist	410.73	4.75	2	1	3
morphine		Unbiased agonist	285.34	0.90	4	2	0
fentanyl		β-arrestin-2-biased agonist	336.47	3.82	2	0	6

* calculated for base compound form; ** determined in InstantJChem. # meaning 'the number of'.

The data gathered in Table 1 draw attention to the relatively high logP value of SR-17018 (4.75) and as many as eight rotatable bonds in PZM21 and six in fentanyl. The high number of possible bond rotations can lead to difficulties in obtaining stable conformation in the binding site (for comparison, there are no rotatable bonds in the morphine structure), whereas logP values affect the ability of a compound to penetrate the blood–brain barrier. Morphine, despite the rigid structure, is also characterized by very low logP (0.90) and the highest number of hydrogen bond acceptors: four.

In this study, we used three μ opioid receptor crystal structures—records with the following PDB codes were used: 4DKL [23], 5C1M [24], and 6DDF [25] (Table 2). The last two crystals refer to the active conformation of the μ opioid receptor, whereas 4DKL is co-crystallized with BF0, which acts as a μ opioid receptor antagonist and keeps the protein in its inactive form. Despite preserved protein activation occurring in 5C1M and 6DDF crystals, these two structures also differ from each other, as the former is activated via a small-molecule agonist, whereas 6DDF activation occurs via the highly selective peptide agonist for the μ opioid receptor, DAMGO. The peptide-like-based activation reflects the naturally occurring process of μ opioid receptor activation; however, the resolution (a very important factor in terms of the application of a particular structure in molecular modeling tasks) of 6DDF (3.5 Å) is significantly worse than the resolution of 5C1M (2.1 Å).

Table 2. Summary of characteristics of crystal structures used in the study.

PDB ID	Receptor State	Resolution (Å)	Co-Crystallized Ligand
4DKL	inactive	2.8	BF0 (Antagonist)
5C1M	active	2.1	BU72 (Agonist)
6DDF	active	3.5	DAMGO (Peptide agonist)

Due to high variation in the residue positions, resolution, and structure of co-crystallized ligands (also influencing the shape of the binding pockets, Figure 1), all calculations conducted within the study were carried out for all three μ opioid receptor crystals.

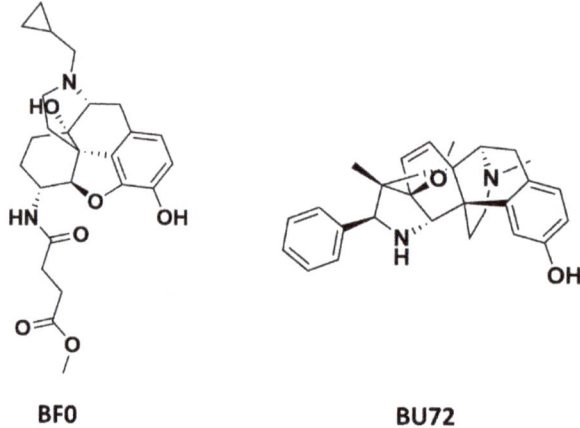

Figure 1. Small molecule ligands co-crystallized with μ opioid receptor crystal structures used in the study.

A comparison of the compound structures presented in Table 1 and Figure 1 indicates that the ligands co-crystallized with μ opioid receptor (BF0 and BU72) are significantly different from the analyzed compounds: PZM21, SR-17018, morphine and fentanyl. To describe these structure variations more formally, the Tanimoto coefficient [26] was calculated for each compound pair using InstantJChem at default settings (detailed numerical values are provided in Table 3). Its highest values were obtained for morphine, and they were equal to 0.764 and 0.595 for BF0 and BU72, respectively. Such high variation between modeled compounds and the co-crystallized ones might lead to changes in the protein structure during simulation with PZM21, SR-17018, morphine and fentanyl to adjust the protein binding site and form energetically favorable ligand–protein complexes.

Table 3. Tanimoto coefficient values between the co-crystallized ligands and the examined compounds.

Modeled Ligand	BF0	BU72
PZM21	0.306	0.318
SR-17018	0.297	0.331
morphine	0.764	0.595
fentanyl	0.289	0.322

2.2. Docking

Before docking the modeled compounds, the validity of the methodology was verified via redocking of BF0 and BU72 to their respective crystal structures. The comparison of the obtained docking poses with crystallized compound conformations is presented in Figure 2. As docking enabled us to obtain orientations similar to the co-crystallized compound fitting (RMSD values between the co-crystallized and docked pose were equal to 1.36 Å and 0.34 Å for BF0, and BU72, respectively), the analogous approach was used for modeling of PZM21, SR-17018, morphine and fentanyl.

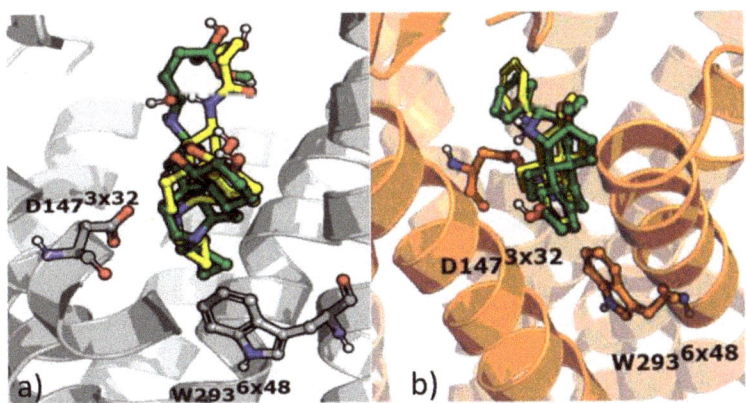

Figure 2. Results of the redocking experiments of co-crystallized ligands BF0 and BU72 to (**a**) 4DKL and (**b**) 5C1M crystal structures—green: co-crystallized conformation, yellow: ligand orientation obtained in docking.

General compound orientations in the µ opioid receptor binding site for different crystals are depicted in Figure 3 and a more detailed analysis of ligand–protein contacts in the form of the interaction matrix is presented in Figure 4.

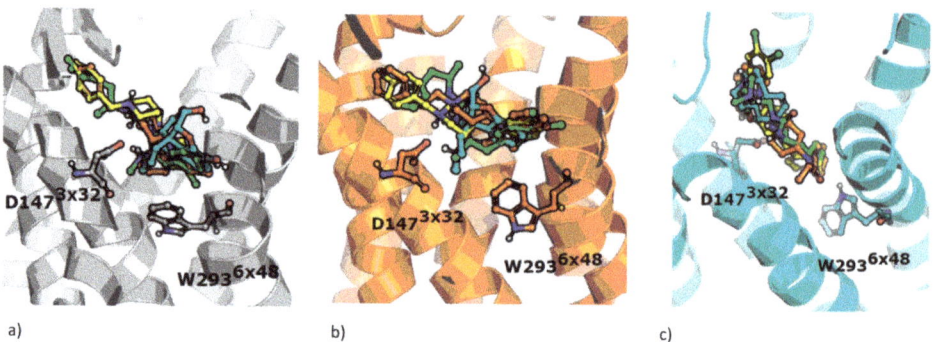

Figure 3. Docking poses of examined compounds at μ opioid receptor crystal structures, (**a**) 4DKL, (**b**) 5C1M, (**c**) 6DDF. PZM21: green; SR-17018: yellow; morphine: cyan; fentanyl: orange. GPCRdb numbering scheme for amino acid labeling is used. Coloring of particular crystal structures is consistent through the whole manuscript.

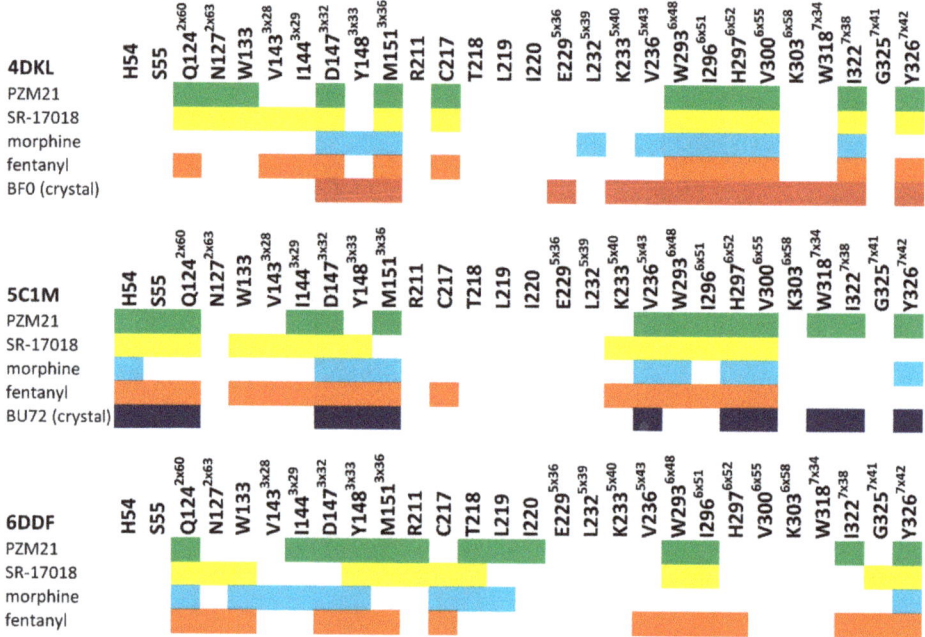

Figure 4. Ligand–protein contacts occurring within complexes obtained in docking to various μ opioid receptor crystal structures. For comparison, interactions of co-crystallized BF0 and BU72 with respective crystal structures are included.

Figure 3 clearly indicates that all the compounds occupy the same region of the binding site, although, due to the structural differences, much less space is taken up by morphine than the other ligands considered. As shown in Figure 4, all ligands consistently make contact with D147^{3x32} and the sixth transmembrane helix (TM6) of the μ opioid receptor for the 4DKL and 5C1M crystal structures. These observations are consistent with the very recent work of Zhao et al. [27], where docking and MD simulations were carried out for PZM21, TRV130 (oliceridine), and morphine using one crystal structure (5C1M) to explain the differences in their functional profiles. On the other hand, the docking poses obtained for 6DDF did not make such frequent contact with TM6—fentanyl made contact with three residues from this protein region, and PZM21 and SR-17018 interacted only with W293$^{6\times48}$ and I296$^{6\times51}$. However, morphine lacked any contact with TM6. Instead, morphine made contact with five amino acids from TM3 when docked to 6DDF, whereas for 4DKL and 5C1M, it interacted only with D147$^{3\times32}$, Y148$^{3\times33}$, and M151$^{3\times36}$ from TM3. For 6DDF-based docking, all the ligands also interacted with Q124$^{2\times60}$, which is unique for this crystal structure (for 4DKL and 5C1M, contact with this residue is missing for morphine). PZM21 and SR-17018 also interacted with more amino acids from TM2 (in comparison to morphine) for 4DKL- and 5C1M-based dockings.

The studied compounds shared interaction patterns presented by Zhao et al., especially in terms of contacts with the set of key residues: D147$^{3\times32}$, Y148$^{3\times33}$, and H297$^{6\times52}$. However, although the compounds occupied the same region of the binding site and were oriented similarly in the binding pockets both in our study and in Zhao's research, there were also some contacts that we did not observe in our poses. For example, morphine lacked contacts with Q124$^{2\times60}$ and I144$^{3\times29}$, K303$^{6\times58}$ and W318$^{7\times34}$, and PZM21 did not interact with W133 or Y148$^{3\times33}$.

The obtained interaction patterns were also confronted with the contact networks formed by the co-crystallized ligands. Antagonist BF0, present in the 4DKL crystal, similarly to modeled compounds, interacted with D147$^{3\times32}$, M151$^{3\times36}$, and a collection of amino acids from TM6. In contrast, BF0 did not come into contact with any residue from TM2 but made interactions with several residues from TM5 (unlike morphine, PZM21, SR-17018, and fentanyl). Contact patterns of the co-crystallized agonist BU72 are more similar to the modeled compounds. BU72 interacted with H54, S55, and Q124$^{2\times60}$ (as for all examined compounds, except morphine), and it possessed the same interaction network with TM3 and TM5 as morphine and with TM7 as PZM21. BU72 also contacted H297$^{6\times52}$, and V300$^{6\times55}$ from TM6, but it did not form an interaction with W293$^{6\times48}$.

The variations in the results obtained in different studies and for different crystal structures indicate the necessity of extending the number of protein structures (either crystal structures or homology models) used in molecular modeling tasks, e.g., during virtual screening. The co-crystallized ligand implies the conformation of the binding site; therefore, the output of docking studies performed for the rigid protein is biased due to the protein adjustment to a co-crystallized agent. The recommendation of using more than one receptor conformation for docking studies was also indicated by Mordalski et al. [28] in the case study of beta-adrenergic receptor type 2.

2.3. Molecular Dynamics and Correlation Studies

As docking captures only one particular moment of interaction between a ligand and protein, it cannot fully explain dependencies between compound behavior towards a given target in relation to its docking pose. The more poses considered, the higher the amount of information provided. To ensure study comprehensiveness, extensive MD simulations with a length of 2000 ns were carried out for each compound–crystal structure combination (12 simulations were run in total). The relative total number of 1000 frames was produced from each simulation, giving a picture of 1000 ligand–protein mutual orientations.

The MD results were analyzed from two perspectives: the stability of compound orientations in the binding site (Figure 5) and changes in ligand–protein contacts that occurred in time (Figure 6).

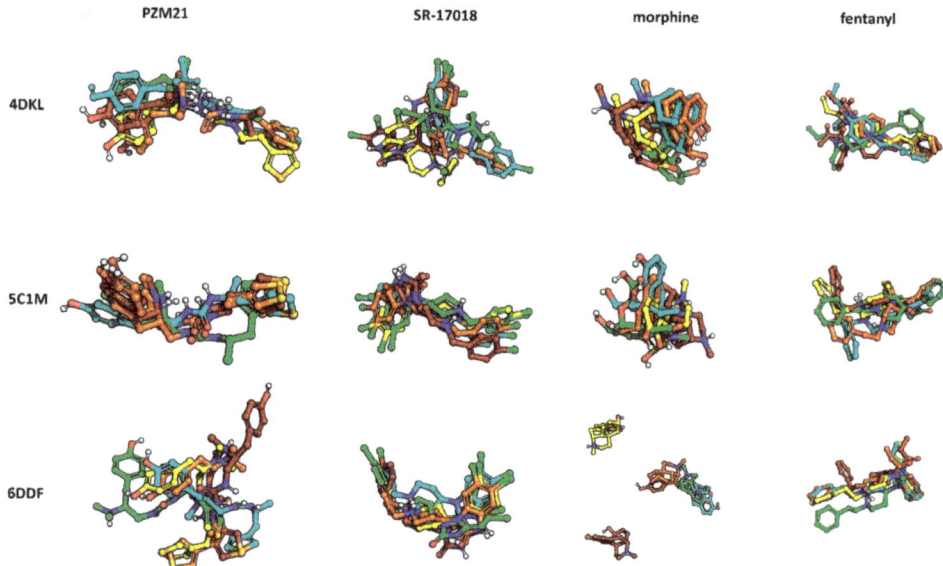

Figure 5. Stability of compound orientations in the binding site during simulations. Green: starting pose; cyan: 250th frame; orange: 500th frame; yellow: 750th frame; red: 1000th frame.

Figure 5 indicates that all of the compounds were most stable when simulated with the 5C1M crystal structure. PZM21 simulated in 5C1M slightly changed its initial position at the beginning and then remained in the adopted conformation. PZM21 in 4DKL was oscillating around its initial pose; however, when 6DDF was taken for simulation, the PZM21 pose varied a lot during the whole simulation time, and the PZM21–6DDF combination resulted in the least stable compound conformation out of all analyzed setups. The highest variation in the compound pose in the binding site was observed for morphine in the 6DDF-based simulation, which changed its initial position and left the binding cavity during the simulation course (after approximately 1000 ns). Fentanyl simulated with 4DKL and 6DDF moved at the beginning of the simulation from its initial position; then, it kept its pose for at least 1500 ns, to slightly change again the conformation when the simulation length approached 2000 ns. In 5C1M-based MDs, fentanyl did not move from the initially occupied region of the binding pocket and the mass center of the compound remained in the same area, with its conformation varying during the whole simulation.

Analyzing the contact patterns presented in Figure 6, one can see that the characteristic MD simulation output is the very strong interaction of PZM21 with $D147^{3\times32}$, even during the simulation with 6DDF, where the compound orientation was in general very unstable (analogous observation also reported by Zhao et al. [27]). Many research studies have indicated this residue as very important for activity towards the μ opioid receptor [29,30]. PZM21 also made consequent contact with $Y148^{3\times33}$, although when simulated with 4DKL, the interaction was formed after approximately 750 ns of simulation. PZM21 changed its orientation very frequently during simulation with 6DDF; however, with $D147^{3\times32}$ and $Y148^{3\times33}$, contact was present during the whole simulation. There was also a set of residues with which it interacted periodically, such as F221, $W293^{6\times48}$, $W318^{7\times34}$, and $Y326^{7\times42}$ (the most frequent contacts between 1000 and 1500 ns of the simulation).

The orientation of PZM21 within the 5C1M binding site was very stable; nevertheless, even in the case of this setup, short contact (occurring only between 250 and 500 ns) with $I296^{6\times51}$ and $H297^{6\times52}$ was observed. Within this period, the intensity of interaction with $W318^{7\times34}$ also strongly increased.

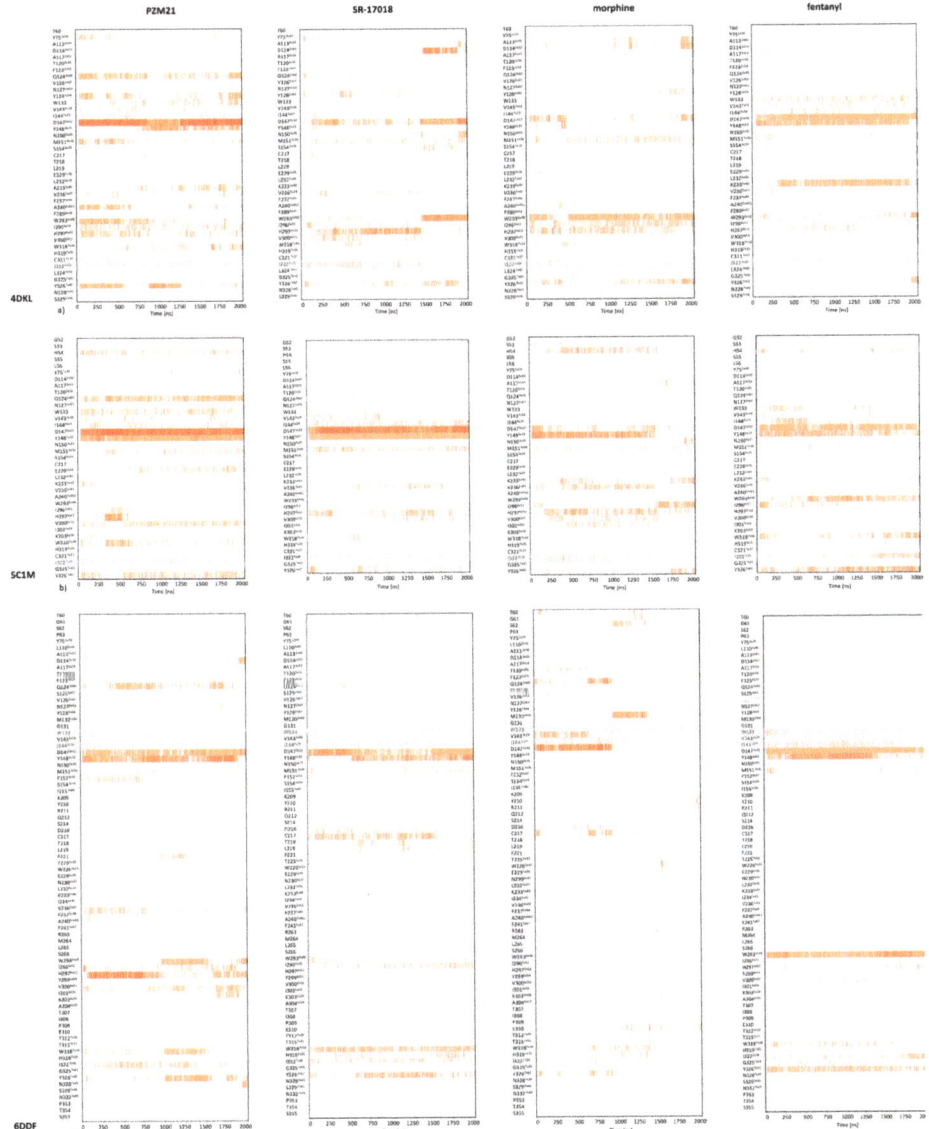

Figure 6. Ligand–protein contacts occurring during molecular dynamics simulations with (**a**) 4DKL, (**b**) 5C1M, and (**c**) 6DDF μ opioid receptor crystal structure. Positions for which the highest correlation between the output of the tail flick experiment and interaction frequency were indicated are shaded.

Consistent contact with D147$^{3\times32}$ is also visible for fentanyl (for all crystal structures), although the interaction is not so strong, as it is in the case of PZM21. This compound also gains interaction with W293$^{6\times48}$ in the simulation with 6DDF, despite its initial lack (the contact occurs constantly during the whole simulation). Fentanyl–W293$^{6\times48}$ contact is also present in MDs with 4DKL and 5C1M, although in the former case, the interactions are relatively sparse.

The last 500 ns of simulation of SR-17018 with 4DKL resulted in the formation of ligand contact with D114$^{2\times50}$, W293$^{6\times48}$, Y326$^{7\times42}$, and an increase in the contact frequency with D147$^{3\times32}$. At the same time, it stopped making contact with $V236^{5\times43}$, $I296^{6\times51}$, $H297^{6\times52}$, $V300^{6\times55}$, and $I322^{7\times38}$. On the other hand, the simulation of SR-17018 with 5C1M and 6DDF resulted in a very consistent and stable interaction pattern over time. Only for 6DDF, an increase in contact intensity with $Y148^{3\times33}$ after 500 ns of simulation and loss of contact with D216 and C217 during the last 500 ns of the simulation were observed. Interestingly, morphine displayed a very unstable conformation when simulated with 6DDF; despite the strong interaction with $D147^{3\times32}$, the contact was lost halfway through the simulation course. In the simulations with 4DKL and 5C1M crystal structures, the contact with $D147^{3\times32}$ occurred during the whole simulation time; however, it was not as frequent and strong as it was in the case of PZM21 and SR-17018.

Strong interaction of the modeled compounds with $D147^{3\times32}$ was also reported by Zhao et al. [27]. This finding is consistent for simulations carried out for all crystal structures. However, there is another observation indicated by Zhao et al., which led to different conclusions when various crystals were considered. Zhao et al. indicated the formation of a strong interaction of morphine with $H297^{6\times52}$, related to its shift deeper into the pocket during the simulation (this effect was not observed for PZM21). Similarly, in our simulations with 5C1M (crystal structure used by Zhao et al.), morphine made contact with $H297^{6\times52}$ after ~200 ns of simulation, which was maintained consistently until the end of the simulation by ~1800 ns. On the other hand, PZM21 also came into short contact with this residue (~300–500 ns), but then the interaction was lost and the compound did not interact with $H297^{6\times52}$, as reported by Zhao et al. [27].

However, similar to the docking studies, MD simulation output also varied depending on the crystal structure, as already discussed. Taking into account the described above interaction with $H297^{6\times52}$, the contact formation with this residue by morphine and its lack for PZM21 was observed only for simulations with 5C1M. For 6DDF-based studies, the situation is reversed, as morphine did not make contact with $H297^{6\times52}$ during the whole simulation, but PZM21 started to interact with this position after ~50 ns of simulation, and the contact was very intense up to ~1000 ns; then, although the interaction was not so strong, it continued until 2000 ns, when the simulation finished. In contrast, in the 4DKL-based studies, both morphine and PZM21 came into contact with $H297^{6\times52}$. For comparison, SR-17018 did not interact with $H297^{6\times52}$ at all for 6DDF; with 5C1M, it continuously came into contact with this residue (although the contact intensity was not very strong), and for 4DKL, the interaction was quite strong at the beginning of the simulation, but after ~1500 ns, the compound changed its conformation and the contact was lost.

These variations in the interaction patterns obtained for different crystal structures, as well as the changes in compound poses after relatively long simulation times (e.g., SR-17018 in 4DKL, which adopted a new pose after 1500 ns), confirm the necessity of applying more protein conformations in structure-based studies and indicate that the simulations should be as long as allowed by computational resources, as some events might not be observed in shorter dynamics.

The interaction schemes obtained in each MD simulation were confronted with selected experimental data produced on examined compounds (see [3,5,31] data gathered in Supporting Information Table S1) to indicate positions that should attract particular attention when developing new ligands of particular activity profiles. This was done by encoding the interactions occurring in each frame from the MD simulation in the form of interaction fingerprints (IFPs) [32] and calculating the Pearson correlation coefficient [33]. The correlation was calculated between the total number of contacts by the particular ligand with a given residue and the experimental parameter value, i.e., the activation of Galphai2 protein (Gai2 activation), activation of G protein-coupled inwardly rectifying (GIRK) potassium channels, recruitment of β-arrestin-2 (bArr2 recruitment), and G protein-activated inward rectifier potassium channel 2 (GIRK2 recruitment). In addition, Galphai-mediated cAMP inhibition value (cAMP inhibition) and efficacy of trafficking of μ opioid receptor to Rab-5 positive endosomes (Rab5 trafficking) were utilized.

The outcome of the studies investigating the correlation between the contact frequency between ligand and a particular amino acid and the outcome of experimental tests is presented in Figure 7 and in Table 4. Cases with the highest values of the Pearson coefficient are presented in the figure, and the remaining highly correlated cases are included in Table 4 (respective charts are presented in the Supporting Information, Figure S1). Frames around each separate chart indicate the crystal structure for which the particular correlation was examined.

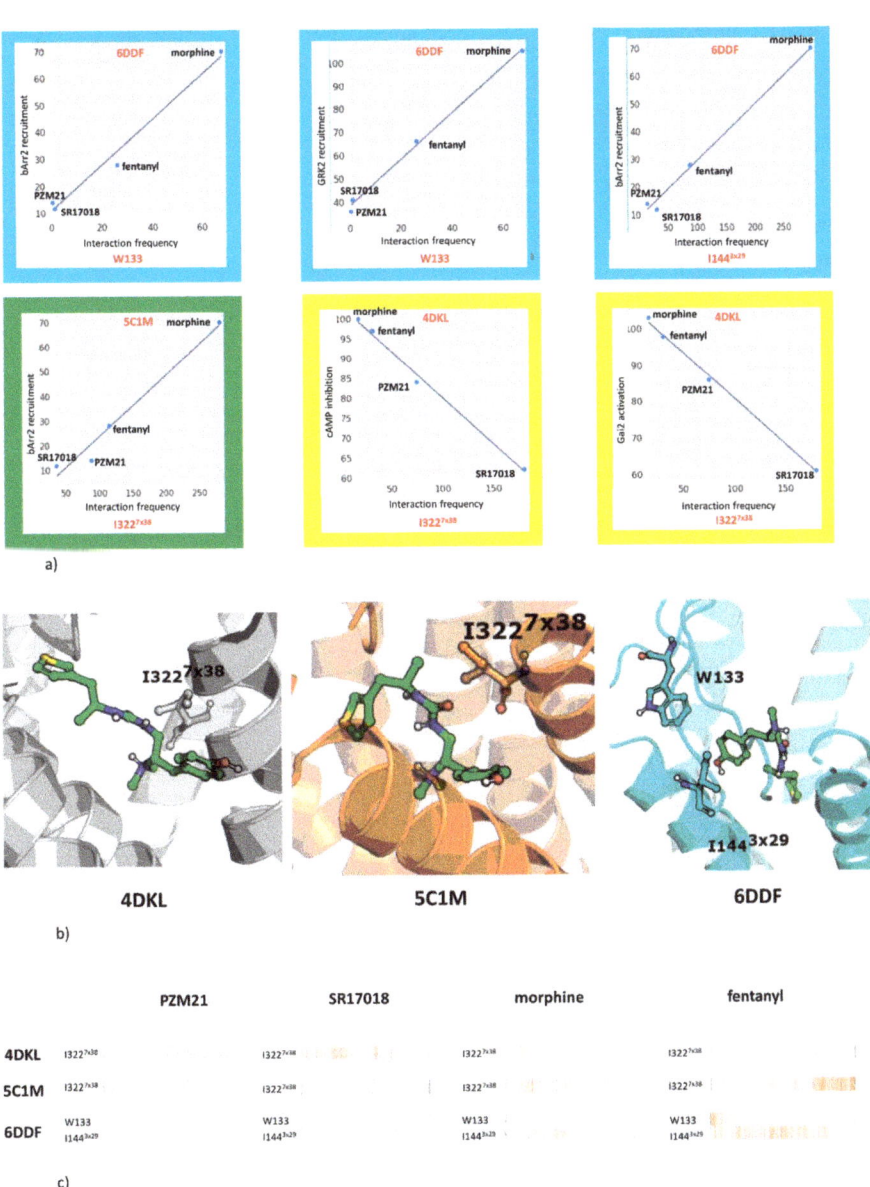

Figure 7. (**a**) Correlation charts between the interaction frequency and outcome of the in vitro experiments (cases with the highest correlation are presented with the Pearson correlation coefficients above 0.98) with frames' color referring to particular crystal structure—yellow: 4DKL, green: 5C1M, blue: 6DDF; (**b**) indication of residues with the highest correlation presented in (**a**), (**c**) ligand–protein interaction diagrams obtained during MD simulations for residues presented in (**a**).

Table 4. Amino acids with the highest values of the Pearson correlation coefficient (above 0.94) between the ligand–residue contact frequency and experimental value (data produced on the basis of the pEC$_{50}$ values of selected agonists for some of the pathways measured at the µ opioid receptor gathered in Gillis et al. [31]).

Crystal Structure/Parameter.	Gai2 Activation	cAMP Inhibition	bArr2 Recruitment	Rab5 Trafficking	GIRK Activation	GRK2 Recruitment
4DKL	T120$^{2\times56}$, I322$^{7\times38}$	T120$^{2\times56}$, V236$^{5\times43}$	F152$^{3\times37}$, R211			
5C1M		I296$^{6\times51}$	L121$^{2\times57}$, I322$^{7\times38}$	Y148$^{3\times33}$		I322$^{7\times38}$
6DDF	W318$^{7\times34}$	W318$^{7\times34}$	L121$^{2\times57}$, W133, I144$^{3\times29}$, C321$^{7\times37}$, G325$^{7\times41}$	W133		W133, I144$^{3\times29}$

Out of the six presented charts with the highest experiment–contact pattern correlations, three were related to simulations with 6DDF, and in the case of three of them, high correlations were found for the β-arrestin-2 recruitment assay. The list of highly correlated amino acids was composed of just one residue for 5C1M and 4DKL (I322$^{7\times38}$). For the former crystal, it was obtained in the β-arrestin-2 recruitment experiment, which led to a Pearson correlation coefficient above 0.98 (it was equal to 0.985), whereas for 4DKL, it was cAMP inhibition and Gai2 activation experiments, which were highly related to the interaction frequency of compounds with I322$^{7\times38}$ during MD simulations (Pearson correlation coefficients were equal to 0.997 and 0.998, respectively). Moreover, 6DDF-based correlations indicated amino acids from different regions of the protein, W133 and I144$^{3\times29}$, with the former related to the β-arrestin-2 recruitment assay and experiments based on GRK2 recruitment.

The results indicate that despite extensive simulation time (2 µs) enabling significant changes in the protein structure, the initial conformation forced by the co-crystallized ligand influenced the results during the whole simulation time. The correlation coefficients between the ligand–contact frequency and the outcome of experimental studies vary significantly for a particular crystal structure. The highest number of experiments with any "highly correlated" residue occurred for 6DDF.

The positions of residues gathered in Table 4 are visualized in the respective crystal structures in Figure 8.

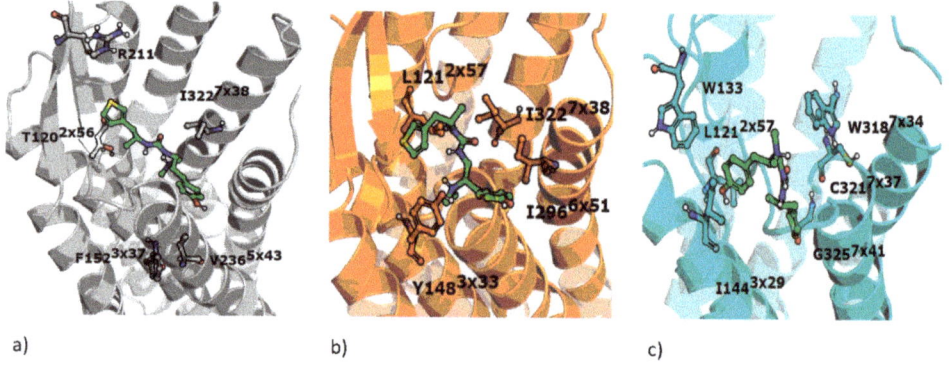

Figure 8. Residues with high correlation between the interaction frequency and experimental tests output obtained for (**a**) 4DKL, (**b**) 5C1M, and (**c**) 6DDF. PZM21 visualized for reference.

When the unbiased morphine is confronted with biased agonists examined in the study, it appears that, in general, morphine interacts less intensively with D147$^{3\times32}$, which is consistently observed for all crystal structures, but this is most visible for 5C1M-based simulations. On the other hand, in 5C1M-based simulations, morphine interacted more frequently with K333$^{5\times40}$, V236$^{5\times43}$, and I301$^{6\times56}$. Simulations with 4DKL revealed more intense interaction of morphine with W293$^{6\times48}$ in comparison to biased ligands, whereas with 6DDF-based studies, PZM21 and SR-17018 interacted more frequently with $I296^{6\times54}$, $I322^{7\times38}$, and $Y326^{7\times42}$. These abovementioned residues should be monitored; however, their discrimination potency between biased and unbiased ligands should be verified for a higher number of compounds, with each activity profile considered.

Zhao et al. indicated $W293^{6\times48}$, $W318^{7\times35}$, $Y326^{7\times42}$, and $Y336^{7\times53}$ as residues that affect the receptor function [27]. These positions were not indicated in our statistical analyses; however, it should be pointed out that the method of residue indication in our study differed from Zhao's approach. We focus on the compound contacts with the protein and analyze its behavior in the binding site, whereas Zhao et al. examined relative positions of particular amino acids and on this basis discussed the role of particular amino acids with reference to the activity profile of examined compounds. Therefore, the conclusions drawn from MD simulations in our study and those obtained by Zhao et al. should be compared cautiously and considering the above-described methodological differences.

To examine the influence of the modeled ligand, as well as to correlate results obtained in the MD simulations with functional activity of the μ opioid receptor, an analysis of the position of $W293^{6\times48}$ (residue important for the activation of opioid receptors [27]) for various setups was carried out (Figure 9). Its conformational changes imply the arrangement of the fifth and sixth transmembrane helices (TM5 and TM6), transmitting a signal to another protein region (intracellular loop).

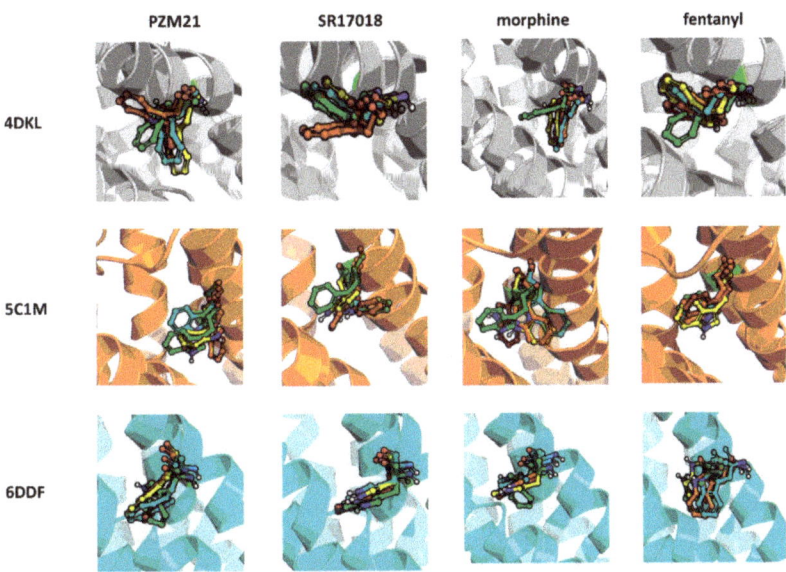

Figure 9. Position of W2936x48 during simulations with various ligands—green: starting pose; cyan: 250th frame; orange: 500th frame; yellow: 750th frame; red: 1000th frame.

The results show that the $W293^{6\times48}$ position changed during the simulations in the majority of cases. When the μ opioid receptor was in its inactive conformation (4DKL crystal), the protein simulation with the agonistic agents resulted in changes in its orientation. Interestingly, the direction of changes varies depending on the ligand. For morphine, $W293^{6\times48}$ moved lower, towards the inner part of the receptor, whereas for fentanyl and SR-17018, it shifted towards the extracellular part of the protein. These events took place at the beginning of the simulations and the residue orientation remained the same until the end of the simulation. PZM21 initially induced a similar change in $W293^{6\times48}$ position as morphine; however, in the middle of the simulation, the residue adopted a similar orientation for a while as in the case of SR-17018 and fentanyl. The activated form of the receptor present in the 5C1M crystal structure also led to variation of the $W293^{6\times48}$ position during simulation: in this case, morphine and SR-17018 led to similar changes in the residue position, and for PZM21, variation in the $W293^{6\times48}$ position occurred which was similar to its simulation with 4DKL. Interestingly, the $W293^{6\times48}$ position did not change during simulation with fentanyl. In simulations fentanyl–6DDF and SR-17018–6DDF, a consistent position of $W293^{6\times48}$ was also observed. Morphine simulated with 6DDF slightly changed its orientation at the beginning of the simulation towards the extracellular part of the receptor, and the PZM21–6DDF simulation resulted only in a minimal change in $W293^{6\times48}$ orientation.

3. Materials and Methods

The compounds were prepared for docking using LigPrep [34] from the Schrödinger Suite: protonation states were generated at pH 7.4+/−0.0, and all possible stereoisomers were enumerated; other settings remained at default. The crystal structures used in the study were fetched from the PDB database [35] and prepared for docking using the Protein Preparation Wizard from the Schrödinger Suite. Mass center of the co-crystallized ligand constituted the grid center in each case, and the grid size was set to 23 Å. The docking was carried out in Glide [36] in extra precision mode. The obtained ligand–receptor complexes with the best docking score constituted an input for MD simulations. They were carried out in Desmond [37], using the TIP3P solvent model [38], POPC (palmitoyl-oleil-phosphatidylcoline) as a membrane model, the OPLS3e force-field under the pressure of 1.01325 bar, and a temperature of 300 K. The box shape was orthorhombic, with a size of +10 Å × +10 Å × +10 Å. In each case, the system was neutralized by addition of the appropriate number of Cl- ions and relaxed before simulation; the duration of each simulation was equal to 2000 ns. The interactions between ligands and the respective proteins during MD simulations were analyzed using Simulation Interaction Diagram from the Schrödinger Suite. Interactions occurring in each frame of the performed simulations were encoded in the form of interaction fingerprints (IFPs) [29]. Then, for each nonzero column, the Pearson correlation coefficient between the total number of contacts formed with a particular ligand by a given residue with the experimental parameter value was determined.

4. Conclusions

In this study, in silico examination of the activity profiles of selected μ opioid receptor agents (PZM21, SR-17018, morphine, and fentanyl) was carried out. Three crystal structures of the target were used for docking and MD simulations and the obtained ligand–protein interaction patterns were confronted with the outcome of selected experimental tests. The variation in the obtained results clearly indicates the necessity of using as much structural data as possible in structure-based studies and not focusing on one receptor conformation. Each computational setup provided new insight into the given problem and indicated a new set of amino acids that should be taken into account when examining compound interaction profiles in silico. Moreover, the study enabled the indication of amino acids that should attract special attention when designing new ligands with particular properties: W133, $I144^{3\times29}$, $I322^{7\times38}$. Apart from these residues, there were over a dozen positions correlated with other experimental output, for single crystal structures, which also should be taken into account during μ opioid receptor ligand modeling.

Supplementary Materials: The following are available online. Table S1. In vitro and in vivo data used in the study (expressed in the form of pEC_{50} values). Figure S1. Correlation charts between the interaction frequency with a particular residue and outcome of experimental tests.

Author Contributions: S.P. and R.P. designed experiments, S.P. carried out in silico studies, S.P., R.B., L.K., A.J.B., R.P. Authors analyzed and discussed the results, as well as prepared, read and agreed to the published version of the manuscript.

Funding: The study was supported by the grant OPUS 2018/31/B/NZ7/03954 funded by the National Science Centre, Poland and statutory activity by Maj Institute of Pharmacology PAS.

Conflicts of Interest: The authors declare no conflict of interest. The funders had no role in the design of the study; in the collection, analyses, or interpretation of data; in the writing of the manuscript, or in the decision to publish the results.

References

1. Grim, T.W.; Acevedo-Canabal, A.; Bohn, L.M. Toward Directing Opioid Receptor Signaling to Refine Opioid Therapeutics. *Biol. Psy.* **2020**, *87*, 15–21. [CrossRef]
2. Manglik, A.; Lin, H.; Aryal, D.K.; McCorvy, J.D.; Dengler, D.; Corder, G.; Levit, A.; Kling, R.C.; Bernat, V.; Hübner, H.; et al. Structure-based discovery of opioid analgesics with reduced side effects. *Nature* **2016**, *537*, 185–190. [CrossRef]
3. Kudla, L.; Bugno, R.; Skupio, U.; Wiktorowska, L.; Solecki, W.; Wojtas, A.; Golembiowska, K.; Zádor, F.; Benyhe, S.; Buda, S.; et al. Functional characterization of a novel opioid, PZM21, and its effects on the behavioural responses to morphine. *Br. J. Pharmacol.* **2019**, *176*, 4434–4445. [CrossRef] [PubMed]
4. Hill, R.; Disney, A.; Conibear, A.; Sutcliffe, K.; Dewey, W.; Husbands, S.; Bailey, C.; Kelly, E.; Henderson, G. The novel μ-opioid receptor agonist PZM21 depresses respiration and induces tolerance to antinociception. *Br. J. Pharmacol.* **2018**, *175*, 2653–2661. [CrossRef] [PubMed]
5. Schmid, C.L.; Kennedy, N.M.; Ross, N.C.; Lovell, K.M.; Yue, Z.; Morgenweck, J.; Cameron, M.D.; Bannister, T.D.; Bohn, L.M. Bias factor and therapeutic window correlate to predict safer opioid analgesics. *Cell* **2017**, *171*, 1165–1175.e13. [CrossRef] [PubMed]
6. Grim, T.W.; Schmid, C.L.; Stahl, E.L.; Pantouli, F.; Ho, J.H.; Acevedo-Canabal, A.; Kennedy, N.M.; Cameron, M.D.; Bannister, T.D.; Bohn, L.M. A G protein signaling-biased agonist at the μ-opioid receptor reverses morphine tolerance while preventing morphine withdrawal. *Neuropsychopharm* **2020**, *45*, 416–425. [CrossRef] [PubMed]
7. Sliwoski, G.; Kothiwale, S.; Meiler, J.; Lowe, E.W. Computational methods in drug discovery. *Pharmacol. Rev.* **2014**, *66*, 334–395. [CrossRef] [PubMed]
8. Rao, V.S.; Srinivas, K. Modern drug discovery process: An in silico approach. *J. Bioinform. Seq. Anal.* **2011**, *2*, 89–94.
9. Reddy, A.S.; Pati, S.P.; Kumar, P.P.; Pradeep, H.N.; Sastry, G.N. Virtual screening in drug discovery—A computational perspective. *Curr. Protein Pept. Sci.* **2007**, *8*, 329–351. [CrossRef]
10. Bittemcourt, J.A.H.M.; Neto, M.F.A.; Lacerda, P.S.; Bittencourt, R.C.V.S.; Silva, R.C.; Lobato, C.C.; Silva, L.B.; Leite, F.H.A.; Zuliani, J.P.; Rosa, J.M.C.; et al. In silico Evaluation of ibuprofen and two benzoylpropionic acid derivatives with potential anti-inflammatory activity. *Molecules* **2019**, *24*, 1476. [CrossRef]
11. Dellafiora, L.; Galaverna, G.; Cruciani, G.; Dall'Asta, C.; Bruni, R. On the mechanism of action of anti-inflammatory activity of hypericin: An in silico study pointing to the relevance of janus kinase inhibition. *Molecules* **2018**, *23*, 3058. [CrossRef] [PubMed]
12. Perez-Aguilar, J.M.; Kang, S.-G.; Zhang, L.; Zhou, R. Modeling and structural characterization of the sweet taste receptor heterodimer. *ACS Chem. Neurosci.* **2019**, *10*, 4579–4592. [CrossRef] [PubMed]
13. Geppert, H.; Vogt, M.; Bajorath, J. Current trends in ligand-based virtual screening: Molecular representations, data mining methods, new application areas, and performance evaluation. *J. Chem. Inf. Model.* **2010**, *2*, 205–216. [CrossRef] [PubMed]
14. Cherkasov, A.; Muratov, E.N.; Fourches, D.; Varnek, A.; Baskin, I.I.; Cronin, M.; Dearden, J.; Gramatica, P.; Martin, Y.C.; Todeschini, R.; et al. QSAR modeling: Where have you been? Where are you going to? *J. Med. Chem.* **2014**, *12*, 4977–5010. [CrossRef] [PubMed]
15. Yang, S.Y. Pharmacophore modeling and applications in drug discovery: Challenges and recent advances. *Drug Discov. Today* **2010**, *15*, 444–450. [CrossRef] [PubMed]
16. Stumpfe, D.; Bajorath, J. Similarity searching. *Wiley Interdiscip. Rev. Comput. Mol. Sci.* **2011**, *2*, 260–282. [CrossRef]
17. Anderson, A.C. The process of structure-based drug design. *Chem Biol.* **2003**, *9*, 787–797. [CrossRef]
18. Sousa, F.; Fernandes, P.A.; Ramos, M.J. Protein—Ligand docking: Current status and future challenges. *Proteins* **2006**, *1*, 15–26. [CrossRef] [PubMed]

19. Daddam, J.R.; Sreenivasulu, B.; Peddanna, K.; Umamahesh, K. Designing, docking and molecular dynamics simulation studies of novel cloperastine analogues as anti-allergic agents: Homology modeling and active site prediction for the human histamine H1 receptor. *RCS Adv.* **2020**, *10*, 4745. [CrossRef]
20. Liu, T.; Lu, D.; Zhang, H.; Zheng, M.; Yang, H.; Xu, Y.; Luo, C.; Zhu, W.; Yu, K.; Jiang, H. Applying high-performance computing in drug discovery and molecular simulation. *Nat. Sci. Rev.* **2016**, *3*, 49–63. [CrossRef]
21. Pándy-Szekeres, G.; Munk, C.; Tsonkov, T.M.; Mordalski, S.; Harpsøe, K.; Hauser, A.S.; Bojarski, A.J.; Gloriam, D.E. GPCRdb in 2018: Adding GPCR structure models and ligands. *Nucleic Acids Res.* **2017**, *46*, D440–D446. [CrossRef] [PubMed]
22. Instant JChem 6.3.0. ChemAxon, 2014. Available online: http://www.chemaxon.com (accessed on 28 September 2020).
23. Manglik, A.; Kruse, A.C.; Kobilka, T.S.; Thian, F.S.; Mathiesen, J.M.; Sunahara, R.K.; Pardo, L.; Weis, W.I.; Kobilka, B.K.; Granier, S. Crystal structure of the {mu}-opioid receptor bound to a morphinan antagonist. *Nature* **2012**, *485*, 321–326. [CrossRef] [PubMed]
24. Huang, W.; Manglik, A.; Venkatakrishnan, A.J.; Laeremans, T.; Feinberg, E.N.; Sanborn, A.L.; Kato, H.E.; Livingston, K.E.; Thorsen, T.S.; Kling, R.C.; et al. Structural insights into mu-opioid receptor activation. *Nature* **2015**, *524*, 315–321. [CrossRef]
25. Koehl, A.; Hu, H.; Maeda, S.; Zhang, Y.; Qu, Q.; Paggi, J.M.; Latorraca, N.R.; Hilger, D.; Dawson, R.; Matile, H.; et al. Structure of the mu-opioid receptor-Giprotein complex. *Nature* **2018**, *558*, 547–552. [CrossRef] [PubMed]
26. Bajusz, D.; Racz, A.; Heberger, K. Why is Tanimoto index an appropriate choice for fingerprint-based similarity calculations? *J. Cheminform.* **2015**, *7*, 20. [CrossRef]
27. Zhao, Z.; Huang, T.; Li, J. Molecular Dynamics Simulations to Investigate How PZM21 Affects the Conformational State of the μ-Opioid Receptor Upon Activation. *Int. I. Mol. Sci.* **2020**, *21*, 4699. [CrossRef]
28. Mordalski, S.; Witek, J.; Smusz, S.; Rataj, K.; Bojarski, A.J. Multiple conformational states in retrospective virtual screening—Homology models vs. crystal structures: Beta-2 adrenergic receptor case study. *J. Cheminform.* **2015**, *7*, 13. [CrossRef]
29. Pasternak, G.W.; Pan, Y.-X. Mu opioids and their receptors: Evolution of a concept. *Pharmacol. Rev.* **2013**, *65*, 1257–1317. [CrossRef]
30. Kaserer, T.; Lantero, A.; Schmidhammer, H.; Spetea, M.; Schuster, D. μ opioid receptor: Novel antagonists and structural modeling. *Sci. Rep.* **2016**, *6*, 21548. [CrossRef]
31. Gillis, A.; Gondin, A.B.; Kliewer, A.; Sanchez, J.; Lim, H.D.; Alamein, C.; Manandhar, P.; Santiago, M.; Fritzwanker, S.; Schmiedel, F.; et al. Low intrinsic efficacy for G protein activation can explain the improved side effect profiles of new opioid agonists. *Sci. Signal.* **2020**, *13*, eaaz3140. [CrossRef]
32. Marcou, G.; Rognan, D. Optimizing fragment and scaffold docking by use of molecular interaction fingerprints. *J. Chem. Inf. Model.* **2007**, *47*, 195–207. [CrossRef] [PubMed]
33. Fisher, R.A. Frequency distribution of the values of the correlation coefficient in samples from an indefinitely large population. *Biometrika* **1915**, *10*, 507–521. [CrossRef]
34. LigPrep. *Schrödinger Release 2020-1*; LLC: New York, NY, USA, 2020.
35. Berman, H.M.; Westbrook, J.; Feng, Z.; Gilliland, G.; Bhat, T.N.; Weissig, H.; Shindyalov, I.N.; Bourne, P.E. The Protein Data Bank. *Nucleic Acids Res.* **2000**, *28*, 235–242. [CrossRef] [PubMed]
36. Glide. *Schrödinger Release 2020-1*; LLC: New York, NY, USA, 2020.
37. *Schrödinger Release 2020-1: Desmond Molecular Dynamics System*; D.E. Shaw Research: New York, NY, USA, 2020.
38. Jorgensen, W.L.; Chandrasekhar, J.; Madura, J.D.; Impey, R.W.; Klein, M.L. Comparison of simple potential functions for simulating liquid water. *J. Chem. Phys.* **1983**, *79*, 26. [CrossRef]

Sample Availability: Not available.

© 2020 by the authors. Licensee MDPI, Basel, Switzerland. This article is an open access article distributed under the terms and conditions of the Creative Commons Attribution (CC BY) license (http://creativecommons.org/licenses/by/4.0/).

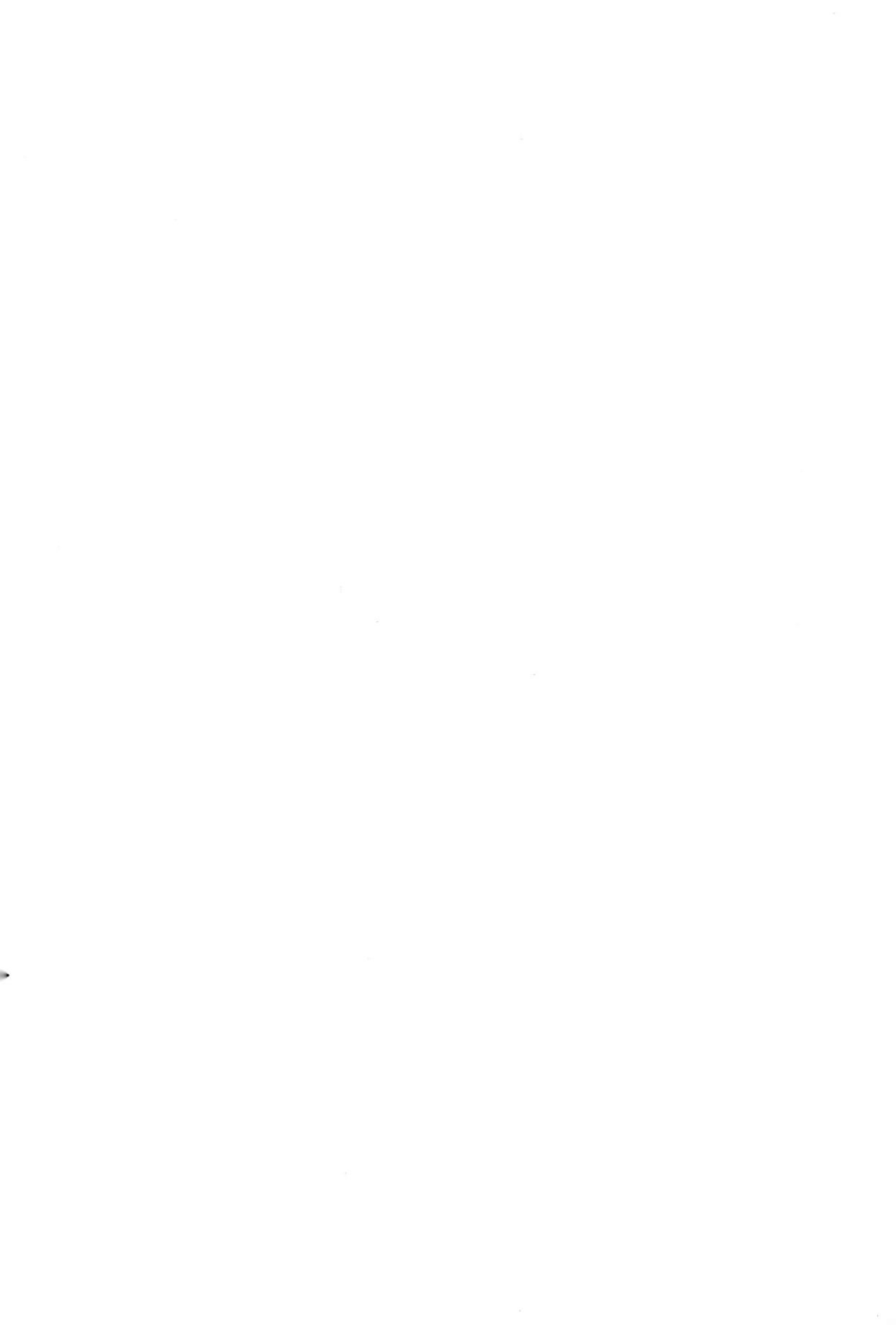